In Vivo MR Techniques **in Drug Discovery and Development**

In Vivo MR Techniques in Drug Discovery and Development

Edited by

Nicolau Beckmann

Taylor & Francis
Taylor & Francis Group
New York London

Taylor & Francis is an imprint of the
Taylor & Francis Group, an informa business

Published in 2006 by
Taylor & Francis Group
270 Madison Avenue
New York, NY 10016

Printed in the United States of America on acid-free paper
10 9 8 7 6 5 4 3 2 1

International Standard Book Number-10: 0-8493-3026-2 (Hardcover)
International Standard Book Number-13: 978-0-8493-3026-1 (Hardcover)
Library of Congress Card Number 2006040352

Library of Congress Cataloging-in-Publication Data

In Vivo MR techniques in drug discovery and development / by Nicolau Beckmann.
p. cm.
ISBN 0-8493-3026-2 (alk. paper)
1. Drug development. 2. Pharmaceutical technology. 3. Magnetic resonance imaging. I. Beckmann, Nicolau.

RM301.25.I5 2006
615'.19--dc22 2006040352

informa
Taylor & Francis Group
is the Academic Division of Informa plc.

Visit the Taylor & Francis Web site at
http://www.taylorandfrancis.com

Dedication

for

智子 *and* 綾和, *with love*

The little girl gave a cry of amazement and looked about her,
her eyes growing bigger and bigger at the wonderful sights she saw…

L. Frank Baum, *The Wizard of Oz*, 1899
(Dorothy upon emerging from her home when she landed in Oz)

Preface

Drug discovery and development is a long and resource-intensive process, confronted with many failures. The basic challenge consists in providing effective and safe therapies at a reasonably low cost. The current hope of achieving this objective relies on the paradigm that, by improving the characterization of compounds and their effects in early and not yet so costly phases, one increases their chance of success in the late phases of development. Intimately linked to this reasoning stands the knowledge about a given disease, and its early diagnosis and characterization. Obviously, the better the mechanism of a disease is known, the higher the probability of finding an appropriate therapy. In addition, the better and earlier a disease can be diagnosed and characterized, the higher the chance of being able to interfere in this process with a chemical entity. This reasoning sets the framework for the use of imaging in pharmaceutical research.

Due to their potential to accelerate the drug discovery and development process, imaging technologies are presently receiving considerable attention in the pharmaceutical area. One of the principal imaging modalities is magnetic resonance imaging (MRI). The multiparametric nature of MRI enables anatomical, functional, metabolic, and even targeted information to be obtained noninvasively from intact organisms at high spatial resolution, thereby allowing a comprehensive characterization of a disease state and the corresponding drug intervention. The noninvasiveness of MRI also strengthens the link between preclinical and clinical drug studies.

This book shows in detail how *in vivo* magnetic resonance (MR) techniques can be or are being used in the drug discovery and development process, from target identification and validation to clinical studies. An introductory chapter on the drug discovery and development process is followed by a general discussion on the use of imaging techniques in this area. The concept of biomarker imaging is also addressed in a following chapter independently from the imaging technique. After this introductory phase, the attention is turned towards MR imaging and spectroscopy. The design of contrast agents with the aim of enabling molecular imaging investigations is the next focus in Chapter 4. This is followed in Chapter 5 by a discussion on strategies for high-throughput imaging aiming at phenotyping transgenic mice used for target validation or as disease models. The book then takes a disease-oriented approach with the following chapters devoted to individual disease areas, in order to better illustrate the fact that every organ demands specific imaging solutions. Each disease area is discussed from the preclinical and clinical points of view, with emphasis on advantages and limitations of the approaches. Chapter 6 to Chapter 12 address the use of MR techniques to characterize neurological disorders. The ensuing three chapters deal with the utilization of MR in cancer studies. Chapter 16 and Chapter 17 discuss cardiac MRI applications, while possible roles of lung MRI in the area of airway diseases are addressed in Chapter 18 and Chapter 19. Chapter 20 and Chapter 21 focus on MR spectroscopy as a tool in diabetes research, and on MRI in obesity related to diabetes. The use of MRI techniques in arthritis is discussed in Chapter 22 and Chapter 23. The next two chapters deal respectively with the utilization of MRI approaches in solid organ transplantation and in stem cell-based therapies. The use of MR techniques in pharmaceutical safety assessments is addressed in Chapter 26. A final discussion on the value of MR in pharmaceutical research is presented in Chapter 27.

I would like to thank all authors who accepted my invitation to share their experiences in a given research area. They had to endure my painstaking comments and in some cases were willing to revise their text a couple of times. Thanks for your patience, dear colleagues. My gratitude also goes to several people who, over many years, supported me in different ways. During my undergraduate studies, Professors Horacio Panepucci, Sérgio Mascarenhas, Mário Schönberg, and Herch Moyses Nussenzweig from the University of São Paulo instilled in me a passion for science. Their view that the pathways of physics is intimately linked to that of biology profoundly influenced my career decisions. Thanks to Professor Seelig from the Biocenter in Basel, I was able to pursue this link in a more systematic way during my graduate studies. It would be impossible to name all further persons who had or are having a positive impact upon my development. However, I am particularly indebted to the following colleagues, who through commitment, support and enthusiasm, provided me invaluable access to expertise, skills, animal models of disease and probes, which have been essential to my daily activities during the past 12 years: François-Xavier Blé, Konrad Bruttel, Catherine Cannet, Dr. John Fozard, Dr. Hans-Ulrich Gremlich, Prof. Robert Hof, Harry Karmouty Quintana, Dr. Rainer Kneuer, Dr. Lazzaro Mazzoni, Elisabeth Schaeublin, Dr. Philipp Schmidt, Dr. Matthias Staufenbiel, Maddeleine Tanner, Dr. Bruno Tigani, and Stefan Zurbruegg from Novartis, Professor Clive Page from the King's College London, and last but not least, Professor Markus Rudin from the ETH/University of Zurich. The management of Novartis is gratefully acknowledged for continuously having supported imaging activities during the past 20 years. My thanks also to Amber Donley, Joette Lynch and Stephen Zollo from Taylor & Francis and Katharine Godfrey from the Alden Prepress Services whose kind support significantly facilitated the edition of this book. Finally, I would like to thank my wife Satoko and our daughter Ayana for their support over the past months, during which a substantial fraction of my attention was devoted to this book rather than to them.

Drug discovery is an undertaking that involves people with substantially different backgrounds. I would be very pleased if this book could contribute a little to improving the understanding between persons working at different stages of this pursuit, but who ultimately are aiming at the same final objective: to help fight disease. I hope also that the text may be useful and provide a small source of inspiration to researchers, technologists, and students interested in the use of imaging technologies in the biomedical and pharmacological areas. The future will tell us if imaging techniques, MRI in particular, will fulfill the expectation within the pharmaceutical community. A great deal of work remains ahead of us. I am convinced that the efforts of many parties in this field, both in industry and in academia, are going to lead at least to more powerful diagnostic tools. In any case, medical practice and public health are going to benefit from this endeavor.

Nicolau Beckmann

Editor

Nicolau Beckmann received a B.Sc. in physics and a M.Sc. in applied physics from the University of São Paulo, Brazil. As an Alexander von Humboldt Fellow he then moved to Europe to become a visiting researcher at Siemens Medical Systems in Erlangen, Germany. This was followed by graduate studies leading to a PhD in Biophysics from the Biocenter of the University of Basel, Switzerland. Dr. Beckmann is a former director of physics at the MR Center of the University of Basel. Currently, he is the head of an MRI laboratory at the Novartis Institutes for BioMedical Research in Basel, Switzerland.

Dr. Beckmann is the author of publications in several peer-review journals and of a book on ^{13}C MR spectroscopy (Academic Press). He has received awards from the Conselho Nacional de Pesquisas (CNPq, Brazil), Fundação de Amparo à Pesquisa do Estado de São Paulo (FAPESP — Brazil), Alexander von Humboldt Foundation (Bonn, Germany), Krupp Foundation (Essen, Germany), Swiss National Foundation (Bern, Switzerland) and 3R Research Foundation (Muensingen, Switzerland). His research interests center on the use of imaging and spectroscopic techniques for *in vivo* biomedical research. Outside of work his family and friends, as well as music, languages, arts, cinema, literature, and traveling play important roles in his life.

Contributors

Ellen Ackerstaff
Russell H. Morgan Department of Radiology and Radiological Science
Johns Hopkins University School of Medicine
Baltimore, Maryland

Silvio Aime
Department of Chemistry IFM and Centre for Molecular Imaging
University of Torino
Torino, Italy

Peter R. Allegrini
Novartis Institutes for BioMedical Research
Discovery Technologies
Basel, Switzerland

Dmitri Artemov
Russell H. Morgan Department of Radiology and Radiological Science
Johns Hopkins University School of Medicine
Baltimore, Maryland

Wolfgang R. Bauer
Medical Clinic
University of Würzburg
Würzburg, Germany

Nicolau Beckmann
Novartis Institutes for BioMedical Research
Discovery Technologies
Basel, Switzerland

Mounia Beloueche-Babari
Cancer Research U.K. Clinical Magnetic Resonance Research Group
Institute of Cancer Research and Royal Marsden NHS Foundation Trust
Surrey, United Kingdom

Cedric Berger
Novartis Institutes for BioMedical Research
Discovery Technologies
Basel, Switzerland

Zaver M. Bhujwalla
Russell H. Morgan Department of Radiology and Radiological Science
Johns Hopkins University School of Medicine
Baltimore, Maryland

François-Xavier Blé
Novartis Institutes for BioMedical Research
Discovery Technologies
Basel, Switzerland

Chas Bountra
Neurology CEDD
GlaxoSmithKline
Harlow, United Kingdom

Jeff W. M. Bulte
Department of Radiology and Institute for Cell Engineering
Johns Hopkins University School of Medicine
Baltimore, Maryland

Elizabeth M. Charles-Edwards
Cancer Research U.K. Clinical Magnetic Resonance Research Group
Institute of Cancer Research and Royal Marsden NHS Foundation Trust
Surrey, United Kingdom

X. Josette Chen
Mouse Imaging Centre
Hospital for Sick Children
Toronto, Ontario, Canada

Yin-Ching Iris Chen
Athinoula A. Martinos Center for Biomedical Imaging
Massachusetts General Hospital and Harvard Medical School
Charlestown, Massachusetts

Ji-Kyung Choi
Athinoula A. Martinos Center for Biomedical Imaging
Massachusetts General Hospital and Harvard Medical School
Charlestown, Massachusetts

David J. Collins
Cancer Research U.K. Clinical Magnetic Resonance Research Group
Institute of Cancer Research and Royal Marsden NHS Foundation Trust
Surrey, United Kingdom

Yannick Crémillieux
Université Lyon
Laboratoire de RMN
Villeurbanne, France

Jeffrey Evelhoch
Amgen, Inc.
Thousand Oaks, California

Jochen B. Fiebach
Department of Neurology
University of Heidelberg
Heidelberg, Germany

Christian Fink
Institute of Clinical Radiology
University of Munich — Campus Grosshadern
Munich, Germany

John R. Fozard
Respiratory Diseases Department
Novartis Institutes for BioMedical Research
Basel, Switzerland

Barjor Gimi
Russell H. Morgan Department of Radiology and Radiological Science
Johns Hopkins University School of Medicine
Baltimore, Maryland

Giovanni B. Giovenzana
Department of Chemical, Food, Pharmaceutical and Pharmacological Sciences
Amedeo Avogadro University of Eastern Piemont
Novara, Italy

Kristine Glunde
Russell H. Morgan Department of Radiology and Radiological Science
Johns Hopkins University School of Medicine
Baltimore, Maryland

Richard Hargreaves
Merck and Co., Inc.
West Point, Pennsylvania

R. Mark Henkelman
Mouse Imaging Centre
Hospital for Sick Children
Toronto, Ontario, Canada

Bruce G. Jenkins
Athinoula A. Martinos Center for Biomedical Imaging
Massachusetts General Hospital and Harvard Medical School
Charlestown, Massachusetts

Beat M. Jucker
Cardiovascular and Urogenital Center of Excellence in Drug Discovery
GlaxoSmithKline
King of Prussia, Pennsylvania

Eric Juettler
Department of Neurology
University of Heidelberg
Heidelberg, Germany

Hans-Ulrich Kauczor
Department of Radiology
German Cancer Center
Heidelberg, Germany

Sebastian Kelle
Department of Internal Medicine/Cardiology
German Heart Institute Berlin
Berlin, Germany

Manish Kothari
Synarc Inc.
San Francisco, California

Didier Laurent
Novartis Institutes for BioMedical Research Inc.
Discovery Technologies
Cambridge, Massachusetts

Martin O. Leach
Cancer Research U.K. Clinical Magnetic Resonance Research Group
Institute of Cancer Research and Royal Marsden NHS Foundation Trust
Surrey, United Kingdom

Dario Longo
Department of Chemistry IFM and Centre for Molecular Imaging
University of Torino
Torino, Italy

Joseph B. Mandeville
Athinoula A. Martinos Center for Biomedical Imaging
Massachusetts General Hospital and Harvard Medical School
Charlestown, Massachusetts

Alex Matter
Novartis Institute for Tropical Diseases Pte. Ltd.
Singapore

Chrit Moonen
Laboratory for Molecular and Functional Imaging
ERT 5543 CNRS
University Victor Segalen Bordeaux
Bordeaux, France

Noriko Mori
Russell H. Morgan Department of Radiology and Radiological Science
Johns Hopkins University School of Medicine
Baltimore, Maryland

Thomas Mueggler
Institute for Biomedical Engineering
ETH Zurich/University of Zurich
Zurich, Switzerland

Eike Nagel
Department of Internal Medicine and Cardiology
German Heart Institute Berlin
Berlin, Germany

Matthias Nahrendorf
Medical Clinic
University of Würzburg
Würzburg, Germany

Detlef Niese
External Relations
Novartis Institutes for BioMedical Research
Basel, Switzerland

Arvind P. Pathak
Russell H. Morgan Department of Radiology and Radiological Science
Johns Hopkins University School of Medicine
Baltimore, Maryland

Geoffrey S. Payne
Cancer Research U.K. Clinical Magnetic Resonance Research Group
Institute of Cancer Research and Royal Marsden NHS Foundation Trust
Surrey, United Kingdom

Iris-Katharina Penner
Department of Cognitive Psychology
University of Basel
Basel, Switzerland

Charles Peterfy
Synarc Inc.
San Francisco, California

Harry Karmouty Quintana
Novartis Institutes for BioMedical Research
Discovery Technologies
Basel, Switzerland

Venu Raman
Russell H. Morgan Department of Radiology and Radiological Science
Johns Hopkins University School of Medicine
Baltimore, Maryland

Martin Rausch
Novartis Institutes for BioMedical Research
Discovery Technologies
Basel, Switzerland

David Reid
Respiratory and Inflammation Centre of Excellence in Drug Discovery
GlaxoSmithKline
Welwyn, United Kingdom

Michael Roden
1.Medical Department
Hanusch Hospital
Karl-Landsteiner Institute for Endocrinology and Metabolism
Vienna, Austria

Markus Rudin
Institute for Biomedical Engineering
ETH Zurich/University of Zurich
Zurich, Switzerland

Peter D. Schellinger
Department of Neurology
University of Heidelberg
Heidelberg, Germany

Petra Schweinhardt
Pain Imaging Neuroscience Group
Centre for Functional Magnetic Resonance Imaging of the Brain
Department of Physiology, Anatomy, and Genetics
Oxford University
Oxford, United Kingdom

Scott A. Small
Department of Neurology
Center for Neurobiology and Behavior
Columbia University School of Physicians and Surgeons
New York, New York

Enzo Terreno
Department of Chemistry IFM and Centre for Molecular Imaging
University of Torino
Torino, Italy

Bruno Tigani
Novartis Institutes for BioMedical Research
Discovery Technologies
Basel, Switzerland

Irene Tracey
Pain Imaging Neuroscience Group
Centre for Functional Magnetic Resonance Imaging of the Brain
Department of Physiology, Anatomy, and Genetics
Oxford University
Oxford, United Kingdom

John A. Wagner
Merck and Co., Inc.
Rahway, New Jersey

Piotr Walczak
Department of Radiology and Institute for Cell Engineering
Johns Hopkins University School of Medicine
Baltimore, Maryland

Abbreviations

5-FC	5-fluorocytosine
5-FU	5-fluorouracil
17AAG	17-allylamino,17-demethoxygeldanamycin
18FDG	18F-fluorodeoxyglucose
AA	adjuvant arthritis
AAZTA	6-amino-6-methylperhydro-1,4-diazepinetetraacetic acid
Aβ	amyloid β-peptide
AChE	acetylcholinesterase
ACL	anterior cruciate ligament
AD	Alzheimer's disease
ADC	apparent diffusion coefficient
ADME	absorption, distribution, metabolism, and excretion
ADMET	absorption, distribution, metabolism, excretion, and toxicology
ADNI	Alzheimer's disease neuroimaging initiative
ADP	adenosine diphosphate
AIA	antigen-induced arthritis
AMPA	alpha-amino-3-hydroxy-5-methyl-isoxazole-4-propionate
ApoE	apolipoprotein E
APP	amyloid precursor protein
ASL	arterial spin labeling
ATP	adenosine triphosphate
ATP_{ase}	ATP synthase
BAL	broncho-alveolar lavage
BBB	blood–brain barrier
BMI	body mass index
BN	brown Norway
BOLD	blood oxygenation level dependent
BPF	brain parenchymal fraction
CA	contrast agent
CAA	cerebral amyloid angiopathy
CAD	coronary artery disease
cAMP	cyclic adenosine monophosphate
CBF	cerebral blood flow
CBV	cerebral blood volume
CCD	charge-coupled device
CD	cytosine deaminase
CE-MRA	contrast-enhanced magnetic resonance angiography
CEST	chemical exchange saturation transfer
CF	cystic fibrosis
CFT	2β–carbomethoxy-3β–(4-fluorophenyl)tropane
CHESS	chemical shift selective
Cho	choline
CIA	collagen-induced arthritis
CMR	cardiac MR
CMRglc	cerebral metabolic rate of glucose consumption
CNR	contrast-to-noise ratio
CNS	central nervous system
COPD	chronic obstructive pulmonary disease
COV	coefficient of variation
Cr	creatine
CRP	C-reactive protein
CsA	cyclosporine A
CSF	cerebrospinal fluid
CSI	chemical shift imaging
CT	computerized tomography
CTA	computerized tomography angiography
CTA-SI	computerized tomography angiography source images
CTEPH	chronic thromboembolic pulmonary hypertension
DA	dark agouti
DAS	disease activity score
DAT	dopamine transporter
DCE-MRI	dynamic contrast-enhanced MRI
deoxy-Hb	deoxyhemoglobin
DG	dentate gyrus
dGEMRIC	delayed gadolinium-enhanced MRI of cartilage
dHB	deoxyhemoglobin
DIAS	desmoplase in acute ischemic stroke
DMEDP	division of metabolic and endocrine drug products
DMPX	3,7-dimethyl-1-propargylaxanthine
DPP-IV	dipeptidylpeptidase IV

DSA	digital subtraction angiography
DSE	dobutamine stress echocardiography
DSMR	dobutamine stress MR
DTI	diffusion tensor imaging
DWI	diffusion-weighted imaging
DWMRI	diffusion-weighted MRI
EAE	experimental autoimmune encephalomyelitis
EC	entorhinal cortex
ECG	electrocardiograph/ electrocardiogram
ECM	extracellular matrix
ECS	extracellular space
EDSS	extended disability status scale
EEG	electroencephalogram
EGFP	enhanced green fluorescent protein
EGP	endogenous glucose production
EMCL	extramyocellular lipids
ENaC	epithelial sodium channels
EPC	endothelial progenitor cell
EPI	echo-planar imaging
EPO	eosinophil peroxidase
ES	embryonic stem cells
FACoA	fatty acyl-CoA
FAD	familial Alzheimer's disease
FCD	fixed charge density
FDA	food and drug administration
FFA	free fatty acid
FLASH	fast low-angle shot
fMRI	functional magnetic resonance imaging
FSE	fast spin-echo
FTPA	perfluorotripropylamine
G6P	glucose-6-phosphate
GABA	γ-amino butyric acid
GAG	glycosaminoglycan
GAPDH	glyceraldehyde-3-phosphate dehydrogenase
GCMS	gas chromatography–mass spectrometry
Gd	gadolinium
Gd-DOTA	gadoterate meglumine
Gd-DTPA	gadolinium diethylenetriamine pentaacetic acid (gadopentate dimeglumine)
Gd-EOB-DTPA	gadolinium ethoxybenzyl diethylenetriamine pentaacetic acid
GDEPT	gene-directed enzyme prodrug therapy
Gd-GRE	gadopentate dimeglumine-enhanced gradient-echo
Gd-MRA	gadolinium-enhanced MR angiography
GFP	green fluorescent protein
GLP	good laboratory practice
GLP-1	glucagon-like-peptide 1
GLUT4	glucose transport protein 4
GMP	good manufacturing practice
GPC	glycerophosphocholine
GPE	glycerophosphoethanolamine
GTP	guanosine triphosphate
HAART	highly active antiretroviral therapy
HASTE	half-Fourier single-shot turbo spin-echo
HbA1	glycosylated hemoglobin A1
HbO2	oxyhemoglobin
HCL	hepatocellular lipids
HD	Huntington's disease
HEP	high energy phosphate
HIF-1	hypoxia inducible factor
HKII	hexokinase II
HMEC	human mammary epithelial cell
HP	hyperpolarized
HRCT	high resolution computerized tomography
HRE	hypoxia response elements
HSA	human serum albumin
HSC	hematopoietic stem cells
Hsp	heat shock protein
HTS	high-throughput screening
IAUGC	initial area under the Gd curve
ICAM	intercellular adhesion molecules
ICH	intracranial hemorrhage
IGF-1	insulin-like growth factor I
IL	interleukin
IMCL	intramyocellular lipids
IMCL-S	intramyocellular lipids, mostly in soleus muscle
IMCL-T	intramyocellular lipids, mostly in tibialis anterior muscle
IMWM	intermediate molecular weight molecule
IR	insulin resistance
IR-HASTE	inversion-recovery single-shot turbo spin-echo

IRON	increased relaxation with iron oxide nanoparticles
IRS	insulin receptor substrate
IRS1	insulin receptor-substrate 1
IVIM	intravoxel incoherent motion
JNK	jun N-terminal kinase
JSN	joint-space narrowing
JSW	joint-space width
LCL	lateral collateral ligament
LDL-C	low density lipoprotein cholesterol
LMWM	low molecular weight molecule
L-NAME	N^G-nitro-L-arginine methyl ester
LOR	line of response
LPS	lipopolysaccharide
LV	left ventricle
mAb	monoclonal antibody
MABP	mean arterial blood pressure
MAO-B	monoamine oxidase-B
MAP	mitogen-activated protein
MBP	myelin basic protein
mBSA	methylated bovine serum albumin
MCA	middle cerebral artery
MCA-O	middle cerebral artery occlusion
MCI	mild cognitive impairment
MCL	medial collateral ligament
MEMRI	manganese enhanced MRI
mGluR	metabotropic glutamate receptor
micro-CT	micro x-ray computed tomography
MMCM	macromolecular contrast molecule
MMP	matrix metalloproteases
MNU	methylnitrosourea
MODY	maturity onset diabetes of the young
MOG	myelin-oligodendrocyte glycoprotein
MPO	myeloperoxidase
MPP^+	N-methyl-4-phenylpyridinium
MPTP	N-methy-4-phenyl-1,2,3,6-tetrahydropyridine
MRA	magnetic resonance angiography
MRI	magnetic resonance imaging
MRS	magnetic resonance spectroscopy
MRSI	MR spectroscopic imaging
MS	multiple sclerosis
MSX-3	3-(3-hydroxypropyl)-8-(m-methoxystyryl)-7-methyl-1-propargylxanthine
MT	magnetization transfer
mTOR	mammalian target of rapamycin
MTP	metatarsophalangeal
MTR	magnetization transfer ratio
MTT	mean transit time
NAA	*N*-acetylaspartate
NCE	new chemical entity
NFκB	nuclear factor κB
NIHSS	National Institutes of Health stroke scale
NIR	near-infrared
NMDA	N-methyl-D-aspartate
NMR	nuclear magnetic resonance
NO	nitric oxide
NOS	nitric oxide synthase
NSAID	nonsteroidal anti-inflammatory drug
NTP	nucleotide triphosphate
NT-pro-BNP	N-terminal pro-brain natriuretic peptide
OA	osteoarthritis
OAI	osteoarthritis initiative
OP	optical pumping
OSA	obstructive sleep apnea
OVA	ovalbumin
PAMAM	polyamidoamide
PC	phosphocholine
PCL	posterior cruciate ligament
PCr	phosphocreatine
PD	Parkinson's disease
PD	pharmacodynamic
PDE	phosphodiester
PDE4	phosphodiesterase type 4
PE	phosphoethanolamine
PE	pulmonary embolism
PET	positron emission tomography
PG	proteoglycans
PGK	phosphoglycerate kinase
pH_e	extracellular pH
phFMRI	pharmacological FMRI
phMRI	pharmacologic MRI
P_i	inorganic phosphate
PK	pharmacokinetics
PKC	protein kinase C
PLL	poly-L-lysine
PLP	proteolipid protein
PME	phosphomonoester

PNA	peptide nucleic acid
PNS	peripheral nervous system
PPAR	peroxisome proliferator activated receptor
PPARγ	peroxisome proliferator activated receptor γ
ppm	part per million
PRESS	point resolved spectroscopy
PS	presenilin
PWI	perfusion-weighted imaging
QD	quantum dot
QSAR	quantitative structure-activity relationship
RA	rheumatoid arthritis
RBV	relative blood volume
rCBV	relative cerebral blood volume
$rCMRO_2$	relative cerebral oxygen consumption
RF	radio frequency
ROI	region of interest
rtPA	recombinant tissue plasminogen activator
RV	right ventricle
SAH	subarachnoid hemorrhage
SAP	square antiprismatic
SAR	structure-activity relationship
SCI	spinal cord injury
SD	standard deviation
SGU	splanchnic glucose uptake
SH	spontaneous hypertensive
siRNA	small interfering RNA
sLex	sialyl Lewis X
SMC	smooth muscle cell
SNP	single nucleotide polymorphism
SNR	signal-to-noise ratio
SNRI	serotonin noradrenaline re-uptake inhibitor
SOP	standard operating procedure
SPAMM	spatial modulation of magnetization
SPECT	single photon emission computed tomography
SPIO	superparamagnetic iron oxide
SSFP	steady-state free precession
SSRI	selective serotonin re-uptake inhibitor
STEAM	stimulated echo acquisition mode
STIR	short inversion time inversion recovery
T_1	longitudinal relaxation time
T_2	transverse relaxation time
T_2^*	effective transverse relaxation time
T1DM	type 1 diabetes mellitus
T2DM	type 2 diabetes mellitus
T4DM	type 4 diabetes mellitus
T1W	T_1-weighted
T2W	T_2-weighted
TA	transfection agent
TBV	total blood volume
TCA	tricarboxylic acid
tCho	total choline
tCr	total creatine
TE	echo time
TG	transgene
TG	triglyceride
TH	tyrosine hydroxylase
TIA	transient ischemic attack
TNF	tumor necrosis factor
TR	repetition time
TSAP	twisted square antiprismatic
TSE	turbo-spin-echo
TTP	time-to-peak
TZD	thiazolidinedione
UBM	ultrasound biomicroscopy
UCP	uncoupling protein
USPIO	ultrasmall superparamagnetic iron oxide
VEGF	vascular endothelium growth factor
VIBE	volumetric interpolated breathhold examination
WAP	waveform analysis protocol
WORMS	whole organ MRI score
ZDF	Zucker diabetic fatty

Table of Contents

1 The Drug Discovery and Development Process: A Brief Overview

Alex Matter

The process of discovering new drugs is positioned at the interface between academic, (i.e., basic research into biological phenomena) and clinical research, defining the efficacy and safety of new drug candidates. In this sense it belongs to the realm of goal-oriented, applied research, and its benchmark is productivity in terms of number of novel, attractive, and technically feasible drug candidates that can be offered to the disciplines of preclinical and clinical research and development, and that have a reasonable chance of success.

This has become a highly structured process that can be divided into several phases (Figure 1.1). A few definitions may be helpful. A drug target is a defined biochemical entity such as an enzyme or a receptor, the function of which is causally related to the initiation and/or maintenance of the disease process. Chemical or biological molecules are able to modify the deregulated function of the target (e.g., excessive activity of an enzyme), resulting in a positive change of the phenotype at the cellular and animal level, and finally, at the disease level. A crucial step is therefore to attain a high degree of certainty about the relevance of a drug target, i.e., its role in the pathophysiology of the disease. Based on this insight, an assay can be developed that reproducibly and accurately measures the activity of the drug target. This allows performance of lead finding activities using a panel of technologies, most frequently, a large library of defined chemical entities in a high throughput screening (HTS). Once a prototype molecule with desirable properties is found (a lead), a so-called lead optimization process refines this molecule to a pharmacological entity that shows well-balanced properties regarding most of the parameters tested. Such a molecule is then examined for efficacy at tolerated and technically feasible doses in relevant disease models before entering preclinical development. These disease models must mirror the processes that occur in patients, in itself a very high technical hurdle. The predictive value of many disease models is questionable, leading to disappointing clinical results; disease models are therefore intensely investigated for their predictive quality, i.e., the probability that any conclusion drawn from the animal models will be borne out in clinical trials.

Also, in order to shorten the length of time when relatively safe statements can be made regarding the tolerability, pharmacokinetic properties, and efficacy of any drug candidate, the search for biomarkers is pursued with great vigor. Biomarkers comprise any changes in serum proteins, easily accessible tissues and noninvasive imaging of organs that allow preliminary conclusions regarding safety and efficacy of a clinical drug candidate in early clinical trials to be drawn. Such statements can lead to early abandonment of projects, thus preserving large amounts of resources. On the other hand, if biomarker activity is positive at tolerated doses, confidence in a drug candidate is markedly increased and the risk decreased. This is of huge importance to pharmaceutical companies, and therefore, biomarker technologies such as noninvasive imaging are central topics of interest.

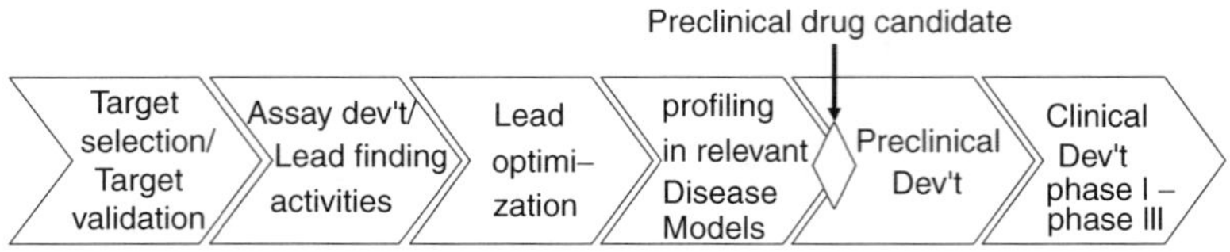

FIGURE 1.1 Phases of the drug discovery process.

The decision to take a drug candidate into development prompts a complex series of activities, defined as preclinical development, and, if successful, the various steps in patient-based studies, known as clinical development, follow with successive phases I, II, and III (see also Chapter 2, Section 2.4).

Preclinical development comprises studies to prove the scaleability of a synthetic process to larger quantities (usually in the kilogram range), activities to optimize the formulation of the compound, testing of the drug in animal models of disease, and a structured program of assays describing the toxicity of the compound in animal species such as rodents, dogs, and monkeys. This is complemented by pharmacokinetic studies measuring absorption, distribution, metabolism, and excretion (ADME) in at least two animal species. All these studies must comply with stringent regulatory guidelines that are described as good laboratory practice (GLP) and good manufacturing practice (GMP). The data produced will allow a decision to be reached as to whether a compound is fit to enter clinical trials. The data must be of a quality to satisfy the regulatory branches of the health authorities.

The clinical phase I trials can start once the necessary permissions of the health authorities and ethical review boards are obtained. Phase I clinical trials are designed to look into the pharmacokinetic behavior of a drug candidate in humans, gaining insight into drug exposure; furthermore, tolerability of the compound is carefully assessed, initially using very low doses followed by increasingly higher, and also multiple, doses. In some cases, effects on biomarkers can provide early information on the pharmacodynamics of the compound. Phase II is largely designed to show efficacy in so-called open clinical trials and to determine an optimal dose and schedule. In phase III trials, incontrovertible evidence is sought for efficacy at tolerated doses, often in double-blind trials, i.e., trials where neither the patient nor the doctor knows whether the active ingredient or a placebo (control substance) has been administered. The whole data package will then be assembled and submitted to health authorities for registration, the final and most important hurdle before marketing of the new medicine can take place.

Risk management in this long and tremendously complex process has become a major driver in drug discovery, and even more so, in drug development. Given the (largely financial) stakes, failure of drug candidates in late-stage clinical trials can have disastrous financial consequences, even for relatively large companies. Risk management is therefore the driver behind initiatives to render the drug discovery process more predictable. The target validation process and the development of molecular diagnostics and biomarkers must be considered in this context. Added to this are competitive pressures to be first in the market. This is in conflict with careful risk management; thus, methods have been sought to reconcile the two demands. Generally speaking, the individual activities are optimized through rigorous quality assurance, automation, robotics, and the like. Once this is accomplished, a further reduction in timelines can only be achieved through telescoping the activities, i.e., these are no longer performed in successive stages, but overlap. This means that certain activities that are dependent on positive outcomes from previous endeavors are started at risk, before the results of those preceding actions are known. This can result in large gains in time, but obviously increases risk. It is the role of experienced project management can balance out these various factors achieving equity between acceptable risk and competitive timelines.

It is evident from the above that the drug discovery process has developed from a purely empirical, almost primitive way of carrying out research, to a highly sophisticated, multidisciplinary, and very expensive area of expertise that is more and more dominated by the latest developments in information technology, robotics, automation, molecular genetics, biochemistry, cell biology, and molecular pharmacology. The changes that have occurred over the last 30 years are truly revolutionary. The pace of technological change is such that often technologies do not reach maturity before they are replaced by the next wave of more advanced ones. It is useful to divide this technological revolution into stages.

The era of 1950 to 1985 was largely dominated by black-box approaches, i.e., studies in intact animals, in perfused organs or tissue slice preparations, bacterial and eukaryotic cell cultures. Relatively crude endpoints such as muscle contraction, lung and cardiac function, tumor shrinkage, minimal inhibitory concentrations, and death rates were recorded in animal studies and used to define a window between efficacy and toxicity.

The period from 1985 to 2000 was characterized by target-driven drug discovery. Drug targets were defined as biochemical entities, such as enzymes, receptors, surface antigens, transcription factors, etc., and validated by three essential components. First, relevant molecular epidemiology needed to demonstrate the presence of the target in a given disease; second, the role of the target in the pathophysiology of the disease needed to be understood, at least in the overall context; third, an understanding of the issues related to drugability needed to be developed. Drugability is defined operationally as the ease with which lead molecules that modify target function in a potent and selective way can be found. This is in many cases very difficult to assess, and remains the hurdle that is most frequently underestimated. Indeed, as it turns out, many putative, relatively well validated targets can simply not be cracked with available technologies. We have learned over the years to recognize hard targets, i.e., targets with low drugability based on structural characteristics such as absence of deep, hydrophobic clefts, or presence of ionic binding sites. The former occurs frequently in protein–protein interaction, the latter is found, for example, in phosphate-binding structures.

The mid-1990s saw the entry of rational drug design, systematic lead optimization guided by structural biology (crystallography and NMR), and HTS of drug targets with increasingly complex libraries, often based on combinatorial approaches. More often now, targeted libraries are being produced that focus on specific targets or target classes such as kinases, proteases and many others, giving raise to so-called platform approaches.

The drug discovery process became more and more structured to reflect the high degree of specialization. Complex multidisciplinary teams had to be formed to deal with this process in a concerted fashion (Table 1.1). Inherently, this process is slow, easily taking 4 to 6 years to be completed. The early stages of the process are relatively cheap but the D3 and D4 stages can cost up to several millions of U.S. dollars per year. Coupled with a success rate that is around 10% for a drug candidate that enters the clinical pipeline, the stakes become truly staggering.

In this environment, the sudden availability of genetic information covering the entire genome of man, and increasingly, of more and more other species, had the effect of a bombshell. Almost overnight, the ambition to study biological systems comprehensively became a realistic perspective. This new era, starting around the 2000, and seriously taking off in subsequent years, witnessed — without any exaggeration — a paradigm shift in thinking about new drugs. With the revelation of the human and several other genomes and the onslaught of new technologies allowing the detailed study of overall gene expression (genomics) and of large-scale translational activity (proteomics), as well as a comprehensive analysis of metabolites (metabolomics), the door has been opened to a systematic and synthetic analysis of biological phenomena. This is a radical departure from the reductionist approaches of the 1980s and 1990s.

Initially, the euphoria created by these technological advances led to statements that we found ourselves in a target-rich landscape, that medical breakthroughs were around the corner, and so on. Clearly, this has not happened until now. The productivity of the pharmaceutical

TABLE 1.1
Stages of Drug Discovery Process before Clinical Testing

Stage	Definition	Time-Lines (Months)	Technologies (Incomplete Selection)
D0	Target discovery/target selection	12 +	Molecular epidemiology, molecular genetics, pathophysiology, biochemistry, knockout/ knockdown technologies, structural biology
D1	Assay development	3	Whole gamut of assay technologies for biochemical and cellular screens that fit criteria such as intended throughput, signal-to-noise ratio, reproducibility, accuracy
D2	Lead finding, high throughput screening/hit-to-lead	6	Screens ranging from several hundreds to several millions of compounds, at various stages of automation and miniaturization, virtual screens, *de novo* drug design, therapeutic models aiming to reproduce some disease parameters
D3	Lead optimization	18–24	Medicinal chemistry, cocrystallization studies, structure-activity relationship (SAR) by NMR, quantitative structure-activity relationship (QSAR), natural product purification or synthesis
D4	Preclinical development	12	Optimization of synthesis, salt selection, upscaling, toxicity studies (acute, subacute, chronic), formulation, stability, purity

industry is stagnant while the costs are skyrocketing, a situation that is not sustainable in the long run. So, where is the difficulty?

It is likely, that at least four factors play an important role in this context:

- Insufficient evidence linking a given drug target causally to a disease process. In most cases, a disease process is not linked to a simple linear causality chain. Expression profiling (transcriptome) quite often delivers confusing and uninterpretable results. We are far from an understanding of disease processes that involve interactions of several genes and environmental factors.
- Hurdles of drugability (see discussion above).
- Lack of predictive quality of cellular and animal models in terms of efficacy as well as toxicity (again, see discussion above).
- Complexity in terms of cost and duration of (pivotal) clinical trials.

Clearly, new ways of thinking and new ways to handle these hurdles are needed. Better means to validate targets, to check the quality of chemical leads, and to make reliable predictions on the efficacy and toxicity profile of drug candidates must be pursued. We have to build a seamless continuum from target to lead to drug candidate and, finally, to a clinical development compound, in a human environment, or if that is not possible, in an environment that reliably mirrors the human context. This must include molecular epidemiology, molecular diagnostics, and biomarker technologies that are applicable both in preclinical and in clinical situations. To achieve this, technologies that work in a cellular context, in intact animals as well as in human patients must become available. Whenever possible we should study living materials.

Noninvasive imaging technologies have been recognized to fulfill many of these requirements. A panel of technologies is now available, ranging from ultrasound to fluorescence and magnetic resonance imaging (MRI), the last being the focus of this book. The common thread is to study noninvasively living cells, tissues, organs, and intact animals in a way that is in many cases directly translatable to the clinical situation. The emergence *of biomarkers* providing mechanistic or at least functional insights into the effects of a new medical entity is permeating the thinking of translational medicine, the field that aims to build a strong bridge between preclinical and clinical research (see Chapter 3 for more details).

It is a realistic hope to expect that noninvasive imaging technologies, such as MRI, will make an important contribution to enhance the predictive quality of cellular and animal models, to shorten the response time to early clinical endpoints, and to diminish thereby the attrition rate of drug candidates. Indeed, out of 12 novel targets only one is truly approachable and attractive for starting the search for drug candidates. Furthermore, on average, one out of ten clinical drug candidates reaches the market. If this huge attrition could be diminished, dramatic effects on the overall productivity of drug discovery as a discipline would be achieved.

2 The Drug Discovery and Development Process: Opportunities and Challenges for MR Techniques

Nicolau Beckmann and Markus Rudin

CONTENTS

2.1 INTRODUCTION

As seen in the previous chapter, development of new drugs requires large amounts of time and resources. Drug development is a formidable undertaking requiring nearly US$ 800 million and 12 years to bring the average drug to market commercialization [1,2]. It is estimated that only one out of 5,000–10,000 compounds tested in preclinical assay is approved as a new medicine [3]. Obviously, it is in the interest of pharmaceutical companies and of consumers that better drugs (more effective, fewer side effects) become available at a lower cost. At first sight, these requirements seem to be mutually exclusive. The current hope of meeting this challenging task is that by improving the characterization of compounds and their effects in early and not yet so costly phases, one would increase their chance of success in late phases of development.

The process of discovering and bringing a drug to market is complex (Figure 2.1). It begins with the identification and validation of a potential drug target. High affinity binders are searched for by using high-throughput screening (HTS). Compounds that have passed some initial selectivity filters are then further evaluated. Approximately 40% of the research costs are charged to the drug discovery effort, as compared with 60% for drug development [2,3]. The high attrition rate of drugs under development coupled with time pressure poses a dilemma. During the last 10 years, the annual research and development expenses for drug discovery have tripled, while the number of new chemical entities (NCEs) launched has remained at the same level of approximately 50 per year [2,3]. Despite significant investments in biology-related areas such as genomics and proteomics and in technology platforms designed to increase the number of compounds assayed, significant problems in development time, patent position, and attrition rate in clinical trials remained unchanged. Some of the problems encountered are:

- The development time after filing a patent and before a drug reaches the market is still unacceptably long, resulting in a limited period to gain from the patent protection.
- Patents are often weak because many companies pursue the same targets and use libraries synthetized utilizing combinatorial or parallel synthesis approaches, or even similar chemical libraries acquired from commercial vendors. The likelihood of obtaining a patent is thus reduced because known compounds and analogues thereof are being tested.
- The attrition rate is unacceptably high — on average, only one out of 10 compounds entered into clinical trials becomes a new drug.

From this, it becomes clear that companies need, on one hand, to invest resources in the early phase of the drug discovery process which encompasses the selection of screening compounds and/or building blocks for combinatorial libraries. For instance, it has been suggested that compounds follow the "Lipinski rules of five" [4]:

1. Molecular weights below 500
2. Log P less than five
3. Number of hydrogen bond donors fewer than five
4. Number of hydrogen bond acceptors fewer than five
5. No more than five fused rings

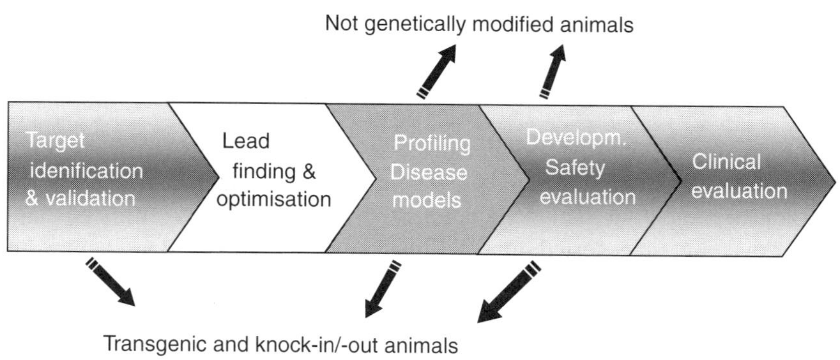

FIGURE 2.1 Simplified view of the drug discovery process. *In vivo* MR techniques may play important roles in several steps, highlighted in gray.

The important features to be considered are absorption, distribution, metabolism, excretion, and toxicology (ADMET) — all associated with the molecular structure. A much better understanding of this structure–performance relationship is needed to develop predictive algorithms that will increase the survival rate of compounds in clinical trials. The challenge is that no single factor can account for NCE success or failure in preclinical and clinical development since factors, such as solubility, pKa (the pH at which the drug is 50% ionized), absorption, metabolism, formulation, pharmacokinetics (PK), toxicity, and efficacy, to name a few, are all interrelated. Nevertheless, it is expected that an appropriate initial investment in the chemistry should reduce the attrition rate, thus increasing the success rate and, perhaps, reducing the development costs at the same time [5].

2.2 IMAGING IN DRUG RESEARCH

Another important attempt in shortening the drug discovery and development process is related to improving the characterization of compounds and their effects in early and not yet so costly phases, and to transferring this knowledge into the clinical phase of testing (Figure 2.1). Intimately linked to this reasoning stands the knowledge about a given disease or disease model, and early diagnosis and characterization. Certainly, the better the etiology of a disease is known, the higher the chance of finding an appropriate therapy. Also, the better a disease can be diagnosed and characterized, the higher the chance to be able to interfere in this process with a chemical entity. Advances in the understanding of disease progression at the cellular and molecular levels that spur the development of drugs that are highly specific for their molecular target, along with progress in bioanalytical assay technologies constitute an attractive basis for choosing, describing, and evaluating new biomarkers.

According to the Food and Drug Administration (FDA), a biomarker is a characteristic that is objectively measured and evaluated as an indicator of normal biological processes, pathogenic processes, or pharmacologic responses to a therapeutic intervention [6]. In our context, a biomarker can be considered a bioanalytical readout with diagnostic and prognostic quality that can be used for the identification of a pathology and for monitoring its progression, and for the evaluation of therapeutic interventions. Criteria for validating biomarkers include considerations of mechanistic plausibility, available methods and technologies, and preclinical and clinical feasibility. Validated biomarkers may be used for identifying patient populations, as well as for providing evidence of drug efficacy and potential toxicity (see Section 2.4). The link between preclinical and clinical studies demands for noninvasive bioanalytical technologies such as imaging.

The development of imaging strategies that meet the requirements for use in a clinical setting will facilitate the translation from animal models to human subjects by minimizing changes in experimental paradigms while the model organism is changed [7–10]. What sets imaging biomarkers apart from, for example, analytes from blood serum and urine used for decades in medicine and in drug development and recently proposed proteomics biomarkers is the fact that imaging readouts tend to be much more closely related to the disease phenotype, thus facilitating direct associations between therapy and effect.

The noninvasive character of imaging enables several questions concerning drug discovery and development to be addressed. Certainly, no single imaging modality can answer all possible questions in this complicated domain. An important initial step is to find out which potential a given imaging modality has in addressing issues regarding a certain disease area. A complete review of imaging within pharmaceutical research is beyond the scope of this chapter. Table 2.1 provides an overview of current imaging modalities of interest for drug research. In this section we briefly discuss the main characteristics of non-MRI techniques.

2.2.1 Computerized Tomography

Computerized tomography (CT) was the first tomographic imaging modality introduced in the late 1960s. In CT, x-rays emitted from a source pass through the tissue and are detected by a detector array on the opposite side of the object. Source and detectors are mounted on a gantry that rotates around the patient, who is moved in the axial direction in a synchronous manner. Back-projection algorithms process the spiral CT scan data to form a series of cross-sectional images which can be assembled into a 3D dataset. Contrast in the images arises from differences in beam attenuation due to tissue specific attenuation coefficients. With the exception of the lung and calcified bone, tissues display similar attenuation coefficients, hence endogenous contrast between soft tissues is low. This determines the principal applications of CT: structural studies of skeletal structures and of the thorax. Gastrointestinal and genitourinary studies require the use of exogenous radio-opaque contrast agents. The image resolution of clinical systems is >0.5 mm. By using thick multiplanar reformation techniques, image quality can be improved while keeping radiation dose low [11].

Although CT is basically a technique that provides anatomical information only, physiological information can be gathered as well. For example, dynamic contrast-enhanced CT allows the analysis of tissue perfusion [12–14]. This technique is based on the peripheral intravenous administration of a bolus of (iodine) contrast medium. Transient changes in blood vessel density can be represented by contrast medium as it makes its first pass in the perfused tissue. Any increase in Hounsfield units is directly proportional to the iodine concentration in the region.

Micro-CT systems providing high-resolution images ($\sim$50 μm) and rapid data acquisition (typically 5 to 30 min) are emerging as a cost-effective means for detecting soft tissue structures, skeletal abnormalities, and tumors in live small animals [15–17]. Use of iodinated contrast agents enhances the weak endogenous contrast between different soft tissues. However, the difficulty in designing CT contrast agents limits the utility of the technique for molecular imaging applications. It is conceivable to generate probes using heavy metals and to improve image contrast by employing methods as K-edge subtraction and x-ray fluorescence imaging [18], but at least in the near future, micro-CT will be rather used to supplement data from other molecular imaging techniques.

Accuracy in the images is determined by the x-ray dose given to the animal. One concern of microCT is therefore radiation dose, which although not lethal, may be high enough to induce changes in the immune response and other biological pathways, so that experimental outcomes could be affected [19,20]. For an ideal scanner, a coefficient of variation (COV) of 1% in the linear attenuation coefficient can be expected for an image with an isotropic voxel size of 135 μm of a mouse exposed to 0.25 Gy. If the same COV is to be achieved in a 65-μm isotropic voxel, a dose of 5.0 Gy would be necessary.

2.2.2 Positron Emission Tomography

Positron emission tomography (PET) produces images of the body by detecting the radiation emitted from radioactive substances injected into the body and labeled with positron emitting radioactive atoms, such as carbon-11, fluorine-18, oxygen-15, or nitrogen-13. These radioactive atoms are formed by bombarding stable chemicals with neutrons to create short-lived radioactive isotopes, for example, ^{15}O ($t_{1/2} = 2.1$ min), ^{11}C ($t_{1/2} = 20$ min), or ^{13}N ($t_{1/2} = 11$ min). PET detects the two gamma rays generated at the site where a positron emitted from the radioactive substance is captured and annihilated by an electron in the tissue. An advantage is that high-energy gamma rays (511 keV) are barely attenuated upon passage through biological tissue. In a PET study, the patient (or animal) is injected with the radiotracer. Gamma photons emitted within a coincidence window are detected by a circular array containing several rings of scintillation crystals connected to position-sensitive photomultiplier tubes. The coincidence detection locates the annihilation event on a so-called line of response (LOR) connecting the two detector elements that have registered the

TABLE 2.1
Summary of Current Imaging Modalities of Interest in Drug Research and Discovery

Technique	Clinical Imaging	Resolution	Animal Imaging	Resolution and Time Scale	Application	Main Characteristics
SPECT (low energy γ-rays)	Yes	6–8 mm; s	Yes	1–2 mm; min	Functional	Radioisotopes have longer half-lives than those used in PET; sensitivity 10 to 100 times smaller than PET
PET (high energy γ-rays)	Yes	4 mm; s	Yes	1–2 mm; min	Metabolic, functional, molecular	High sensitivity (picomolar concentrations); cyclotron needed
CT	Yes	0.5 mm; s	Yes	50–100 μm; min	Anatomical, functional	Poor soft tissue contrast
Ultrasound	Yes	300–500 μm; s	Yes	50 μm; min	Anatomical, functional	Difficulties to image through bone or lungs; microbubbles used for contrast enhancement
MRI	Yes	1 mm; s to min	Yes	80–100 μm; s to h	Anatomical, functional, molecular	High spatial resolution and soft tissue contrast
Bioluminescence	No	—	Yes	1–10 mm; s to min	Molecular	High sensitivity; transgene-based approach; light emission prone to attenuation with increased tissue depth
Near infrared fluorescence imaging	No	—	Yes	1–3 mm; s to min	Molecular	Excitation and emission light prone to attenuation with increased tissue depth

events. Measurement of a sufficient number of LORs allows image reconstruction. Thin cross-sectional images over a region of interest can thus be generated. Similarly to SPECT, PET provides physiological (e.g., blood flow) images, but also yields detailed metabolic information (glucose utilization, DNA and protein synthesis). Highly attractive is the option to label organic compounds with ^{11}C: as isotopic substitution does not affect the physicochemical and binding properties of a compound, PET is the method of choice for pharmacokinetic studies of biologically active compounds (e.g., drugs or drug candidates). However, the short half-life of PET radionuclides implies that PET scanners have to be located near particle accelerators (cyclotrons) that produce the radioisotopes.

PET imaging is one of the most sensitive approaches and picomolar amounts of radiolabel can be readily detected and quantified *in vivo*, irrespective of tissue depth. For comparison, SPECT and MRI require, respectively, 10^1 to 10^2 and 10^7 to 10^8 higher amounts of probe. Recent advances in radionuclide labeling allow the design and development of a large variety of radiopharmaceuticals including macromolecular structures [21]. The availability of such tools enables *in vivo* target-specific studies of label biodistribution, pharmacokinetics, and excretion, as well as the visualization and quantification of target expression levels and target function.

Preclinical PET studies using small laboratory animals demand high spatial resolution provided by dedicated micro-PET systems. Smaller voxel volumes are achieved by decreasing the size of lutetium oxyorthosilicate scintillation crystals while increasing their number. For instance, the latest generation of PET instruments contains between 18,000 and 24,000 crystals of approximate volume $1 \times 1 \times 12$ mm^3 each, arranged in contiguous rings [22,23]. Volumetric image resolution also depends on both the statistical reconstruction and modeling algorithm employed [22,24]. Typical voxel volumes reported are between 1.1 and 1.5 mm^3, rendering the systems adequate for studies in mice, rats, and nonhuman primates. Such resolutions also demand optimized correction schemes, in particular those addressing Compton scattering as the dominant source of registration errors in PET, which impacts the quality of reconstructed images and the accuracy of quantitative analysis [25]. Ultimately the physics of the decay process (positron range and deviations from photon colinearity) imposes limits on the spatial resolution possible with PET.

2.2.3 Single Photon Emission Computed Tomography

Single photon emission computed tomography (SPECT) is a nuclear imaging technique recording 3D datasets (allowing the reconstruction of cross-sectional images) that display the distribution of gamma ray emitting radiopharmaceuticals. Multiple views of the body part to be imaged are acquired by rotating the Anger camera detector head(s) around a craniocaudal axis. Using a backprojection algorithm, the 3D distribution of the radionuclide is then computed with the axial field of view determined by the axial field of view of the detecting device. SPECT detectors consist either of a standard gamma camera head, which is rotated around the patient's axis, or of two or even three heads, enabling reduction of the acquisition time. Data reconstruction has to take into account that emitted rays are attenuated by tissue. While in CT this beam attenuation is the origin of image contrast, in SPECT it leads to degradation of the image quality [26]. For instance, uncorrected SPECT data of the human head will show substantial artificial enhancement of the peripheral brain structures relative to the deep ones, which might be misinterpreted as high radiolabel concentration in cortical areas. This problem can be accounted for by filtering the data before reconstruction using a depth-dependent filter function. A more elegant but elaborate method for triple head cameras uses a gamma-ray line source between two camera heads, and the transmitted radiation is detected by the opposing camera head after passage through the patient. These transmission data allow the direct determination of correction factors to be used in the image reconstruction.

SPECT radionuclides (xenon-133, technetium-99, iodine-123) are characterized by relatively long half-lives. They stabilize by emission of single gamma rays as compared to two in PET.

SPECT is used to collect physiological information (e.g., blood flow) and to measure the biodistribution of radioactive substances. Its images have less sensitivity and are less detailed than PET images, but the SPECT technique is less expensive than PET. Also, SPECT centers do not have to be located near a particle accelerator.

The resolution of SPECT is basically limited by the geometry of the collimating device and not by the underlying physics as in PET. A modern SPECT camera has a spatial resolution of only 6 to 8 mm. When the standard (cylindrical) collimator is replaced by a pinhole device, resolutions of the order of 1 mm may be achieved, however, at the expense of a dramatic loss in sensitivity. In addition, a number of issues related to the physics of pinhole imaging must be taken into account. For instance, gamma rays penetrate the edges of the pinhole, thereby increasing the effective diameter of the hole and reducing the resolution. Also, because of the depth of the interaction of the photon in the crystal, gamma rays that pass through the pinhole and hit the crystal at an oblique angle might be mis-assigned by the Anger logic. Since pinhole SPECT does not fully sample the object space, unlike a conventional parallel-hole collimator, incomplete projection data are acquired with implications for image reconstruction [27]. Multiple pinholes may resolve some of these issues.

Commercial small animal SPECT systems capable of measuring mice typically use pixelated crystal arrays coupled to position-sensitive photomultiplier tubes and a pinhole collimator [28,29]. A less expensive alternative consists of adapting a pinhole collimator to a clinical system [30,31]. Although the intrinsic resolution of a conventional Anger-type camera is lower than that of pixellated crystal arrays, the larger detector allows for a significant magnification effect, resulting in enough resolution in the images.

2.2.4 Ultrasound

Today, ultrasound imaging comprises the use of small hand-held devices that provide basic structural and functional information, as well as complex 3D procedures that yield dynamic information on regional myocardial function. Spatial resolution in human ultrasound imaging devices is limited to 300 to 500 μm due to the frequencies of operation (7.5 to 15 MHz). Of particular importance is the use of ultrasound imaging for cardiac studies (echocardiography), for which it is used as imaging modality of choice due to its simplicity and low cost. Nevertheless, compared to MRI assessments, echocardiographic techniques tend to underestimate end-diastolic left vetricular volume and concomitantly overestimate left ventricular mass, which also affects estimates of ejection fractions [32,33]. These deviations might be attributed in part to issues in image quality affecting automated volumetric measurements. Tissue Doppler myocardial velocities have been suggested to provide an objective quantitative assessment of myocardial function. [34,35]. Moreover, myocardial contrast echocardiography can be used to determine myocardial perfusion in the experimental assessment of therapies designed to limit infarct size and restore function after infarction [36,37].

Contrast in ultrasound arises from different compressibilities of tissues. As the compressibility of gases is orders of magnitude higher than that of fluids (tissues), gas-filled microbubbles are sensitive ultrasound contrast agents. Technologically, microbubbles consisting of compressible liquids with high vapor pressure, such as perfluorocarbons, encapsulated by lipid membranes are easier to handle. While the use of these ultrasound contrast agents is established in diagnostic echocardiography [38], their effective impact has been more predominant in the detection and characterization of focal hepatic lesions. Distinctive disease states can be probed by targeting microbubbles through the attachment of specific proteins, e.g., antibodies. Alternatively microbubbles are used as carriers of bioactive substances for the site-specific delivery of gene therapy and drug [39,40]. By application of ultrasound, the microbubbles can be destroyed at a specific site to deliver the contents to the targeted tissues.

An important method to image the cardiovascular system in small animals is 2D directed M-mode echocardiography employing linear array broadband transducers operating at 12 to 15 MHz. New generation scanners with high frame rates permit high spatial resolution real-time tomographic imaging in multiple planes, making it possible to calculate 2D left ventricular volume and mass [41,42]. Recent advances in ultrasound biomicroscopy (UBM)-Doppler echocardiography have enabled cardiovascular function analyses in embryonic mice *in utero* [43,44]. UBM systems employing 20 to 55 MHz ultrasound transducers with axial and lateral resolutions as good as 30 and 60 μm, respectively, are commercially available.

2.2.5 Optical Imaging

The development of highly sensitive light detection systems coupled with advancements in the design and use of optical reporter systems, such as green fluorescent protein, luciferase, and cyanine dyes has allowed biologists to use optical imaging for studying *in vivo* biological processes at the cellular and molecular levels. *In vivo* optical imaging exploits the near-infrared (NIR) window of tissue absorbance, i.e., it takes advantage of the low absorbance of tissue chromophores such as oxy- and deoxy-hemoglobin, water, melanin, and fat for light of wavelengths between 650 and 900 nm. At these wavelengths scattering of photons is a more significant attenuation factor than absorption.

2.2.5.1 Bioluminescence

The development of the first transgenic tobacco plant expressing the firefly luciferase (*luc*) gene [45] demonstrated the feasibility of using bioluminescent reporter genes to monitor gene expression *in vivo*. Bioluminescence refers to the generation of (visible) light by living organisms, commonly due to an enzymatic reaction [46,47]. Reporter genes are used to study the expression of a gene of interest. This is achieved by inserting into the host cell genome a gene cassette containing the reporter gene construct under the control of the target gene. Bioluminescent reporters yield exquisite sensitivity as there is no endogenous background signal in mammalian cells, resulting in high signal-to-background ratios. Using sensitive detection devices, such as photomultiplier tubes or cooled charge-coupled devices (CCD), sensitivity is sufficient to count only a few emitted photons.

A prerequisite for bioluminescence imaging is genetic engineering of the tissue cells of interest, i.e., the incorporation of an exogenous reporter gene. The most common bioluminescent reporter is luciferase from the North American firefly. Luciferases are oxygenases that catalyze the transformation of D-luciferin (injected, for example, intraperitoneally) into oxyluciferin in the presence of both O_2 and Mg^{2+}-ATP. Significant portions of the emission spectrum of firefly luciferase are at wavelengths larger than 600 nm [48], i.e., they fall into the window of reduced tissue absorption, thereby increasing detectability under *in vivo* conditions. Reporter gene assays have been demonstrated to yield fundamental biological information on, for example, transcriptional regulation, signal transduction, protein–protein interactions, cell trafficking, and targeted drug action [49,50].

A difficulty of bioluminescence imaging and optical imaging in general is spatial resolution: the light intensity distribution measured at the surface critically depends on the depth of the light source within the tissue. A population of luciferase-expressing cells near the surface of the skin will appear both brighter and more focused than the same number of cells growing at deeper tissue sites. This drawback can be accounted for by devising tomographic approaches that are critical to improve data quantification [51].

2.2.5.2 Near-Infrared Fluorescence Imaging

Related to bioluminescence imaging is NIR fluorescence imaging, an attractive tool due to its operational simplicity, safety, and cost-effectiveness. Exogenous fluorochromes (dyes or genetically engineered fluorescent proteins) are excited by, for example, laser diodes operating at a frequency close to that of the detected light; the emitted fluorescent light (wavelength ≥ 700 nm) is then detected in a spatially resolved manner by a CCD camera. Due to obvious reasons, the NIR window has been shown to be particularly suitable for *in vivo* investigations.

Various labeling strategies can be followed. Coupling of fluorochromes (cyanine dyes, such as Cy5, Cy6 or Cy7) to biologically relevant molecules allows the study of their uptake and biodistribution. However, it has to be kept in mind that the attachment of a bulky fluorescent reporter may significantly influence the properties of the carrier molecule. The measured signal intensity is a function of several parameters: the receptor density, the binding affinity, and the pharmacokinetic properties of the construct (uptake rate, clearance kinetics from the interstitial space, and nonspecific cellular uptake). In general, both bound and unbound reporter fraction will contribute to the signal degrading the signal-to-background ratio. Therefore, imaging studies using fluorescent reporters (similar to SPECT studies) are usually carried out several hours after probe administration assuming that the unbound and nonspecifically bound probe had been largely cleared at this time point.

An alternative attractive method to increase signal-to-background ratios are the so-called "smart" probes that change their physical properties after specific molecular interactions with their target. For instance, Weissleder and collaborators developed NIR smart probes for the detection of protease activity based on a quenching–dequenching paradigm. The probes are optically silent in their native (quenched) state and become highly fluorescent after enzyme-mediated release of fluorochromes, resulting in signal amplification of up to several 100-fold [52–54]. Quenching results from fluorescence resonance energy transfer, due to the spatial proximity of fluorophors in the bound state. Proteolytic probe cleavage separates the donor–acceptor pair leading to dequenching. Introduction of protease-specific cleavage motifs between two fluorophor groups yield protease-specific probes. Smart probes have several advantages over passive targeting: (1) background signal is reduced since the probe is optically inactive upon injection and remains so until activated by its target; (2) specific enzyme activities can be addressed; (3) signal amplification is achieved as a single enzyme cleaves multiple fluorochromes. This probe design has been applied to pharmacological proof-of-concept studies, demonstrating, for example, the efficacy of protease inhibition in tumor xenografts [55] and in a model of rheumatoid arthritis [56].

Organic dyes have two significant disadvantages: their fluorescence spectrum is broad rendering multiplexed experiments difficult, and they tend to photobleach. Nanosized photonic crystals termed quantum dots (QDs) comprise a new class of fluorescent labels not limited by these restrictions and, hence, having great potential to image multiple biological processes concurrently *in vivo* [57–59]. Emission wavelengths (from visible to near-infrared portions of the spectrum) are directly proportional to the size of the photo-excitable core and hence tunable; emission bands are relatively narrow and characterized by a remarkable photostability. Biocompatible QD cores are typically composed of CdSe or CdTe encased by an inert protective shell and a layer of organic material that enables direct conjugation of the reporter moiety to biological targeting molecules such as antibodies. QDs of different colors tuned to target different biological process by coupling to corresponding carrier molecules will potentially enable multiplexed imaging *in vivo*. However, feasibility of this concept needs yet to be demonstrated. A potential drawback of QDs is their large size with corresponding issues concerning probe delivery.

Currently, the majority of *in vivo* fluorescence imaging approaches is based on planar detection of fluorescent light, with obvious limitations with regard to deriving quantitative information. This is currently being addressed by developing fluorescence molecular tomography approaches with improved signal quantification [60].

In the following section, we will discuss the use of MR techniques in drug research, which is the focus of our attention in this book.

2.3 BENEFITS AND LIMITATIONS OF MRI/S

The principal assets of MRI are noninvasiveness, high spatial resolution, of the order of 100 μm for rodent studies, and excellent soft tissue contrasting capabilities. The MR signal is governed by a number of parameters, e.g., proton density, relaxation times (T_1, T_2, T_2^*), proton exchange rates, water diffusion, macroscopic motion (blood flow), which depend on the biophysical properties of the tissue. This wealth of information renders MRI a valuable tool for diagnosis, tissue staging, and *in vivo* morphometry, for obtaining physiological and functional readouts, and for deriving metabolic and, to some extent, target-specific tissue characteristics (see Section 2.6 below) in a noninvasive manner.

A major limitation of MR is its low sensitivity, which significantly determines the possible roles of the technique in pharmaceutical research. A simple calculation illustrates the fact that MR is, generally speaking, not suited for directly assessing the distribution of drugs in the organism [61]. A compound of molecular mass 500 administered at a dose of 1 mg/kg and evenly distributed throughout the body will result in an approximately 2 μM tissue concentration (neglecting drug elimination). Nuclear medicine techniques, such as SPECT or PET and, more recently, NIR fluorescence imaging, provide the required sensitivity to detect compounds in micromolar concentrations. Yet, these methods are hampered by a relatively low spatial resolution (in best cases, of about 1 mm), which although acceptable in clinical applications turns out to be limiting when studying small animals, and a lack of chemical specificity, being therefore unable to distinguish whether the emitting reporter group is attached to the parent drug molecule or a metabolite. *In vivo* MR methodologies on the other hand require tissue concentrations in the millimolar range. The signals of a few endogenous metabolites can be observed and until now in exceptional cases only the fate of a drug in the target organ could be monitored using MRS. For instance, ^{19}F MRS has been successfully applied to assess the pharmacokinetics of fluorinated drugs [62–65] and ^{13}C MRS to detect the distribution of ^{13}C-labeled compounds in tumors [66,67] (see also Chapter 13, Section 13.3.5 and Chapter 14, Section 14.3.2). These examples have been essentially limited to cancer therapeutics administered at high concentrations [68]. How many of such compounds can be administered at doses sufficiently high to be detectable *in vivo* by MR is unknown. Moreover, spatial resolution in these studies is poor, significantly inferior to nuclear approaches. Therefore, in general terms, the role of MRI/S in pharmacological research is to study the effects of a drug on tissue morphology, physiology, and biochemistry rather than to follow the fate of the drug itself in the organism; in other words MR methods yield pharmacodynamic and not pharmacokinetic readouts [69–72].

Another limitation of MR methods is quantification. While absolute values of structural parameters (e.g., volumes of organs) are readily attainable, assessments of absolute physiological parameters from MRI data or absolute concentrations of metabolites are not straightforward. Complex tissue models involving multiple assumptions and approximations are required to translate MRI parameters into relevant biomedical information. For instance, assessment of absolute rates of tissue perfusion requires knowledge of the arterial input function [73,74]. Hence, the majority of physiological MRI applications use semiquantitative analysis (i.e., parameter values in the region of interest in relation to a reference tissue). An exemption remains cardiological applications, in which absolute values of functional parameters like stroke volume and ejection fraction can be derived by MRI, which is essentially based on morphometric measurements [75] (see also Chapter 16 and Chapter 17).

2.4 *IN VIVO* MR TECHNIQUES IN DRUG RESEARCH

In a simplified view, the drug discovery and development process can be divided in several steps (Figure 2.1). *In vivo* MR techniques allow relevant problems to be addressed almost throughout the process.

2.4.1 Target Identification and Validation

The first task in drug discovery is target identification and validation. Target selection, defined as the decision to focus drug discovery efforts on a specific (molecular) mechanism that is plausibly related to the disease process and, hence, anticipated to be of therapeutic value, is influenced by considerations related to the underlying scientific rationale, medical need, and strategic/commercial aspects [76,77] (see also Chapter 1). Today, all drugs on the market target about 500 biological entities: receptors (~45%), enzymes (~28%), hormones (~11%), ion channels (~5%), nuclear receptors and nucleic acids (each ~2%), the rest (~7%) being of unknown nature [78]. With the publication of the human genome, the number of potential new targets has increased dramatically [79–81]. Various technologies are helping to identify and validate targets at a high-throughput, for instance microarrays technologies for gene/protein expression profiling at the tissue or cell level, bioinformatics, antisense technologies, and chemical genomics to name just a few (for reviews, see Refs. [82–84]).

Target validation requires a causative link between a molecular/mechanistic drug target and a phenotype readout of the targeted disease. Genetically engineered animals are being increasingly used for this task. Since mouse and man display striking similarities at the genetic level, it is likely that disease parameters observed in humans might be reproduced in mice. Correspondingly, phenotypic readouts in genetically altered mice might allow the prediction of relevant pharmacological effects in man. Indeed, retrospective evaluation of the knockout phenotypes for the targets of the 100 best-selling drugs indicates that effects in these murine models of human disease correlate well with known clinical drug efficacy, illuminating a productive path forward for discovering future drug targets. Prospective mining of the druggable genome is being catalyzed by large-scale mouse knockout programs combined with phenotypic screens focused on identifying targets that modulate mammalian physiology in a therapeutically relevant manner [85–87].

Evidently, characterization of transgenic animals in a noninvasive manner is an important task for MRI techniques, which are particularly suited to analyze the structural and functional consequences of genotype expression. Hopes, strategies, and difficulties in phenotyping mice with MRI/S are extensively discussed in Chapter 5 and Chapter 6. The current lack of routine strategies to characterize transgenic animals on a broader basis should be a stimulus to invest in large scale mouse imaging, an area which still is in its infancy.

2.4.2 Lead Finding, Validation, and Optimization

Once a target has been identified and validated, identification of a lead compound is the starting point for the development of new drug candidates. Today large compound libraries of typically 10^6 compounds are screened using biochemical and cellular assays that have been made compatible for highly automated HTS. Primary hit compounds displaying activity exceeding a set threshold are further evaluated in secondary screening assays. The most promising hits are then selected for an often lengthy lead optimization program involving the synthesis and testing of compound analogues, during which issues such as target affinity, physicochemical properties and aspects of compound safety are addressed.

Hit identification by HTS is relatively efficient; nevertheless, false-positive hits can be selected, which may lead to drastic consequences for a certain project. MR spectroscopic techniques play a central role in hit validation. They are specific and less prone to false positives, a problem often encountered when using classic spectrophotometric assays (see Ref. [88] for a recent review). *In vivo* MR techniques, on the other hand, do not have any function in this phase.

2.4.3 Profiling Compounds in Animal Models of Diseases

Lead optimization results in drug candidate compounds that need to be thoroughly evaluated in animal models of human disease. The basic aim here is to obtain relevant information concerning drug efficacy, absorption, distribution, efficacy, metabolism, and elimination. Both wildtype and transgenic animals, mostly small rodents, are used.

In view of a potential translation of methods to clinical drug testing, noninvasive readouts of drug efficacy are preferable at this stage, yet not mandatory. In fact, the majority of pharmacological studies use invasive procedures. Nevertheless, there is an ethical motivation to use noninvasive methods, such as imaging techniques, which contribute to the three Rs (reduce, refine, replace) principles enforced by animal ethics committees in the governance of animal experimentation [89]. The use of imaging might be attractive from both an animal welfare and an economical point of view, since the number of animals required for a study can be reduced by up to 80% [69,72], a fact that is especially interesting in chronic studies, and in experiments involving transgenic species. Study designs furthermore allow the reduction of interindividual variances by using each animal as its own control, thereby enhancing the statistical power of experiments.

In the past, MR techniques have most extensively been used during compound profiling [69,71,72]. An extensive review of such studies and their value for different disease areas is given in the following chapters. The general flow of activities is summarized in Figure 2.2. For many diseases/disease models, a potential endpoint for the evaluation of the disease status or therapy efficacy is not readily accessible requiring the identification of a biomarker, which is indicative of the disease status. Such biomarkers should have a clear disease relevance and should have predictive quality both with regard to spontaneous disease progression and potential therapy response (see Chapter 3). In addition, in order to facilitate translational activities, biomarkers used for preclinical studies should also be relevant for the human disease and clinical drug efficacy. Validation/qualification of MR biomarker involves extensive comparison with established, usually invasive, readouts, in particular histology. Furhermore, they should correctly reproduce the well-described effects of reference compounds. Only then may they be applied for noninvasive testing of novel drug candidate compounds.

It should be borne in mind that in animal experimentation, MR methods are in competition with established, highly developed analysis tools. In pharmaceutical research, only MR applications that offer substantial advantages over existing approaches will be successful in the long term. It is the task of imaging researchers to demonstrate to their colleagues in the pharmacological laboratories the advantages and, whenever applicable, superiority of noninvasive imaging readouts.

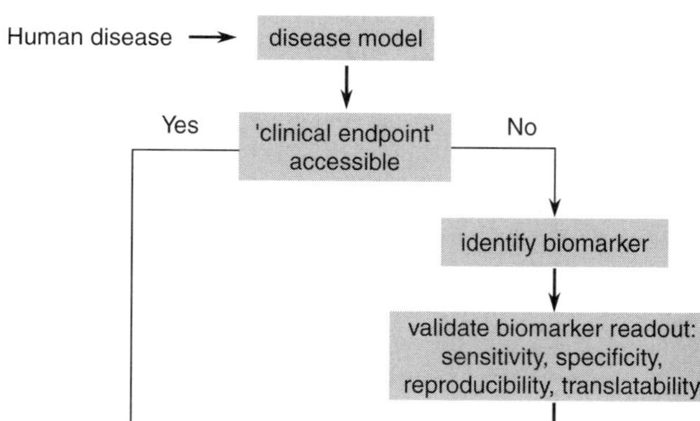

FIGURE 2.2 General flow of activities for testing therapy efficacy, from animal models of diseases to humans.

2.4.4 Safety Evaluation

The same MR techniques used for evaluation of treatment efficacy in preclinical models of human diseases can also be applied to detect potential safety issues. The advantages of using MRI (and other noninvasive technologies) for toxicological studies are that effects can be studied *in vivo* (or *post mortem*) without the need for tissue dissection, sectioning, and staining. Also, the occurrence and progression of potentially harmful structural and functional tissue alterations can be monitored in a longitudinal manner. Despite this attractive profile, the use of MRI, and of imaging technologies in general, in drug safety studies has received little attention up to now. As will be discussed in Chapter 26, a main reason is the fact that toxicological studies used for regulatory authorities must be carried out following the guidelines for good laboratory practice (GLP). Incorporation of MR techniques into routine toxicology programs running under GLP conditions will most likely require separate installations, since GLP compliance is usually not guaranteed in standard biological imaging laboratories. On the other hand, application of imaging techniques in experimental toxicology does not fall under these restrictions: studies in separate groups of animals aimed at establishing novel toxicological readouts or for internal decision-making can be carried out in a straightforward manner. Such studies should be of great value to pharmacological research and will ultimately show whether imaging techniques might be used in a broader sense for evaluation of drug safety.

2.4.5 Clinical Studies

The aim of a novel therapy is to improve the patient's clinical status (endpoint). Clinical drug studies, in particular those addressing chronic disease, are time-consuming and expensive. Similarly to the preclinical phase, biomarkers are a means to obtain early information on drug effectiveness and safety in clinical studies, which can lead to a substantial reduction in costs and development time [90,91]. More important is patient management: the time lost for a patient, who is not responsive to treatment, can be significantly reduced. A biomarker that substitutes a clinical endpoint is called a surrogate endpoint [92–95]. The most important criteria for valid surrogates are biological plausibility, a documented statistical relationship between the surrogate and an accepted clinical endpoint in epidemiological studies, and demonstration that treatment effects on the surrogate correspond to the clinical outcome.

In early clinical trials, biomarkers can be used to demonstrate proof-of-concept of the pharmacological principle and to identify appropriate dose regimens for efficacy studies. Both preclinical and clinical investigations are necessary to show a link between disease, pharmacological mechanism, and clinical endpoints.

The acceptance of biomarkers in general, and of imaging biomarkers in particular, by regulatory agencies is increasing [90], especially for oncology [96,97]. For example, for the 71 oncology drug approvals by the FDA in the period 1990–2002, endpoints other than survival were the basis for approval in 68% (39 of 57) of applications granted regular approval and for all 14 applications granted accelerated approval [97]. The most common surrogate endpoint used was tumor response as determined by changes in tumor volume assessed by MRI or CT.

The use of noninvasive readouts to assess therapy efficacy facilitates the translation from preclinical to clinical drug development. In this regard, the noninvasive character of MR is a major asset. The potential of using the same readout in the preclinical and clinical phases of drug testing enhances the value of MR in pharmaceutical research. With the recent advances in the field of medical imaging, it is not surprising that the use of imaging biomarkers for the assessment of drug therapies is becoming more common. An imaging readout able to diagnose and characterize a disease state better than conventional methods will sooner or later be incorporated into clinical drug trials. Provided that imaging has improved diagnostic capacity (sensitivity, specificity, quantitation) for a given disease, then shorter studies with fewer patients should become feasible, which may lead to savings of the order of hundreds of millions of US dollars because of a faster time-to-market [98].

A clinical trial, which is a prospective, organized, systematic exposure of subjects to a drug in order to answer some question about a compound, is divided into phases 1 to 4:

1. Phase 1 represents the first test of a drug in a human population. Phase 1 trials examine whether the pharmacological effects seen in experimental animals are reproduced in humans. These trials also designed to determine toxicity, absorption, metabolism, and safe dose range of a compound, are limited to relatively few healthy (male) subjects (typically 20 to 80) and often involve dose escalation until the maximum tolerated dose is established. In case of cancer, studies may also be performed in patients. During phase 1, sufficient information about the drug's pharmacokinetics and pharmacological effects should be obtained to permit the design of well controlled, phase 2 studies.
2. Phase 2 studies are well-controlled, closely monitored, and conducted in a relatively small number of patients (usually involving several hundred people). In phase 2a, the primary aim is the assessment and confirmation of proof of therapeutic concept (efficacy), as well as determination of acute tolerability, maximum safe dose and plasma concentration, and lack of acute safety issues in patients. Phase 2b aims at gaining further evidence of efficacy and at exploring dose regimens for the general target population in phase 3.
3. Phase 3 is an expanded trial (several thousand patients), designed to gain additional evidence on efficacy, long-term toxic effects, and tolerability. Studies are carried out in multicenter, double-blind, placebo-controlled studies. Superiority to established therapies (if there are any) has to be demonstrated. Phase 3 studies form the basis for the registration documentation.
4. Phase 4 is a postmarketing study of an approved drug in order to obtain more information, e.g., to elucidate the incidence of a specific adverse reaction or to determine the long-term effects of the drug on morbidity and mortality.

2.5 MEASURING AT DIFFERENT SCALES

The criteria imaging biomarkers must meet in order to be accepted by regulatory agencies are extensively discussed in Chapter 3. The validation/qualification process may involve not only clinical activities, but also extensive animal experimentation. Hence, transferability of images and protocols from small animal to human scanners and vice versa becomes an issue. Sharing images from different platforms and manufacturers is necessary (see also Section 2.6). The use of similar acquisition consoles in small animal and whole body systems is an option being evaluated by many manufacturers. Although this is an attractive approach for translational research, since it would considerably simplify the comparison of data obtained in different systems, it remains to be shown that protocol optimizations for human imaging are also applicable to, for example, mouse imaging. Some characteristics specifically related to the anatomy and physiology of every species could render this transition more challenging than a mere change of dimensional parameters in the acquisition protocols.

Spatial resolution constitutes a challenge when performing studies in small rodents. Voxel volumes have to be scaled with anatomical scales in order to accurately represent structures. Typical voxel volumes for a mouse brain study are about 3 nl ($100 \times 100 \times 300\ \mu m^3$), while a corresponding voxel in studies of human brain is 2 μl ($1000 \times 1000 \times 2000\ \mu m^3$). The reduction in voxel volume by almost three orders of magnitude leads to a sensitivity issue: the signal-to-noise ratio in the mouse image is reduced by a factor of 25 (square root of the ratio of voxel volumes) provided all other experimental parameters including the detector coil are identical. Additionally, artifacts may be more severe when studying small structures. For example, effects of magnetic field inhomogeneities at tissue interfaces (bone/soft tissue), which are governed by the magnetic field strength and the change in magnetic susceptibility, but not by the anatomical dimension of the study object, will be more serious in mouse than in human images. Also, small rodents have higher respiratory and cardiac rates, which pose additional challenges when studying the thorax or abdominal viscera (see Chapter 16 and Chapter 18).

Technological and methodological adaptations allow some of the above-mentioned issues to be addressed:

- High magnetic fields. Most MR systems for animal imaging employ magnetic field strengths of 4.7 T and higher. In general, sensitivity increases with field strength, yet prolonged longitudinal relaxation times and larger susceptibility effects render these systems not trivial.
- Gradient systems. Actively shielded gradients generating magnetic field gradients of 200 mT/m are typically available for animal systems. Gradient sets with improved design and smaller dimensions, capable of generating gradient fields up to 650 mT/m, have been reported recently [99,100].
- The most critical factor with regard to sensitivity is the use of optimal rf coils. Although solenoid and birdcage coils are commonly used in animal systems, several approaches have been proposed for the design of more specialized coils aiming at MR microimaging applications (for a review, see Ref. [101]). For instance, implantable and surface coils have been designed for fields as high as 9.4 T [102]. Microfabricated small-volume probes consisting of electroplated planar microcoils integrated on a glass substrate with etched microfluidic channels have also been constructed [103]. The challenge for coils in which the diameter of the conductor is of the order of the dimensions of the electrical skin depth is the accurate determination of coil performance [104]. Another approach consists of using high-temperature superconducting probes [105].
- Anesthesia and physiological control. Small animal imaging requires expertise in anesthesia and animal physiology. The choice of anesthesia, physiological monitoring, acquisition gating and ventilation requirements will depend on the animal model and the question being addressed. Halothane and isoflurane are inhalation anesthetics commonly used for rats and mice. Injectable agents include pentobarbital and ketamine, which are administered intraperitonially or intramuscularly. Any physiological intervention might interfere with the process to be investigated; this is particularly relevant for metabolic or functional studies of the brain (see Chapter 6, Section 6.3.2, and Chapter 10). Agents applied via inhalation are preferred for longitudinal studies because they are easy to administer and rapidly adjustable, and animals recover rapidly. During the studies, body temperature should be kept constant, and heart rate/ECG and respiratory rate continuously monitored. Specialized physiologic support and monitoring equipment for cardiac and lung MRI may ensure consistency of biological motion and permit synchronization of imaging with the cardiac and respiratory cycles [106,107] (see also Chapter 5, Chapter 16, and Chapter 18).

As pointed out above, in many cases, acquiring high quality images requires long examination times and interference with the animals' physiology. This is often incompatible with the reality of *in vivo* pharmacological studies in animals, in which the disease model and/or a compound may profoundly influence the physiology. The primary purpose of MRI in preclinical research is not to generate images of ultimate quality, but to allow the acquisition of data from which useful biomedical information can be derived with good reproducibility (and with a reasonable throughput). Obviously, MR techniques must be adapted to the biological situation, rather than to enforce the physiology for the sake of facilitating image acquisition. Since an MRI session always represents a certain burden for an animal, starting from the anesthesia, a careful balance between image quality and biological constraints should be envisaged [108]. As a general rule, the duration of an imaging session, including animal preparation, should be shorter than 1 h.

2.6 MOLECULAR IMAGING

Questions asked by drug developers are:

- Where do drugs act in the body?
- Do they reach their target?
- At what dose do side or even toxicological effects occur?
- What organs are affected?
- What are the optimal routes for drug delivery?
- What is the receptor occupancy at a given dose level?
- For how long does a compound stay bound?

Addressing such questions demands methods that allow visualization and quantification of molecular interactions in the intact organism, so-called molecular imaging approaches [109–111]. Although the field is still in its infancy, novel imaging modalities and molecular probes are being developed at a rapid pace. It is therefore to be anticipated that drug researchers will profit from such developments in a near future.

The most important imaging techniques potentially suited for providing molecular information in small animals are summarized in Table 2.1. In many respects the techniques are complementary; there is no all-in-one imaging modality providing optimal sensitivity, specificity, and temporospatial resolution. Due to its limited sensitivity, MRI is of restricted value for detecting molecular processes *in vivo*. Nevertheless, its high spatial resolution provides the exquisite anatomical reference for molecular data obtained with high sensitivity, low resolution imaging modalities. This can be achieved by postprocessing of data obtained in different imaging sessions or by simultaneous multimodality small animal imaging, such as PET-MRI [112,113] and PET-CT [114]. Combining imaging data requires compatibility of data formats for the various modalities as well as sophisticated software tools for image coregistration (fusion), data visualization, and integration across modalities. The integration of multimodal imaging information into bioinformatics platforms comprising nonimaging data (gene/protein expression data, pharmacodynamic, pharmacokinetic, and pharmacogenetic databases, histological data, atlases) will be mandatory in the near future for handling of the ever-increasing complexity of biomedical information.

Besides the imaging technique *per se*, a critical aspect of molecular imaging applications concerns the synthesis of appropriate target-specific probes. Two important avenues are pursued in the context of drug research:

- Imaging the drug biodistribution. As already discussed, early information on drug biodistribution and pharmacokinetic properties is essential during lead optimization and profiling. Conventionally, such data are obtained in rodents by blood and tissue sampling, or by autoradiography requiring isotopically (^{14}C, ^{3}H) labeled compounds. In nonhuman primates and in humans, this information is derived using nuclear imaging methods, in particular PET [115,116]. With the development of small animal PET scanners analogous studies may be carried out in small rodents. Isotopic substitution using ^{11}C or ^{18}F does not affect the physicochemical properties of the compound [115,116]. However, radiolabeling methods suffer from the disadvantage that it cannot be differentiated whether the signal originates from the parent compound or from a metabolite. Another significant limitation is the short lifetime of the radionuclide, as the timescale of the biological process to be studied must be of the same order of magnitude. As outline above (Section 2.3), fluorinated and ^{13}C-labeled compounds can, under special circumstances, be detected *in vivo* using MRS techniques. The advantage here is the ability of the approach to distinguish the compounds from metabolites thereof.

- Imaging the target distribution. The visualization of a target requires specific reporter probes and amplification strategies in order to differentiate target information from nonspecific background signals and to cope with the low (subnanomolar) target concentrations. Minimization of background signals requires elimination of the unbound and possibly of the nonspecifically bound fraction of the label, which implies a waiting period following the administration of the reporter probe. Modulations of the signal from the reporter probe following administration of a drug candidate can be used to assess the compound binding to the target (receptor occupancy). Reporter probes include targeted agents, for example, small molecules, peptides, metabolites, antibodies, or other molecules labeled with (1) ^{11}C and ^{18}F for PET; (2) ^{111}In or ^{99m}Tc for nuclear imaging; (3) fluorochromes for optical imaging; or (4) magnetic reporter probes [117–119] and activatable probes. The latter undergo chemical or physicochemical changes upon interacting with their target. Examples include caged near-infrared fluorochromes [52,120], protease-activatable dequenching probes [121], paramagnetic agents that change spin-lattice relaxivity on activation [122], or superparamagnetic sensors [123].

Most probes synthetized for molecular imaging will be limited to experimental research, since the approval process for human use involves similar hurdles as those for registering drugs [124]. Nevertheless, concerning target validation and assessments of drug distribution in animals, molecular imaging is going to play a relevant role in drug discovery. In order to take advantage of multimodality small animal imaging, the development of multimodal probes (e.g., for optical and MR imaging) is desirable [125]. The design of MR contrast agents for molecular imaging *in vivo* is extensively discussed in Chapter 4.

2.7 CONCLUDING REMARKS

The impact that MR techniques may exert on the complex drug discovery process is basically determined by three factors:

1. The multiparameteric contrast is of high diagnostic value increasing the chances to detect pathological transformation of tissue. Early disease detection enhances the probability of a successful therapeutic intervention.
2. Accurate *in vivo* morphometric measurements allow sensitive and reproducible assessments of drug effects.
3. Noninvasiveness allows the design of longitudinal study designs with increased statistical power.

There are significant differences with regard to opportunities and challenges for using MRI/S for the various disease areas/organs. This is accounted for in the individual chapters of this volume.

Due to insufficient sensitivity, visualization of the drug *per se* is not feasible, i.e., questions concerning drug biodistribution, pharmacokinetic profiles, and drug–target interaction can, in general, not be addressed. Hence, MRI/S provides pharmacodynamic rather than pharmacokinetic information. Combined pharmacokinetic/pharmacodynamic studies, which would be of high relevance for pharmaceutical research and development, might be carried out by combining MR with more sensitive molecular imaging approaches, such as PET or optical imaging. A crucial step for imaging to be fully integrated in drug research concerns the systematic and rigorous qualification of biomarkers via extensive correlation with well-characterized and accepted reference data. Finally, standardization of imaging acquisition protocols and processing procedures, which will facilitate the comparison of data acquired at different sites, has to be propagated.

These huge tasks are going to keep researchers and clinicians busy for quite some time. The impact of their work will be the establishment of even more powerful diagnostic and prognostic tools that should translate into shortened drug development times. Not only will the pharmaceutical industry profit from such an effort, but also so will the larger medical community and, ultimately, the patients.

ACKNOWLEDGMENTS

We are gratefully indebted to Dr. Pierre Acklin from the Novartis Institutes for BioMedical Research for critically reading the manuscript.

REFERENCES

1. Dickson, M. and Gagnon, J. P., Key factors in the rising cost of new drug discovery and development, *Nat. Rev. Drug Discov.*, 3, 417, 2004.
2. Rawlins, M. D., Cutting the cost of drug development?, *Nat. Rev. Drug Discov.*, 3, 360, 2004.
3. Preziosi, P., Science, pharmacoeconomics and ethics in drug R&D: a sustainable future scenario?, *Nat. Rev. Drug Discov.*, 3, 521, 2004.
4. Lipinski, C. A., Chris Lipinski discusses life and chemistry after the Rule of Five, *Drug Discov. Today*, 8, 12, 2003.
5. Kassel, D. B., Applications of high-throughput ADME in drug discovery, *Curr. Opin. Chem. Biol.*, 8, 339, 2004.
6. NIH-FDA Conference: biomarkers and surrogate endpoints: advancing clinical research and applications, Abstracts, *Disease Markers*, 14, 187, 1998.
7. Duyk, G., Attrition and translation, *Science*, 302, 603, 2003.
8. Seddon, B. M. and Workman, P., The role of functional and molecular imaging in cancer drug discovery and development, *Br. J. Radiol.*, 76(Suppl. 2), S128, 2003.
9. Stahl, A. et al., Positron emission tomography as a tool for translational research in oncology, *Mol. Imaging Biol.*, 6, 214, 2004.
10. Horig, H. and Pullman, W., From bench to clinic and back: Perspective on the 1st IQPC Translational Research conference, *J. Transl. Med.*, 2, 44, 2004.
11. Prokop, M., Multislice CT: technical principles and future trends, *Eur. Radiol.*, 13(Suppl. 5), M3, 2003.
12. Miles, K. A. and Griffiths, M. R., Perfusion C.T: a worthwhile enhancement?, *Br. J. Radiol.*, 76, 220, 2003.
13. Hoeffner, E. G., Cerebral perfusion CT: technique and clinical applications, *Radiology*, 231, 632, 2004.
14. Koyama, Y., Mochizuki, T., and Higaki, J., Computed tomography assessment of myocardial perfusion, viability, and function, *J. Magn. Reson. Imaging*, 19, 800, 2004.
15. Badea, C., Hedlund, L. W., and Johnson, G. A., Micro-CT with respiratory and cardiac gating, *Med. Phys.*, 31, 3324, 2004.
16. Cavanaugh, D. et al., *In vivo* respiratory-gated micro-CT imaging in small-animal oncology models, *Mol. Imaging*, 3, 55, 2004.

17. Ritman, E. L., Micro-computed tomography — current status and developments, *Annu. Rev. Biomed. Eng.*, 6, 185, 2004.
18. Ritman, E. L., Molecular imaging in small animals — roles for micro-CT, *J. Cell. Biochem.*, (Suppl. 39), 116, 2002.
19. Ford, N. L., Thornton, M. M., and Holdsworth, D. W., Fundamental image quality limits for microcomputed tomography in small animals, *Med. Phys.*, 30, 2869, 2003.
20. Boone, J. M., Velazquez, O., and Cherry, S. R., Small-animal X-ray dose from micro-CT, *Mol. Imaging*, 3, 149, 2004.
21. Duatti, A., *In vivo* imaging of oligonucleotides with nuclear tomography, *Curr. Drug Targets*, 5, 753, 2004.
22. Yang, Y. et al., Optimization and performance evaluation of the microPET II scanner for in vivo small-animal imaging, *Phys. Med. Biol.*, 49, 2527, 2004.
23. Tay, Y. C. et al., Performance evaluation of the microPET focus: a third-generation microPET scanner dedicated to animal imaging, *J. Nucl. Med.*, 46, 455, 2005.
24. Weber, S. and Bauer, A., Small animal PET: aspects of performance assessment, *Eur. J. Nucl. Med. Mol. Imaging*, 31, 1545, 2004.
25. Zaidi, H. and Koral, K. F., Scatter modelling and compensation in emission tomography, *Eur. J. Nucl. Med. Mol. Imaging*, 31, 761, 2004.
26. Ogawa, K., Image distortion and correction in single photon emission CT, *Ann. Nucl. Med.*, 18, 171, 2004.
27. Vanhove, C. et al., Interest of the ordered subsets expectation maximization (OS-EM) algorithm in pinhole single photon emission tomography reconstruction: a phantom study, *Eur. J. Nucl. Med.*, 27, 140, 2000.
28. MacDonald, L. R. et al., Pinhole SPECT of mice using the LumaGEM gamma camera, *IEEE Trans. Nucl. Sci.*, 48, 830, 2001.
29. McElroy, D. P. et al., Performance evaluation of A-SPECT: a high resolution desktop pinhole SPECT system for imaging small animals, *IEEE Trans. Nucl. Sci.*, 49, 2139, 2002.
30. Acton, P. D. et al., Quantification of dopamine transporter in mouse brain using ultra-high resolution single photon emission tomography, *Eur. J. Nucl. Med.*, 29, 691, 2002.
31. Booij, J. et al., Imaging of dopamine transporters in rats using high resolution pinhole single photon emission tomography, *Eur. J. Nucl. Med.*, 29, 1221, 2002.
32. Jenkins, C. et al., Reproducibility and accuracy of echocardiographic measurements of left ventricular parameters using real-time three-dimensional echocardiography, *J. Am. Coll. Cardiol.*, 44, 878, 2004.
33. Kuhl, H. P. et al., High-resolution transthoracic real-time three-dimensional echocardiography: quantitation of cardiac volumes and function using semi-automatic border detection and comparison with cardiac magnetic resonance imaging, *J. Am. Coll. Cardiol.*, 43, 2083, 2004.
34. Vogel, M. et al., Noninvasive assessment of left ventricular force–frequency relationships using tissue Doppler-derived isovolumic acceleration: validation in an animal model, *Circulation*, 107, 1647, 2003.
35. Hashimoto, I. et al., Tissue Doppler-derived myocardial acceleration for evaluation of left ventricular diastolic function, *J. Am. Coll. Cardiol.*, 44, 1459, 2004.
36. Hansen, A. et al., Evaluation of cardioprotective effects of recombinant soluble P-selectin glycoprotein ligand-immunoglobulin in myocardial ischemia-reperfusion injury by real-time myocardial contrast echocardiography, *J. Am. Coll. Cardiol.*, 44, 887, 2004.
37. Kunichika, H. et al., Effects of glycoprotein IIb/IIIa inhibition on microvascular flow after coronary reperfusion: a quantitative myocardial contrast echocardiography study, *J. Am. Coll. Cardiol.*, 43, 276, 2004.
38. Leen, E., Moug, S. J., and Horgan, P., Potential impact and utilization of ultrasound contrast media, *Eur. Radiol.*, 14(Suppl. 8), P16, 2004.
39. Leong-Poi, H. et al., Noninvasive assessment of angiogenesis by ultrasound and microbubbles targeted to alpha(v)-integrins, *Circulation*, 107, 455, 2003.
40. Bekeredjian, R., Grayburn, P. A., and Shohet, R. V., Use of ultrasound contrast agents for gene or drug delivery in cardiovascular medicine, *J. Am. Coll. Cardiol.*, 45, 329, 2005.
41. Collins, K. A. et al., Accuracy of echocardiographic estimates of left ventricular mass in mice, *Am. J. Physiol. Heart Circ. Physiol.*, 280, H1954, 2001.

42. Kiatchoosakun, S. et al., Assessment of left ventricular mass in mice: comparison between two-dimensional and m-mode echocardiography, *Echocardiography*, 19, 199, 2002.
43. Phoon, C. K. L. and Turnbull, D. H., Ultrasound biomicroscopy-Doppler in mouse cardiovascular development, *Physiol. Genomics*, 14, 3, 2003.
44. Hoit, B. D., Murine physiology: measuring the phenotype, *J. Mol. Cell. Cardiol.*, 37, 377, 2004.
45. Ow, D. W. et al., Transient and stable expression of the firefly luciferase gene in plant cells and transgenic plants, *Science*, 234, 856, 1986.
46. Contag, C. et al., Visualizing gene expression in living mammals using a bioluminescent reporter, *Photochem. Photobiol.*, 66, 523, 1997.
47. Zhang, W. et al., Rapid *in vivo* functional analysis of transgenes in mice using whole body imaging of luciferase expression, *Transgenic Res.*, 10, 423, 2001.
48. Rice, B. W., Cable, M. D., and Nelson, M. B., *In vivo* imaging of light-emitting probes, *J. Biomed. Opt.*, 6, 432, 2001.
49. Choy, G., Choyke, P., and Libutti, S. K., Current advances in molecular imaging: noninvasive *in vivo* bioluminescent and fluorescent optical imaging in cancer research, *Mol. Imaging*, 2, 303, 2003.
50. Piwnica-Worms, D., Schuster, D. P., and Garbow, J. R., Molecular imaging of host-pathogen interactions in intact small animals, *Cell. Microbiol.*, 6, 319, 2004.
51. Wang, G., Li, Y., and Jiang, M., Uniqueness theorems in bioluminescence tomography, *Med. Phys.*, 31, 2289, 2004.
52. Weissleder, R. and Ntziachristos, V., Shedding light onto live molecular targets, *Nat. Med.*, 9, 123, 2003.
53. Kircher, M. F., Weissleder, R., and Josephson, L., A dual fluorochrome probe for imaging proteases, *Bioconjug. Chem.*, 15, 242, 2004.
54. Pham, W. et al., Developing a peptide-based near-infrared molecular probe for protease sensing, *Bioconjug. Chem.*, 15, 1403, 2004.
55. Bremer, C. et al., Imaging of differential protease expression in breast cancers for detection of aggressive tumor phenotypes, *Radiology*, 222, 814, 2002.
56. Wunder, A. et al., *In vivo* imaging of protease activity in arthritis: a novel approach for monitoring treatment response, *Arthritis Rheum.*, 50, 2459, 2004.
57. Ballou, B. et al., Noninvasive imaging of quantum dots in mice, *Bioconjug. Chem.*, 15, 79, 2004.
58. Ozkan, M., Quantum dots and other nanoparticles: what can they offer to drug discovery?, *Drug Discov. Today*, 9, 1065, 2004.
59. Michalet, X. et al., Quantum dots for live cells, in vivo imaging, and diagnostics, *Science*, 307, 538, 2005.
60. Ntziachristos, V. et al., Looking and listening to light: the evolution of whole-body photonic imaging, *Nature Biotechnol.*, 23, 313, 2005.
61. Rudin, M., Beckmann, N., and Rausch, M., Magnetic resonance imaging in biomedical research: imaging of drugs and drug effects, *Methods Enzymol.*, 385, 240, 2004.
62. Klomp, D. W. et al., Optimization of localized 19F magnetic resonance spectroscopy for the detection of fluorinated drugs in the human liver, *Magn. Reson. Med.*, 50, 303, 2003.
63. van Laarhoven, H. W. et al., *In vivo* monitoring of capecitabine metabolism in human liver by 19fluorine magnetic resonance spectroscopy at 1.5 and 3 Tesla field strength, *Cancer Res.*, 63, 7609, 2003.
64. Hamstra, D. A. et al., The use of 19F spectroscopy and diffusion-weighted MRI to evaluate differences in gene-dependent enzyme prodrug therapies, *Mol. Ther.*, 10, 916, 2004.
65. Kamm, Y. J. et al., 19F-magnetic resonance spectroscopy in patients with liver metastases of colorectal cancer treated with 5-fluorouracil, *Anticancer Drugs*, 15, 229, 2004.
66. Griffiths, J. R. and Glickson, J. D., Monitoring pharmacokinetics of anticancer drugs: non-invasive investigation using magnetic resonance spectroscopy, *Adv. Drug Deliv. Rev.*, 41, 75, 2000.
67. Artemov, D., Solaiyappan, M., and Bhujwalla, Z. M., Magnetic resonance pharmacoangiography to detect and predict chemotherapy delivery to solid tumors, *Cancer Res.*, 61, 3039, 2001.
68. Rudin, M., Beckmann, N., and Sauter, A., *In vivo* pharmacokinetics using MRS, *NMR Biomed.*, 12, 404, 1999.
69. Rudin, M. et al., *In vivo* magnetic resonance methods in pharmaceutical research: current status and perspectives, *NMR Biomed.*, 12, 69, 1999.

70. Rudin, M. et al., Noninvasive imaging in drug discovery and development, *Ernst Schering Res. Found. Workshop*, 48, 47, 2004.
71. Beckmann, N. et al., From anatomy to the target: contributions of magnetic resonance imaging to preclinical pharmaceutical research, *Anat. Rec.*, 265, 85, 2001.
72. Beckmann, N. et al., Magnetic resonance imaging in drug discovery: lessons from disease areas, *Drug Discov. Today*, 9, 35, 2004.
73. Weisskoff, R. M. et al., Pitfalls in MR measurement of tissue blood flow with intravascular tracers: which mean transit time?, *Magn. Reson. Med.*, 29, 553, 1993.
74. Rudin, M., Beckmann, N., and Sauter, A., Analysis of tracer transit in rat brain after carotid artery and femoral vein administrations using linear system theory, *Magn. Reson. Imaging*, 15, 551, 1997.
75. Rudin, M. et al., Determination of rat heart morphology and function in vivo in two models of cardiac hypertrophy by means of magnetic resonance imaging, *Basic Res. Cardiol.*, 86, 165, 1991.
76. Stein, R. L., A new model for drug discovery — meeting our societal obligation, *Drug Discov. Today*, 8, 245, 2003.
77. Knowles, J. and Gromo, G., A guide to drug discovery: Target selection in drug discovery, *Nat. Rev. Drug Discov.*, 2, 63, 2004.
78. Bleicher, K. H. et al., Hit and lead generation: beyond high-throughput screening, *Nat. Rev. Drug Discov.*, 2, 369, 2003.
79. Walke, D. W. et al., *In vivo* drug target discovery: identifying the best targets from the genome, *Curr. Opin. Biotechnol.*, 12, 626, 2001.
80. Hopkins, A. L. and Groom, C. R., The druggable genome, *Nature Rev. Drug Discov.*, 1, 727, 2002.
81. Drews, J., Stategic trends in the drug industry, *Drug Discov. Today*, 8, 411, 2003.
82. Lindsay, M. A., Target discovery, *Nat. Rev. Drug Discov.*, 2, 831, 2003.
83. Wang, S. et al., Tools for target identification and validation, *Curr. Opin. Chem. Biol.*, 8, 371, 2004.
84. Jackson, P. D. and Harrington, J. J., High-throughput target discovery using cell-based genetics, *Drug Discov. Today*, 10, 53, 2005.
85. Tornell, J. and Snaith, M., Transgenic systems in drug discovery: from target identification to humanized mice, *Drug Discov. Today*, 7, 461, 2002.
86. Zambrowicz, B. P., Turner, C. A., and Sands, A. T., Predicting drug efficacy: knockouts model pipeline drugs of the pharmaceutical industry, *Curr. Opin. Pharmacol.*, 3, 563, 2003.
87. Zambrowicz, B. P. and Sands, A. T., Knockouts model the 100 best-selling drugs — will they model the next 100?, *Nat. Rev. Drug Discov.*, 2, 38, 2003.
88. Pellecchia, M. et al., NMR-based techniques in the hit identification and optimisation processes, *Expert Opin. Ther. Targets*, 8, 597, 2004.
89. Schuppli, C. A., Fraser, D., and McDonald, M., Expanding the three Rs to meet new challenges in humane animal experimentation, *Altern. Lab. Anim.*, 32, 525, 2004.
90. Frank, R. and Hargreaves, R., Clinical biomarkers in drug discovery and development, *Nat. Rev. Drug Discov.*, 2, 566, 2003.
91. Smith, J. J., Sorensen, A. G., and Thrall, J. H., Biomarkers in imaging: realizing radiology's future, *Radiology*, 227, 633, 2003.
92. Colburn, W. A., Optimizing the use of biomarkers, surrogate endpoints, and clinical endpoints for more efficient drug development, *J. Clin. Pharmacol.*, 40, 1419, 2000.
93. Lesko, L. J. et al., Optimizing the science of drug development: opportunities for better candidate selection and accelerated evaluation in humans, *J. Clin. Pharmacol.*, 40, 803, 2000.
94. Lesko, L. J. and Atkinson, A., Use of biomarkers and surrogate endpoints in drug development and regulatory decision making: criteria, validation, strategies, *Ann. Rev. Pharmacol. Toxicol.*, 41, 347, 2001.
95. Pien, H. H. et al., Using imaging biomarkers to accelerate drug development and clinical trials, *Drug Discov. Today*, 10, 259, 2005.
96. Kelloff, G. J. and Sigman, C. C., New science-based endpoints to accelerate oncology drug development, *Eur. J. Cancer*, 41, 491, 2005.
97. Johnson, J. R. et al., End points and United States Food and Drug Administration approval of oncology drugs, *J. Clin. Oncol.*, 21, 1404, 2003.
98. DiMasi, J. A., The value of improving the productivity of the drug development process: faster times and better decisions, *Pharmacoeconomics*, 20(Suppl. 3), 1, 2002.

99. Dodd, S. J. and Ho, C., Short planar gradient coils for MR microscopy using concentric return paths, *J. Magn. Reson.*, 156, 1, 2002.
100. Leggett, J., Crozier, S., and Bowtell, R. W., Actively shielded multi-layer gradient coil designs with improved cooling properties, *J. Magn. Reson.*, 165, 196, 2003.
101. Webb, A. G., Radiofrequency microcoils in magnetic resonance, *Progr. Nucl. Magn. Reson. Spectrosc.*, 31, 1, 1997.
102. Bilgen, M., Simple, low-cost multipurpose RF coil for MR microscopy at 9.4 T, *Magn. Reson. Med.*, 52, 937, 2004.
103. Massin, C. et al., Planar microcoil-based microfluidic NMR probes, *J. Magn. Reson.*, 164, 242, 2003.
104. Peck, T. L., Magin, R. L., and Lauterbur, P. C., Design and analysis of microcoils for NMR microscopy, *J. Magn. Reson. B*, 108, 114, 1995.
105. Hurlston, S. E. et al., A high-temperature superconducting Helmholtz probe for microscopy at 9.4 T, *Magn. Reson. Med.*, 41, 1032, 1999.
106. Brau, A. C., Hedlund, L. W., and Johnson, G. A., Cine magnetic resonance microscopy of the rat heart using cardiorespiratory-synchronous projection reconstruction, *J. Magn. Reson. Imaging*, 20, 31, 2004.
107. Hedlund, L. W. et al., MR-compatible ventilator for small animals: computer-controlled ventilation for proton and noble gas imaging, *Magn. Reson. Imaging*, 18, 753, 2000.
108. Colby, L. A. and Morenko, B. J., Clinical considerations in rodent bioimaging, *Comp. Med.*, 54, 623, 2004.
109. Rudin, M. and Weissleder, R., Molecular imaging in drug discovery and development, *Nat. Rev. Drug Discov.*, 2, 123, 2003.
110. Massoud, T. F. and Gambhir, S. S., Molecular imaging in living subjects: seeing fundamental biological processes in a new light, *Genes Dev.*, 17, 545, 2003.
111. Hildebrandt, I. J. and Gambhir, S. S., Molecular imaging applications for immunology, *Clin. Immunol.*, 111, 210, 2004.
112. Slates, R. et al., Design of a small animal MR compatible PET scanner, *IEEE Trans. Nucl. Sci.*, 46, 565, 1999.
113. Benveniste, H. et al., Maternal and fetal 11C-cocaine uptake and kinetics measured in vivo by combined PET and MRI in pregnant nonhuman primates, *J. Nucl. Med.*, 46, 312, 2005.
114. Fahey, F. H., Instrumentation in positron emission tomography, *Neuroimaging Clin. N. Am.*, 13, 659, 2003.
115. Fischman, A. J., Alpert, N. M., and Rubin, R. H., Pharmacokinetic imaging: a noninvasive method for determining drug distribution and action, *Clin. Pharmacokinet.*, 41, 581, 2002.
116. Phelps, M. E., Positron emission tomography provides molecular imaging of biological processes, *Proc. Natl Acad. Sci. U.S.A*, 97, 9226, 2000.
117. Weissleder, R. et al., *In vivo* magnetic resonance imaging of transgene expression, *Nat. Med.*, 6, 351, 2000.
118. Hogemann, D. et al., High throughput magnetic resonance imaging for evaluating targeted nanoparticle probes, *Bioconjug. Chem.*, 13, 116, 2002.
119. Sipkins, D. A. et al., Detection of tumor angiogenesis in vivo by $\alpha V\beta 3$-targeted magnetic resonance imaging, *Nature Med.*, 4, 623, 1998.
120. Bornhop, D. J. et al., Advance in contrast agents, reporters, and detection, *J. Biomed. Opt.*, 6, 106, 2001.
121. Tung, C. H. et al., *In vivo* imaging of proteolytic enzyme activity using a novel molecular reporter, *Cancer Res.*, 60, 4953, 2000.
122. Louie, A. Y. et al., *In vivo* visualization of gene expression using magnetic resonance imaging, *Nature Biotechnol.*, 18, 321, 2000.
123. Perez, J. M. et al., Magnetic relaxation switches capable of sensing molecular interactions, *Nature Biotechnol.*, 20, 816, 2002.
124. Jaffer, F. A. and Weissleder, R., Molecular imaging in the clinical arena, *JAMA*, 293, 855, 2005.
125. Doubrovin, M. et al., Multimodality in vivo molecular-genetic imaging, *Bioconjug. Chem.*, 15, 1376, 2004.

Editorial Comments

The rising costs and duration of drug discovery and development processes pose a great challenge to the pharmaceutical industry. It is estimated that merely about 5% of the molecules identified in discovery make it to clinical trials, and of these, only one of ten compounds reaches complete regulatory approval. Within this context, the view that availability of good biomarkers for assessing drug efficacy and safety should positively impact the drug discovery process by reducing attrition rates and/or development times is well-accepted within industry.

The concept of markers is not new and covers various molecular signatures including genes (and their expression levels), proteins, metabolites, and labeled substrates. It includes as well the detection of signs of disease at the intact organ level, an arena in which imaging biomarkers come into play. The rationale behind the use of imaging in pharmaceutical research is based on the idea that the better and earlier a disease can be diagnosed and characterized, the higher the chance one has to interfere in the pathological process with a chemical entity. As readouts are obtained *in situ* in a noninvasive manner, imaging has the potential to provide a connection between disease mechanisms and therapy. Furthermore, through its ability to directly and quantitatively observe effects of therapeutic interventions in intact organs, imaging plays a fundamental role in modern drug research, especially in view of translational medicine aiming at transforming a candidate compound displaying *in vitro* potency into a high value and well-characterized drug candidate for clinical trials.

Notwithstanding this overall positive appreciation of the capabilities of imaging, its readouts need to be properly validated and/or qualified in order to become accepted biomarkers that can be used for drug testing. Richard Hargreaves and John Wagner review in Chapter 3 some of the key points concerning biomarkers in general and the challenges for the development of imaging biomarkers.

3 Imaging as Biomarker for Decision-Making in Drug Development

Richard Hargreaves and John A. Wagner

CONTENTS

3.1 INTRODUCTION

There is a clear need to change drug discovery paradigms fundamentally to meet today's healthcare needs. There are epidemics in obesity-related type 2 diabetes and metabolic syndromes as well as an ever increasing burden from chronic diseases of aging. Drug discovery is becoming increasingly focused on early treatment with disease modifying drugs. Genomics, proteomics, rapid analog synthesis, and high throughput screening have yielded many more candidate targets and molecules for drug discovery and development than ever before, yet it is likely that only a tiny fraction of these will result in useful drug products. The path of traditional outcomes-based drug discovery and development within these confines can be long, expensive, and uncertain [1] without early knowledge that validates the therapeutic concept, endorses the candidate molecule, and facilitates dose selection.

Small improvements in decisive clinical trials' outcomes can translate to large financial savings, and importantly, a faster time to bring new medicines to patients [2–6]. Importantly too, there are safety and ethical reasons to improve decision-making in drug discovery since absence of such early indicators could result in large numbers of human subjects (healthy volunteers and patients) being exposed to experimental drugs with little or no therapeutic potential while being deprived of current best therapeutic care. One of the greatest values of a biomarker strategy is therefore to improve early decision-making on safety and efficacy in drug discovery and this can sometimes outweigh the more difficult task of qualifying biomarkers as surrogate endpoints for drug approval.

Fortunately today the necessity for biomarkers is balanced by the practicality of a diverse biomarker toolbox in which biomedical imaging is a key component alongside genomics, blood and other fluid biomarkers, and experimental clinical models. Biomarkers can accelerate drug development by providing translational research strategies from the laboratory to the clinic, rapid progress from first human dose to first patient dose, and fast proof of principle testing. In later stage testing, the use of biomarkers makes it possible to be highly discriminating during development, by defining optimal patient populations to enrich clinical efficacy trials and by providing clear criteria for dose selection.

Biomarker activities cover discrete applications in drug discovery. Target- and mechanism-specific biomarkers that inform on the pharmacodynamics of drug candidates, thereby facilitating proof of concept in information-rich early clinical trials, are most often used to optimize drug discovery and development decision-making processes. The use of patient, disease, and toxicity biomarkers can also have great impact on the efficiency and success of drug development (for additional comprehensive reviews see Refs. [4,7–11]).

Biomarkers can be conceptualized as detector systems. Novel drugs and their targets are likely to require novel biomarkers that are rarely qualified. Indeed, it has been said that in biomarker science innovation is almost always inversely proportional to validation. It is therefore often necessary to invest off the critical path of drug discovery to develop biomarkers in advance of drug candidates in order for them to be available in time to impact key decision-making processes during clinical trials. The most important biomarkers, but those that are most difficult to achieve, are disease biomarkers with cross-mechanism utility that can form surrogate end points for clinical outcomes. Importantly, the U.S. Food and Drug Administration (FDA) has recognized the potential value of surrogate endpoints to accelerating the registration of drugs in its 1997 modernization act [12] when it was given authority to approve drugs for the treatment of serious or life-threatening conditions upon determination that a product has an effect on a clinical endpoint or on a surrogate endpoint that is reasonably likely to predict clinical benefit [13]. However, given the complexity of many pathological processes, surrogate endpoint qualification and development can be as hard as drug discovery itself. Indeed, it is an especially high hurdle for a single biomarker to become a universal surrogate endpoint where change is independently predictive of outcome (benefit or increased risk or no effect) across all drugs and mechanistic targets. In fact it is debatable whether this can ever really be achieved.

The research and development of biomarkers in many respects follows a classical drug development paradigm (Table 3.1). After objective and hypothesis setting, basic research establishes the feasibility and proof of concept for a biomarker in small experimental medicine trials. This may be enough for decision-making if the biomarker is for target or mechanism of action and not outcome based. Further development of a biomarker involves evaluation of cost, practicality, and performance, and careful management of its application. If the biomarker is to be used for outcomes then extensive development is required before integration into clinical trials. The methodologies need to be standardized, highly reproducible, and useable at multiple sites, and decision criteria that consider all sources of signal to noise variability need to be established *a priori*.

The use of imaging as a biomarker has accelerated in recent years in line with advances in minimally or noninvasive medical imaging technologies (MRI, x-ray computerized tomography (CT), positron emission tomography (PET), single photon emission computed tomography (SPECT), ultrasound, intravascular ultrasound) and their miniaturization to evolve a science of microimaging that can be used as a translational research bridge from the laboratory to the clinic. This article will review some of the key points regarding biomarkers in general, and particular

TABLE 3.1
Clinical Trials: What Is Done, When, and Why

Phase 1: First in humans; 6 months to 1 year

- Limited number (20 to 80) healthy volunteers
  - Exception cancer when patients are studied
- Safety and tolerability, pharmacokinetics, and pharmacodynamics
  - Single doses and multiple dosing to steady state
  - Probe drug interaction liability, food effects
- Biomarker use: Proof of concept for molecule and mechanism
  - Target occupancy, evaluate activity

Phase II: 100 to 500 patients with disease: 1 to 3 years

- Clinical efficacy proof of concept
  - Blinded, randomized
  - Controlled: placebo or active comparator
- Selection of therapeutic dose range and regimen
  - Inform phase III design: power and selection of endpoints
  - Increased safety experience

Biomarker use: Development of exposure–response relationships

Phase III: 2500 to 15,000 patients: 1 to 3 years

- So-called "pivotal" studies for registration and labeling
  - Blinded, randomized, controlled
  - Long-term safety and efficacy
  - Usually worldwide at many study sites
- Biomarker uses
  - Identify and stratify and track study populations
  - Support for regulatory approval

Phases IV and V: Thousands of patients; lifetime of the product

- Postapproval studies
  - Expand safety data in chronic use
  - Strategic: differentiate from other drugs
  - Additional age groups, patient types, or indications
  - Prove value to healthcare and payers

challenges for the use of imaging biomarkers (see also Ref. [11]), taking some examples from cardiovascular and neuroscience drug discovery and development.

3.2 BIOMARKER LEXICON

Central to the discussion of a roadmap for biomarkers, including those that are based on imaging, is a clear understanding and agreement on the definitions and terminology that will be used. This remains very much a work in progress although there have been important recent initiatives that have laid a framework for ongoing discussions between the regulators and industry [14,15].

The issues that have been extensively discussed surround the different systems of biomarker nomenclature that have evolved based on different types of biomarkers and their diverse uses. Indeed, the use of biomarkers, utilizing different technology platforms extending from immunologic assays to expression profiling to imaging, ranges from hypothesis generation to definitive go/no-go decision-making in late-phase clinical development.

Different strategies are employed for the validation (assay or method validation) and qualification (clinical validation) of biomarkers and these require careful distinction. There is often confusion between what is a target biomarker vs. a mechanism or pharmacodynamic marker and what really constitutes a true surrogate endpoint. A major goal of the more recent initiatives has been to foster development of a vocabulary to provide a consistent framework within which to develop a productive dialogue on biomarker science.

3.2.1 Terminology

Biomarker — a characteristic that is objectively measured and evaluated as an indicator of normal biological processes, pathogenic processes, or pharmacological responses to a therapeutic intervention.

Three common terms are used to classify biomarkers as they are currently employed in drug development:

1. Target biomarker informs on physical or biological interactions with the molecular target of the drug.
2. Mechanistic or pharmacodynamics biomarkers inform on biological effects that form a pharmacological response and that are assumed to be downstream of the interaction with the molecular target.
3. Outcome or disease biomarkers where the change in marker predicts clinical benefit (independently of mechanism or target).

Surrogate Endpoint — a biomarker intended to substitute for a clinical endpoint (a characteristic or variable that reflects how a patient feels, functions, or survives). The surrogate biomarker should be a plausible, clinically meaningful intermediate in human pathophysiology that is supported by population studies, epidemiology, or experiments of nature as being predictive of risk with changes that are clearly and independently predictive of clinical benefit (or harm, or lack of benefit or harm). Under accelerated approval regulations, a surrogate endpoint has potential use as a basis for approval of a new drug if it is "reasonably likely to predict clinical benefit."

Validation — the scientific controlled measurement of the characteristics of a biomarker that enables quantification of important clinical protocol metrics such as test–retest variability, precision, and specificity taking account of confounding variables (e.g., fasting, diurnal, gender, and age); the term preclinical relates to animal data and clinical to human.

Qualification (clinical validation) — measurement of the biomarker's ability to reflect a pharmacological modification of the physiological or biochemical process. The biomarker parameter changes in proportion to the physiology and biochemistry. Clinical validation should also include an independent measure of activity.

3.2.2 Progression from Validation to Qualification

At face value it appears trivial to distinguish validation from qualification but there is clearly the opportunity for an iterative interaction between validation and qualification as biomarker development progresses. Validation can be viewed as the process of evaluating performance characteristics of the assay or measurement whereas qualification is the evidentiary process of linking a biomarker with biological and clinical endpoints. The purpose of validation is to produce reliable biomarker data that show the biomarker to have characteristics capable of meeting an experimental or study objective. For example, the most crucial components of validation are accuracy, precision, and reproducibility (test–retest variability), with specificity, sensitivity, range, and stability becoming important as qualification ensues. There is progression in validation and it can be staged dependent on use or level of qualification. In contrast, the purpose of qualification is to produce reliable biomarker data that are scientifically and clinically meaningful. There can be progression in the qualification process based on the evidentiary status of the biomarker (Figure 3.1).

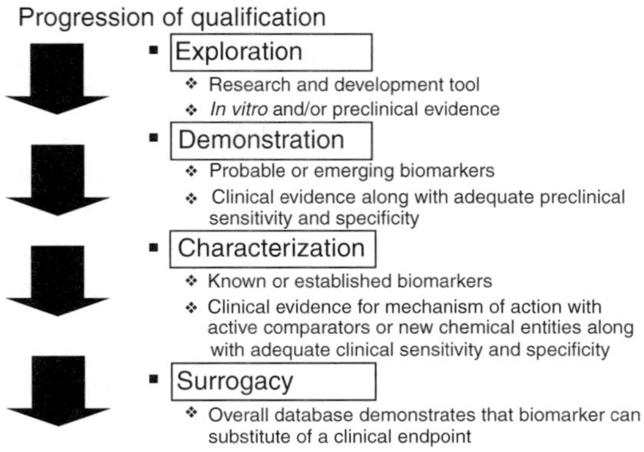

FIGURE 3.1 Progression for the qualification of biomarkers.

Recently a simplified three-tier categorization of biomarkers based on their proven linkage to efficacy or safety has been proposed:

1. Low: may have been shown in nonclinical studies studies but not demonstrated in humans
2. Medium: demonstrated in humans, but not reproducibly in clinical trials
3. High: reproducibly linked to outcome in two or more clinical trials

Preliminary characterization of the biomarker may be all that is needed for decision-making in early phase 1 and 2 clinical trials. Indeed, it has been argued that investment in the development of a true surrogate (other than perhaps as part of a consortium of competing parties) makes little sense as it can enable fast follower competition producing second-generation drugs acting through the same mechanism as a novel therapeutic candidate.

The reasons for the failure of surrogate endpoints has been extensively reviewed previously [4,15–17].

3.2.3 Biomarker Nomenclature

Many different systems of nomenclature have been used to describe the use of biomarkers at different stages of clinical trials. For example, in AIDS research:

- Type 0 markers chart natural history
- Type 1 markers assess biologic activity
- Type 2 markers act as surrogate endpoints for clinical outcome of therapy

A more detailed nomenclature was proposed after the European Federation of Pharmaceutical Sciences Conference on Optimizing Drug Development [15] where biomarker types were based on mechanism. Thus:

- Type 0 = phenotype/genotype
- Type 1 = concentration (drug, metabolite)
- Type 2 = molecular target occupancy
- Type 3 = molecular target activation
- Type 4 = physiological measures
- Type 5 = pathological measures
- Type 6 = clinical scales

This schema could clearly be useful to describe the use of many imaging biomarkers.

While industry groups have recognized the need to find early decision points to speed cost-effective discovery of safe and effective medicines, the regulators too have responded to this healthcare challenge by issuing guidance on how they view exposure–response relationships and the use of biomarkers in drug discovery [18,19]. Biomarkers can include a wide variety of normal physiologic, pathologic, or anatomic measurements that suggest the etiology of, the susceptibility to, or the progress of disease that are in turn related to the mechanism of response to treatments and actual clinical responses to therapeutic interventions. In this setting biomarker types are classified by their relationship to the intended therapeutic response or clinical benefit endpoints. Examples of these are:

1. Valid surrogates for clinical benefit (such as blood pressure, cholesterol, viral load)
2. Candidate surrogates reflecting the pathologic process (brain structure in Alzheimer's disease, brain infarct size in stroke, or radiographic and isotopic tests of function
3. Measurement of drug action but of uncertain relation to clinical outcome (e.g., inhibition of ADP-dependent platelet aggregation or even angiotensin converting enzyme inhibition in hypertension)
4. Biomarkers that are remote from the clinical benefit endpoint (e.g., degree of binding to a receptor or inhibition of an agonist provoked response)

The FDA have also provided insight into their view of biomarkers through guidance on pharmacogenomic data submissions (www.fda.gov/cder/guidance/6400fnl.htm), that show they are likely to distinguish further into probable valid biomarkers and known valid biomarkers depending on the weight of supporting evidence.

3.3 IMAGING BIOMARKERS

Having set the framework for a biomarker discussion, the issues facing the use of imaging as a biomarker can now be considered. The challenges to the use of imaging as a biomarker arise from the change in expectations when its primary use changes from being diagnostic. Thus, classically imaging as diagnostic utilizes binary images, is discontinuous, cross-sectional and looks at conversion or threshold structural events in primary/local lesions that are read with a view to symptomatic therapy. In contrast, imaging as a biomarker needs to produce highly quantitative longitudinal data that can assess a continuum or rate of change in total as well as primary lesion loads. Imaging as a biomarker also needs to embrace structure, function, and molecular specificity and be responsive to disease modification so that it can drive evaluation and use of presymptomatic or secondary prevention disease modifying agents as well as symptomatic therapy.

3.3.1 Application and Qualification of Imaging Biomarkers

Application of imaging biomarkers into clinical trials requires enormous attention to detail and close coordination between multidisciplinary imaging and therapeutic area experts to ensure drug development teams are always fully informed. Ideally, the imaging technologies that generate the imaging marker must be widespread across clinical centers conducting the therapeutic efficacy trials (sometimes a subset of those participating). The marker needs to be measurable using standardized protocols that can be readily implemented at the technical centers. Centralized core laboratories are valuable for image archiving, quality assurance, and control, and their oversight ensures cross-site consistency and rapid turn around of data.

The initial qualification of imaging endpoints for novel drug therapies ideally first requires studies using a known clinically active drug or on the background of a known clinically effective drug with documented or plausible effect on the imaging marker. If the effect of the novel drug on the marker is greater than that with the established agent alone then there is potentially a beneficial effect. For any imaging modality and time course of study, it is important to establish what level of change is actually clinically significant. Thus, the minimum change associated with either a clinically meaningful change in a proven biomarker or with a proven clinically effective dose of an existing drug agent should be determined. It is important to remember that for any imaging biomarker the signal (its value and bandwidth) will be determined by the balance between biological signal, biological noise, and technical noise, and it is only the technical noise that can be effectively managed.

In order to infer efficacy for a new drug it must be established that any change in an imaging endpoint is similar to or better than that observed with a proven effective drug or validated biomarker. Indeed, even if imaging biomarker changes are correlated with events in the context of an endpoint study, it has been argued that it is still a leap of faith that a single marker could be a universal surrogate for outcome since it would need to be proven that the marker was not drug, mechanism, disease stage, and population dependent by additional series of studies. Evidently, qualification of a novel imaging biomarker is facilitated by the availability of effective drugs. Many study proposals, however, actually have two unknowns — an unqualified novel imaging biomarker endpoint and a novel unproven drug candidate — but fail to recognize that this is a difficult (if not impossible) long and risky path to take as traditional outcomes will be required and the biomarker may in this case not help speed the drug development process.

Perhaps the most extensive use of surrogate endpoints for regulatory approval today is in oncology where tumor size (or permeability) measured using imaging is a common endpoint. This has been the subject of recent reviews and so will not be covered here [20–22]. In the following sections examples have been chosen from the diverse imaging modalities used in neuroscience and cardiovascular medicine to show how imaging can be an excellent proximal biomarker of drug activity, yet highlight that the road to validation of an imaging as a surrogate endpoint may be long. For imaging endpoints to become surrogates for outcome, rather than early phase proof of concept markers, will require considerable investment of resources and time. It is worth considering that the best path forward may be through collaboration rather than competition. Industry, academia, and government could come together in key high-impact therapeutic areas to reach consensus on the best imaging methods to qualify and validate rather than creating confusion through diverse advocacy of disparate techniques that have rarely been compared for their sensitivity and specificity in the evaluation of clinical benefit and risk. Let us decide where and what the goal is, collaborate, share the costs between industry, government, and academia, and let our chemists and biologists compete to produce novel therapies that can be judged by a consensus best criterion.

3.4 IMAGING IN CARDIOVASCULAR DISEASE

Biomarkers have been used for decades as surrogates to support the approval of drugs for the treatment of atherosclerotic cardiovascular disease. A considerable body of corroborative angiographic and carotid ultrasound imaging data show that drugs which diminish low density lipoprotein cholesterol (LDL-C), nonHDL-C and atherogenic triglycerides can slow plaque progression and cause plaque regression, which has been demonstrated in outcome studies to lead to reduced morbidity and mortality. Recent progress in the pathophysiology and pharmacology of atherosclerosis has resulted in novel drug molecules with mechanisms of action that directly target specific processes happening in the vessel wall. As a result, there has been a surge in research to validate and qualify novel vessel wall imaging biomarkers that could potentially be used as surrogates, alongside soluble biomarkers, to increase the efficiency of selection and subsequent speed of registration of safe and effective new medicines without waiting for the outcome of extensive long-term trials [23–27].

The time-dependent biology of atherosclerotic progression in the vessel wall has been well-characterized creating the opportunity to target therapeutic intervention by stage of disease and tailor the selection of imaging technologies for the evaluation of drug effects. It has been suggested that in the formative stages endothelial function could be evaluated, in the adaptive stages subclinical plaque shown by wall thickening and plaque volume, and in the clinical stage frank coronary disease through measurements of myocardial function and perfusion. The extent and reversal of disease may be studied noninvasively in the carotid blood vessels using ultrasound [28, 29] or invasively in the coronary arteries employing intravascular techniques [30–32]. MRI [33] and high resolution CT [34,35] may also be used. Myocardial perfusion can be studied using SPECT or PET [36] (the latter gives sensitive measures of microvascular perfusion). All these imaging modalities can also be used to study experimental models of atherosclerosis and so provide excellent translational research tools. The opportunity to apply a diverse range of imaging techniques to this important medical problem first seemed to be a strength but unfortunately has become somewhat of a weakness as competition rather than consensus on the best technique to use for registration of drugs has occurred.

3.4.1 Cardiovascular Imaging Biomarkers

Recent consensus meetings of academia, industry, and regulatory agencies have considered the use of cardiovascular biomarkers including imaging to speed drug discovery and development.* At the outset, it should be noted that before using imaging to support registration claims it will be necessary to define *a priori* the magnitude of clinically meaningful change in the vessel wall for each imaging modality that is to be used, so that studies can be adequately statistically designed and powered. For example, the effects could be benchmarked using the minimum magnitude change associated with a clinically meaningful alteration in another fluid biomarker-say LDL-C-or even the minimum magnitude change associated with a clinically effective dose of a statin or other antiatherosclerosis marker regardless of effects on any biomarker. Three scenarios in which cardiovascular imaging biomarkers might hypothetically be used for the registration of new drugs or claims for treatment of atherosclerosis were considered by Orloff, when giving the current position of the Division of Metabolic and Endocrine Drug Products (DMEDP) at the FDA on surrogate imaging endpoints for registration [37], providing an excellent framework for discussion. These were:

1. First approval of a new drug or first approval for a population at risk of cardiovascular disease
2. Broadening the claim for approved agents
3. A new claim for a drug already approved for a different indication, perhaps within the spectrum of metabolic disease (obesity/diabetes)

In the first scenario, it was suggested that two modalities, two vascular beds, two studies together with an effect on an established or plausible fluid marker will be required along with a large safety experience and commitment to extensive phase 4 monitoring of hard endpoints. Here, for example, the new agent could be studied in the presence and absence of an established therapeutic agent, such as a statin, and the vessel wall imaged using intravascular ultrasound in the coronaries and B-mode ultrasound in the carotids could be used to look for additional benefits of

*Cardiovascular Biomarkers and Surrogates Symposium, Bethesda MD September 10–11, 2004 and September 23–24, 2005.

the combination over the monotherapy regime alongside positive effects on lipid profile. It is a salutary lesson that drug registration by this route has not yet been achieved.

In the second scenario, the hurdle is potentially much lower in that one imaging modality, such as intima-media thickness measurement, could be sufficient as clinical effects have already been demonstrated using traditional outcomes. In the third scenario, it is debatable whether one or two imaging modalities could be used, and this perhaps depends on the magnitude of the changes observed and on the level of confidence in the validity of the biomarker in the context of the other actions of the drug. Any unique safety issues in the new population would have to be addressed as well as making sure hard endpoints are collected in phase 4. Clearly, to register a drug using imaging alone will be very challenging indeed (see also Chapter 17).

3.5 IMAGING IN NEUROSCIENCE

In central nervous system (CNS) research noninvasive imaging acts best because of the inaccessibility of the brain. Imaging has been extensively used in several different ways in the CNS field:

1. To help translate and interpret preclinical data and select optimal molecules for development
2. For early concept validation
3. To select and optimize dosing

MRI has also played a central role in the registration of drugs for the treatment of multiple sclerosis but this will not be reviewed here except to say that with time it now seems that the surrogate imaging endpoint of MR bright plaques may be more sensitive to therapeutic modulation than the disease symptoms [38,39] (see also Chapter 12). This makes this imaging endpoint good for no-go decisions if no effect is seen; however, it still leaves a requirement for traditional clinical outcome measures even if an imaging response to treatment is observed.

The CNS field is unique in that despite there being a large number of potential drug targets only a few are exploited by current CNS therapeutics. In the field of psychiatry, for example, nonclinical model predictability is weak and tests are often biased towards known mechanisms [40,41]. The indications for the drugs are chronic, making clinical studies long, complex, and expensive. In clinical trials, as currently designed, outcomes are based on rating scales that are subjective and suboptimal, and there are high placebo response rates. The chances of mechanistic failure are therefore very high, making it imperative to get early proof of concept before embarking on late-stage development.

3.5.1 Positron Emission Tomography

PET has been an invaluable imaging tool in the development of CNS drugs [42]. It is a dynamic imaging technique that uses low-dose, high specific activity, short half-life positron emitting radionuclides. The tracers are usually radiolabeled antagonist drugs (^{11}C and ^{18}F). The mass of compound dosed in PET studies is very low (50 ng/kg) — and by definition pharmacologically inactive. PET provides a unique bridge from laboratory to clinic and is currently the optimal way to measure receptor (pM to nM levels) pharmacology quantitatively *in vivo* in animals and humans in a minimally invasive manner.

PET can help focus proof of concept studies by establishing the relationship between drug exposure in plasma and occupancy of the therapeutic target by drugs, this being especially important when other surrogate endpoints for drug action are lacking. It should always be remembered, however, that occupancy is not efficacy. A valid proof of concept requires adequate receptor occupancy at safe and well-tolerated doses. Thus, if there is no target occupancy and no efficacy it is absolutely not surprising — a new molecule is needed! Whereas with full occupancy and no efficacy it is clear that the concept is flawed and it is time to do something else! In later stages of development knowing receptor occupancy can also help dose selection for pivotal efficacy trials and open the therapeutic window.

The development of novel PET tracers alongside clinical CNS therapeutic programs is a key strategy for success in the pharmaceutical industry. The use of [^{18}F] SPA-RQ at Merck for the development and dose setting of Aprepitant (Emend®, Merck) for the prevention of chemotherapy-induced nausea and vomiting [43–45] is a good example (Figure 3.2).

3.5.2 Alzheimer's Disease Imaging: A Multimodality Challenge

In Alzheimer's disease (AD) drug target identification of the γ and β-secretases to prevent production of β-amyloid has come from an understanding of disease mechanisms [46–48]. Given

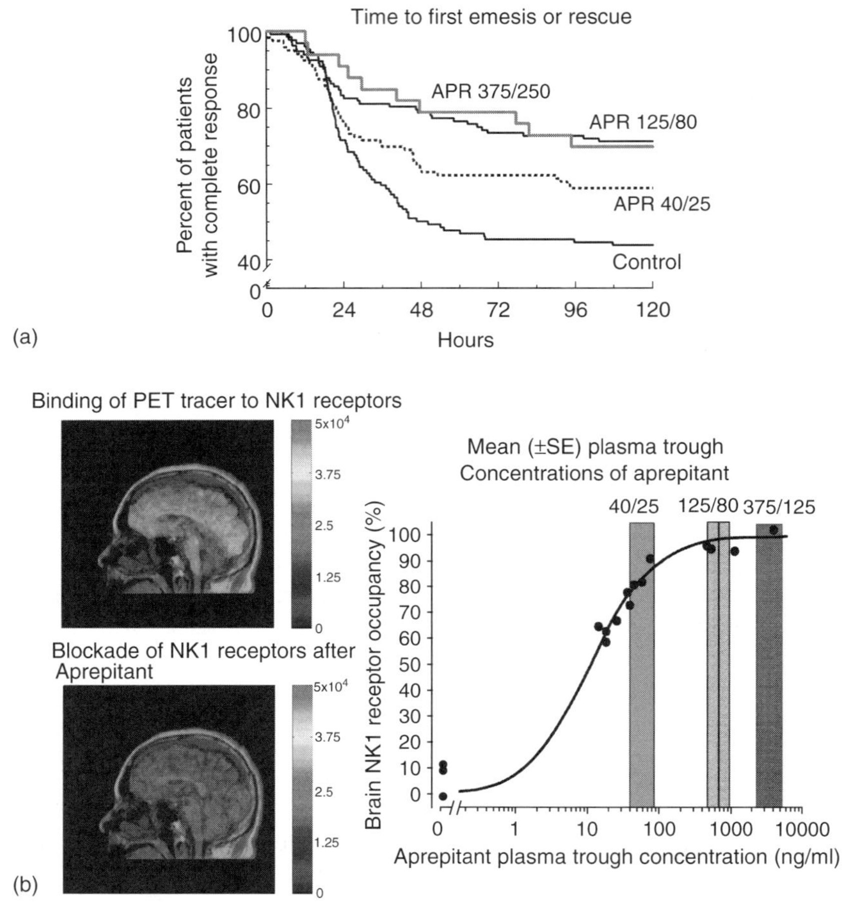

FIGURE 3.2 (See color insert for (b) following page 328.) (a) Survival plot showing the percent of patients given cisplatin who had a complete response (no vomiting, no rescue) after administering Aprepitant at different dose levels (figures in mg/dose day 1 and days 2 to 5) in combination with standard antiemetic therapy with dexamethasone and a 5-HT3 receptor antagonist (control). The most favorable profile was shown by the 125/80 mg dose regimen. (Adapted from Chawla, S. P. et al., *Cancer*, 97, 2290, 2003. With permission of American Cancer Society Copyright 2003.) (b) PET plasma concentration CNS NK1 receptor occupancy for Aprepitant. It is clear that the dose response against emesis is likely to be related to CNS occupancy with the best dose being 125/80 mg as this achieves essentially the same therapeutic response as the higher dose of 375/2125 mg with lower drug exposure, thereby opening the therapeutic window. (Adapted from Bergstrom, M. et al., *Biol. Psychiat.*, 55, 1007, 2004. With permission of the Society of Biological Psychiatry Copyright 2004.)

the time course of the disease and the likely protracted timescale that will be required to evaluate drugs that modify the time course of the disease, it has been widely suggested that brain imaging could play a central role in proof of concept studies (see Chapter 7). Recently, the National Institute of Aging in the U.S.A. has launched a five-year study (ADNI, Alzheimer's Disease Neuroimaging Initiative; www.nia.nih.gov/NewsAndEvents/PressReleases/PR20041013ADNI.htm) to establish baselines for the natural history of the disease in today's patient population in order to provide imaging and fluid biomarker metrics to facilitate therapeutic trial design [49]. It is instructional, therefore, to consider how imaging technologies might be used to help develop safe and effective medicines for this debilitating disorder:

1. PET could be used to study binding of drugs to secretase inhibitory sites (e.g., [50]) to ensure adequate delivery and occupancy.
2. [^{18}F] FDG PET has a unique signal in AD compared with other dementias and could be used for diagnosis enabling the identification of appropriate subjects for trials and it has recently been covered for AD identification and reimbursement by Centers for Medicare and Medicaid Services in the U.S.A. (http://www.cms.hhs.gov/mcd/viewdecisionmemo.asp?id = 104).
3. Amyloid PET tracers could provide minimally invasive assessment of CNS amyloid burden again facilitating patient stratification and recruitment.
4. Pharmacological proof of concept if amyloid tracers are sensitive enough to detect changes in central β-amyloid levels.
5. Brain function measurements ([^{18}F] FDG PET, MRS, functional MRI; [51–55]) can be used to assess the therapeutic effects of amyloid modifying therapies yet would be expected to improve both with palliative and disease modifying approaches.
6. Neurodegeneration (structural MRI) prevention or slowing of atrophy of whole brain or specific brain regions (entorhinal cortex and hippocampus) may discriminate disease modification from palliatives without withdrawal of active agent.

What then are the pros and cons of these imaging endpoints for AD? [^{18}F]FDG PET is widely available and now reimbursed for some individuals for the diagnosis of AD. It has clear value to identify early disease and exclude confounding dementias from trial populations. The case for amyloid PET tracers is multifaceted. Tracers such as the Pittsburgh Compound-B [56], the stilbene derivative SB-13 [57], FDDNP [58] and novel styrylbezoxazole derivatives, [59] may identify patients with high amyloid load to help enrich proof of concept trials with amyloid lowering therapies and perhaps later identify those suitable for preventive treatment. The question is whether they add value to [^{18}F]FDG or effectively give the same information since it can be argued that their distribution in areas of high lesion load mirrors the hypometabolism detected by [^{18}F]FDG [56,58]. It remains to be proved what the putative amyloid tracers are actually imaging in life. Tracer validation for proof of concept paradoxically needs an effective Aβ lowering therapy. It is currently unknown how long it might take to see treatment effects on brain amyloid load, and whether any change in tracer signal precedes, parallels, or follows improvement that can be more easily followed clinically with neuropsychiatric tests of working memory. Do we really want to image plaque? Is plaque burden related to clinical presentation of disease [60]? Should we try to image inflammation [61,62]?

Finally, there are high hopes for structural imaging being a fast read out for disease modification [63–68], yet recent studies of the brains of patients from the AN1792 active immunization trials showed that brain atrophy was observed to be greater in individuals apparently responding to therapy, and interestingly, this was accompanied by preliminary pathological findings that plaque burden was also reduced to lower levels than would have been expected given the stage of the disease [69]. It was suggested that removal of amyloid plaques could be a possible explanation (total amyloid plaque volume is thought to be 2 to 4% of whole brain volume). The structural MRI endpoint is thus now somewhat controversial and absolutely requires scientific validation through integrated trials such as ADNI, that include neuropsychiatric measures and simultaneous measurement of other known antecedent and putative fluid biomarkers of AD [49,70,71].

3.6 SUMMARY

Biomarkers have great value without being surrogate endpoints. The requirements for imaging as biomarker do not differ in general from any other biomarkers but have some unique challenges in implementation across sites as instruments can vary widely. Imaging biomarkers can undoubtedly play a role in guiding key decision-making through drug development yet it is important to judge the level of validation and qualification required to match resource investment to the intended use of the data. Imaging biomarkers will undoubtedly become more widely used, especially if agreement can be reached on standardized, validated, and qualified paradigms with cross-mechanism utility that can help speed registration of safe and effective new medicines.

REFERENCES

1. Reichert, J. M., Trends in development and approval times for new therapeutics in the United States, *Nat. Rev. Drug Discovery*, 2, 695, 2003.
2. DiMasi, J. A., The value of improving the productivity of the drug development process: faster times and better decisions, *Pharmacoeconomics*, 20(Suppl. 3), 1, 2002.
3. DiMasi, J. A., Hansen, R. W., and Grabowski, H. G., The price of innovation: new estimates of drug development costs, *J. Health Econ.*, 22, 151, 2003.
4. Frank, R. and Hargreaves, R., Clinical biomarkers in drug discovery and development, *Nat. Rev. Drug Discovery*, 2, 566, 2003.
5. Kola, I. and Landis, J., Can the pharmaceutical industry reduce attrition rates?, *Nat. Rev. Drug Discovery*, 3, 711, 2004.
6. Innovation or stagnation? Challenge and opportunity on the critical path to new medical products, United States Food and Drug Administration, 2004.
7. Rudin, M. and Weissleder, R., Molecular imaging in drug discovery and development, *Nat. Rev. Drug Discovery*, 2, 123, 2003.
8. Beckmann, N. et al., Magnetic resonance imaging in drug discovery: lessons from disease areas, *Drug Discovery Today*, 9, 35, 2004.
9. Rudin, M. et al., Non-invasive imaging in drug discovery and development, *Ernst Schering Res. Found. Workshop*, 48, 47, 2004.
10. Jaffer, F. A. and Weissleder, R., Molecular imaging in the clinical arena, *JAMA*, 293, 855, 2005.
11. Pien, H. H. et al., Using imaging biomarkers to accelerate drug development and clinical trials, *Drug Discovery Today*, 10, 259, 2005.
12. Congress US, *Food and Drug Administration: Modernization Act of 1997, Public Law 105–115, 105th Congress*, 1997.
13. Peck, C. C., Rubin, D. B., and Sheiner, L. B., Hypothesis: a single clinical trial plus causal evidence of effectiveness is sufficient for drug approval, *Clin. Pharmacol. Ther.*, 73, 481, 2003.
14. Biomarkers Definitions Working Group, Biomarkers and surrogate endpoints: preferred definitions and conceptual framework, *Clin. Pharmacol. Ther.*, 69, 89, 2001.
15. Rolan, P., Atkinson, A. J., and Lesko, L. L., Use of biomarkers from drug discovery through clinical practice. Report of the ninth federation of pharmaceutical sciences conference on optimizing drug development, *Clin. Pharmacol. Ther.*, 73, 284, 2003.
16. Fleming, T. R. and DeMets, D. L., Surrogate endpoints in clinical trials: are we being misled?, *Ann. Intern. Med.*, 125, 605, 1996.
17. Temple, R., Are surrogate markers adequate to assess cardiovascular disease drugs?, *JAMA*, 282, 790, 1999.
18. Aurecchia, S., Orloff, D., and Sobel, S., Regulatory concerns at various phases of drug development, *Am. J. Cardiol.*, 81(8A), 2F, 1998.

19. Isaacsohn, J. L., Troendle, A. J., and Orloff, D. G., Regulatory issues in the approval of new drugs for diabetes mellitus, dyslipidemia and the metabolic syndrome, *Am. J. Cardiol.*, 93(11A), 49C, 2004.
20. Johnson, J. R. et al., End Points and United States food and drug administration approval of oncology drugs, *J. Clin. Oncol.*, 21, 1404, 2003.
21. Stroobants, S. et al., 18FDG Positron emission tomography for the early prediction of response in advanced soft tissue sarcoma treated with imatinib mesylate (Glivec), *Eur. J. Cancer*, 39, 2012, 2003.
22. Kelloff, G. J. et al., Progress and promise of FDG-PET imaging for cancer patient management and oncologic drug development, *Clin. Cancer Res.*, 11, 2785, 2005.
23. Orloff, D. G., Use of surrogate endpoints: a practical necessity in lipid altering and atherosclerosis drug development, *Am. J. Cardiol.*, 87(Suppl.), 35A, 2001.
24. Rajaram, V. et al., Role of surrogate markers in assessing patients with diabetes mellitus and the metabolic syndrome and in evaluating lipid lowering therapy, *Am. J. Cardiol.*, 93, 32C, 2004.
25. Patel, S. N. et al., Emerging noninvasive surrogate markers of atherosclerosis, *Curr. Atheroscler. Rep.*, 60, 2004.
26. Choudhury, R. P., Fuster, V., and Fayad, Z. A., Molecular, cellular and functional imaging of atherothrombosis, *Nat. Rev. Drug Discovery*, 3, 913, 2004.
27. Jaffer, F. A. and Weissleder, R., Seeing within: molecular imaging of the cardiovascular system, *Circ. Res.*, 94, 433, 2004.
28. Spence, J. D., Ultrasound measurement of carotid plaque as a surrogate outcome for coronary artery disease, *Am. J. Cardiol.*, 89(Suppl.), 10B, 2002.
29. Fenster, A. et al., 3D ultrasound imaging of the carotid arteries, *Curr. Drug Targets Cardiovasc. Haematol. Disord.*, 4, 161, 2004.
30. Nissen, S. E., Application of intravascular ultrasound to characterize coronary artery disease and assess progression or regression of atherosclerosis, *Am. J. Cardiol.*, 89(Suppl.), 24B, 2002.
31. Klingensmith, J. D. et al., Automated three dimensional assessment of coronary artery anatomy with intravascular ultrasound scanning, *Am. Heart J.*, 145, 795, 2003.
32. Nissen, S. E. et al., Effect of intensive compared with moderate lipid lowering therapy on the progression of coronary atherosclerosis: a randomized controlled trial, *JAMA*, 291, 1071, 2004.
33. Conti, R. et al., Lipid lowering by simvastatin induces regression of human atherosclerotic lesions. Two years follow up using high resolution non-invasive magnetic resonance imaging, *Circulation*, 106, 2884, 2002.
34. Nieman, K. et al., Reliable non-invasive coronary angiography with fast submillimeter multislice spiral computed tomography, *Circulation*, 106, 2051, 2002.
35. Schoepf, U. J. et al., Multislice CT angiography, *Eur. Radiol.*, 13, 1946, 2003.
36. Takalkar, A. et al., PET in cardiology, *Radiol. Clin. N. Am.*, 43, 107, 2005.
37. Orloff, D. G., *DMEDP View of Surrogates, Presentation at 2004 Cardiovascular Biomarkers and Surrogate Endpoints Symposium Bethesda MD USA September 10th and 11th 2004*, (proceedings scheduled to be published by Am. J. Cardiol. in 2005).
38. McFarland, H. F. et al., The role of MRI as a surrogate outcome measure in multiple sclerosis, *Mult. Scler.*, 8, 40, 2002.
39. Frank, J. A. et al., Interferon beta-1b slows progression of atrophy in RRMS: three year follow up in Nab − and Nab + patients, *Neurology*, 62, 719, 2004.
40. Seong, E., Seasholtz, A. F., and Burmeister, M., Mouse models for psychiatric disorders, *Trends Genet.*, 18, 643, 2002.
41. Cryan, J. F. and Mombereau, C., In search of a depressed mouse: utility of models for studying depression-related behavior in genetically modified mice, *Mol. Psychiat.*, 9, 326, 2004.
42. Burns, H. D. et al., PET ligands for assessing receptor occupancy in vivo, *Ann. Rep. Med. Chem.*, 36, 267, 2001.
43. Hargreaves, R. J., Imaging substance P (neurokinin 1) receptors in the living human brain using positron emission tomography, *J. Clin. Psychiat.*, 63(Suppl. 1), 18, 2002.
44. Bergstrom, M. et al., Human positron emission tomography studies of brain neurokinin 1 receptor occupancy by aprepitant, *Biol. Psychiat.*, 55, 1007, 2004.
45. Chawla, S. P. et al., Establishing the dose of the oral NK1 antagonist aprepitant for the prevention of chemotherapy-induced nausea and vomiting, *Cancer*, 97, 2290, 2003.

46. Nussbaum, R. L. and Ellis, C. E., Alzheimer's disease and Parkinson's disease, *New Engl. J. Med.*, 348, 1356, 2003.
47. Cummings, J. L., Alzheimer's disease, *N. Engl. J. Med.*, 351, 56, 2004.
48. Nestor, P. J., Scheltens, P., and Hodges, J. R., Advances in the early detection of Alzheimer's disease, *Nat. Rev. Neurosci.*, S34, 2004, Neurodegeneration supplement July.
49. Frank, R. A. et al., Biological markers for therapeutic trials in Alzheimer's disease, *Proceedings of the Biological Markers Working Group. NIA Initiative on Neuroimaging in Alzheimer's Disease, Neurobiol. Aging*, 24, 521, 2003.
50. Yan, X. X. et al., Binding sites of g-secretase inhibitors in rodent brain; distribution, postnatal development and effect of deafferentation, *J. Neurosci.*, 24, 2942, 2004.
51. Cummings, J. L. et al., The role of positron emission tomography in the diagnosis of Alzheimer's disease, *J. Am. Geriatr. Soc.*, 52, 467, 2004.
52. Small, G. W., What does imaging add to the management of Alzheimer's disease?, *CNS Spectr.*, 9(7 Suppl. 5), 20, 2004.
53. Krishnan, K. R. et al., Randomized controlled trial of the effects of Donepezil on neuronal markers and hippocampal volumes in Alzheimer's disease, *Am. J. Psychiat.*, 160, 2003, 2003.
54. Sperling, R. A. et al., fMRI studiers of associative encoding in young and elderly controls and Alzheimer's disease, *J. Neurol. Neurosurg. Psychiat.*, 74, 44, 2003.
55. Machulda, M. M. et al., Comparison of fMRI response among normal, MCI and Alzheimer's patients, *Neurology*, 61, 500, 2003.
56. Klunk, W. E. et al., Imaging brain amyloid in Alzheimer's disease with Pittsburgh Compound-B, *Ann. Neurol.*, 55, 306, 2004.
57. Verhoeff, N. P. et al., In vivo imaging of Alzheimer's disease beat amyloid with 11C SB-13 PET, *Am. J. Geriatr. Psychiat.*, 12, 584, 2004.
58. Shoghi-Jadid, K. et al., Localization of neurofibrillary tangles and beta amyloid plaques in the brains of living patients with Alzheimer's disease, *Am. J. Geriatr. Psychiat.*, 10, 24, 2002.
59. Okamura, N. et al., Styrylbenzoxazole derivatives for in vivo imaging of amyloid plaques in the brain, *J. Neurosci.*, 24, 2535, 2004.
60. Stege, G. J. and Bosman, G. J., The biochemistry of Alzheimer's disease, *Drugs Aging*, 14, 437, 1999.
61. Cagnin, A. et al., In vivo measurement of activated microglia in dementia, *Lancet*, 358, 461, 2001.
62. Halks-Miller, M. et al., CCR1 is an early and specific marker of Alzheimer's disease, *Ann. Neurol.*, 54, 638, 2003.
63. Fox, N. C. et al., Using serial magnetic resonance imaging to measure disease progression in Alzheimer's disease. Power calculations and estimates of sample size to detect treatment effects, *Arch. Neurol.*, 57, 339, 2000.
64. Bradley, K. M. et al., Serial brain MRI at 3–6 month intervals as surrogate marker for Alzheimer's disease, *Brit. J. Radiol.*, 75, 506, 2002.
65. Resnick, S. M. et al., Longitudinal imaging studies of older adults: a shrinking brain, *J. Neurosci.*, 23, 3295, 2003.
66. Du, A. T. et al., Atrophy rates of entorhinal cortex in AD and normal aging, *Neurology*, 60, 481, 2003.
67. Jack, C. R. et al., MRI as a biomarker of disease progression in a therapeutic trial of milameline for AD, *Neurology*, 60, 253, 2003.
68. Mani, R. B., The Evaluation of disease-modifying therapies in Alzheimer's disease; a regulatory viewpoint, *Stat. Med.*, 23, 305, 2004.
69. Fox, N.C. et al., Effects of Abeta immunization (AN1792) on MRI measures of cerebral volume in Alzheimer disease, *Neurology*, 64, 1563, 2005.
70. Hampel, H. et al., Core biological marker candidates of Alzheimer's disease — perspectives for diagnosis, prediction of outcome and reflection of biological activity, *J. Neural Transm.*, 111, 247, 2004.
71. De Leon, M. J. et al., MRI and CSF studies in the early diagnosis of Alzheimer's disease, *J. Intern. Med.*, 256, 205, 2004.

Editorial Comments

Elucidation of the molecular mechanisms responsible for disease development and progression is boosting the elaboration of tools for early diagnosis, including molecular imaging techniques with targeted contrast agents. Nuclear and optical imaging, based on the use of dedicated probes to produce a signal, are molecular imaging techniques par excellence because of their high sensitivity and the lack of background signal from living tissues.

A clear strength of magnetic resonance imaging (MRI) is its ability to explore native mechanisms to modulate image contrast, a feature that is possible because the signal depends on multiple parameters. Contrast material is used to increase the signal difference between an area of interest (e.g., a pathological region or the blood pool) and the remaining tissue. MRI contrast agents (for instance, gadolinium-diethylenetriaminepentaacetic acid, Gd–DTPA) administered systemically normally change the signal intensity in a passive and nonspecific manner. Despite the main challenges concerning low sensitivity on the one hand and the high level of inherent tissue signal on the other, efforts are also being made to develop targeted MRI approaches. The potential of combining high resolution anatomical images with molecular information from targeted contrast agents using a single imaging system justifies such efforts.

In Chapter 4, Silvio Aime and colleagues discuss the synthesis of targeted MRI agents designed to localize to a specific cell type or tissue via a passive or active mechanism. Specific binding is stimulated through the use of biomolecules such as antibodies or small peptides. These developments are likely to significantly impact drug discovery and development, since they may enable one to derive more precise information on drug mechanisms related to a given disease and to select more appropriate molecular biomarkers that will serve as objective end points of treatment efficacy, as well as facilitate the development of new target-specific therapeutics.

Medical imaging agents are generally governed by the same regulations as other drugs and biological products. However, because contrast agents are used solely to diagnose and monitor diseases or conditions as opposed to treat them, and therefore are not intended to affect any bodily functions, development programs for such agents can be tailored to reflect their particular uses [1]. Indeed, review methods and approaches to required clinical data, outcomes and endpoints are different from those traditionally necessary for drug registration. Despite this somewhat favorable situation, development of new agents for clinical application takes several years. Therefore, it is expected that most targeted contrast agents are going to remain exclusively for preclinical use in animal models of diseases. This should not be a limitation within the realm of pharmaceutical research, as targeted imaging may stimulate improvements in early discovery research that might contribute to decrease the high attrition in late-stage drug development. Also, it cannot be excluded that some targeted agents, without undergoing registration procedures, be used in limited proof-of-concept studies of new drugs in humans. Obviously, such a possibility could only be taken in consideration after performing proper safety assessments, in close consultation with health authorities [1].

REFERENCE

1. U.S. Food and Drug Administration, Center for Biologics Evaluation and Research, Guidance for Industry, Developing Medical Imaging Drug and Biological Products, http://www.fda.gov/cber/gdlns/medimagesaf.htm

4 Design of Contrast Agents for Molecular Imaging *In Vivo*

Silvio Aime, Giovanni B. Giovenzana, Dario Longo, and Enzo Terreno

CONTENTS

4.1 INTRODUCTION

The outstanding achievements in molecular and cellular biology are continuously providing new information on the factors determining the cause and the progression of the most important diseases. In this scenario, a new field has emerged, i.e., molecular imaging that pursues the *in vivo* visualization of molecular events occurring at cellular and subcellular level [1]. The possibility of visualizing a molecule that represents the signature of a given disease is an outstanding breakthrough in the diagnostic protocols currently followed in clinical settings.

Basically, any molecular imaging procedure requires an imaging probe that is specific for a given molecular event. Magnetic resonance imaging (MRI) is a relatively poor-sensitive imaging technique and, therefore, the development of MRI contrast agents for molecular imaging protocols requires: (1) the design of probes characterized by a very high contrasting ability, and (2) the identification of an efficient route for the delivery/accumulation of a high number of contrast agent units at the site of interest [2].

MRI contrast agents are chemicals able to markedly alter the relaxation times of water protons in the region where they are distributed. Depending on whether the dominant effect occurs mainly on T_1 or T_2, MRI contrast agents are classified as positive or negative agents, respectively. Paramagnetic complexes of Gd(III) or Mn(III) ions represent the T_1-positive agents, whereas iron oxide particles represent the most used class of T_2-negative agents.

4.2 PARAMAGNETIC Mn(II) AND Gd(III) COMPLEXES

The effectiveness of a paramagnetic metal complex to act as an MRI contrast agent is first assessed by measuring its relaxivity, i.e., the relaxation enhancement of water protons observed for a 1 mM solution of the contrast agent.* The theory of paramagnetic relaxation provides the basis for understanding the relationship between the structural and dynamic properties of a given paramagnetic complex and its relaxivity [3]. Mn(II) and Gd(III) represent the ions with the highest number of unpaired electrons among the transition metals and the lanthanide series, respectively. Moreover, they display relatively long electronic relaxation times. As far as Mn(II) is concerned, being an essential element in living systems, it has been accepted that the administered agent acts as a releaser of Mn(II) ions which are then taken up by endogenous biomolecules. Therefore, the contrast enhancement has to be mainly ascribed to large Mn(II)-containing macromolecules. The only approved Mn(II) containing system is represented by Mn–DPDP (Teslascan®, Chart 4.1).

Recently, there have been several applications of the contrast enhancement promoted by Mn(II) ions to investigate organ functionality and signal pathway transduction. The procedure sometimes called MEMRI (manganese enhanced MRI), relies on the fact that Mn^{2+} competes with Ca^{2+} for entry from the extracellular compartment to the cytosol and from the cytosol to the mitochondria [4]. MEMRI is a powerful preclinical tool for studying the structure and function of white matter in the central nervous system (CNS): assessment of the brain function is based on the assumption that intracellular uptake of Mn(II) is an indirect measure of neuronal activity [5].

In most studies, Mn(II) ions are provided by the injection of $MnCl_2$ in very small amounts to minimize its toxicity. Using spin–echo/inversion–recovery sequences to enhance the contrast between the manganese accumulation regions, it is possible to visualize CNS pathways by exploiting the trans-synoptic paramagnetic tracing capacities. A marked contrast enhancement arises from structures characterized by high Mn uptake, such as the olfactory bulb, amygdaloid complex, hippocampal formation, and cerebellum. This Mn(II)-based magnetic staining enables the recording of anatomical brain images that reports on the neuronal activation patterns after stimulation.

Besides the interesting application of MEMRI, most of the work is still in the field of Gd(III) complexes [6]. Currently, about one third of the MRI scans recorded in clinical settings make use of Gd-based contrast agents. They are chelates of polyaminocarboxylate ligands, either linear or macrocyclic molecules (Chart 4.2). All act as octadentate ligands and yield very stable Gd(III) complexes, thus strongly limiting any risk associated to the release of the harmful Gd^{3+} ions (Table 4.1).

The currently used Gd-based contrast agents distribute in the vascular and extravascular space and are particularly useful to report about lesions in the CNS [7]. A very active area of investigation deals with the dynamic use of contrast agents since the kinetics of their distribution in the extravascular space is related to the vascular permeability [8]. For instance, newly formed vessels functional to the tumor growth display permeability much higher than normal capillaries, an issue that is tackled also by assessing the changes in the expression of vascular endothelium growth factor (VEGF) receptors. Thus, research in the field of dynamic contrast enhancement has a strong synergism with the development of molecular imaging procedures aimed at reporting a direct visualization of the expression of VEGF receptors (see also Chapter 13, Section 13.3.2 and Chapter 14, Section 14.2.2).

Over the last 10 to 15 years, much attention has been devoted to the development of angiographic agents. For such applications it is required that the agent is confined in the blood pool

*Although most of the clinical tomographs work at 1.5–3.0 T and the preclinical research is carried out at even higher fields (4.7–7 T), it is still customary to refer to the relaxivity measured at 20 MHz, i.e. at 0.5 T. This is due to the fact that in neat water the relaxivity of paramagnetic agents does not change significantly as the field strength is increased from 0.5 to 7 T.

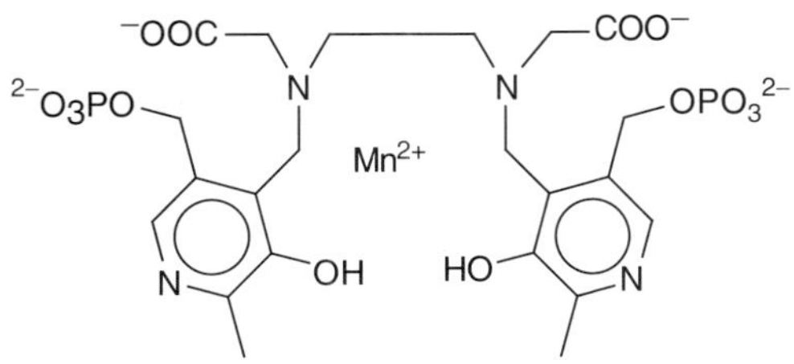

CHART 4.1 Mn-DPDP complex. (Teslascan. With permission.)

with a relatively constant concentration for the time of measurement. One successful approach consists of designing functionalized Gd chelates displaying high binding affinity to human serum albumin (HSA). In blood, HSA has a concentration of about 0.6 mM and its main physiological role deals with the transport of a number of substrates [9]. For many of them, the binding regions have been identified on the basis of extensive competitive assays and this information has been useful in addressing the design of Gd(III)-based blood-pool agents [10].

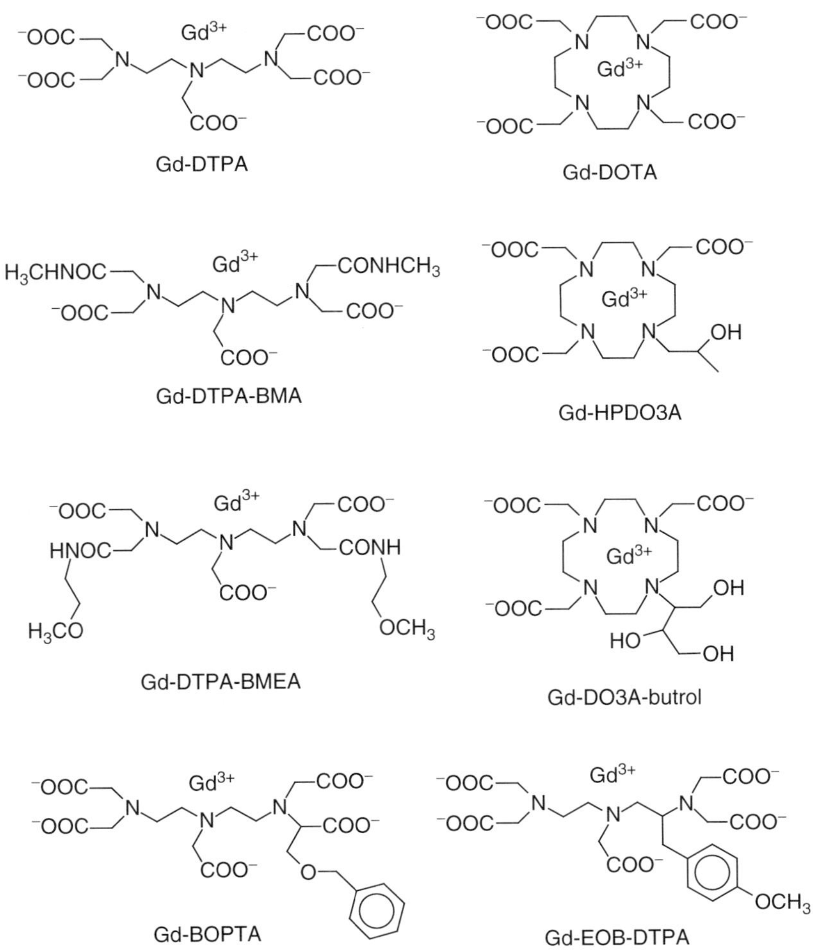

CHART 4.2 Gd(III) complexes approved for clinical use.

TABLE 4.1
Thermodynamic Stability Constant of the Clinically Approved Gd(III)-Based MRI Contrast Agents

Complex	Commercial Name	Company	Log K_{GdL}
$[GdDTPA(H_2O)]^{2-}$	Magnevist®	Schering	22.5
$[GdDOTA(H_2O)]^{-}$	Dotarem®	Guerbet	24.7
$[GdHPDO3A(H_2O)]$	ProHance®	Bracco	23.8
$[GdDO3A\text{-}butrol(H_2O)]$	Gadovist®	Schering	20.8
$[GdDTPA\text{-}BMA(H_2O)]$	Omniscan®	Nycomed-Amersham	16.8
$[GdDTPA\text{-}BMEA(H_2O)]$	OptiMARK®	Mallinckrodt	16.8
$[GdBOPTA(H_2O)]^{2-}$	MultiHance®	Bracco	22.6
$[GdEOB{-}DTPA(H_2O)]^{2-}$	Eovist®	Schering	23.5

Among several systems acting as good angiographic reporters, two agents, MS325 and B22956 (Chart 4.3), are currently in advanced clinical stage [11,12]. Figure 4.1 shows results obtained with B22956 aiding the visualization of the coronary arch.

Upon formation of the supramolecular adduct between a Gd(III) chelate and HSA, a marked relaxation enhancement takes place that is primarily related to the increase of the molecular reorientational time, τ_r, on going from the free to the bound form. An additional contribution to the observed relaxivity arises from exchangeable protons and water molecules on the surface of the protein in close proximity with the binding site of the paramagnetic agent [13]. The theory of the paramagnetic relaxation foresees relaxivities up to 100 $s^{-1}mM^{-1}$ and more (calculated at 20 MHz) for complexes containing one water molecule ($q = 1$) bound to HSA [14]. However, the values reported until now for Gd(III) complexes bound to HSA are significantly lower than the predicted ones [10]. The primary reason for the quenching of the relaxation enhancement is often associated with the occurrence of a long exchange lifetime, τ_M, of the coordinated water. Therefore, efforts have been made to get a better understanding of the determinants of the exchange rate of a water molecule coordinated to a lanthanide(III) ion [15]. The rationale which accounts for the water exchange rate in linear and cyclic polyaminocarboxylate Gd(III) complexes relies on the difference in energy between the ground state (coordination number = 9) and the intermediate state (coordination number = 8) corresponding to the dissociation of the water ligand. It follows that fast exchange rates can be obtained by introducing proper structural modifications on the ligand in order to decrease the activation energy for the water dissociation process. In the case of DOTA-like systems, it was found that there is a subtle structural effect on the exchange rate of coordinated water. In fact, these types of complexes exist in solution as a mixture of two structural isomers, namely the square antiprismatic (SAP) and the twisted square antiprismatic (TSAP) isomer (Figure 4.2) [16]. The latter form displays a water exchange rate that is approximately 50 times faster than the corresponding rate in the SAP isomer [17]. On this basis, the attainment of very high relaxivities have to be pursued by means of systems based on Gd(III) chelates characterized by a fast exchange of the coordinated water. Recently, we undertook an investigation with two GdL complexes (GdL1 and GdL2, Chart 4.4) aimed at getting more insight into the reason why the relaxivities values of paramagnetic Gd–L adducts with HSA are significantly lower than the theoretically expected ones [18]. The two Gd-DOTMA-like complexes display exchange lifetimes of their coordinated water with optimal values for the attainment of high relaxivities. They bind quite strongly to HSA ($K_A = 2.7 \times 10^3 M^{-1}$ and $9.5 \times 10^4 M^{-1}$ for Gd–L1 and Gd–L2, respectively) at the binding site of

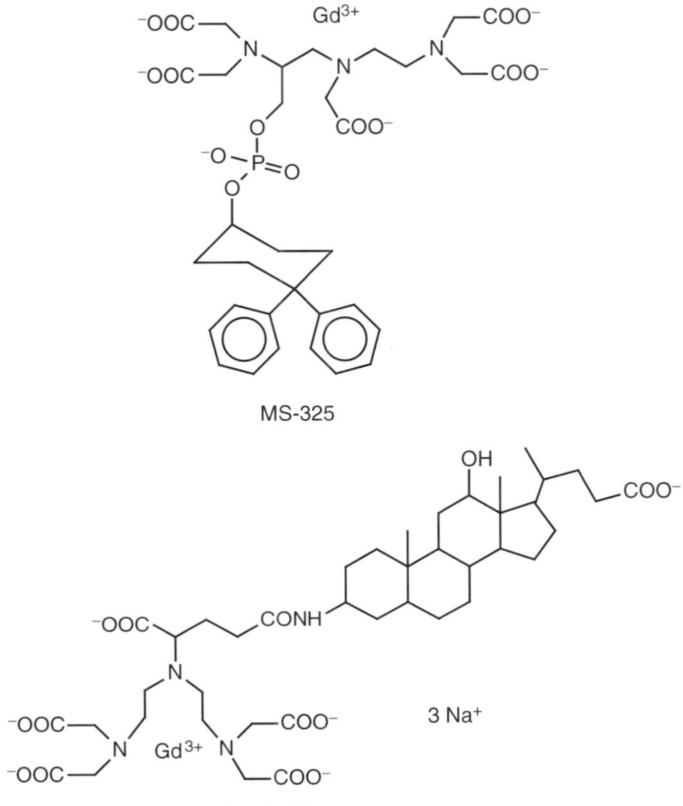

CHART 4.3 Gd(III) complexes currently in advanced clinical trials as angiographic MR agents. (From Perreault, P. et al., *Radiology*, 229, 811, 2003; La Noce, A., et al., *Acad., Radiol.*, 9, S404, 2002. With permission.)

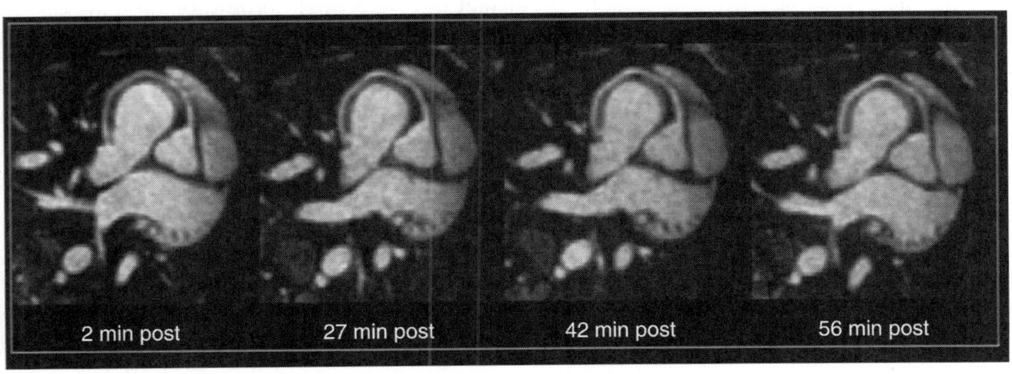

FIGURE 4.1 Multiplanar reconstruction, obtained from inversion-recovery 3D contrast enhanced MR angiography (at 2.0 T), showing the right coronary artery of a micropig after administration of B22956/1 (0.1 mmol/kg). B22956/1 binds strongly to human serum albumin, thus its distribution is only in the intravascular compartment (experimental parameters: TR/TE/TI/α: 3.5 msec/1.81 msec/180 msec/22°, matrix size: $256 \times 168 \times 48$).

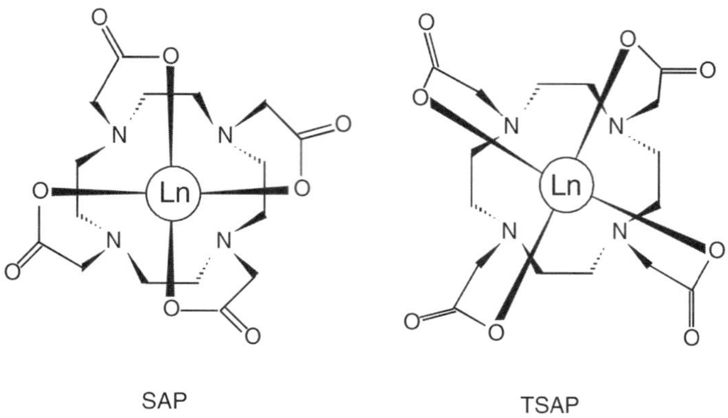

FIGURE 4.2 Schematic representation of the square antiprismatic/twisted square antiprismatic (SAP/TSAP) diastereoisomers of DOTA-like complexes. (From Parker, D. et al., *Chem. Rev.*, 102, 1977, 2002. With permission.)

ibuprofen (Sudlow's site II). As the structural characterization of site II is well defined, it has been possible to pursue accurate molecular modeling studies to dock the binding interaction of Gd–L1 and Gd–L2 on HSA. It has been found that for Gd–L1, the aromatic substituent is well embedded inside the hydrophobic pocket thus leaving the Gd-containing cage just out of its rim at a binding distance to a glutamic residue (Figure 4.3). For Gd–L2, the longer hydrophobic moiety leads the coordination cage to be more spaced out from the surface of the protein in respect of Gd–L1.

The findings from molecular modeling studies yield a strong support to the different behavior shown by Gd–L1 and Gd–L2 as far as concerns the exchange of their coordinated water when the complexes are bound to HSA. In fact, in the case of Gd–L1, binding to HSA causes the quenching of the contribution to the observed relaxivity arising from the inner sphere water molecule likely because its exchange is frozen by the interaction with the glutamic residue. On the other hand, Gd–L2 displays a higher relaxivity because the increased size of the tris-phenyl moiety allows protruding the Gd-chelate far off from the intervention of the glutamic residue to interfere with the exchange of the coordinated water molecule. A further caveat has been obtained from these studies. In fact the ^{1}H NMRD profile of the Gd–L2/HSA

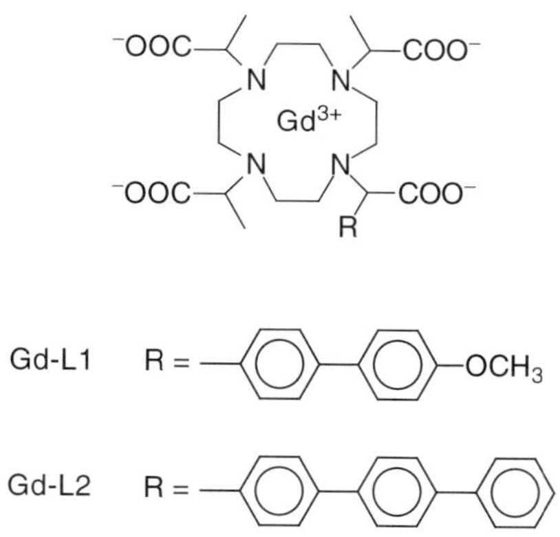

CHART 4.4 GD(III) complexes investigated for their binding to HSA. (From Aime, S. et al., *Chem. Bio. Chem.*, 6, 818, 2005.)

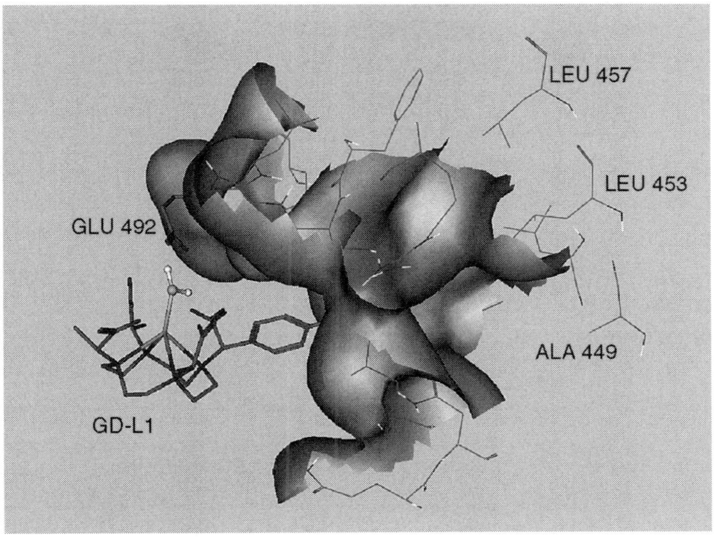

FIGURE 4.3 Results of the docking procedure applied to the interaction of GdL1 to fatted human serum albumin (HSA).

adduct is fitted with a τ_r value that is much shorter than that one would expect for such a macromolecule (1.2 vs. 30 nsec). The shortening of τ_r may be due to the superimposition of the internal rotation of the coordinated water to the overall molecular reorientation of the macromolecular adduct [19]. If this interpretation is correct, a challenging question is posed to chemists for the achievement of the theoretically predicted relaxivities: how to design a Gd-chelate whose coordinated water is in fast exchange with the bulk (short τ_M) and rigid inside the coordination cage?

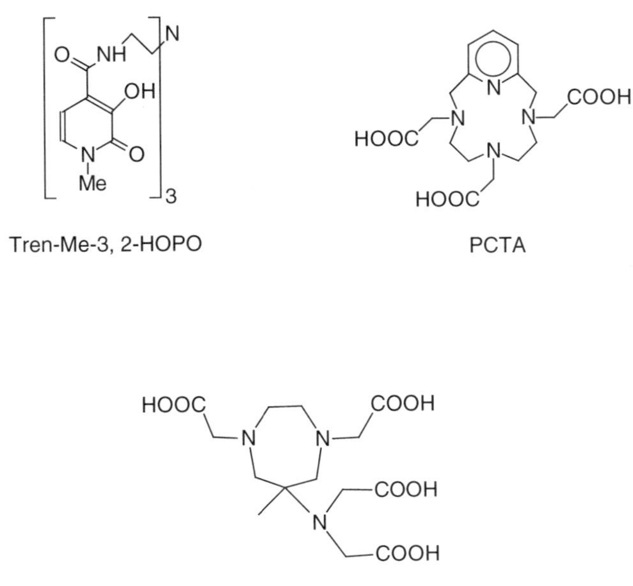

CHART 4.5 Some ligands forming $q = 2$ Gd(III) complexes.

Actually, promising routes to high relaxivities may be envisaged by the use of Gd chelates containing two or even three water molecules. Upon addressing such systems, attention has to be devoted to avoid Gd-chelates that form ternary complexes with endogenous ligands such as carbonate, phosphate or Asp or Glu residues on proteins. If this happens, it will cause a decrease in the hydration of the Gd(III) ion with the consequent loss of the expected relaxation enhancement [20]. A few interesting structures with $q = 2$ have already been identified (Chart 4.5) that show either a high thermodynamic stability or the preservation of their hydration state in the presence of endogenous ligands.

Among them an interesting class is represented by Gd–HOPO complexes developed by Raymond and co-workers at Berkeley. HOPO ligands are based on the 4-carboxylamido-3,2-hydroxypyridinone structure and act as heptadentate ligands towards Gd(III), thus leaving two water molecules in the inner coordination sphere. The peculiar coordination geometry of Gd–HOPO complexes does not allow an easy replacement of the two water molecules by other ligands [21].

Another system that looks very interesting in this regard is constituted by the Gd(III) complexes of AAZTA (6-amino-6-methylperhydro-1,4-diazepinetetraacetic acid). AAZTA is readily obtained in high yields and its Gd(III) complex displays good relaxivity (7.1 $s^{-1}mM^{-1}$ at 20 MHz and 298K), a relatively fast exchange of the coordinated water molecules, a high thermodynamic stability and a nearly complete inertness towards the influence of bidentate endogenous anions [22].

4.3 IRON OXIDE PARTICLES

Iron oxide particles of nanosize dimensions display the phenomenon of superparamagnetism, i.e., thanks to the cooperativity effect, the individual spins of iron ions build up a superspin S [23]. Thus, the relaxation enhancement shown by superparamagnetic iron particles is much higher than that provided by the same number of paramagnetic ions. The size of the Fe_3O_4 crystals strongly affects the magnetic properties. Moreover, the magnetic core is embedded in a coating that prevents agglomeration of particles. According to the size of the particles, the iron oxide particulates are classified as SPIO (superparamagnetic iron oxide) and USPIO (ultrasmall superparamagnetic iron oxide) (Figure 4.4). Larger aggregation (particle size $> 1\ \mu m$) have also been investigated, but their practical use appears to be limited to *in vitro* cellular labeling and *in vivo* exploration of the gastrointestinal tract [24,25]. A common coating of the magnetic cores is represented by dextran, but other substrates have also been used [26]. The surface is obviously very important for the conjugation of the targeting vectors necessary for molecular imaging applications.

In Table 4.2, representative examples of commercially available USPIO and SPIO products are reported along with their characteristic properties. The $1/T_1$ NMRD profiles of USPIO and SPIO systems show a relaxivity bump at approximately 5 to 10 MHz. The interpretation of the relaxation enhancement curves is not straightforward, as several parameters have to be taken into account.

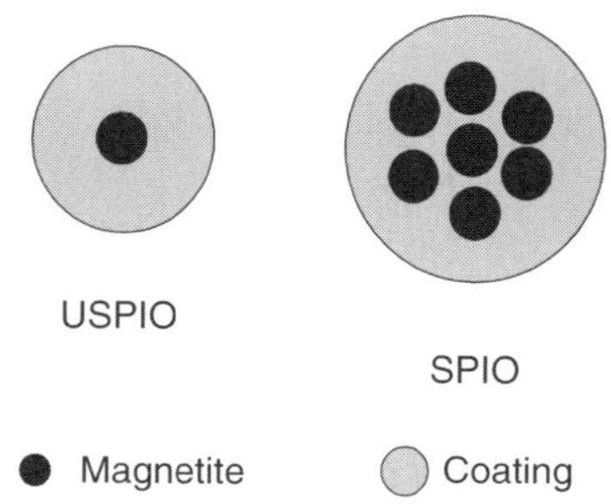

FIGURE 4.4 Schematic representation of SPIO and USPIO particles.

TABLE 4.2
Some General Characteristics of the Clinically Approved USPIO and SPIO Particulates

Commercial name	Sinerem®	Endorem®	Resovist®
Company	Guerbet	Guerbet	Schering
Classification	USPIO	SPIO	SPIO
Crystal size (nm)	4.3–4.9	4.3–4.8	4.2
Mean particle size(nm)	50	200	62
r_1 ($s^{-1}mM^{-1}$)	22.7	24	20
r_2 ($s^{-1}mM^{-1}$)	53.1	107	190

In principle, the systems are analyzed in terms of the classical outer-sphere relaxation theory, i.e., the observed longitudinal and transverse relaxation rates of water protons arise from their diffusion in the proximity of the unpaired electrons responsible for the particle magnetization. However, Curie relaxation for such systems with large magnetic moments is very important, especially at high field. Thus, different timescales have to be considered for the modulation of water diffusion in the inhomogeneous fields around the surface of the particles and for the modulation arising from the fluctuations of the magnetic moment of the particle itself. In general, one may expect that these contrast agents (in particular the USPIO systems) act as both T_1 and T_2 relaxation enhancers. However, in most cases, the presence of iron oxide particles is essentially detected in the corresponding MR images as T_2 or T_2^* effect. Furthermore, it is worth noting that in the presence of some clustering processes, one would expect an elongation of T_1 and a T_2 shortening. Therefore, a T_1 effect in T_1-weighted images can be observed only in the presence of low concentrations of the agent, as it has been shown to occur in blood vessels. After i.v. administration, the fate of superparamagnetic particles is mainly determined by their size, i.e. the largest ones are captured by the Kupffer cells in the liver, whereas the smaller ones may escape them thus remaining in the blood circuit for a much longer time [27–29]. When captured by macrophages of the reticular endothelial system, the particles are found mainly in the liver (60 to 80%) and in the spleen (5 to 7%) [30]. The macrophages entrap the iron-containing particles into phagolysosomes from where they are then slowly recycled in the pool of the physiological iron. The entrapment into the liposomic vesicles affects the overall magnetic properties of the particles; in particular, it has been reported that the increase of the internalized particles leads to a quenching of the observed relaxivity as a result of the limited exchange of water among compartments separated by the bilayered membrane [31]. This behavior is shared with the Gd(III) chelates internalized by the pynocitotic route and it will be discussed in more detail later in this chapter.

4.4 MAIN ROUTES FOR THE CONJUGATION OF IMAGING PROBES TO TARGETING VECTORS

Conjugation of imaging probes to targeting vectors relies on the formation of a covalent bond between the paramagnetic compound and the targeting molecule.

In this session the main routes to the conjugation of imaging probes to targeting moieties are described. Most of the published work addressed the conjugation of Gd(III) chelates. This is still a tricky task: usually these compounds are designed to be highly stable to reduce the *in vivo* toxicity, leaving few or no free functional groups. The need for a linking moiety is then satisfied by: (1) sacrificing one of the pendant coordinating arms; (2) designing the ligand structure with a remote free functional group (so called bifunctional chelators). The ligands DTPA and DOTA (Chart 4.2) have been the candidates of choice for the set-up of conjugation procedures.

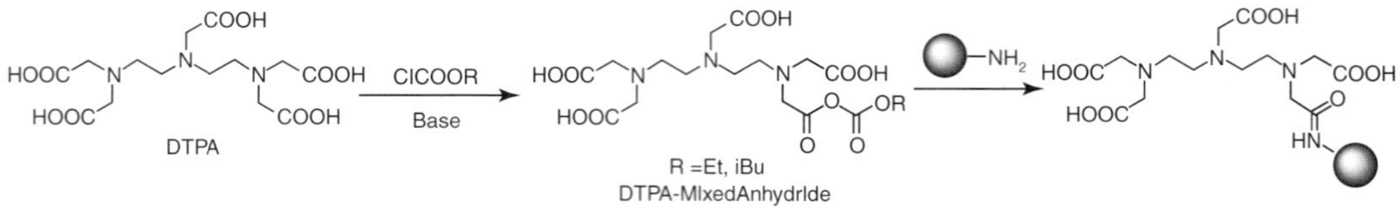

SCHEME 4.1 Activation of DTPA through formation of the mixed monoanhydride. (From Sieving, P. F., Watson, A. D., and Rocklage, M., *Bioconjugate Chem.*, 1, 65, 1990; Arano, Y. et al., *Bioconjugate Chem.*, 8, 442, 1997. With permission.)

The linking of DTPA to targeting molecules may be accomplished directly, through activation of the carboxyl moiety. The activation is performed by conversion of one (or more) carboxyl group to the mixed anhydride by mean of a chloroformate and a scavenger of hydrochloric acid. The anhydride is then reacted *in situ* with an amino group (also an alcoholic hydroxyl group may be used) of peptides or other targeting molecules, affording the corresponding amido-conjugate (Scheme 4.1) [32–34].

Although the low cost of reagents and the rapid one-pot assembly of the conjugate are appealing, this method is plagued by the lack of selectivity in the activation step, leading eventually to a mixture of isomeric (by activation of the two types of carboxyl groups) and multiple conjugates (by activation of more than one carboxyl group per molecule of DTPA).

The most common strategy for DTPA activation is its conversion to a bis-anhydride, commercially available or easily attainable by heating DTPA in the presence of acetic anhydride in pyridine [35].

The bis-anhydride can form one or two amide bonds with one or two amino groups of the targeting molecule, depending on the experimental conditions and in particular on the stoichiometric ratio (Scheme 4.2).

This method has been applied to the conjugation of DTPA to peptides [34,36], antibodies [37], polysaccharides [38,39], oligonucleotides [40] and to the preparation of polyamides DTPA/diamino-PEG [41]. The general applicability of this approach is further exemplified by the extension to other DTPA derivatives; for instance, benzyl-DTPA and EOB-DTPA (Chart 4.6) are efficiently coupled with amino-compounds through their bis-anhydrides [42].

Nevertheless, the unavoidable formation of mono- and bis-amide by the bis-anhydride route frequently leads to mixtures of hardly separable conjugates. To overcome this limitation, partially protected DTPA derivatives have been synthesized in which three or four carboxyl moieties are protected by esterification with *t*-butyl groups (Chart 4.7).

The residual free carboxyl group of DTPA-(tBu)$_4$ is activated through the mixed anhydride method or by other activating agents (DCC,cBOP) [34,43,44], while the two carboxyl groups of

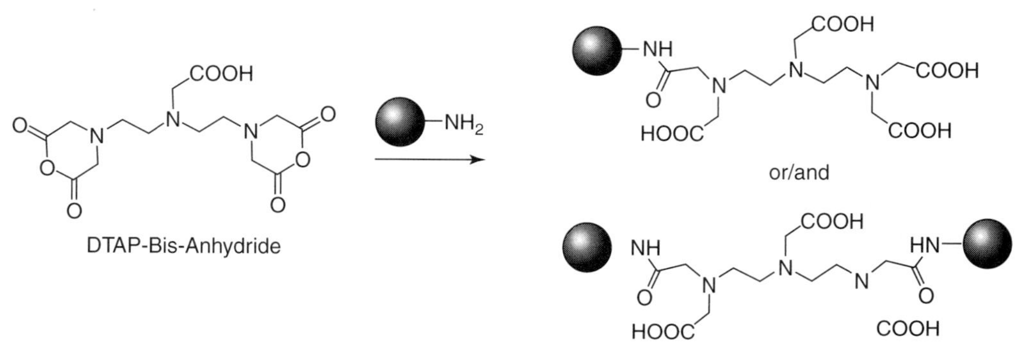

SCHEME 4.2 DTPA-Bis-Anhydride as starting material for conjugations.

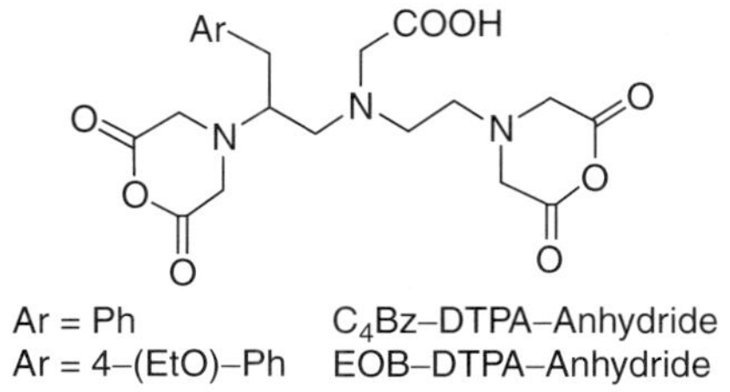

CHART 4.6 Substituted DTPA-Bis-Anhydrides. (From Laurent, S. et al., *Eur. J. Inorg. Chem.*, 463, 2004. With permission.)

DTPA-(tBu)$_3$ are converted to the intramolecular anhydride [45]. The anhydrides are then coupled with an amino-moiety of the targeting moiety; the *t*-butyl esters are finally removed by simple treatment with trifluoroacetic acid to give the desired conjugate, ready to host the paramagnetic metal.

The synthesis of DTPA conjugates through one or more carboxyl groups leads to the conversion of the latter into amides, whose coordinating ability is significantly reduced with negative consequences for the potential *in vivo* application. However, the synthesis of DTPA derivatives embodying a remote functionality allows the linkage of the ligand to the targeting molecule with no effect on the coordinating groups, which are left unchanged in the conjugation step. The functional group must be remote to avoid any interference with the coordination sphere of the resulting chelate, and selective in its reaction with a specific functional group of the targeting molecule.

On this basis DTPA derivatives have been developed, mostly based on the isothiocyanato functional group. The latter reacts selectively with amino groups in aqueous solution, where it is reasonably stable even at slightly basic pH.

In Scheme 4.3 the conjugation scheme for isothiocyanato-benzyl substituted DTPA derivatives to afford stable thioureido linkage is reported. The dashed lines represent the isomeric linkages of the isothiocyanatobenzyl substructure in the various derivatives that may be prepared [46–50].

The versatility of this route is further witnessed by the reported synthesis of a number of modified DTPA derivatives, where the polyaminic backbone is functionalized with a methyl group (Mx–DTPA) [51] or the central pendant arm bears a phosphinic acid group in place of the carboxylic acid (ITC–Bn–DTTAP) [52].

Fully esterified DTPA derivatives bearing a side chain with a free carboxyl or amino group (Chart 4.8) are useful compounds for conjugations to peptides and other targeting molecules by means of the well-known methods of peptide synthesis. The t-butyl protection is preferred due to its compatibility with peptide-synthesis protocols [53–55].

An alternative strategy to link a targeting molecule is based on the selective reaction between a substituted maleimide and thiol group. This route is particularly attractive for the linkage to cysteine residues of peptides and proteins (Scheme 4.4) [44].

The routes for conjugating cyclic ligands such as DOTA are similar to those of DTPA. DOTA may be directly conjugated with targeting molecules by activation through the mixed anhydride method (Scheme 4.5). Unfortunately, up to now no intramolecular anhydride or bis-anhydride of DOTA has been reported.

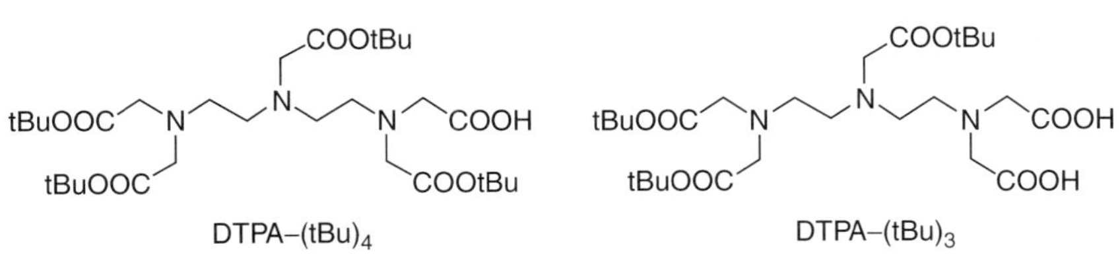

CHART 4.7 Partially esterified DTPA derivatives.

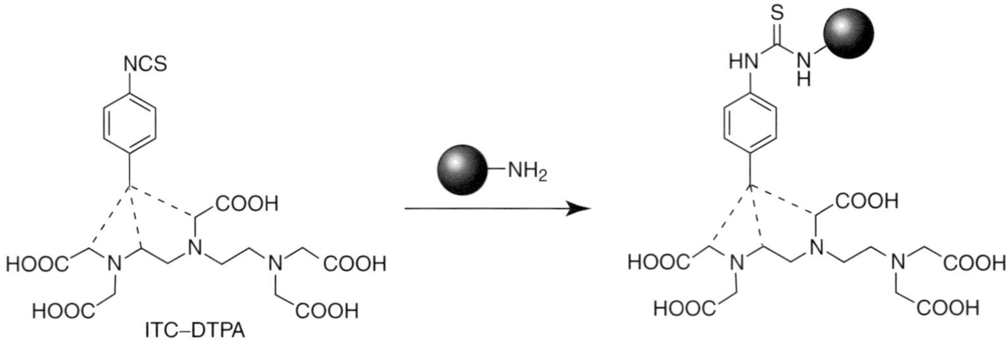

SCHEME 4.3 Isothiocyanato-functionalized DTPA derivatives. (Brechbiel, M. W. et al., *Inorg. Chem.*, 25, 2772, 1986; Westerberg, D. A. et al., *J. Med. Chem.*, 32, 236, 1989. With permission.)

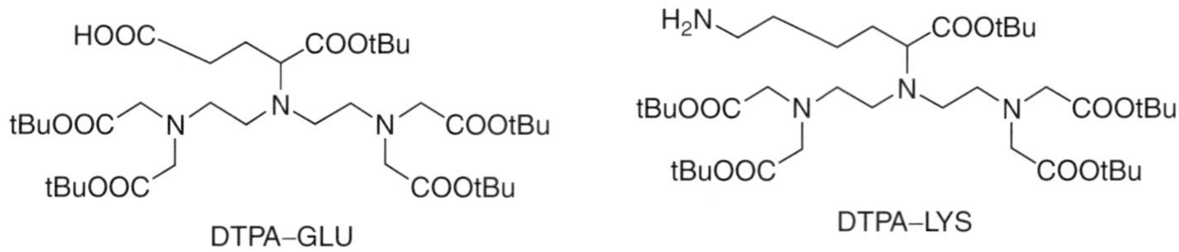

CHART 4.8 Fully esterified DTPA with carboxyl- or amino-functionalized side chains.

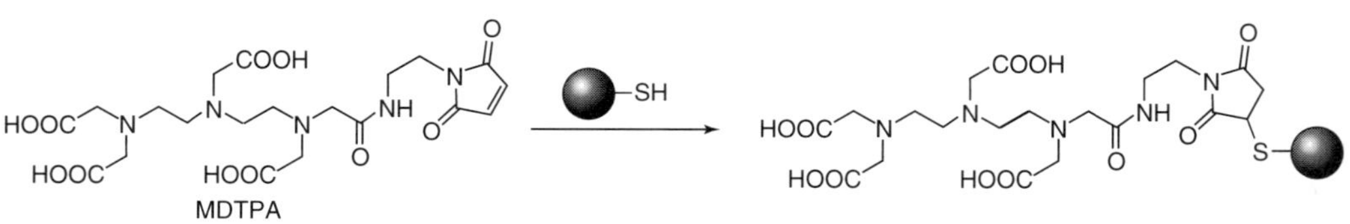

SCHEME 4.4 Maleimido-functionalized DTPA. (From Arano, Y. et al., *J. Med. Chem.*, 39, 3451, 1996. With permission.)

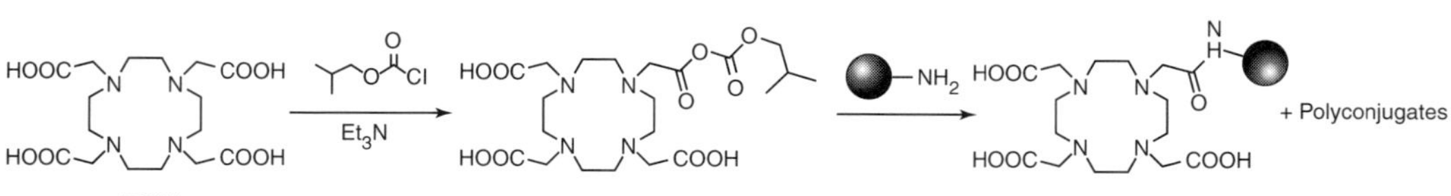

SCHEME 4.5 Activation of DOTA through mixed anhydride formation.

DOTA is reacted with isobutyl chloroformate in the presence of an acid scavenger and the mixed anhydride is then ready to react with a free amino group of the targeting molecule [33]. As with DTPA, the reaction is plagued by byproducts deriving from multiple activation processes.

Partially protected DOTA derivatives have then been reported to overcome the formation of multiple conjugation byproducts and to simplify the purification processes. Probably the most popular compound of this class is the triprotected *t*-butyl ester DOTA(tBu)$_3$, even if the tribenzyl DOTA(Bn)$_3$ is known as well (Scheme 4.6).

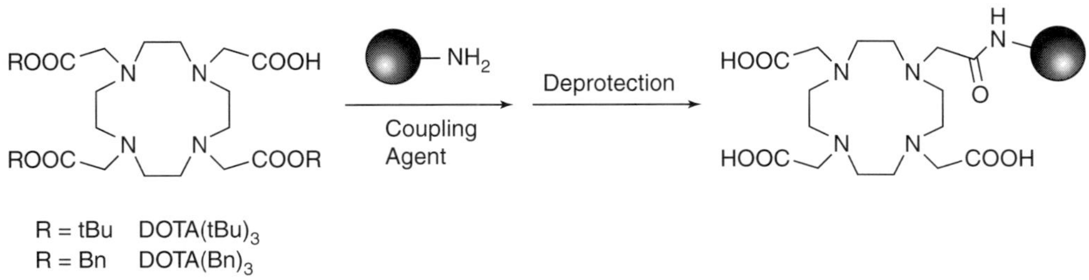

SCHEME 4.6 DOTA triesters as starting materials for conjugations.

DOTA(tBu)$_3$ may be coupled to a variety of amino compounds, by means of the usual methods of peptide synthesis. The t-butyl protection warrants the monoconjugation while being fully compatible with peptide synthesis protocols [54,56–59]. Deprotection is accomplished with trifluoroacetic acid, while DOTA(Bn)$_3$ may be debenzylated after conjugation by catalytic hydrogenolysis [60].

Coupling to one of the nitrogen atoms of the macrocyclic ring is another possibility. This approach makes use of the DO3A(tBu)$_3$ ligand (tri-t-butyl 1,4,7,10-tetraazacyclododecan-1,4,7-triacetate), that is easily obtained from the corresponding polyazamacrocycle and may be bound to targeting molecules upon a prederivatization with halogenoalkyl moieties or epichlorhydrin (Scheme 4.7) [54].

Alternatively, the NH-group of DO3A(tBu)$_3$ can be activated by a reaction with diethyl squarate (3,4-diethoxy-3-cyclobutene-1,2-dione) to give DO3ASQ(tBu)$_3$. The latter reacts efficiently in basic aqueous–alcoholic solutions or in the free acid form in aqueous solutions with amino compounds to give the corresponding conjugates (Scheme 4.8) [61,62].

As the linking of the targeting molecules occurs in the proximity of the metal coordination sphere, some interactions may arise due to the coordinating groups or steric requirements of the targeting molecule itself. For these reasons, the NH group of DO3A may be functionalized giving

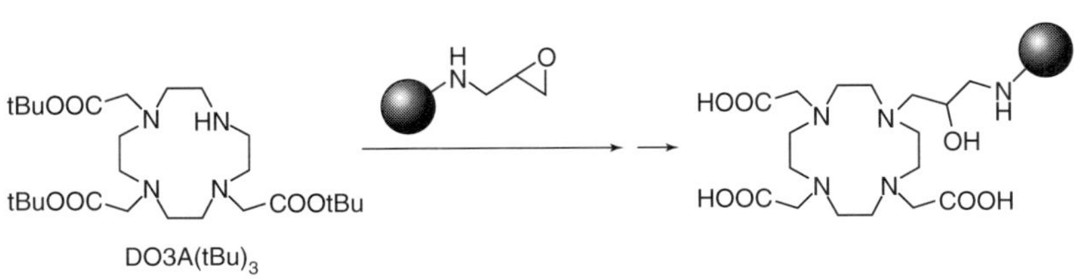

SCHEME 4.7 DO3A(tBu)$_3$ as starting material for conjugations. (From Anelli, P. L. et al., *J. Med. Chem.*, 47, 3629, 2004. With permission.)

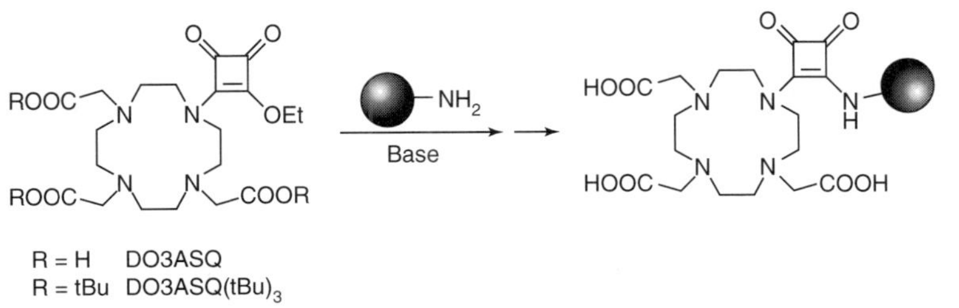

SCHEME 4.8 Squarate as a linker for conjugation of DO3A derivatives. (From Aime, S. et al., *J. Am. Chem. Soc.*, 121, 5762, 1999; Corsi, D. M. et al., *Chem. Eur. J.*, 1, 64, 2001. With permission.)

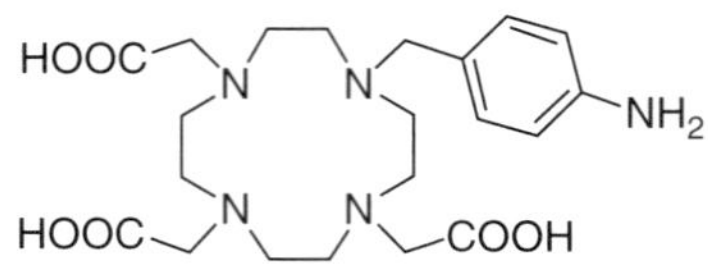

CHART 4.9 Aminobenzyl-DO3A ligand. (From Mishra, A. K. et al., *Tetrahedron Lett.*, 37, 7515, 1996. With permission.)

DO3A derivatives bearing an additional amino group on a suitable spacer, as in aminobenzyl-DO3A (Chart 4.9) [63].

Even though macrocyclic chelates of DOTA are highly stable, the conversion of one carboxyl group to amide or the substitution of an entire carboxymethyl pendant arm negatively affects the stability of the complex. Furthermore, Gd–DOTA–monoamides may show a reduced relaxation enhancement due to slow exchange of the coordinated water molecule, usually found in this type of neutral complex. To overcome this drawback, the coordinating groups of DOTA should be left unchanged, moving the linking site on the macrocyclic backbone or in the α-position of a carboxymethyl pendant arm that does not interfere with the coordination cage. Isothiocyanato functional groups are again one of the better choices to link DOTA to a targeting molecule with a stable thioureido moiety.

Some ready to link isothiocyanato-DOTA derivatives (ITC–Bn–DOTA [64] and PA–DOTA [65]) are known and reported in Chart 4.10, together with macrocyclic analogues derived from ligand TETA [64] (1,4,8,11-tetraazacyclotetradecane-1,4,8,11-tetraacetic acid) and NOTA [64] (1,4,7-triazacyclononane-1,4,7-triacetic acid).

Thiol-linking moieties have also been introduced on the ligand backbone as in BABnDOTA [66] (Chart 4.11), or bound via amidic bond to a carboxymethyl side arm as in VinylSulfonDOTA [67] (Scheme 4.9).

The maleimide affinity for –SH groups is well known, and it has been introduced in the phosphinic analogues of DOTA depicted in Chart 4.12 [68].

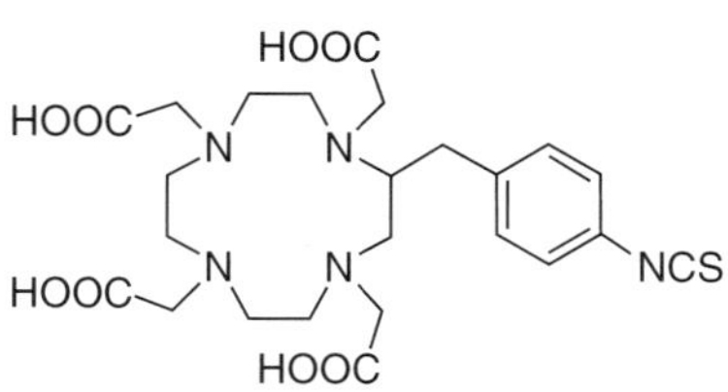

ITC–Bn–DOTA

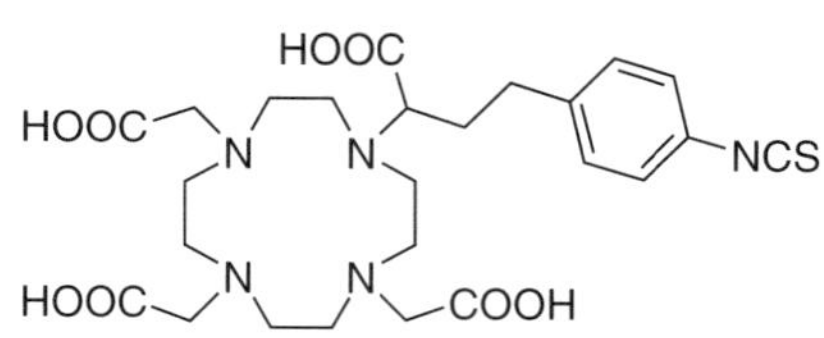

PA–DOTA

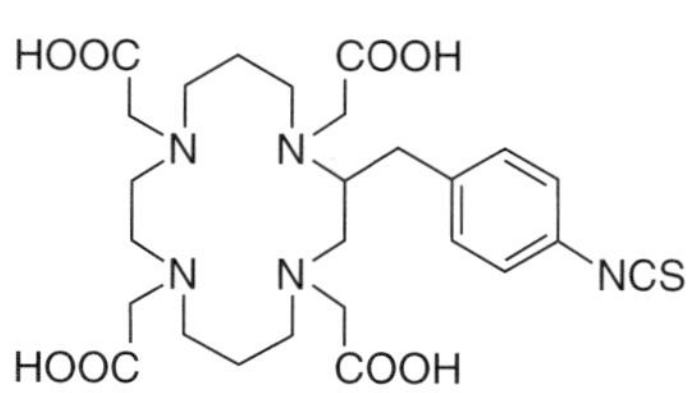

ITC–Bn–TETA

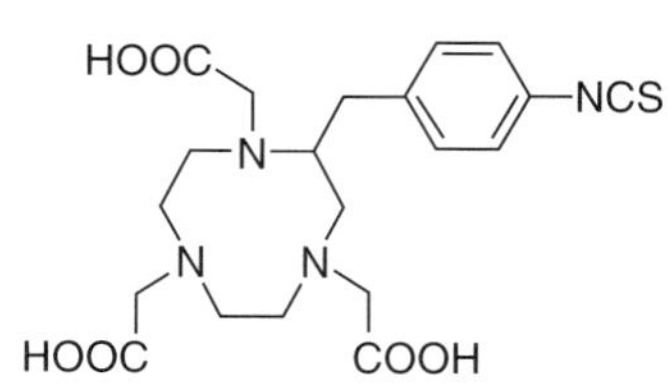

ITC–Bn–NOTA

CHART 4.10 Isothiocyanato-functionalized macrocyclic ligands. (From McMurry, T. J. et al., *Bioconjugate Chem.*, 3, 108, 1992; Chappell, L. L. et al., *Bioorg. Med. Chem.*, 7, 2313, 1999. With permission.)

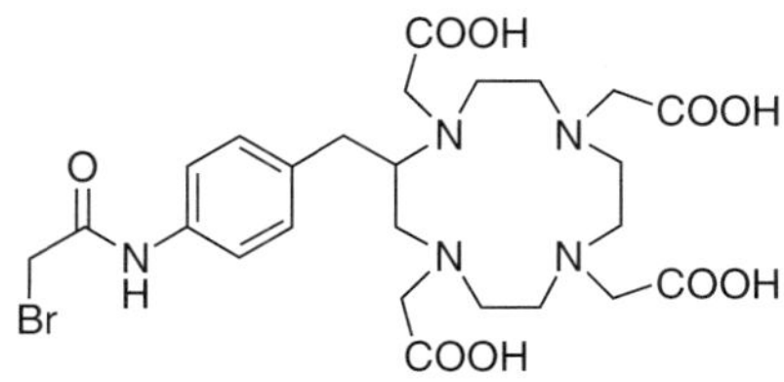

CHART 4.11 Bromoacetamidobenzyl (BABn)-DOTA ligand. (From Whetstone, P. A. et al., *Bioconjugate Chem.*, 15, 3, 2004. With permission.)

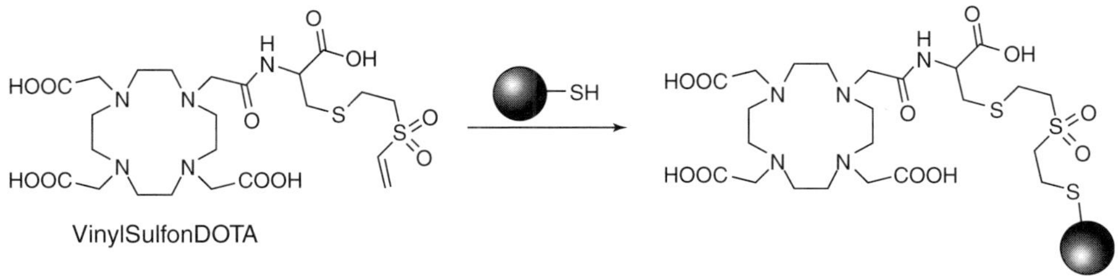

SCHEME 4.9 Vinylsulfone-functionalized DOTA for conjugation to thiols. (From Li, L. et al., *Bioconjugate Chem.*, 13, 110, 2002. With permission.)

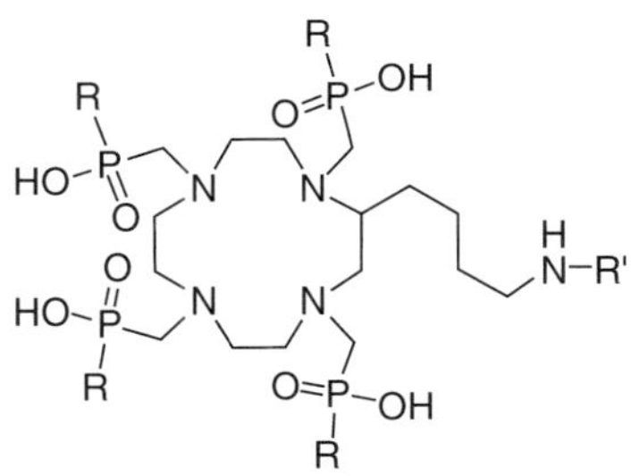

CHART 4.12 Functionalized DOT(R)P derivatives. (From Broan, C. J. et al., *Synthesis*, 63, 1992. With permission.)

In spite of the number of successful derivatives reported up to now, the need for more efficient routes for the conjugation of imaging probes is still evident. The direct conjugation is usually rapid and cheap, but selectivity and purification protocols may cause problems. Bifunctional chelators appear to be the candidates of choice, especially ready to link systems that are able to react with functional groups other than free amines or thiols, not always available on the targeting molecules.

4.5 ACCUMULATION OF IMAGING PROBES AT THE TARGET SITE

As mentioned above, MRI agents are much less sensitive than nuclear or optical imaging probes. Therefore, molecular imaging applications using MRI invariably involve the need for accumulating a high number of contrast-enhancing units at the site of interest. The sensitivity issue is more acute for contrast agents based on paramagnetic complexes rather than on iron oxide particles. Several approaches have been proposed to tackle this problem. A straightforward approach is to recur to polymeric derivatives containing a high number of covalently bound Gd-chelates [10]. It was shown early on that the Gd(III) poly(aminocarboxylate) moiety can be easily conjugated to the ε-amino group of the lysine backbone (see Scheme 4.2) [37]. Analogously, dextran has been used as substrates to bind DTPA or DOTA residues to yield a highly hydrophilic macromolecular carrier [69].

Other systems under intense scrutiny are represented by dendrimers which deal with highly rigid and monodisperse systems. A representative, widely studied example is given by polyamidoamide (PAMAM) dendrimers that have been shown to be nontoxic, nonimmunogenic, and degradable. According to the generation of the dendrimer, a variable number of Gd-chelates can be bound to the NH_2 moieties exposed on the surface (Figure 4.5) [70,71]. As far as the molecular imaging applications are concerned, these macromolecular Gd-loaded carriers need to be further conjugated with one or more targeting vectors. In principle, one may reach very high relaxivities when calculated for carrier unit; for instance, a relaxivity of 66960 $s^{-1}mM^{-1}$ has been reported for generation 10, Gd-DOTA-loaded, PAMAM dendrimers [70].

A further route to design the delivery of a large number of contrast-enhancing units relies on the use of mixed micelles, liposomes and other form of lipophilic aggregates. The overall size attainable with these systems may limit their accessibility to targets located on the endothelial walls. Wickline and co-workers at Washington State University have widely explored the MRI visualization of targeting molecules by using lipidic microemulsions containing several thousands of Gd-chelates [72]. Recently, they showed that targets at picomolar concentrations on a single layer of cells can be visualized by their imaging probe containing 96,400 Gd units [73].

Another example is provided by the work of Sipkins et al. [74] who developed a procedure for the visualization of $\alpha_v\beta_3$ integrins as markers of angiogenesis. The target is first bound by a biotinylated antibody against $\alpha_v\beta_3$, which is successfully recognized by an avidin moiety on the surface of a liposome loaded with Gd-chelates. By this procedure, they were able to provide an enhanced detection of a rabbit carcinoma through the imaging of the angiogenetic vasculature. The exploitation of the outstanding binding affinity between biotin and avidin ($K_A = 10^{15}$) appears to be increasingly used in MR-molecular imaging applications. Bhujwalla and co-workers have recently applied this recognition path for the visualization of HER-2/c-neu receptors (a member of the epidermal growth factor family hyperexpressed in multiple cancers) [75]. They addressed the extracellular domain of the receptors by means of a biotinylated monoclonal antibody (mAb). After clearance of the unbound mAb, Gd-labeled avidin is administered and binds, with a high affinity, to the biotinylated mAb (Figure 4.6). The expression level of the receptor was estimated at

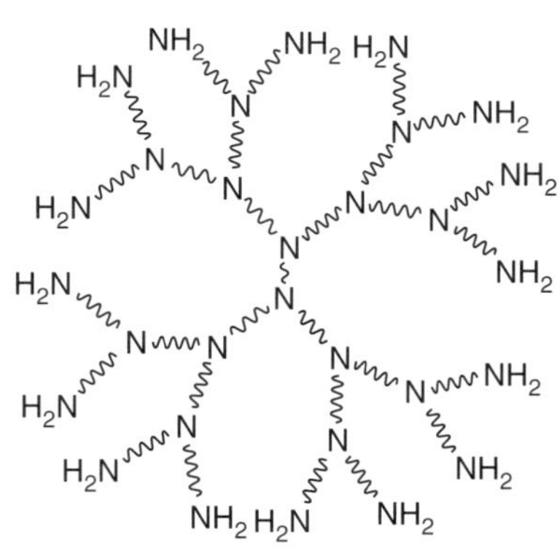

FIGURE 4.5 Core (generation 0) of PAMAM dendrimers. (From Bryant, L. H. et al., *J. Magn. Res. Imaging*, 9, 348, 1999; Wiener, E. C. et al., *Magn. Res. Med.*, 31, 1, 1994. With permission.)

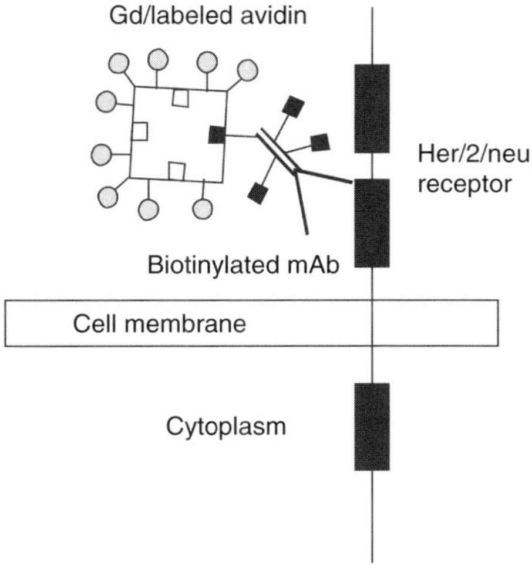

FIGURE 4.6 Schematic representation of the Gd-labeling of Her-2/neu receptors by a biotinylated monoclonal antibody (mAb)-avidin linker.

7×10^5 receptors/cell and the averaged number of Gd–DTPA units per avidin molecule was 12.5. The method has been successfully applied in an experimental mouse model of breast carcinoma.

Another example based on the recognition properties of the biotin/avidin pair has been reported by Kobayashi and Brechbiel [76] who investigated the uptake of a macromolecular construct comprised of avidin and a biotinylated dendrimer bearing 254 Gd–DTPA chelates into SHIN3 cells (a cell line obtained originally from human ovarian cancer). The internalization process is driven by the avidin molecule, a glycoprotein that recognizes β-D-galactose receptors, which are present in either normal hepatocytes or cancer cells (especially ovarian and colorectal adenocarcinoma cells).

We have further developed this approach by using mono- and bis-biotinylated Gd-chelates. By proper addition of avidin and the two chelates it is possible to build up, at the avidin receptor sites, multilayered structures containing a number of Gd(III) ions sufficient for the MRI detection (Figure 4.7) [77].

Once the recognition synthon has delivered the imaging probe to the proper site at the membrane surface, an internalization process may take place that leads to the intracellular entrapment of the imaging probe. As receptor proteins represent the most frequent targets, the vector is often designed on the structure of the ligand for a given receptor. However, the extensive structural modification induced by conjugating the contrast-enhancing moiety may alter dramatically the internalization pathway available for the simple ligand. Actually, the receptor-mediated endocytosis appears a likely route for an imaging probe to be accumulated inside the cell. In such cases, the stimulation of the receptors may cause their migration on the cellular membrane to reach regions where the intracellular side is rich in clathrin, an important mediator of endocytosis. Upon crowding in such regions, a process starts with the introflection of a portion of a cellular membrane followed by the welding of its extremities. Through this process, the imaging probe and its receptor remain entrapped in the endosomic vesicles. The small endosomes may eventually fuse into larger lysosomes. Entrapment into the endosomes appears to be a quite safe method for reducing the toxicity of such endogenous materials in living cells.

Actually, internalization of high amounts of imaging probes into endosomes can be easily attained by exploiting the normal pynocytosis activity of cells (the drinking of the cells). In fact, it has been found that incubating a cell culture in the presence of relatively high concentrations of harmless Gd-based contrast agents like Gd–HPDO3A (Pro-Hance®) or Gd–DTPA (Magnevist®) for a few hours, one may accumulate enough agent for MRI visualization of the treated cells. An

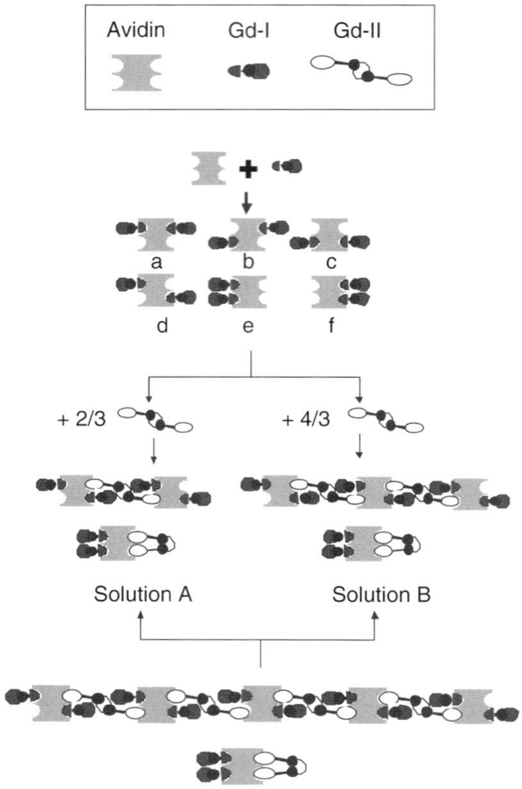

FIGURE 4.7 Routes to the formation of avidin/biotinylated Gd(III)-based adducts. In addition to multilayered adducts, also simple, mono-avidin-based systems are formed. (From Geninatti Crich, S. et al., *J. Biol. Inorg. Chem.*, 10, 78, 2005. With permission.)

example is provided in Figure 4.8, which reports the MRI visualization of stem cells. As a representative example of stem cell labeling, we have considered blood-derived endothelial progenitor cells (EPCs) whose infusion is expected to increase the neovascularization at ischemic sites. In a typical experiment of uptake by pynocytosis, a few million EPCs were incubated in a medium containing Gd–HPDO3A in the mM concentration range (10 to 50 mM) [78]. No saturation effect was detected and the amount of entrapped Gd(III) was proportional to the concentration of the contrast agent in the incubation medium. The proof that the imaging probe accumulated into endosomic vesicles was obtained by replacing the Gd-chelate with the corresponding Europium (Eu)-chelate, as Eu owns good fluorescent properties. In fact, images at the confocal microscope clearly showed that the imaging probe was confined into endosomic vesicles in the perinuclear region.* Then, EPCs were implanted subcutaneously, within a matrigel plug, to a mouse model of angiogenesis. After 7 days, matrigel plugs were vascularized by a capillary network formed by EPCs and connected to the circulation as shown by histological analysis. The process could be followed in the living animal as the presence of Gd-labeled EPCs induced the appearance of hyperintense spots in T_1-weighted images. The detection of hyperintense

*The need for double-labeling procedures in order to validate molecular imaging protocols by multi-modality approaches will certainly increase in the near future. This opens a new area of chemical research to address the synthesis of imaging probes endowed by double detection capabilities; i.e. MRI and optical imaging, MRI and PET or SPECT, etc...Likely, efforts will also be devoted on the technological side to design hybrid tomographs.

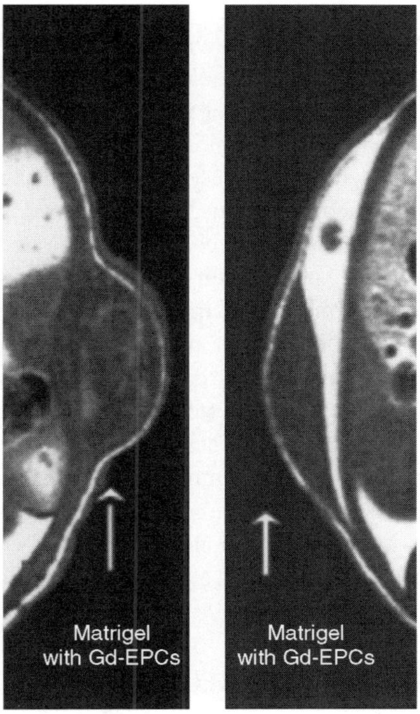

FIGURE 4.8 *In vivo* T_1-weighted spin echo images (at 7 T) of Gd-labeled endothelial progenitor cells dispersed into a subcutaneous matrigel plug 7 days after the implantation to a mouse model of angiogenesis (experimental details: TR/TE/NEX: 120 msec/4.4 msec/42, FOV 2.7 cm, slice thickness 1 mm).

signals in MR images of EPCs 14 days after their grafting on matrigel structures shows that Gd-complexes can be competitive with iron oxide particles for *in vivo* tracking of stem cells.

Actually, SPIO nanoparticles are the most used systems for labeling stem cells or other cells (see Chapter 25). In general, their cellular uptake is mediated by the formation of supramolecular adducts with suitable carriers. Polycationic transfection agents proved to be particularly suitable for this purpose. More recently, Frank and co-workers have shown that this type of magnetic labeling may be obtained by using two FDA approved agents, ferumoxides and protamine sulfate. The two species combine by electrostatic interaction on the surface of the cells and their uptake proceeds by endosomal incorporation. Neither short- or long-term toxicity, nor changes in function, differentiation capacity, or phenotype occur when compared to unlabeled cells [79].

Internalization into the cytoplasm appears possible when the receptor uptake is carried out on a substrate that maintains the recognition properties of the endogenous ligand unaltered. We found that the use of Gd-loaded apoferritin represents a good model to investigate the cell internalization of Gd-chelates via the receptor route [80]. In fact, apoferritin can be loaded by entrapping Gd-chelates inside its internal cavity, which is naturally devoted to store iron under the form of polymeric oxide. The exterior of such Gd-loaded apoferritin is unaltered and therefore still suitable to be recognized by receptors devoted to the transport of ferritin. Since it is known that intravenously administered ferritin is cleared up by the liver in a few minutes, *in vitro* experiments have been carried out on rat hepatocytes. It has been found that the amount of Gd-loaded apoferritin internalized into rat hepatocytes is similar to the values reported for the native ferritin (6.5×10^6 molecules per cell in 6 h). The contrast induced by Gd-loaded apoferritin is very good because the relaxivity shown by these systems is one of the highest reported up to now (approximately 80 $s^{-1}mM^{-1}$). We found that the *in vitro* visualization of labeled hepatocytes is possible when each cell has taken up approximately 5×10^7 Gd–HPDO3A units [2].

Another route that appears promising for accumulating large amounts of imaging probes inside the target cells is represented by the transmembrane transporter system because this is the way the cells intrinsically use for the uptake of large quantities of substrate molecules. An example of efficient uptake is given by the internalization of suitable functionalized Gd-chelates into normal hepatocytes via transporters like the organic anion transport protein [81]. Although a number of transporting systems may be considered, in the case of tumor cells, the transporters of choice appear to be those involved in the transport of nutrients and pseudonutrients. In fact, during cell proliferation, the altered metabolism of tumor cells determines a much higher demand of these substances and therefore an increase of their uptake efficiency with upregulation and/or overexpression of the corresponding membrane transporters.

Finally, it is worth mentioning the use of membrane translocation peptides. Through the binding to these peptides, imaging probes may cross the cellular membrane. In this context, an interesting development has been recently reported by Heckl et al. who synthesized an imaging probe made of a Gd-complex, a peptide nucleic acid (PNA) sequence and a transmembrane carrier peptide [82]. The system accumulated only in tumor cells because of the specific binding of the PNA moiety for the mRNA specifically upregulated in those cells. Thus, the recognition motif between the PNA sequence and given regions of the mRNA yields the formation of a supramolecular adduct that accumulates in the cells.

4.6 UNDERSTANDING THE *IN VIVO* RELAXATION EFFICACY OF MR-IMAGING PROBES

With the commercially available Gd-based extracellular agents, it may be stated that a 50% contrast enhancement is observed when the local concentration of the agent is of the order of 50 μM [83]. Clearly, this threshold can be lowered by using systems characterized by higher relaxivities and the chemists are actively seeking for new structures endowed with enhanced sensitivities. However, as far as the molecular imaging applications are concerned, additional issues related to the *in vivo* location of the imaging probe, have to be considered.

4.6.1 NONUNIFORMLY DISTRIBUTED TARGETS

The sensitivity of the imaging probe may be limited when sparse epitopes are not distributed uniformly in the voxel. This situation may be met when the target molecules are on the endothelial wall. The decrease of sensitivity relies on the limited walking path of the water molecule during the acquisition protocol, for which a given voxel does not appear as a hyperintense spot in a T_1-weighted image if the contrast agent is not uniformly distributed, i.e., if it is confined only in a small region of the acquired voxel. Recently, Morawski et al. reported an interesting experiment that appears to rule out this issue [73]. They succeeded in the MRI visualization of a single cell layer exposing, on their outer surface, epitopes at approximately 10^2 pM concentration by anchoring to each target site, an imaging probe containing approximately 10^5 Gd-chelates. At 1.5 T, the relaxivity of the imaging probe was $17.9 \pm 0.6\ s^{-1}mM^{-1}$ when referred to Gd(III) unit, and $1.69 \times 10^6 \pm 6 \times 10^4\ s^{-1}mM^{-1}$ when referred to the concentration of the whole probe. With the use of a standard 3D imaging technique, they were able to observe substantial contrast between the voxels containing the labeled cell monolayer and the corresponding voxels containing unlabeled cells. From their results the authors concluded that: (1) picomolar binding is sufficient to achieve diagnostic contrast to noise level if high payload particles are employed; (2) sparse molecular epitopes, such as tissue factors, can be imaged on cells at clinical field strengths under certain reasonable conditions; and (3) model-based predictions of the local concentrations of targeted paramagnetic agents are accurate if the fundamental characteristics of the agents are known.

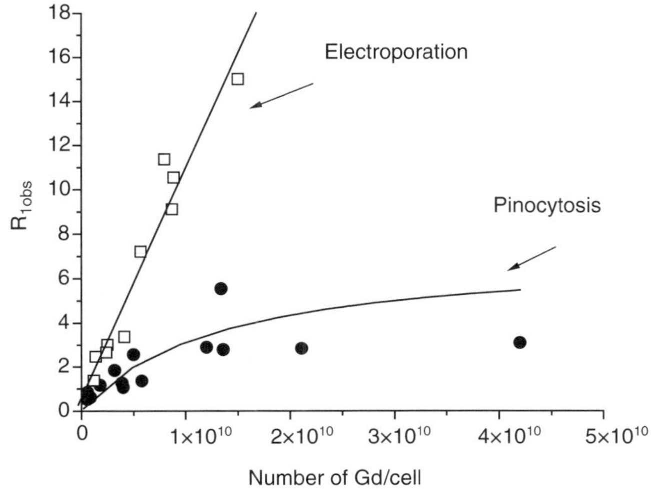

FIGURE 4.9 Longitudinal relaxation rate ($1/T_1$) measured at 20 MHz and 25°C of cell pellets labeled with Gd–HPDO3A by pinocytosis or by electroporation.

4.6.2 Intracellular Distribution of the Imaging Probe

When the imaging probe is internalized into the cell, its effect may depend upon its location. To improve our insight into this issue, we have compared the relaxation enhancement measured for Gd–HPDO3A internalized in HTC (post-hepatocarcinoma cell line) by pynocytosis and by electroporation, respectively, [84]. Whereas the former route causes the entrapment of the contrast agent into endosomic vesicles, the latter one leads to its dispersion into the cytoplasm. Electroporation consists of the formation of transient hydrophilic pores on the cell membrane upon the application of suitable electric pulses between the two electrodes placed in the cell suspension [85]. As shown in Figure 4.9, the relaxation rate of the cells labeled by pynocytosis shows a saturation effect upon increasing the amount of the internalized Gd–HPDO3A with limiting R_1 values of approximately 3 s^{-1}. Conversely, the R_1 values for the cellular pellets labeled by electroporation are markedly higher, and even more importantly, they are linearly dependent upon the amount of the internalized complex. A cellular pellet (and a portion of tissue as well) can be considered as a multisite system where the water molecules are distributed in the extra- and in the intracellular (or cytosolic) compartments. Such compartments are separated by the cellular membrane, whose water permeability is crucial for determining the relaxometric behavior of the whole pellet. The behavior observed in Figure 4.9 may be explained in terms of a three-site water exchange model when the imaging probe is entrapped into endosomes (extracellular/cytoplasm/endosome compartments) and in terms of a two-site exchange model when the paramagnetic agent is only dispersed into the cytoplasm. On this basis, the quenching effect of the exchange on the relaxation rate of cytosolic water protons is the responsible factor for the saturation of the relaxation rate observed at high concentrations of the internalized probe for the HTC pellets labeled by pynocytosis. The results obtained note the importance of the procedure used for labeling cells and demonstrate that the cytosol confinement of the probe yields higher relaxing efficiency, in turn allowing the MRI detection of a smaller number of cells with respect to the entrapment into endosomes.

4.7 FUTURE PERSPECTIVES

Although a number of interesting results have been already achieved with the available classes of contrast agents, it is expected that the development of novel imaging probes will bring a further improvement in the use of the MRI modality in the field of molecular imaging applications. For instance, as far as the cellular labeling is concerned, the use of chemical exchange saturation transfer (CEST) agents might allow the tracking of more than one ensemble of labeled cells in the same animal [86]. This experiment is precluded to the currently available contrast agent based on Gd(III) or on iron oxide particles and would bring the *in vivo* MRI technique closer to the *in vitro* hystochemical procedures used in cellular biology laboratories. In fact, CEST agents are systems that respond only if the proper frequency (that is specific for each agent) is irradiated. A CEST agent is a chemical containing one or more pools of exchangable protons that, upon proper irradiation, transfer saturated magnetization to the water signal [87]. Therefore, they act as negative agents but their action is detected at will only when the irradiation frequency is set at the absorption frequency of the exchangable protons.

Likely, relevant advances may also be expected in the field of paramagnetic systems. Whereas most of the work carried out until now relies on the optimization of the determinants of the paramagnetic relaxation processes in terms of classical Solomon–Bloembergen–Morgan theory for isolated paramagnetic centers, interesting insights have been gained to suggest that much higher relaxivities may be attained by tackling new avenues. In this context, it was found that the relaxivity of Gd–HPDO3A could be increased by a factor of approximately 20 when the agent was entrapped in the apoferritin cavity [81]. This finding may be accounted for in terms of: (1) the contribution arising from exchangable protons and water molecules on the inner protein surface that acts as an amplification proton pool upon the interaction with the paramagnetic agent; and (2) the contribution arising from the multiple interactions a single water molecule may have with several Gd–HPDO3A units before escaping the apoferritin cavity. It is possible that analogous relaxation enhancement mechanisms may be found in other compartmentalized systems. Much attention is currently devoted to systems based on Gd–fullerene and its derivatives [88].

In summary, in spite of the low sensitivity intrinsically associated with the use of MR imaging probes, the huge versatility of these tools makes us confident that MRI should keep an important role in the armoury of the modalities available for tackling the challenges of cellular and molecular imaging.

Finally, an impressive improvement of sensitivity has been obtained by the use of hyperpolarized ^{13}C-containing molecules [89]. In theory, enhancement of the NMR signal up to 10^5 is expected for these systems. The hyperpolarization of ^{13}C or other nuclei may be obtained by the irradiation of the electron paramagnetic resonance absorption of a stable organic radical mixed to the substrate of interest, when such a solid state solution is kept at very low temperature (liquid He). An alternative method to hyperpolarized molecules (although not so general) is based on the use of para-hydrogen [90]. The availability of hyperpolarized molecules that have crucial roles in metabolic signaling pathways may be used to elucidate the upsurge of a pathological behavior. Of course, as the ^{13}C-polarization lasts only a few minutes, there is an intrinsic limitation in the types of processes that can be investigated. Nevertheless, it is likely that this approach of spectroscopic imaging with the hyperpolarized molecules might be of outstanding relevance for the future applications of molecular imaging by NMR.

REFERENCES

1. Weissleder, R. and Mahmood, U., Molecular imaging, *Radiology*, 219, 316, 2001.
2. Aime, S. et al., Insights into the use of paramagnetic Gd(III) complexes in MR-molecular imaging investigations, *JMRI*, 16, 394, 2002.
3. Banci, L., Bertini, I., and Luchinat, C., *Nuclear and Electron Relaxation*, VCH, Weinheim, 1991.
4. Hu, T. C. C. et al., Manganese-enhanced MRI of mouse heart during changes in inotropy, *Magn. Res. Med.*, 46, 884, 2001.

5. Pautler, R. G., Mongeau, R., and Jacobs, R. E., In vivo trans-synaptic tract tracing from the murine striatum and amygdala utilizing manganese enhanced MRI (MEMRI), *Magn. Res. Med.*, 50, 33, 2003.
6. Caravan, P. et al., Gadolinium(III) chelates as MRI contrast agents: structure, dynamics, and applications, *Chem. Rev.*, 99, 2293, 1999.
7. Brady, T. J. and Reimer, P., Contrast agents in whole body magnetic resonance: an overview, In *Methods in Biomedical Magnetic Resonance Imaging and Spectroscopy*, Vol. 1, Young, I. R., Ed., John Wiley & Sons, Chichester, chap. 9, 2000.
8. Padhani, A. R., Dynamic contrast-enhanced MRI in clinical oncology: current status and future directions, *JMRI*, 16, 407, 2002.
9. Peters, T. J., *All About Albumin: Biochemistry, Genetics and Medical Applications*, Academic Press, San Diego, CA, 1996.
10. Aime, S. et al., Protein-bound metal chelates, In *The Chemistry of Contrast Agents in Medical Magnetic Resonance Imaging*, Merbach, A. E. and Tóth, E., Eds., John Wiley & Sons, Chichester, chap. 5, 2001.
11. Perreault, P. et al., MR angiography with gadofosveset trisodium for peripheral vascular disease: phase II trial, *Radiology*, 229, 811, 2003.
12. La Noce, A. et al., B22956/1, a new intravascular contrast agent for MRI: first administration to humans—preliminary results, *Acad. Radiol.*, 9, S404, 2002.
13. Aime, S. et al., Towards MRI contrast agents of improved efficacy. NMR relaxometric investigations of the binding interaction to HSA of a novel heptadentate macrocyclic triphosphonate Gd(III) complex, *J. Biol. Inorg. Chem.*, 2, 470, 1997.
14. Aime, S. et al., Lanthanide(III) chelates for NMR biomedical applications, *Chem. Soc. Rev.*, 27, 19, 1998.
15. Tóth, E., Helm, L., and Merbach, A. E., Relaxivity of gadolinium(III) complexes: theory and mechanism, In *The Chemistry of Contrast Agents in Medical Magnetic Resonance Imaging*, Merbach, A. E. and Tóth, E., Eds., John Wiley & Sons, Chichester, chap. 2, 2001.
16. Parker, D. et al., Being excited by lanthanide coordination complexes: aqua species, chirality, excited-state chemistry, and exchange dynamics, *Chem. Rev.*, 102, 1977, 2002.
17. Aime, S. et al., NMR relaxometric, and structural studies of the hydration and exchange dynamics of cationic lanthanide complexes of macrocyclic tetraamide ligands, *J. Am. Chem. Soc.*, 121, 5762, 1999.
18. Aime, S. et al. New insights for pursuing high relaxivity MRI agents from modeling the binding interaction of Gd(III) chelates to HSA, *Chem. Biol. Chem.*, 6, 818, 2005.
19. Dunand, F. A., Borel, A., and Merbach, A. E., How does internal motion influence the relaxation of the water protons in Ln(III)DOTA-like complexes? *J. Am. Chem. Soc.*, 124, 710, 2002.
20. Aime, S. et al., Ternary Gd(III)L-HSA adducts: evidence for the replacement of inner-sphere water molecules by coordinating groups of the protein. Implication for the design of contrast agents for MRI, *J. Biol. Inorg. Chem.*, 5, 488, 2000.
21. Xu, J. et al., Gadolinium(III) 1,2-hydroxypyridonate-based complexes: toward MRI contrast agents of high relaxivity, *Inorg. Chem.*, 43, 5492, 2004.
22. Aime, S. et al., [Gd-AAZTA](−): a new structural entry for an improved generation of MRI contrast agents, *Inorg. Chem.*, 43, 7588, 2004.
23. Muller, R. N. et al., Particulate magnetic contrast agents, In *The Chemistry of Contrast Agents in Medical Magnetic Resonance Imaging*, Merbach, A. E. and Tóth, E., Eds., John Wiley & Sons, Chichester, chap. 10, 2001.
24. Yeh, T. C. et al., *In-vivo* dynamic MRI tracking of rat T-cells labeled with superparamagnetic iron-oxide particles, *Magn. Res. Med.*, 33, 200, 1995.
25. Johnson, W. K. et al., Superparamagnetic iron oxide (SPIO) as an oral contrast agent in gastrointestinal (GI) magnetic resonance imaging (MRI): comparison with state-of-the-art computed tomography (CT), *Magn. Res. Imaging*, 14, 43, 1996.
26. Fleige, G. et al., *In vitro* characterization of two different ultrasmall iron oxide particles for magnetic resonance cell tracking, *Investig. Radiol.*, 37, 482, 2002.
27. Weissleder, R. and Reimer, P., Application of a stable cell culture assay for the functional assessment of novel MR contrast agents, *Eur. Radiol.*, 4, 527, 1997.
28. Bach-Gansmo, T. et al., Superparamagnetic iron oxide for liver imaging. Comparison among three different preparations, *Investig. Radiol.*, 29, 339, 1994.

29. Weissleder, R. et al., Ultrasmall superparamagnetic iron oxide: an intravenous contrast agent for assessing lymph nodes with MR imaging, *Radiology*, 175, 494, 1990.
30. Majumdar, S., Zoghbi, S. S., and Gore, J. C., Ultrasmall superparamagnetic iron oxide: an intravenous contrast agent for assessing lymph nodes with MR imaging, *Investig. Radiol.*, 25, 771, 1990.
31. Colet, J. M. et al., Intravascular and intracellular hepatic relaxivities of superparamagnetic particles: an isolated and perfused organ pharmacokinetics study, *J. Magn. Res.*, 134, 199, 1998.
32. Sieving, P. F., Watson, A. D., and Rocklage, M., A macromolecular Gd(III) complex as pH-responsive relaxometric probe for MRI applications, *Bioconjugate Chem.*, 1, 65, 1990.
33. Uzgiris, E. E. et al., Conformation and structure of polymeric contrast agents for medical imaging, *Biomacromolecules*, 5, 54, 2004.
34. Arano, Y. et al., Conventional and high-yield synthesis of DTPA-conjugated peptides, application of a monoreactive DTPA to DTPA-D-Phe1-octreotide synthesis, *Bioconjugate Chem.*, 8, 442, 1997.
35. Eckelmann, W. C., Karesh, S. M., and Reba, R. C., New compounds: fatty acid and long chain hydrocarbon derivatives containing a strong chelating agent, *J. Pharm. Sci.*, 64, 704, 1975.
36. Bakker, W. H. et al., [^{111}In-DTPA-D-Phe^{1}]-octreotide, a potential radiopharmaceutical for imaging of somatostatin receptor-positive tumors: synthesis, radiolabeling, and in vitro validation, *Life Sci.*, 49, 1583, 1991.
37. Hnatowich, D. J. et al., Radioactive labeling of antibody: a simple and efficient method, *Science*, 220, 613, 1983.
38. Armitage, F. E., Richardson, D. E., and Li, K. C. P., Polymeric contrast agents for magnetic resonance imaging: synthesis, characterization, and preliminary in-vivo evaluation of gadolinium-DTPA conjugated to polysaccharides, *Bioconjugate Chem.*, 1, 365, 1990.
39. Sun, G. et al., Synthesis and evaluation of novel polysaccharide-Gd-DTPA compounds as contrast agent for MRI, *Magn. Magn. Mater.*, 265, 123, 2003.
40. Hines, J. V. et al., Paramagnetic oligonucleotides: contrast agents for magnetic resonance imaging with proton relaxation enhancement effects, *Bioconjugate Chem.*, 10, 155, 1999.
41. Ladd, D. L. et al., Polymeric gadolinium chelate magnetic resonance imaging contrast agents: design, synthesis, and properties, *Bioconjugate Chem.*, 10, 361, 1999.
42. Laurent, S. et al., New bifunctional contrast agents: bisamide derivatives of C-substituted Gd-DTPA, *Eur. J. Inorg. Chem.*, 463, 2004.
43. Leclercq, F. et al., Design, synthesis, and evaluation of gadolinium cationic lipids as tools for biodistribution studies of gene delivery complexes, *Bioconjugate Chem.*, 14, 112, 2003.
44. Arano, Y. et al., Reassessment of diethylenetriaminepentaacetic acid (DTPA) as a chelating agent for indium-111 labeling of polypeptides using a newly synthesized monoreactive DTPA derivative, *J. Med. Chem.*, 39, 3451, 1996.
45. Achilefu, S. et al., A new method for the synthesis of tri-tert-butyl diethylenetriaminepentaacetic acid and its derivatives, *J. Org. Chem.*, 65, 1562, 2000.
46. Brechbiel, M. W. et al., Synthesis of 1-(p-isothiocyanatobezyl)derivatives of DTPA and EDTA. Antibody labeling and tumor-imaging studies, *Inorg. Chem.*, 25, 2772, 1986.
47. Westerberg, D. A. et al., Synthesis of novel bifunctional chelators and their use in preparing monoclonal antibody conjugates for tumor targeting, *J. Med. Chem.*, 32, 236, 1989.
48. Corson, D. T. and Meares, C. F., Efficient multigram synthesis of the bifunctional chelating agent (S)-1-p-isothiocyanatobenzyl-diethylenetetraminepentaacetic acid, *Bioconjugate Chem.*, 11, 292, 2000.
49. Keana, J. F. W. and Mann, J. S., Chelating ligands functionalized for facile attachment to biomolecules. A convenient route to 4-isothiocyanatobenzyl derivatives of diethylenetriaminepentaacetic acid (DTPA) and ethylenediaminetetraacetic acid, *J. Org. Chem.*, 55, 2868, 1990.
50. Deal, K. A. et al., Evaluation of the stability and animal biodistribution of gadolinium(III) benzylamine-derivatized diethylenetriaminepentaacetic acid, *J. Med. Chem.*, 39, 3096, 1996.
51. Brechbiel, M. W. and Gansow, O. A., Backbone-substituted DTPA ligands for yttrium-90 radioimmunotherapy, *Bioconjugate Chem.*, 2, 187, 1991.
52. Lebdušková, P. et al., A gadolinium(III) complex of a carboxylic-phosphorus acid derivative of diethylenetriamine covalently bound to inulin, a potential macromolecular MRI contrast agent, *Bioconjugate Chem.*, 15, 881, 2004.
53. Anelli, P. L. et al., L-Glutamic acid and L-lysine as useful building blocks for the preparation of bifunctional DTPA-like ligands, *Bioconjugate Chem.*, 10, 137, 1999.

54. Anelli, P. L. et al., Conjugates of gadolinium complexes to bile acids as hepatocyte-directed contrast agents for magnetic resonance imaging, *J. Med. Chem.*, 47, 3629, 2004.
55. Accardo, A. et al., Physicochemical properties of mixed micellar aggregates containing CCK peptides and Gd complexes designed as tumor specific contrast agents in MRI, *J. Am. Chem. Soc.*, 126, 3097, 2004.
56. DeLeón, L. M. et al., Solid phase synthesis of DOTA-peptides, *Chem. Eur. J.*, 10, 1149, 2004.
57. DeLeón, L. M. et al., Magnetic resonance imaging detects a specific peptide–protein binding event, *J. Am. Chem. Soc.*, 124, 3514, 2002.
58. Lu, Z.-R. et al., Poly(L-glutamic acid) Gd(III)-DOTA conjugate with a degradable spacer for magnetic resonance imaging, *Bioconjugate Chem.*, 14, 715, 2003.
59. Mier, W. et al., Synthesis of peptide conjugated chelator oligomers for endoradiotherapy and MRT, *Tetrahedron Lett.*, 45, 5453, 2004.
60. Anelli, P. L. et al., DOTA tris(phenylmethyl) ester: a new useful synthon for the synthesis of DOTA monoamides containing acid-labile bonds, *Bioconjugate Chem.*, 12, 1081, 2001.
61. Aime, S. et al., A macromolecular Gd(III) complex as pH-responsive relaxometric probe for MRI applications, *Chem. Commun.*, 1577, 16, 1999.
62. Corsi, D. M. et al., Inulin as a carrier for contrast agents in magnetic resonance imaging, *Chem. Eur. J.*, 1, 64, 2001.
63. Mishra, A. K. et al., A convenient, novel approach for the synthesis of polyaza macrocyclic bifunctional chelating agents, *Tetrahedron Lett.*, 37, 7515, 1996.
64. McMurry, T. J. et al., Convenient synthesis of bifunctional tetraaza macrocycles, *Bioconjugate Chem.*, 3, 108, 1992.
65. Chappell, L. L. et al., Improved synthesis of the bifunctional chelating agent 1,4,7,10-tetraaza-N-(1-carboxy-3-(4-nitrophenyl)propyl)-N′,N″,N‴-tri s(acetic acid)cyclododecane (PA-DOTA), *Bioorg. Med. Chem.*, 7, 2313, 1999.
66. Whetstone, P. A. et al., Element-coded affinity tags for peptides and proteins, *Bioconjugate Chem.*, 15, 3, 2004.
67. Li, L. et al., Vinyl sulfone bifunctional derivatives of DOTA allow sulfhydryl- or amino-directed coupling to antibodies. Conjugates retain immunoreactivity and have similar biodistributions, *Bioconjugate Chem.*, 13, 110, 2002.
68. Broan, C. J. et al., Synthesis of new macrocyclic aminophosphinic acid complexing agents and their C-and P-functionalized derivatives for protein linkage, *Synthesis*, 63, 1992.
69. Meyer, D. et al., Paramagnetic dextrans as magnetic-resonance contrast agents, *Investig. Radiol.*, 26, S50, 1991.
70. Bryant, L. H. et al., Synthesis and relaxometry of high-generation ($G = 5$, 7, 9, and 10) PAMAM dendrimer-DOTA-gadolinium chelates, *J. Magn. Res. Imaging*, 9, 348, 1999.
71. Wiener, E. C. et al., Dendrimer-based metal-chelates—a new class of magnetic-resonance-imaging contrast agents, *Magn. Res. Med.*, 31, 1, 1994.
72. Winter, P. M. et al., Molecular imaging of angiogenesis in nascent vx-2 rabbit tumors using a novel alpha(v)beta(3)-targeted nanoparticle and 1.5 tesla magnetic resonance imaging, *Cancer Res.*, 63, 5838, 2003.
73. Morawski, A. M. et al., Targeted nanoparticles for quantitative imaging of sparse molecular epitopes with MRI, *Magn. Res. Med.*, 51, 480, 2004.
74. Sipkins, D. A. et al., Detection of tumor angiogenesis in vivo by alpha(v)beta(3)-targeted magnetic resonance imaging, *Nat. Med.*, 4, 623, 1998.
75. Artemov, D. et al., Magnetic resonance molecular imaging of the HER-2/neu receptor, *Cancer Res.*, 63, 2723, 2003.
76. Kobayashi, H. and Brechbiel, M. W., Dendrimer-based macromolecular MRI contrast agents: characteristics and application, *Mol. Imaging*, 2, 1, 2003.
77. Geninatti Crich, S. et al., MRI visualization of targeted cells by the internalization of supramolecular adducts formed between Avidin and Biotinylated Gd^{3+} chelates, *J. Biol. Inorg. Chem.*, 10, 78, 2005.
78. Geninatti Crich, S. et al., Improved route for the visualization of stem cells labeled with a Gd-/Eu-chelate as dual (MRI and fluorescence) agent, *Magn. Res. Med.*, 51, 938, 2004.
79. Arbab, A. S. et al., Efficient magnetic cell labeling with protamine sulfate complexed to ferumoxides for cellular MRI, *Blood*, 104, 1217, 2004.

80. Aime, S., Frullano, L., and Geninatti Crich, S., Compartmentalization of a gadolinium complex in the apoferritin cavity: a route to obtain high relaxivity contrast agents for magnetic resonance imaging, *Angew. Chemie Int. Ed.*, 41, 1017, 2002.
81. Pascolo, L. et al., Molecular mechanisms for the hepatic uptake of magnetic resonance imaging contrast agents, *Biochem. Biophys. Res. Commun.*, 257, 746, 1999.
82. Heckl, S. et al., Intracellular visualization of prostate cancer using magnetic resonance imaging, *Cancer Res.*, 63, 4766, 2003.
83. Ahrens, E. T. et al., A model for MRI contrast enhancement using T-1 agents, *Proc. Natl. Acad. Sci. USA*, 95, 8443, 1998.
84. Terreno, E. et al., Effect of the intracellular localization of a Gd-based imaging probe on the relaxation enhancement of water protons, *Magn. Res. Med.*, DOI: 10.1002/mrm.20793.
85. Neumann, E., Kakorin, S., and Toensing, K., Fundamentals of electroporative delivery of drugs and genes, *Bioelectrochem. Bioenerg.*, 48, 3, 1999.
86. Aime, S. et al., Light-on/light-off of cells labeled with MRI-PARACEST agents, *Angew. Chemie Int. Ed.*, 44, 1813, 2005.
87. Ward, K. M., Aletras, A. H., and Balaban, R. S., A new class of contrast agents for MRI based on proton chemical exchange dependent saturation transfer (CEST), *J. Magn. Res.*, 143, 79, 2000.
88. Okumura, M. et al., Evaluation of water-soluble metallofullerenes as MRI contrast agents, *Acad. Radiol.*, 9, S495, 2002.
89. Golman, K. et al., Molecular imaging with endogenous substances, *Proc. Natl. Acad. Sci. USA*, 100, 10435, 2003.
90. Golman, K. et al., Parahydrogen-induced polarization in imaging: subsecond C-13 angiography, *Magn. Res. Med.*, 46, 1, 2001.

Editorial Comments

Genetically engineered mice are routinely used in pharmaceutical research, for target validation, as disease models, and in toxicological studies. Since mice and humans are similar at the genetic level so that most pathways are likely to be conserved between them, it is often possible to measure similar disease parameters in both species. Importantly, genetic alterations in the mouse often result in functional changes through which relevant pharmacological effects in man can be predicted.

Phenotyping transgenic mice in a noninvasive manner is a very important task for MR techniques. When performing such work, the main issue to be considered is throughput. In Chapter 5, Josette Chen and Mark Henkelman discuss ways by which the throughput of MRI for mice imaging can be increased. They address in particular technical requirements for imaging multiple animals simultaneously, an undertaking of considerable complexity from the perspectives of data acquisition and analysis. The ability to automatically assess volumes of organs or of certain organ regions from whole body images acquired at high throughput, although not yet feasible in a routine manner, would be highly desirable. However, one needs to keep in mind that the concept of high throughput imaging may become somewhat challenged when dealing with functional assessments needing special animal preparation, as shown in Chapter 6.

As a consequence of the improvements in mouse imaging, more and more *in vivo* pharmacological studies are going to be performed in this species. This will certainly be appreciated by chemists, since lower amounts of compounds are needed compared to rat studies.

5 Rapid Phenotyping of Mice with MRI

X. Josette Chen and R. Mark Henkelman

CONTENTS

5.1 INTRODUCTION

The mouse was the first live animal to be imaged using magnetic resonance imaging (MRI) [1], but it has not been utilized extensively in small animal imaging experiments. Historically, rats and guinea pigs have been better studied due to their larger size. This allows for easier manipulation and more signal available for imaging. However, because both the draft sequences of the human and mouse genome have been completed in the last few years, the field of mouse MRI is rapidly expanding as biologists need new tools to both discover models of human disease and to test responses to different drug therapies administered to large numbers of mice.

The assessment of reactions to different drug regimes, especially in preclinical trials, has to be quick and decisive. Upon administration of a new drug, a mouse is characterized by looking for changes in anatomy, physiology, behavior and function. Many of these tests can be undertaken *in vivo*, but the final step is to perform histopathology to look for organ and biochemical abnormalities — a slow and laborious step. Furthermore, given the large numbers of mice studied, it is difficult for mouse pathologists to characterize each mouse in depth. By adapting the techniques and tools of MRI, which is inherently noninvasive, we are able to take detailed images of the inside of a mouse without conventional slicing and dicing. This way, anatomical, physiological and functional measurements can be made in the same living mouse.

As researchers have become aware of the power of MRI, the methods for imaging have become more sophisticated. Early approaches used fairly simple MRI techniques in conjunction with other phenotyping tests [2–4]. More recently, MRI physicists have started to develop methodologies to enhance mouse phenotyping through hardware enhancements [5–7] and physiological assays [8–11].

In this chapter, we will discuss how the methods of MRI have to change to phenotype mice; what sort of animal handling is required for *in vivo* imaging; what special considerations are required for focusing on different organ systems; and address *post mortem* imaging. Finally, image analysis tools are described with the concept of a digital atlas introduced as an automated tool to look for anatomic variants.

Typically, easy entry into this field is gained by using available clinical scanners and associated hardware and software. However, this chapter will focus primarily on using higher field magnets, specifically 7 T, for higher resolution studies. The descriptions about animal handling and imaging applications are independent of the magnet choice except where noted.

5.2 HOW MRI CHANGES FOR MOUSE PHENOTYPING

5.2.1 HARDWARE

MRI uses a static magnet field, nonionizing radio frequency (RF) pulses and magnetic gradients to give exquisite images of soft tissues. In the clinic, MRI is essential in both research and routine diagnosis. Evidence of Alzheimer's disease, multiple sclerosis, strokes and tumors can all be detected with MRI. To scale the technology down to small animals — mice ranging in size from 25 to 40 g — requires a number of changes. Since there is less signal in mice, higher magnetic field strengths are better suited as useful signal scales with field strength; 7, 9.4, and 11.7 T are usual field strengths as compared to 1.5 or 3 T for clinical systems. For comparison, the earth's magnetic field is only 0.5×10^{-4} T. Correspondingly, the RF power and frequency also increases as do the gradient field strengths to obtain higher resolutions. The net result is the ability to image under a hundred microns (μm) instead of the usual millimeters on clinical scanners.

In general, two types of RF coils are used: volume and surface coils. Volume coils (either solenoid or birdcage coils) are used to excite and receive signal evenly over a large volume. Solenoid coils are perpendicular to the main magnetic field and are typically used for imaging specimens. In contrast, birdcage coils are coaxial with the magnetic field, which makes them suited for *in vivo* studies in horizontally oriented magnets. Surface coils are more sensitive and excite a more localized area but usually with a nonuniform profile. Hence, they are useful for tumor studies that are close to the surface of the body.

5.2.2 PULSE SEQUENCES

A pulse sequence is a series of user-controllable commands that drives the gradients and the RF to obtain images. Different pulse sequences can exploit varying contrast mechanisms highlighting different anatomy [12]. For high fields, pulse sequences typically used are T_2-weighted or

T_1-weighted with a contrast agent. The major drawbacks of imaging at high fields are that the T_1s (spin–lattice relaxation times) of tissues increase and converge to the same value. This results in increased imaging times (unless a contrast agent is used) and lack of tissue contrast using T_1-weighted imaging. So if no contrast agent is employed, researchers typically use T_2-weighted imaging or fast-spin echo techniques. Another problem at high fields is susceptibility, which makes gradient-echo techniques and fast imaging techniques like spiral trajectories difficult to use. The key thing to keep in mind when performing a phenotyping project is to maintain not only the same type of imaging sequence but also parameters from subject to subject for consistency.

Another factor that also results in increased imaging time is that phenotyping usually requires full 3D images, as opposed to multiple 2D slices. Most importantly, it is only with isotropic 3D imaging that true volumes of structures can be measured. Isotropy also leads to the ability to digitally slice and dice in any direction, even at oblique angles. Finally, 3D images allow the viewer to see the relationship of organ systems in real 3D space.

5.2.3 Increasing Throughput

When performing biological research, the ability to find conclusive results requires studying multiple subjects — sometimes on the order of dozens — to improve the statistics of the experiment and account for biological variation. In the context of analyzing genetically manipulated mice, if no previous information on the possible outcome of a given genetic modification is available, as for example in random mutation, having information on the whole body is mandatory. In this case, using MRI as a phenotyping tool becomes problematic since acquisition times for imaging the whole body of one mouse can be on the order of hours. If previous information is available concerning the organ of target primarily affected by a given genetic manipulation, the complexity of the task is reduced by concentrating efforts to image that organ.

For whole body phenotyping, a number of groups have begun to investigate various methods to image multiple mice, thereby increasing throughput [5,13–15]. In general, there are two sorts of multiple mouse imaging methods, each with its costs and benefits. The easier method involves placing several mice into clinical RF coils and using a clinical scanner. However, because the majority of clinical scanners are low field (1.5 and 3 T), the image resolution will be poorer than at high field. In addition, because the coil is so much bigger than the mouse, the so-called filling factor is low, leading to even lower signal-to-noise ratio (SNR). The more difficult method uses separate RF coils for each mouse in the same magnet. While the implementation is more difficult, there is no loss of sensitivity compared to single mouse imaging. The theories behind these methods are fully discussed in Ref. [5].

Imaging four mice at a time in a cancer screen has been accomplished in our laboratory [16]. Prototypical four-mouse imaging systems are now commercially available (Varian NMR, Palo Alto, CA, U.S.A.). We have more recently increased our throughput to seven live mice and 16 fixed mice. At the time of writing, live multiple mouse imaging is limited to seven animals due to the lack of monitoring channels and independent receivers. By solving these engineering problems, there should no problem extending the numbers to 19 at a time. The limitation in going to numbers beyond this is with animal preparation. As discussed below, we have devised several shortcuts to speed up animal preparation, but an experiment is ultimately limited to how long the first mouse is under anesthesia while the rest are being prepared.

5.3 ANIMAL PREPARATION FOR *IN VIVO* IMAGING

One of the advantages of MRI is the ability to image living animals, which allows for longitudinal studies in the same subject. In other words, instead of performing histology on different mice at different time points, progress of disease or tumor in the same animal can be followed over time.

The survival of the animal is especially important when studying valuable mutants that can be one of a kind, as well as being expensive and difficult to produce.

5.3.1 Anesthesia and Monitoring

To perform *in vivo* imaging requires maintaining and monitoring the physiology of the mouse during imaging sessions. Anesthesia affords more control over the subject and a recent review discusses usage of different anesthetics for MRI [17]. Injection anesthetics (e.g., ketamine/xylazine, avertin) are commonly used in animal studies. However, the length of time a mouse stays under anesthesia can be variable with the possibility of the animal waking up during the scanning session. Alternatively, it is possible to maintain a catheter in the tail vein during the imaging session but this adds significant complication. In general, inhalation anesthetics, such as isoflurane and halothane, are employed as they are easy to control and are fairly gentle to the animal. Anesthetic induction of the mouse is typically done at 3 to 4% with maintenance at $\leq 1\%$ isoflurane in 100% oxygen. After induction, mice are intraperitoneally injected with saline to prevent dehydration. Because anesthesia causes the animal's temperature to drop, a heating system is necessary. In fact, Qiu et al. have demonstrated that image quality improves with tighter temperature control [18], although a few degrees of control is generally sufficient. Heating is usually done with forced, heated air or circulating water baths with feedback control. A water bath is usually not desirable as it is needs to be in close proximity to the mouse, thus necessitating a larger volume coil. This reduces the filling factor and hence the SNR. If a small, localized surface coil is used then a water bath need have no impact on SNR.

Monitoring of the physiologic state can involve any or all of the following: electrocardiograph (ECG), temperature, ventilation, exhaled CO_2, and blood pressure. However, the more interfaces with the mouse requires more preparation time. In general, the first two measurements are usually sufficient to observe the status of the mouse. Since the monitoring of the mouse will be taking place inside a magnetic field, all connections need to be nonmagnetic. Furthermore, to prevent interference from the gradients, either fiberoptic connections [19] or analog filters are necessary.

ECG connections can be made with copper tape, ECG pads, or silver needle electrodes. If using tape or pads, hair from the contact points (chest or limbs) must be removed. Applying ECG gel helps improve electrical contact. Internal temperature of the mouse can be monitored with a rectal probe.

Beyond simple monitoring of the mouse, some experiments require gating on either or both of the cardiac and respiratory signals. Usually with the ECG connections arranged across the mouse's chest, the respiratory signal can be seen superimposed with the cardiac signal (see also Chapter 16, Section 16.2). The two signals can be separated electronically but for a cleaner signal, a respiratory bellows system should be used to measure the breathing separately. In the future, MRI-based monitoring of heart and breathing motions will be developed for multiple mice. Current prospective techniques [20,21] cannot be done with multiple mice; hence our laboratory is developing retrospective gating techniques.

While most of the monitoring equipment can be developed in house with basic electronics equipment, commercial packages are available. Two of the most popular vendors that provide MR-compatible animal monitoring equipment are SA Instruments (Stony Brook, NY, U.S.A.) and Rapid Biomedical (Wuerzburg, Germany).

5.3.2 Considerations for Multiple Mice

Animal handling is exacerbated when dealing with multiple mice. Since it is important to minimize the time the mouse is under anesthesia — sometimes up to 3 h for whole-body imaging — every attempt should be made to streamline the process of preparing the individual mice. This ensures that the mouse prepared first is not under anesthesia for too long as the other mice are being prepared.

In our laboratory, we have devised several shortcuts to reduce preparation of seven mice to less than half an hour [22]. The MRI we use is a 7 T, 40 cm clear bore magnet (Magnex, Oxford, U.K.) driven by a UnityINOVA console (Varian, Palo Alto, CA, U.S.A.) with four parallel receivers. The steps can be broken down into three categories described below.

5.3.2.1 The Mouse Loading System

The mouse loading system consists of two major parts: the "mouse hive" and the "loading array" (Figure 5.1). The mouse hive's main function is to position up to 19 Millipede RF coils [7] in a hexagonal array inside the magnet bore. The loading array is designed to hold and transport multiple mice housed in 50-mL centrifuge tubes with holes drilled through their tips to allow entry of anesthetic gas. After the mice are anesthetized in an induction chamber in the vicinity of the magnet, they are inserted into the modified centrifuge tubes and mounted on to the loading array. After mounting all mice, the loading array is transported and inserted into the magnet where it is positioned on a rail system, which allows the array to couple with the mouse hive when pushed down bore of the magnet.

When fully inserted into the magnet, the centrifuge tubes dock on to the anesthetic delivery system within the RF coils (Figure 5.2). Isoflurane mixed with oxygen is supplied from the mouse hive end to the animal through a tube along the axis of each individual coil. The anesthetic gas mixture flows into the tubes, past the mice, and is collected by a passive scavenging unit attached to the back of the loading array.

5.3.2.2 The Induction Chamber

The custom induction chamber creates a single environment for both induction and handling of multiple mice (Figure 5.3). Constructed from clear acrylic, the induction chamber features self-closing silicone iris ports to minimize anesthetic leakage and allows the user to access the internal environment without the need for special gloves. Compared to conventional mask and circuits for a single mouse, the induction chamber is large enough to house up to 20 mice and allows for free manipulation of the mice without the attachment of cumbersome tubes and masks. The unit is supplied with a constant flow of anesthetic gas which is collected using a passive scavenging system. Resistive heating elements are used to heat the floor of the chamber to maintain the animals' body temperature during preparation. Instead of custom building an induction chamber, a commercially available glove box can be modified to suit these purposes.

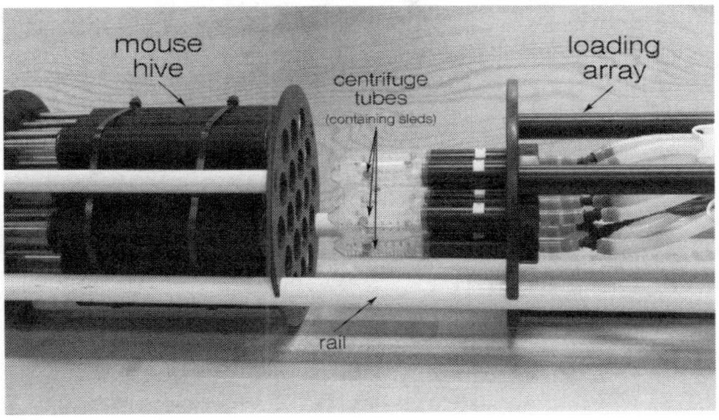

FIGURE 5.1 The mouse loading system. The loading array and mouse hive are connected with a common fiberglass rail system. (From Dazai, J. et al., *Magn. Reson. Med.*, 52, 709, 2004. Courtesy of Jun Dazai. With permission of Wiley-Liss, Inc. Copyright 2004.)

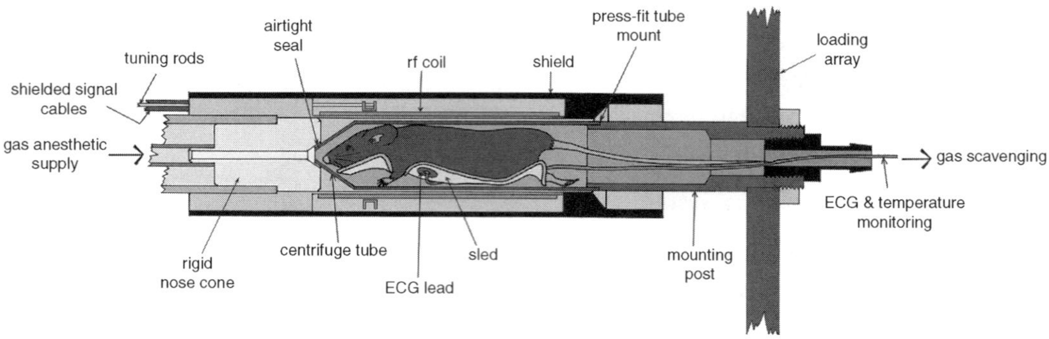

FIGURE 5.2 Cross-sectional diagram illustrating the integration between the loading array and mouse hive. (From Dazai, J. et al., *Magn. Reson. Med.*, 52, 709, 2004. Courtesy of Jun Dazai. With permission of Wiley-Liss, Inc. Copyright 2004.)

5.3.2.3 The Sled

One of the most awkward and time-consuming aspects of preparing mice for the MRI is the application of ECG electrodes and rectal temperature probes. In addition, many of the conventional electrodes, such as cuff and needle electrodes can distort the animal's posture making it difficult to standardize positioning. Therefore, we devised a custom form-fitted positioning platform with embedded ECG and temperature probes called the sled (Figure 5.4) (U.S. Proposal patent serial #60/485, 727).

The sled was constructed by generating a precise physiological plaster facsimile of a representative specimen in a favorable position. Polypropylene sheets were then vacuum-formed and cut around the plaster facsimile to create thin, lightweight, autoclavable sleds. Nonmagnetic neonatal/pediatric ECG electrodes were embedded into the sled to contact the chest, and a thermocouple was mounted in a similar fashion to measure skin temperature at the abdomen. A nonmagnetic electrical connector mounted on each sled allows for easy sensor connection to the loading system. Motion restraints made from Velcro® fasteners were used to limit movement of the head.

After removing the hair from a mouse's chest, the mouse is positioned on a sled (Figure 5.4b) and loaded into a modified 50-mL centrifuge tube. The sleds are electrically connected to the monitoring system. Once the mice are all loaded, the loading array can be docked into the RF coils within the magnet bore.

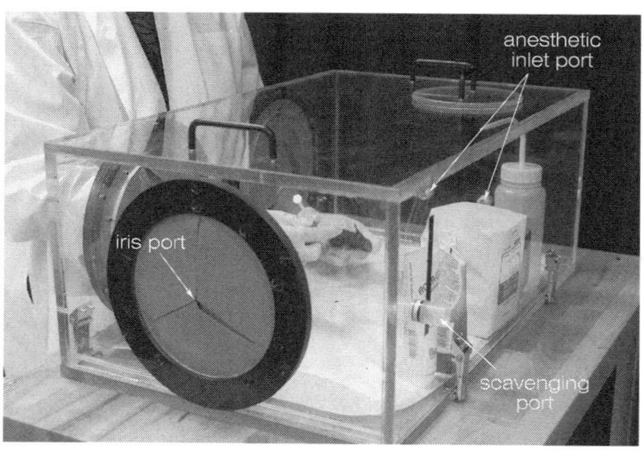

FIGURE 5.3 The induction chamber. (From Dazai, J. et al., *Magn. Reson. Med.*, 52, 709, 2004. Courtesy of Jun Dazai. With permission of Wiley-Liss, Inc. Copyright 2004.)

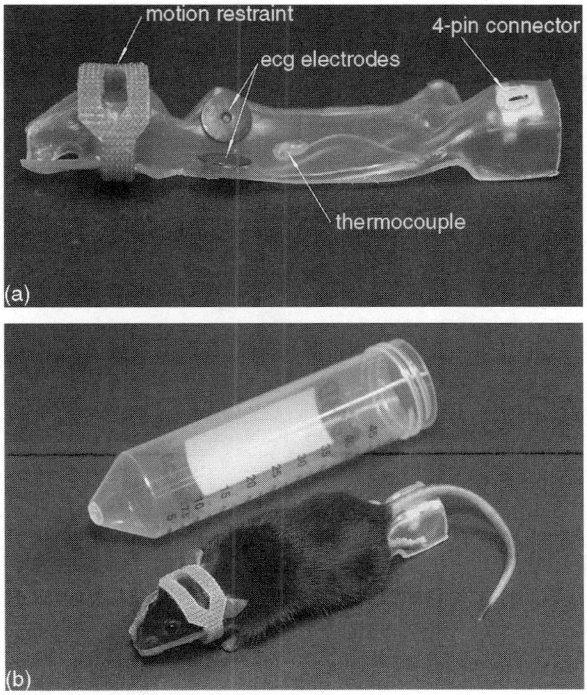

FIGURE 5.4 (a) The sled, showing embedded monitoring sensors and head restraint. (b) An anesthetized mouse on a sled with the head restraint attached. The sled assembly easily slides into the centrifuge tube. (From Dazai, J. et al., *Magn. Reson. Med.*, 52, 709, 2004. Courtesy of Jun Dazai and Lori Davidson. With permission of Wiley-Liss, Inc. Copyright 2004.)

An added benefit in using the sled is that the position of the animal is standardized, making it easier for comparisons of animals either by observer or with post-processing algorithms. An example of multiple mice imaging is provided in Figure 5.5, which shows seven mice imaged simultaneously and arranged in the same configuration as in the mouse loading array. The full 3D data set is volume rendered and a cutaway shows a single slice from the brain.

5.4 IMAGING SPECIFIC ORGANS

As pointed out earlier, in many phenotyping experiments the anatomical region of interest is known so imaging can focus to that area. Currently, major developments have been for the brain and heart, though other organ systems are studied as well.

5.4.1 Brain

When the mouse is anesthetized, the head still moves, especially with inhalation anesthetics. Typically, most groups employ stereotaxic holders to fix the head position in place [10,23,24]. This type of approach is best when using surface coils or sufficiently large volume coils. Since we use birdcage coils that optimize filling factor, more form-fitting head restraints are utilized (Figure 5.4b). Figure 5.6 displays high resolution images from the brain of a live mouse obtained using our approach for restraining movements.

Successful use of MRI to help phenotype mouse models of human disease include Alzheimer's disease [25], Canavan's disease [26], megencephaly [27], hydrocephalous [28,29], as well as other

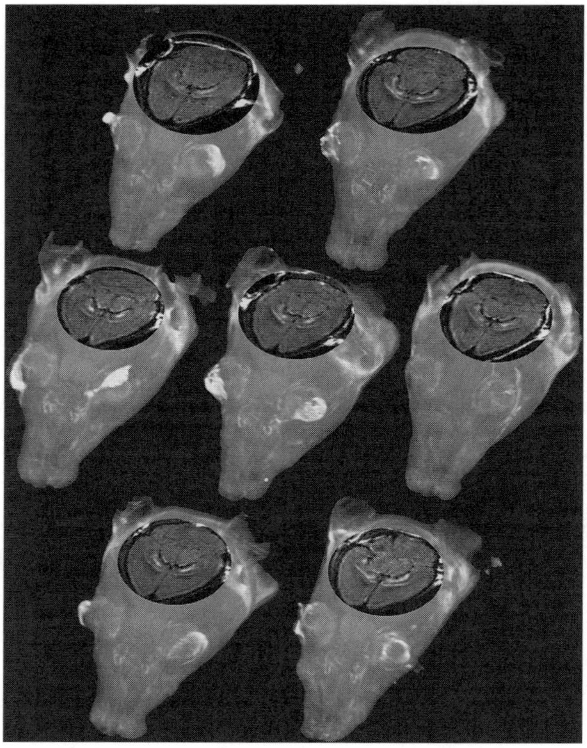

FIGURE 5.5 Seven live mice imaged simultaneously. The full 3D data is volume rendered with a horizontal slice shown in the cut-away. These mice were injected with $MnCl_2$ 48 h prior to imaging [11]. Spin echo sequence with $TR = 300$ ms, $TE = 7.7$ ms, $NEX = 2$, $FOV = 20 \times 20 \times 40$ mm, and matrix $= 128 \times 128 \times 256$, resulting in a pixel size of 156 μm^3 and imaging time of 2.75 h. (Courtesy of Nicholas A. Bock.)

CNS mutations [30,31]. Recently, mouse brain phenotyping has also been used to follow the growth of brain tumors [16,32–36]. Any study that involves following a growth progression requires careful attention to be paid to ensure reproducibility of position and imaging parameters in all scans.

5.4.2 Heart

Since the mouse heart rate is between 300 and 500 beats per minute, accounting for motion is a necessity to prevent artifacts in the images. Recently, several groups have investigated various gating strategies — where the ECG signal from the mouse is used to trigger the MRI acquisition — and imaging paradigms [20,37–39]. Cardiac imaging in small rodents is described in more detail in Chapter 16.

5.4.3 Other Organs

Organs that are in the vicinity of the thorax typically require respiratory gating. Respiration produces motion around the diaphragm in the superior-inferior direction. For example, studies of the liver require respiratory gating [39,40] whereas kidney and hindlimb studies only need securing of the region of interest with tape [41–43].

As mentioned in above, a consequence of imaging at high fields means that relaxation times (T_1) can be on the order of seconds. By lowering these times with a contrast agent, scans can be

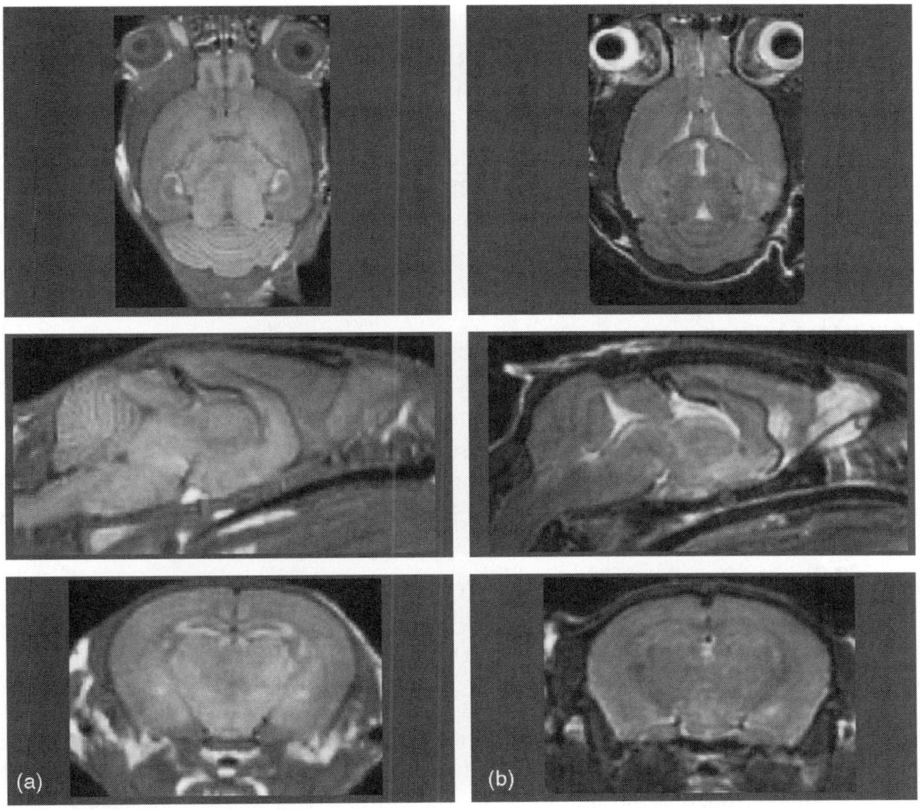

FIGURE 5.6 Two examples of different contrast weighting in the brains of two different live mice. Three orthogonal views are shown for each mouse. (a) 48 h after i.p. injection of $MnCl_2$, spin echo sequence with TR = 300 ms, TE = 7.7 ms, NEX = 2, FOV = 20 × 20 × 40 mm, matrix = 128 × 128 × 256 for resolution of 156 μm^3 and imaging time of 2.75 h. (b) T_2-weighting with a fast spin echo sequence and 40° flip angle, TR = 900 ms, 8 echoes, effective TE = 36 ms (single echo TE = 12 ms), NEX = 2, FOV = 24 × 24 × 40 mm, matrix = 208 × 208 × 384 for a resolution of 115 × 115 × 104 μm and imaging time of 2.7 h. (Courtesy of Brian Nieman and Nir Lifshitz.)

accomplished in a shorter amount of time. The most popular form of contrast agent is a chelated gadolinium compound, such as gadopentetate dimeglumine. To lower the T_1s across almost all tissues, an i.p. injection of contrast agent is given 20 min prior to imaging. For brain imaging, a contrast agent that crosses the blood-brain barrier is necessary; typically $MnCl_2$ is used as the Mn^{2+} behaves as a Ca^{2+} analogue.

5.4.4 Whole Body Imaging

The ultimate goal in phenotyping with MRI is to image the whole body of a mouse. Since gene expression and the effects of treatments can occur in a number of organ systems, imaging the entire mouse is highly desirable. Recently, Fink et al. have performed whole-body magnetic resonance angiography at 1.5 T [44], but to our knowledge no-one has yet demonstrated anatomical whole-body live imaging. Current work in our laboratory indicates that for high resolutions, a fast spin echo is required along with motion compensation.

5.5 POST MORTEM IMAGING

Without a doubt, *in vivo* imaging is an extremely useful aspect of MRI. However, MR images can approach microscopic resolutions when obtained *post mortem*. This is because animal motion and imaging time are no longer issues. Since the scan times can approach tens of hours, it is necessary to fix the mice as some tissue degradation occurs during the first few hours after death. Despite such long imaging times, acquiring a 3D data set is still much shorter than conventional histology, which is very labor intensive. The 3D aspect of the data also allows the researcher to study the organ from any angle; this is impossible with histology.

5.5.1 Excised Organs

To image individual organs like the brain, kidneys, and liver, the mouse is first fixed by conventional perfusion, which involves a midline incision followed by a left ventricular puncture and drainage through the right atrium. A contrast agent can be mixed with the fixative solution to reduce the imaging time. The organ of interest is then excised, immersed in a proton-free, susceptibility matching fluid (e.g., Flourinert, 3M Canada, London, Canada) and imaged. The benefit of excision is to use smaller RF coils, which give better sensitivity. Figure 5.7 shows examples of MR images of fixed spine and heart.

5.5.2 Whole Body Perfusion

Recently, there has been interest in preserving and imaging the entire mouse for phenotyping purposes [9,45]. The usual procedure to perfuse and fix the entire mouse is the same as for excised organs. However, the opening of the chest disturbs the integrity of the thoracic and abdominal cavity. To circumvent opening up the body, Johnson et al. use a multiple perfusion method that fixes all the organ systems with cannulations and drainages through various points in the body [9,45]. Alternatively, we have used an ultrasound-guided ventricular puncture and fixed the mouse via the beating heart [46], as described below.

Mice are anesthetized using a mixture of ketamine/xylazine. When adequately anesthetized, the mouse is secured with tape in the supine position in a custom-built mold designed to maintain the mouse's natural body shape after fixation (Figure 5.8). The hair on the chest wall is removed with a chemical depilatory hair remover (Nair, Church and Dwight Co., Princeton, NJ, U.S.A.). Ultrasound gel is spread over the precordial region and the ultrasound biomicroscope with a 30-MHz transducer is used to visualize the left ventricle (Figure 5.9a). When the cross-section with the largest left ventricular chamber dimension is located, an i.v. catheter with needle is placed at the precordial area on the chest wall, with the longitudinal axis of the needle in the ultrasound imaging plane (Figure 5.9b). Under real-time image guidance, the needle is inserted into the left ventricle (Figure 5.9c). The needle is then removed, and the catheter secured in place by tape (Figure 5.9d) and connected to a peristaltic pump via a plastic tube.

A mixture of saline, heparin and 10 m*M* gadopentetate dimeglumine (Magnevist®) is then infused at a flow rate of 0.125 ml/min. This slow infusion with high concentration of the contrast agent is performed for about 5 min, to avoid rapid build-up of blood volume that could cause heart failure, and to ensure that the whole mouse is thoroughly perfused with contrast agent while the heart is beating. The jugular and femoral veins are cut to drain the blood and perfusate, and the mouse is flushed with a mixture of saline, heparin, Magnevist (1 m*M*) and blue dye (to monitor the progress of the perfusion) at a flow rate of 1.25 mL/min. Typically the heart stops beating after 2 to 3 min with this faster perfusion procedure. When the draining fluid runs clear blue, a mixture of 10% buffered formalin phosphate, Magnevist (1 m*M*), and blue dye is pumped through at a flow rate of 1.25 ml/min for approximately 15 min to fix the whole mouse. The perfusion and fixation procedure from puncturing the left ventricle to the end of fixation takes less than 30 min. During the

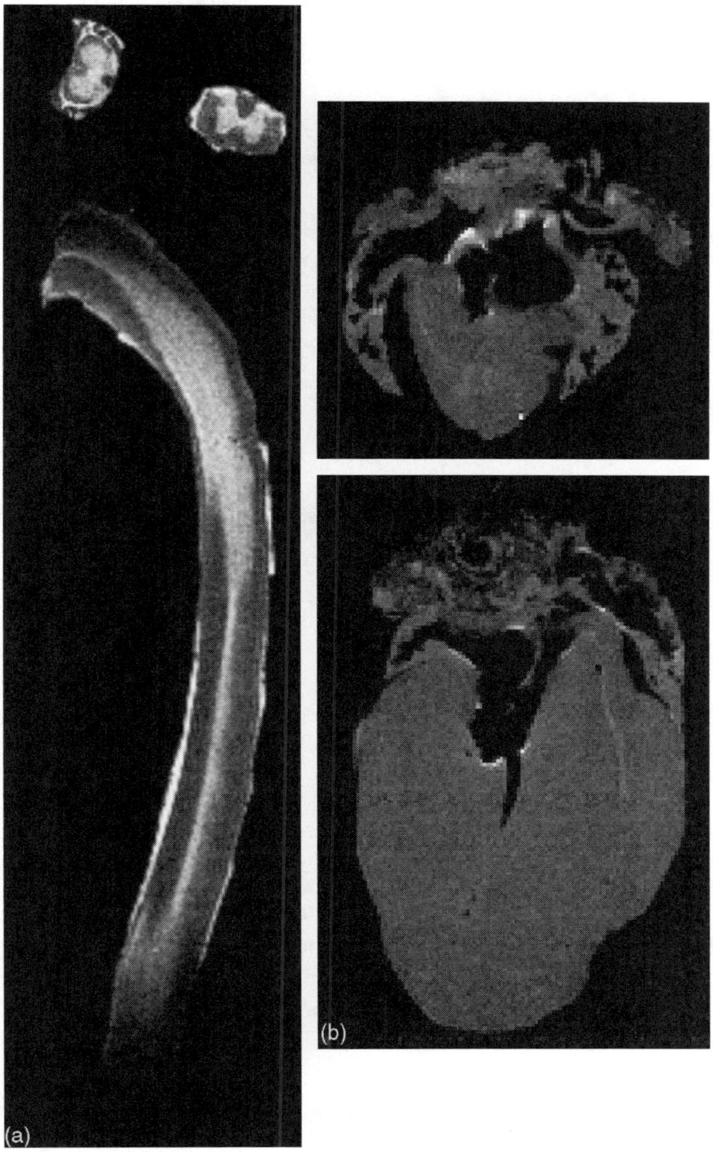

FIGURE 5.7 Two examples of fixed specimens. (a) Cross-sectional views and the side view (bottom) of a fixed spine cut into pieces so that it could fit into a coil. Spin echo sequence with TR = 1600 ms, TE = 35 ms, NEX = 1, FOV = 6 × 13.8 × 13.8 mm, matrix = 100 × 230 × 230 for pixel size of 60 μm^3 and imaging time of 10.2 h. (b) Short axis view (top) and long axis view (bottom) through a fixed heart. Spin echo sequence with TR = 300 ms, TE = 9.2 ms, NEX = 1, FOV = 2.8 × 2.8 × 12 mm, matrix = 420 × 420 × 1800 for resolution of 67 μm^3 and imaging time of 14.7 h. (Courtesy of Brian Nieman and Nir Lifshitz.)

perfusion, the proximal and distant ends of the right jugular vein and the right femoral vein are closed alternatively by hemostat to force the perfusate through the head, thorax, and abdomen.

Figure 5.10 demonstrates a typical 3D data volume of a whole mouse MRI (Figure 5.10a), and two-dimensional cross-sections showing specific organs (Figure 5.10b–f). The integrity of the thorax, the natural shape and spatial relation of the organs in the chest are well preserved

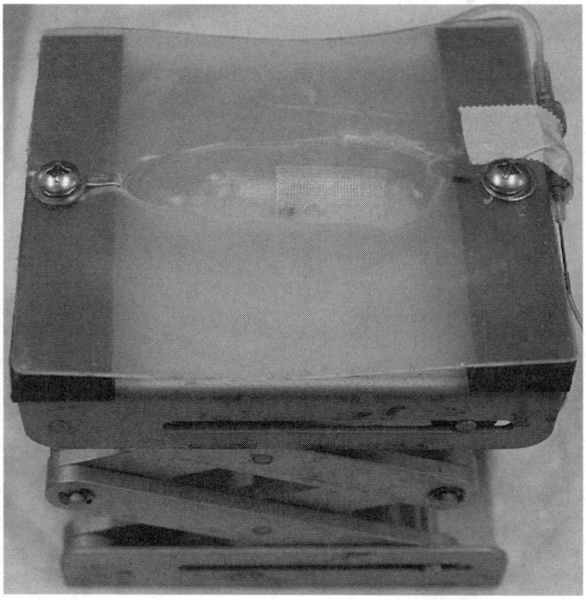

FIGURE 5.8 The custom-built mold to preserve the shape of the mouse after whole-body perfusion-fixation.

(Figure 5.10b–Figure 5.10d), except for a small hole through the chest and the left ventricular wall due to the catheterization (Figure 5.10b).

5.6 IMAGE ANALYSIS AND ATLASES

After acquisition of the images for a given study, the big question that faces the investigator is how to analyze all the data. The most straightforward method is to use an image processing package to segment the volumes of interest (e.g., NIH Image and Analyze). This then allows for quantitative comparisons between mutant and wildtype mice or between diseased and normal mice. Figure 5.11 shows an example of a whole brain that has been segmented from a 3D image of a live mouse. Three internal structures have also been segmented and the volumes are easily calculated by voxel counting.

However, the image data contain much more information beyond simple volumetrics. A mutant can differ from a wildtype through different shapes in structures or appearance of the tissue. This type of analysis requires more sophisticated image processing and leads to the concept of a normal mouse as represented in an MR image. The idea of average or normal is relatively easy to comprehend when considering measurements such as heart rate or blood pressure: these are simple numbers that can be averaged over a number of mice. This is not the case when dealing with anatomies in three-dimensional space.

At the Mouse Imaging Centre, we have developed a variational excised brain atlas in which a number of normal age-, weight-, and sex-matched mice are imaged and then processed to provide an unbiased average atlas and estimates of its variation [47]. A number of tools developed in human brain registration have been adapted for our purposes [48,49]. Figure 5.12 shows our initial results from the averaging together of brains excised from nine 8-week-old, male inbred 129S1/SvImJ mice. We have found the variability in this strain of mice at this particular age to be low. For example, the mean volume and standard deviation of the cerebral cortex and corpus callosum were 109 ± 2 and 13 ± 0.3 mm^3, respectively. Since the variability is so small, we believe that our variational atlas can serve as a yardstick against which mutants with anatomical anomalies can be measured.

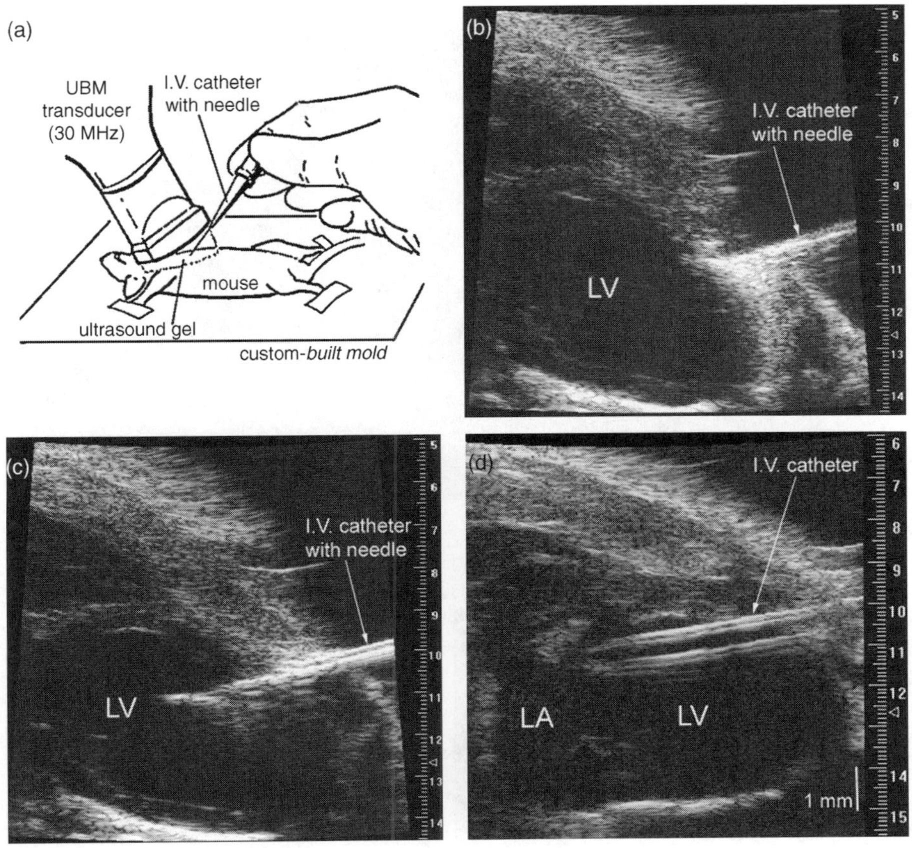

FIGURE 5.9 Ultrasound-guided left ventricular catheterization of an anesthetized mouse. (a) Sketch showing the spatial relation among the mouse chest, ultrasound transducer and the i.v. catheter with needle. (b) Two-dimensional ultrasound image showing the left ventricle (LV), and the tip of the needle on the surface of the chest. (c) Ultrasound image showing the needle punctured through the chest into the LV chamber. (d) Ultrasound image showing the catheter in the LV chamber after the needle was pulled out. (From Zhou, Y. Q. et al., *Lab. Invest.*, 84, 385, 2004. Courtesy of Yu-Qing Zhou. With permission of Nature Publishing Group Copyright 2004.)

5.7 CONCLUSIONS

MRI can be extended to provide high throughput for mouse phenotyping of live mice and fixed whole body or organ specimens. *Post mortem* imaging of individual organs provides data that are of lower resolution than conventional histology, but the relative speed and their nondestructive nature allow researchers to rapidly assess results and to digitally slice and dice in any direction. *Post mortem* whole-body imaging affords information from the entire organ system, which is crucially important for random mutagenesis studies and genetic experiments that affect multiple organs.

The ultimate limit of live, multiple, whole-body mouse imaging has currently not yet been reached. The approach at our laboratory uses a large gradient set to allow for several individual RF coils, but we then suffer from slow gradient performance times and currently need to use spin-echo type sequences. Improved performance of large gradient sets for multiple mouse imaging is going to enable the use of faster sequences, such as gradient-echo. Therefore, it can be expected that the throughput is going to increase significantly in the near future. Being able to anatomically phenotype 10,000 mice per year is a goal that should be reachable.

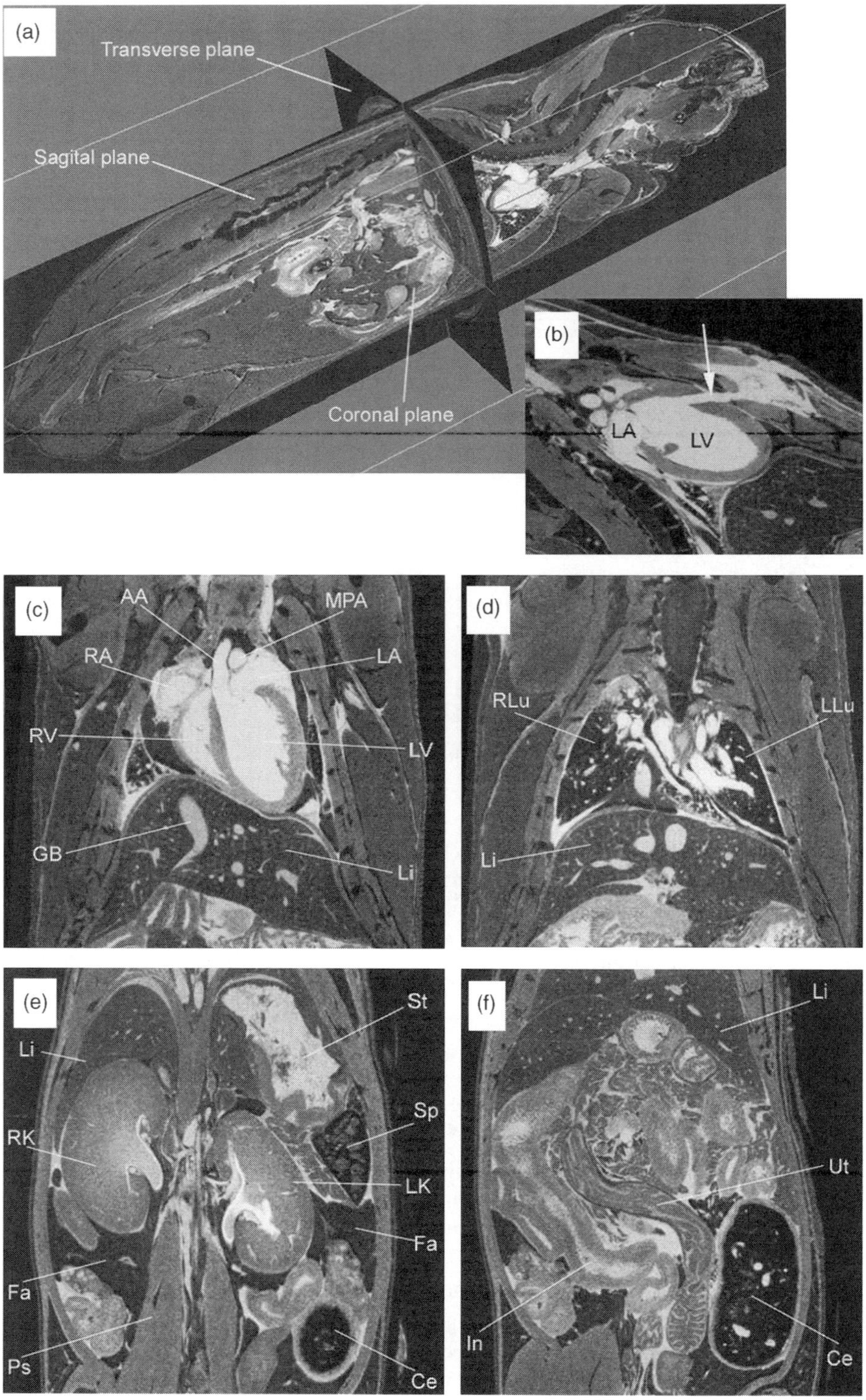

FIGURE 5.10 Typical MR images of a mouse perfused with gadopentetate dimeglumine (see text for details). (a) The three-dimensional (3D) data volume of the whole-body MR imaging. (b) An oblique cross-section showing the left atrium (LA) and left ventricle (LV), and the hole (arrow) through the ventricular and the chest walls caused by the catheterization. (c) A coronal cross-section showing the cardiac structures such as the

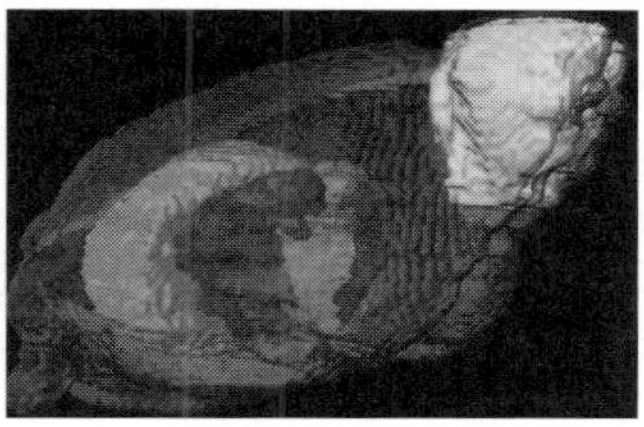

FIGURE 5.11 Surface renderings of a wildtype brain and three internal structures: lateral ventricles, olfactory bulbs, and hippocampus. (Courtesy of Nir Lifshitz.)

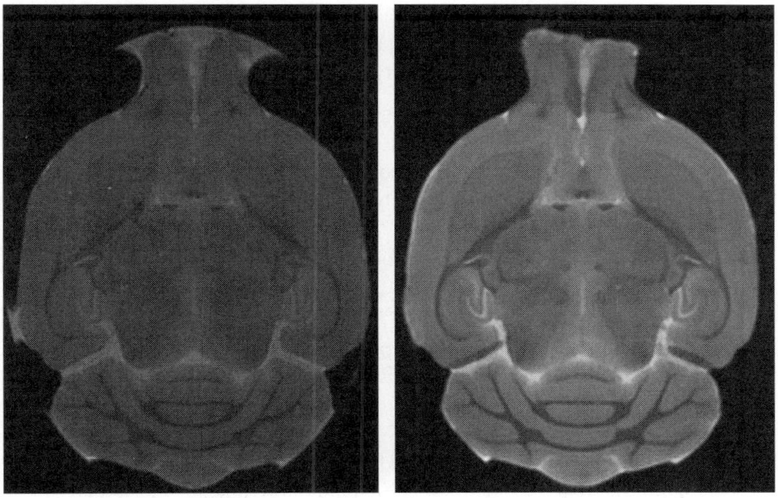

FIGURE 5.12 Horizontal images from an individual excised brain (left) in comparison with the average atlas (right). The individual image suffers from image artifacts like remnant fixative. The average brain shows overall improvement in the visibility and delineation of large anatomical structures but loss of definition in smaller structures such as the blood vessels in the striatum. Spin echo sequence with TR = 1600 ms, TE = 35 ms, NEX = 1, FOV = 12 × 12 × 24 mm, matrix = 200 × 200 × 400 for resolution of 60 μm^3 and imaging time of 18 h. (From Kovacevic, N. et al., *Cereb. Cortex*, 15, 639, 2005. (Courtesy of Natasa Kovacevic.)

LA, LV, ascending aorta (AA), right atrium (RA), right ventricle (RV), and main pulmonary artery (MPA) in the thoracic cavity, and the liver (Li) with gallbladder (GB). (d) A coronal cross-section showing the right lung (RLu) and left lung (LLu) and the pulmonary vasculature. (e) A coronal cross-section showing right kidney (RK) and left kidney (LK), spleen (Sp), stomach (St), cecum (Ce), fat (Fa), and psoas (Ps) in the abdomen. (f) A slightly oblique coronal cross-section showing small and large intestines (In) and one horn of uterus (Ut). Spin echo sequence with TR = 200 ms, TE = 10 ms, NEX = 1, FOV = 28 × 28 × 120 mm, matrix = 420 × 420 × 1800 for resolution of 67 μm^3 and imaging time of 9.8 h. Note that these parameters are specific to 7 T and the dosage of contrast agent. For higher fields, lower doses of contrast agent are used and the sequence timings will change [50]. (From Zhou, Y. Q. et al., *Lab. Invest.*, 84, 385, 2004. Courtesy of Yu-Qing Zhou. With permission of Nature Publishing Group Copyright 2004.)

Realizing robust high-throughput MR imaging of mice is stepping stone to many areas of biological research. The tight anatomical similarity among mice from inbred strains allows for easy recognition of mutant outliers and noninvasive imaging of cohorts of live mice allow for time-course studies of development and also disease progression.

ACKNOWLEDGMENTS

The authors gratefully acknowledge the staff and students of the Mouse Imaging Centre. In addition, Dr. Benoit Bruneau and Dr. Jeffrey Henderson are acknowledged for providing mouse samples. This work is part of the Mouse Imaging Centre (MICe) at the Hospital for Sick Children and the University of Toronto. The infrastructure has been funded by the Canada Foundation for Innovation (CFI) and Ontario Innovation Trust (OIT). The research has been funded by an Ontario Research and Development Challenge Fund (ORDCF) grant to the Ontario Consortium for Small Animal Imaging (OCSAI).

REFERENCES

1. Lauterbur, P. C., Magnetic resonance zeugmatography, *Pure Appl. Chem.*, 40, 149, 1974.
2. Clapham, J. C. et al., Mice overexpressing human uncoupling protein-3 in skeletal muscle are hyperphagic and lean, *Nature*, 406, 415, 2000.
3. Jalanko, A. et al., Mice with an aspartylglucosaminuria mutation similar to humans replicate the pathophysiology in patients, *Hum. Mol. Genet.*, 7, 265, 1998.
4. Jones, M. E. et al., Aromatase-deficient (ArKO) mice have a phenotype of increased adiposity, *Proc. Natl. Acad. Sci. USA*, 97, 12735, 2000.
5. Bock, N. A., Konyer, N. B., and Henkelman, R. M., Multiple-mouse MRI, *Magn. Reson. Med.*, 49, 158, 2003.
6. Graf, H. et al., Inductively coupled rf coils for examinations of small animals and objects in standard whole-body MR scanners, *Med. Phys.*, 30, 1241, 2003.
7. Wong, W. H. and Sukumar, S., Millipede imaging coil design for high field micro imaging applications, *Proceedings of Eighth Annual Meeting of the ISMRM, Denver*, 2000, p. 1399.
8. Cha, S. et al., Dynamic, contrast-enhanced perfusion MRI in mouse gliomas: Correlation with histopathology, *Magn. Reson. Med.*, 49, 848, 2003.
9. Johnson, G. A. et al., Morphologic phenotyping with MR microscopy: the visible mouse, *Radiology*, 222, 789, 2002.
10. Natt, O. et al., High-resolution 3D MRI of mouse brain reveals small cerebral structures in vivo, *J. Neurosci. Methods*, 120, 203, 2002.
11. Pautler, R. G. and Koretsky, A. P., Tracing odor-induced activation in the olfactory bulbs of mice using manganese-enhanced magnetic resonance imaging, *Neuroimage.*, 16, 441, 2002.
12. Natt, O. et al., Magnetization transfer MRI of mouse brain reveals areas of high neural density, *Magn. Reson. Imaging*, 21, 1113, 2003.
13. Matsuda, Y. et al., Super-parallel MR microscope, *Magn. Reson. Med.*, 50, 183, 2003.
14. Schmiedl, U. P., Maravilla, K. R., and Nelson, J. A., Improved method for in vivo magnetic resonance contrast media research, *Invest. Radiol.*, 26, 65, 1991.
15. Xu, S. et al., In vivo multiple-mouse imaging at 1.5 T, *Magn. Reson. Med.*, 49, 551, 2003.
16. Bock, N. A. et al., High-resolution longitudinal screening with magnetic resonance imaging in a murine brain cancer model, *Neoplasia*, 5, 546, 2003.
17. Lukasik, V. M. and Gillies, R. J., Animal anaesthesia for in vivo magnetic resonance, *NMR Biomed.*, 16, 459, 2003.
18. Qiu, H. H. et al., Automated feedback control of body temperature for small animal studies with MR microscopy, *IEEE Trans. Biomed. Eng.*, 44, 1107, 1997.
19. Brau, A. C. et al., Fiber-optic stethoscope: a cardiac monitoring and gating system for magnetic resonance microscopy, *Magn. Reson. Med.*, 47, 314, 2002.

20. Streif, J. U. et al., In vivo time-resolved quantitative motion mapping of the murine myocardium with phase contrast MRI, *Magn. Reson. Med.*, 49, 315, 2003.
21. Wiesmann, F. et al., Cardiovascular phenotype characterization in mice by high resolution magnetic resonance imaging, *MAGMA*, 11, 10, 2000.
22. Dazai, J. et al., Multiple mouse biological loading and monitoring system for MRI, *Magn. Reson. Med.*, 52, 709, 2004.
23. Benveniste, H. et al., Magnetic resonance microscopy of the C57BL mouse brain, *Neuroimage*, 11, 601, 2000.
24. Tada, T. et al., A head holder for magnetic resonance imaging that allows the stereotaxic alignment of spontaneously occurring intracranial mouse tumors, *J. Neurosci. Methods*, 116, 1, 2002.
25. Beckmann, N. et al., Age-dependent cerebrovascular abnormalities and blood flow disturbances in APP23 mice modeling Alzheimer's disease, *J. Neurosci.*, 23, 8453, 2003.
26. Matalon, R. et al., Adeno-associated virus-mediated aspartoacylase gene transfer to the brain of knockout mouse for Canavan disease, *Mol. Ther.*, 7, 580, 2003.
27. Diez, M. et al., MRI and in situ hybridization reveal early disturbances in brain size and gene expression in the megencephalic (mceph/mceph) mouse, *Eur. J. Neurosci.*, 18, 3218, 2003.
28. Cohen, A. R. et al., Characterization of a model of hydrocephalus in transgenic mice, *J. Neurosurg.*, 91, 978, 1999.
29. Mueggler, T. et al., Age-dependent impairment of somatosensory response in the amyloid precursor protein 23 transgenic mouse model of Alzheimer's disease, *J. Neurosci.*, 23, 8231, 2003.
30. Xue, M. et al., Periventricular/intraventricular hemorrhage in neonatal mouse cerebrum, *J. Neuropathol. Exp. Neurol.*, 62, 1154, 2003.
31. Lin, T. et al., A central nervous system specific mouse model for thanatophoric dysplasia type II, *Hum. Mol. Genet.*, 12, 2863, 2003.
32. Nelson, A. L. et al., Magnetic resonance imaging of patched heterozygous and xenografted mouse brain tumors, *J. Neurooncol.*, 62, 259, 2003.
33. Moats, R. A. et al., Micro-MRI at 11.7 T of a murine brain tumor model using delayed contrast enhancement, *Mol. Imaging*, 2, 150, 2003.
34. Rubin, J. B. et al., A small-molecule antagonist of CXCR4 inhibits intracranial growth of primary brain tumors, *Proc. Natl. Acad. Sci. USA*, 100, 13513, 2003.
35. Weissfloch, L. et al., Comparison study of oxygen-induced MRI-signal changes and pO2 changes in murine tumors, *Adv. Exp. Med. Biol.*, 530, 461, 2003.
36. Yang, Y. S., Guccione, S., and Bednarski, M. D., Comparing genomic and histologic correlations to radiographic changes in tumors: a Murine SCC VII Model Study, *Acad. Radiol.*, 10, 1165, 2003.
37. Nahrendorf, M. et al., Cardiac magnetic resonance imaging in small animal models of human heart failure, *Med. Image Anal.*, 7, 369, 2003.
38. Schneider, J. E. et al., Fast, high-resolution in vivo cine magnetic resonance imaging in normal and failing mouse hearts on a vertical 11.7 T system, *J. Magn. Reson. Imaging*, 18, 691, 2003.
39. Cassidy, P. J. et al., Assessment of motion gating strategies for mouse magnetic resonance at high magnetic fields, *J. Magn. Reson. Imaging*, 19, 229, 2004.
40. Thomas, C. D. et al., Morphological and carbogen-based functional MRI of a chemically induced liver tumor model in mice, *Magn. Reson. Med.*, 50, 522, 2003.
41. Checkley, D. et al., Dynamic contrast-enhanced MRI of vascular changes induced by the VEGF-signalling inhibitor ZD4190 in human tumour xenografts, *Magn. Reson. Imaging*, 21, 475, 2003.
42. Kostourou, V. et al., Effects of overexpression of dimethylarginine dimethylaminohydrolase on tumor angiogenesis assessed by susceptibility magnetic resonance imaging, *Cancer Res.*, 63, 4960, 2003.
43. Raghunand, N. et al., Renal and systemic pH imaging by contrast-enhanced MRI, *Magn. Reson. Med.*, 49, 249, 2003.
44. Fink, C. et al., High-resolution three-dimensional MR angiography of rodent tumors: morphologic characterization of intratumoral vasculature, *J. Magn. Reson. Imaging*, 18, 59, 2003.
45. Johnson, G. A. et al., Magnetic resonance histology for morphologic phenotyping, *J. Magn. Reson. Imaging*, 16, 423, 2002.
46. Zhou, Y. Q. et al., Ultrasound-guided left-ventricular catheterization: a novel method of whole mouse perfusion for microimaging, *Lab. Invest.*, 84, 385, 2004.

47. Kovacevic, N. et al., A three-dimensional MRI Atlas of the mouse brain with estimates of the average and variability, *Cereb. Cortex*, 15, 639, 2005.
48. Collins, D. L. and Evans, A. C., Animal: validation and applications of nonlinear registration-based segmentation, *Int. J. Pattern Recognit.*, 11, 1271, 1997.
49. Woods, R. P. et al., Automated image registration: II. Intersubject validation of linear and nonlinear models, *J. Comput. Assist. Tomogr.*, 22, 153, 1998.
50. Nieman, B. J. et al., The relaxation effects of gadolinium concentration at 1.5 T and 7.0 T in fixed mice, *Proc. Intl. Soc. Magn. Reson. Med.*, 11, 808, 2003.

Editorial Comments

Because of its homogeneous structure, the brain is the ideal organ for *in vivo* MR studies. Whole organ and regional volumes are remarkably similar in individuals of the same age, facilitating the comparison of data and the creation of average atlases. Also, movements can be basically suppressed by appropriate fixation of the head. Functional MRI of the brain has become a routine in the clinics and, following proper control of anesthesia, is making its way in animal studies as well. Despite the fact that the tightness of the blood–brain barrier in the healthy brain makes the delivery of contrast material into the parenchyma very difficult, leakiness of the barrier can be immediately associated to a diseased status, thus providing opportunities for diagnosis. The central role played by the brain in the functioning of the body and its well-protected location in the skull render it basically inaccessible to conventional analysis means based on biopsies. Therefore, the brain is the organ which par excellence requires noninvasive imaging techniques for tissue staging in the context of diagnosis. Taking all these factors together, it is not surprising that the largest fraction of *in vivo* MR studies is performed on the brain. This situation is also reflected in the way the role of imaging within pharmaceutical research is perceived. The value of imaging for studies of neurological disorders is rarely questioned, since there are basically no alternatives for brain tissue analysis. In order to be accepted in other disease areas, noninvasive imaging readouts need to demonstrate their ability to provide additional value compared to that derived using conventional, often invasive, procedures.

Chapter 6 to Chapter 12 introduce different MR approaches to assess brain structure, function, and metabolism, with the scope of diagnosing neurological disorders and of probing drug efficacy in animal models of these diseases, as well as in humans suffering from them.

6 Magnetic Resonance Imaging and Spectroscopy in Transgenic Mice Modeling Alzheimer's Disease

Thomas Mueggler

CONTENTS

6.1 INTRODUCTION

At present, the only definitive diagnosis of Alzheimer's disease (AD), the major cause of late-onset dementia, is made *post mortem*, being based on the verification of the pathological hallmarks: extracellular aggregates of β-amyloid (Aβ) peptide (amyloid plaques) and intracellular neurofibrillary tangles (reviewed in Ref. [1]). By processes not completely understood, the accumulation of Aβ and neurofibrillary tangles produces neurodegeneration, which ultimately accounts for the clinical signs of the disease. Mild memory impairment at the early stage is followed by a more global cognitive deficit leading to generalized behavioral impairments and, ultimately, death. Exactly when the neuropathological changes are manifested clinically is uncertain. There are several lines of evidence that the neural dysfunction associated with the disease starts several years before the first clinical phenotypes can be validated or even detected at a time when the degenerative process has already progressed to an advanced stage with massive cell loss. The diagnostic value of the levels of the Aβ peptide species (a decrease of soluble monomeric species), increases of specifically phosphorylated tau protein in cerebrospinal fluid (CSF) and the ApoE genotype are currently being assessed [2,3].

Although symptomatic treatments are available (acetylcholinesterase inhibitors), there are no mechanism-based, disease-modifying agents that slow the course of the disease in susceptible individuals. The identification of mutations in specific genes implicated in the inherited forms of AD (amyloid precursor protein [APP], presenilin [PS] 1 and 2) has provided new opportunities to explore pathogenic mechanisms using transgenic approaches. The growth of research on murine models of AD is documented in a number of reviews that chronicle early stages of the field and recent advances [4,5]. Based upon this foundation, these model systems provide a highly useful tool to assess candidate therapies and expedite the path to clinical trials [6–9]. A comprehensive phenotyping of these models is needed to establish robust paradigms involving correlative biomarkers and predictive endpoints for preclinical disease-modification studies.

The pathophysiological status of transgenic animals is usually assessed by *post-mortem* analysis of brain tissue samples. It is obvious that noninvasive, quantitative readouts would be highly desirable as they would allow monitoring disease progression in longitudinal studies providing information on intra-individual disease evolution, and could be combined with more classical readouts (e.g., behavioral assessments). For this purpose, different imaging modalities are being currently investigated, namely optical imaging, nuclear imaging (e.g., PET), computed tomography (CT), and MRI.

This chapter outlines the role of MR techniques for phenotyping of transgenic mouse models of AD. Focusing on their potential as surrogate biomarkers or endpoints for therapeutic intervention, morphological and functional MRI (fMRI), as well as MRS readouts will be discussed.

6.2 TRANSGENIC MODELS OF ALZHEIMER'S DISEASE

6.2.1 ALZHEIMER'S DISEASE: PATHOLOGICAL HALLMARKS

AD is characterized by progressive cognitive decline and is defined pathologically by the occurrence of amyloid plaques [10,11]. As a second neuropathological feature, many neurons in the brain regions typically affected in AD (e.g., hippocampus) contain neurofibrillary tangles, composed of filamentous aggregates of hyperphosphorylated tau protein [12]. AD is a complex, multifactorial disease in which several genes (APP, PS) act independently or in concert with each other and/or with environmental agents resulting in amyloid deposition in the brain, in neurofibrillary tangle formation and in cell death. The deposition of amyloid follows a specific spatial and temporal pattern.

According to the amyloid hypothesis [13], elevated cerebral levels of Aβ peptides, particularly those ending at amino acid 42 (Aβ 1–42), which is particularly prone to aggregation [14], are an early and invariant feature of all forms of AD driving the pathogenesis. Downstream events of the disease process including neurofibrillary tangles have been proposed to result from an imbalance between Aβ production, fibrillogenesis, and Aβ clearance [1].

6.2.2 TRANSGENIC APPROACH TO MODEL AD PATHOLOGY

One of the major difficulties in studying the relationship between the production and deposition of Aβ, the onset of dementia and the neuritic abnormalities, synaptic dysfunction and neuronal cell death that occurs in AD, has previously been the paucity of mouse models of the disease. Designing experimental models of AD is a complex task since the disease manifests with alterations at the molecular, subcellular, neurophysiological and cognitive levels. However, the early-onset form of AD shows strong genetic linkage, being clustered within families (familial AD, FAD) and transmitted as autosomal dominant traits with almost 100% penetrance. Therefore, it is well suited to induce a disease phenotype in transgenic animals.

Several transgenic lines to date mimic individual or multiple alterations found in AD (Table 6.1). Although they do not recapitulate the full phenotype of AD, some of the mutant APP and APP + PS mice represent excellent models of Aβ amyloidosis. These models will increasingly allow the preclinical evaluation of potential therapeutics, given that drugs interfere at different levels of the disease processes.

Various approaches have been used to characterize the mice: behavioral readouts, *in vitro*/*in vivo* electrophysiology, biochemical analysis either *post mortem* or using *in vivo* microdialysis methods, and histology. An in-depth description of all characterized models to date is far beyond the scope of this chapter, but has been the subject of several reviews [4,5,15–17]. The focus here is on the main pathological alterations of AD transgenic lines that have been investigated using MRI and MRS in addition to more classical methods (Table 6.1).

The PDAPP [18], Tg2576 [19], and APP23 [20] lines, single-transgenic models of AD, have been extensively characterized and show pathological alterations closely resembling those observed in AD. The development of typical neuritic plaques (Figure 6.1a), dystrophic neurites, loss of presynaptic terminals, and gliosis has been reported [19–22]. Earliest amyloid deposits can be found at around 6 months of age (Table 6.1). Crossing of the Tg2576 with the hPS1M146L transgenic line [23] resulted in a novel mouse line (PSAPP) that showed greatly accelerated plaque pathology and concomitant gliosis [24]. Mice from the double-transgenic lines PSAPP (coexpressing mutated hAPP and PS1) and PS2APP [25] do, in general, recapitulate many of the features reported for single-transgenic APP mice.

AD is characterized by neuronal loss affecting areas including the enthorhinal cortex, the CA1 region of the hippocampus, the amygdala, and the neocortex. Disappointingly, even considering both APP and APP + PS double-transgenic mice, only one of the published AD models (TgAPP23) exhibits cell loss, restricted to hippocampal CA1 neurons [26]. A further feature of the TgAPP23 mouse model is the fact that amyloid deposition can also be found in the cerebral vasculature in APP23 mice beyond the age of 1 year [27]. This is remarkable since neither cells of the vasculature express detectable amounts of APP nor can Aβ be measured in the plasma. Due to the neuron-specific promoter the Aβ deposits must originate from APP made by neurons. In adult APP23 mice cerebral amyloid angiopathy (CAA) leads to local perivascular neurodegeneration, synaptic abnormalities, and microhemorrhages [27–30].

Clinically AD is characterized by a progressive decline in cognitive performance with compromised learning, memory, and speed of problem-solving. Thus, cognitive testing of AD mice is obviously a subject of great importance, given the goal of applying therapies that deal with the earliest manifestations of the disease. TgAPP and TgAPP + PS1 mice that progress to deposit of amyloid often exhibit cognitive dysfunction [19,25,31–36]. However, inconsistencies are apparent regarding the relationship between cognitive impairment and pathology. Some of the cognitive changes described in behavioral studies seem to be age-related, others are age-unrelated and hence do not correlate with amyloid burden. In fact, in some cases compromised performance is seen at the preplaque stage, and may be accompanied by changes in synaptic activity [31, 36–38], an observation readily compatible with the concept of diffusible toxic forms of Aβ (protofibrils, Ref. [39]) and highlighting a growing awareness that, in APP transgenic mice at least, the accumulation of soluble Aβ species may be a significant contributory factor in the expression of cognitive impairment. Differences in the relative amounts (or forms) of soluble vs. insoluble Aβ may therefore also contribute to the variable observations across different AD models.

TABLE 6.1
APP-Based Transgenic Mouse Models of AD Investigated Using MRI/MRS[a]

		Phenotype							
Transgenic Line	Transgene[b] (Mutation)	AP	Aβ Deposits (Age of onset)	Glia[c]	NFT[d]	ND[e]	Cog[f]	Initial References	MRI/MRS Study References
PDAPP	$APP_{695,751,770}$ (V717F)	✓	✓ (6 months)	✓	—		✓	[18]	[54,73,76]
Tg2576	APP_{695} (Swedish)	✓	✓ (9–12 months)	✓	—		✓	[19]	[53,56,57,81]
APP23	APP_{751} (Swedish)	✓	✓ (6 months)	✓	—	✓	✓	[20]	[51,71,75,78,92,93]
PSAPP	APP_{695} (Swedish), PS1 (M146L)	✓	✓ (3 months)	✓	—		✓	[24]	[52,53,55–57,74]
PS2APP	APP_{751} (Swedish), PS2 (N141I)	✓	✓ (4–5 months)	✓	—		✓	[25]	[72]

Abbreviations: APP, amyloid precursor protein; AP, amyloid plaques; Cog, cognitive impairment; ND, neurodegeneration; NFT, neurofibrillary tangles; PS1,2, Presenilin 1 and 2.

[a] Modified after Higgins, G.A. and Jacobsen, H., *Behav. Pharmacol.*, 14, 419, 2003 and Hock, B.J.J. and Lamb, B.T., *Trends Genet.*, 17, S7, 2001.
[b] cDNA-based transgenic approach including various APP isoforms expressed from the construct (695, 751, or 770 amino acids). APP FAD Swedish: K670N/M671L.
[c] identified by presence of microglia around Aβ deposits and various inflammatory cytokines, as well as astrocytosis.
[d] No NFTs in any model; presence of hyperphosphorylated tau has been documented (positive to phosphorylation-specific antibody AT8).
[e] Documented by cell counts in various brain regions; in APP23: 25% reduction in CA1 at 14 months.
[f] Behavioral impairments as documented by the Morris water maze, spatial alternation, and other specific tasks.

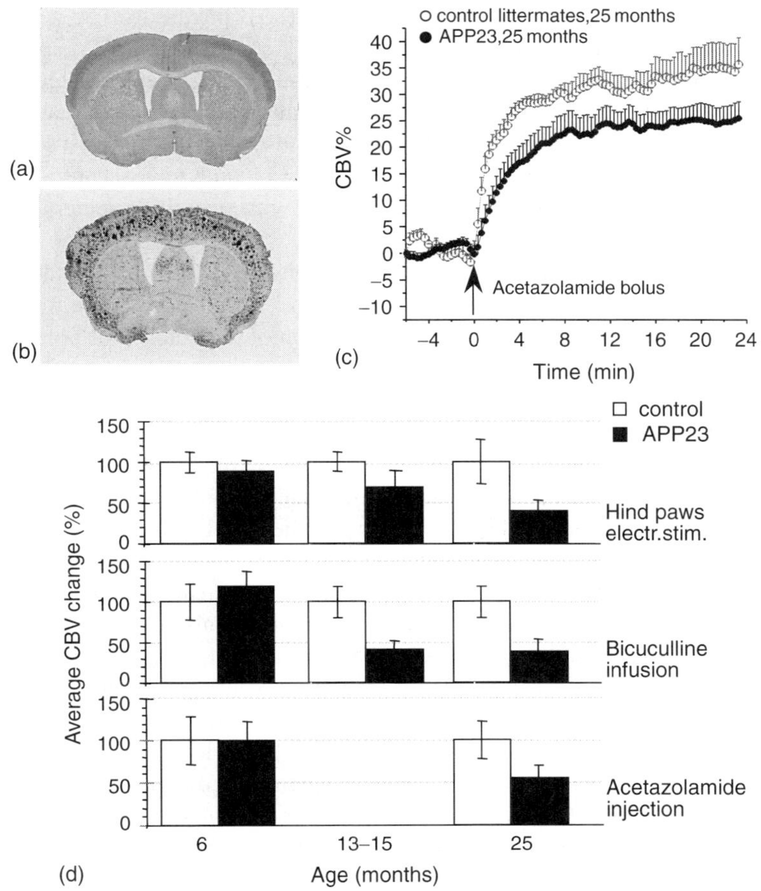

FIGURE 6.1 Presence of amyloid plaques in the cortex and functional MRI characterization of APP23 mice. Ab immunostaining with the NT12 antibody shows no amyloid deposits in aged control littermates (a) and massive amyloid plaques predominantly in the neocortex of aged APP23 (b). The temporal CBV profile (c) after intravenous injection of acetalzolamide (arrow) for 25-month-old APP23 mice and age-matched controls revealed significantly lower DCBV% changes in transgenic animals compared with their littermates. Summary of fMRI characterization of the APP23 model using electrical stimulation of the hindpaws, infusion of the $GABA_A$ antagonist bicuculline, and injection of acetazolamide at various ages (d). Young APP23 show a normal hemodynamic response to the stimuli, whereas in older transgenic animals (13–15 and 25 months, respectively) the CBV changes are clearly decreased. For more details, see Refs. [94,95].

6.3 PHENOTYPING AD MOUSE MODELS USING MRI/MRS

6.3.1 Structural MRI and MRS in Transgenic Models of AD

6.3.1.1 Detection of β-Amyloid Deposits Using MRI

From the foregoing account it seems clear that generation of Aβ is a critical step in the disease process and direct visualization and quantification of the plaque load is considered highly attractive for diagnosis, disease staging, and therapy evaluation. However, considerable controversy exists as to whether the extent of Aβ accumulation correlates with dementia. Evidence suggests that the Aβ-plaque burden correlates with the clinical severity of the disease [40–42]. Deposition, particularly of Aβ1–42, occurs very early in the disease process, even before AD is diagnosed [42].

Considerable effort has been thus undertaken to visualize Aβ plaque load *in vivo* using imaging techniques such as MRI, PET, or optical imaging.

In aged AD transgenics neuritic plaques can reach up to 200 μm in diameter, averaging 80 to -120 μm [43,44]. In comparison, human AD compact plaques are classified as "burned-out" or "naked core" plaques and classical plaques [45,46]. Burned-out plaques consist simply of a central amyloid core 10 to -20 μm in diameter, whereas classical plaques have a central core surrounded by an empty region with a halo of fluorescent material, with overall diameters averaging 60 to -80 μm.

Thus, MRI theoretically provides the spatial resolution needed to resolve neuritic plaques. The ability to detect such amyloid-positive brain lesions *in vivo* using noninvasive imaging modalities would allow disease progression to be tracked and to monitor the efficacy of potential therapies in clinical trials and in disease-modifying studies using transgenic models resembling AD pathology. However, assuming that adequate signal-to-noise ratio (SNR) is attainable with MRI, plaque visualization still may be constrained by an insufficient contrast-to-noise ratio. Mechanisms by which plaques might affect MR contrast and thus become visible are still unknown.

Early MRI studies based on T_1- or T_2-contrast mechanisms did not reveal plaques in formalin-fixed hippocampi from AD patients [47]. Plausibility studies predicted that, because some neuritic plaques contain iron particles [48], they might have a different magnetic susceptibility than the surrounding tissue. In fact, using formalin-fixed tissue from human brain samples, large neuritic plaques of 100 μm could be successfully detected as hypo-intense areas in T_2^*-weighted images recorded with a voxel size of 5.9E-5 μm^3 (i.e., $39 \times 39 \times 39$ μm^3) at 7 T [49]. This study did not detect the more numerous small plaques. More recently, a similar number of hypo-intense areas were found in MR images obtained from AD specimens using a related T_2^* gradient echo sequence, but a more than four times finer spatial resolution at 11.7 T [50]. However, almost all of them could be matched with blood vessels in corresponding histological sections and were probably caused by the iron-rich cell aggregates within the vessels. These authors suggested that susceptibility effects are not associated with neuritic plaques and do not provide a mechanism to differentiate them from surrounding tissue [50].

Several similar MRI studies have been carried out investigating the detection of plaques in formalin-fixed brain tissue from single-transgenic APP23, Tg2576, and $PS1_{M146L}$ mice, or from double-transgenic PSAPP mice, using T_2- and T_2^*-weighted images [51–53]. First attempts to visualize Aβ plaques in the intact animal [54] have shown that these MR microscopy approaches cannot be easily transferred into the *in vivo* situation due to prohibitive measurement times and different contrast characteristics. Recently, methods to optimize visualization of plaques *in vivo* in mice at 9.4 T have been reported. Using a spin-echo sequence based on adiabatic pulses, Jack et al. [55] successfully visualized plaques with diameters as small as 50 μm in aged PSAPP double-transgenic mice [24]. Scanning time has been reduced below 2 h approaching a range acceptable to *in vivo* imaging. However, besides the difficulty in perfectly matching histological sections and MRI slices, all these studies have to cope with the problem of classification of observable hypo-intense areas in T_2 and T_2^*-weighted images. For example, areas bearing microhemorrhages or heavily myelinated fiber tracts may also appear dark on T_2-weighted images [56]. Moreover, such a classification can not only be based on the 3D pattern of the hypo-intense structure because it has been shown that blood clots that lead to hypo-intense spots in T_2^*-weighted images may spread out in the vascular system leading to spheric shapes (ovoid forms) originally proposed only for plaques. In consistency with these observations the numerous hypo-intense spots observed in T_2^*-weighted images obtained *in vivo* in a study carried out in APP23 mice might be rather classified as vessels than as parenchymal plaques (^Beckmann N., personal communication).

Strategies to improve the specificity have therefore been investigated. Plaque-specific MR contrast agents such as labeled Aβ peptides to enhance contrast-to-noise ratio have been applied [56,57]. Some of these agents did not cross the blood–brain barrier [57]. However, experiments carried out in Tg2476 and PSAPP mice document the feasibility of labeling amyloid plaques *in vivo* with a probe, putrescine-gadolinium-amyloid-β peptide (PUT-Gd-Aβ), which due to the presence of the polyamine moiety is transported across the blood–brain barrier following intravenous injection, causing specific plaque enhancement in T_1-weighted images [56]. Surprisingly, the modified peptide bound almost exclusively to the dense amyloid cores of neuritic plaques, not to the innumerable "diffuse" deposits of Aβ in AD brain that appear to represent immature, precursor lesions. Thus, further experiments using increased amounts of labeled Aβ, mixtures of Aβ1–42 and Aβ1–40 (or fragments thereof) have to clarify the additive value of this approach in an early diagnosis of AD or its potential as an early biomarker of AD pathology in transgenic mice, providing a direct measure of the efficacy of antiamyloid therapies. However, considering the inherently low sensitivity of MRI the additive value of such target-specific approaches have to be evaluated in comparison with other imaging modalities.

Scintigraphic probes conjugated to various agents targeted for Aβ-peptides, or histological dyes such as Congo red or thioflavin S, have been used to label plaques in animal and human specimens *in vitro* and *in vivo* in mice (for review see Refs. [58,59]) and in Alzheimer's patients [60]. Optical imaging of individual probe labeled plaques has also been demonstrated [61,62]. Recently an MR-compatible, F19-containing amyloidophilic Congo red-type compound, which crosses the blood–brain barrier has been synthetized [63]. Amyloid plaque visualization has been demonstrated by detecting the F19 nucleus derived MR signal in the brain of living APP transgenic mice (Tg2576) after intravenous injection of this compound [64]. Very low tissue background noise and the high specificity of this approach provides a new direction for *in vivo* amyloid imaging. However, MR sensitivity of F19 is lower than that of 1H. Thus sensitivity remains a limited factor of any target-specific MR approach and new strategies have to be evaluated in comparison with other imaging modalities.

One of the main conditions for plaque-specific MR contrast agents has to be their ability to cross the blood–brain barrier nondestructively. Furthermore, the toxicity of MR contrast reagents has yet to be established; hence their application in the clinics is currently not possible. As a consequence, other MRI approaches have been used both clinically and preclinically to provide secondary structural readouts, such as measurements of brain atrophy or indicators of microstructural changes of brain parenchyma using diffusion-weighted MRI (DWI).

6.3.1.2 Assessment of Brain Atrophy

When assessing a demented subject, conventional structural CT and MRI are the most powerful investigation for excluding other pathologies, such as tumor, normal-pressure hydrocephalus, and multiple vascular lesions [65] and is recommended for the routine evaluation of AD [66] (see also Chapter 7). Besides this traditional, exclusionary role, structural neuroimaging is increasingly being used to add positive prognostic information in the differential diagnosis of patients with cognitive impairment [67,68].

For this purpose, rates of change of brain atrophy can be assessed using both volumetric and voxel subtraction MR techniques [69–71]. Recent data support the use of different brain atrophy rate measures (hippocampus, entorhinal cortex, whole brain, and ventricles) from serial MRI studies in addition to standard clinical measures as markers of disease progression in AD [72].

To determine brain volumetric changes in APP23 mice and assess the time-point of morphological alteration in this model, we have determined the ventricle size in mutant and age-matched littermates [73]. In 24-month-old APP23 mice, a significant increase in brain ventricle size ($18 \pm 4\%$) has been measured compared to age-matched littermates. In younger, 14-month-old transgenic animals, no significant difference has been found between APP23 and wildtype mice, suggesting that an enlargement of CSF volume, which might indicate global or regional brain atrophy, occurs at later stages in the disease progression. These results are consistent with the findings reporting that, in 14- to 18-month-old APP23 mice, no global neuron loss occurs despite a high amyloid plaque load [26]. Therefore, at least for APP23 mice, assessments of ventricle size would be of little prognostic value for evaluating pharmaceutical interventions.

In a similar study carried out in APP/PS double transgenic mice, a statistically significant, albeit small, difference in the volume of the ventricles between PS2APP and control mice has been found [74]. No difference in the volume of the whole brain was detected between the two groups. In contrast to the human situation, the brain grew continually and linearly throughout the life span. A change in the growth rate over time, which potentially would indicate the progression of the pathology, has not been observed.

In perfusion-fixed brains of 100-day-old PDAPP mice, a significant reduction of hippocampal volume has been measured and confirmed by stereological analysis [75], opening a highly specific and surprisingly early temporal window (i.e., clearly before first appearance of Aβ deposits) for the detection of an inferred onset of pathology. The hippocampal volume deficit in 100- and 630-day-old PDAPP mutants is not progressive and is due to a continued postnatal increase in hippocampal volume in wildtype mice that does not occur in the mutant mice. More longitudinal prospective *in vivo* MRI studies are needed to assess volumetric changes and their exact time-point of appearance, which may differ from model to model depending on the corresponding FAD mutation.

6.3.1.3 Brain Tissue Relaxation Times, Diffusion Properties, and Cerebrovascular Flow Abnormalities

Alternative structural MRI approaches are based on the quantitative assessment of MRI parameters determining image contrast. For instance, the occurrence of microstructural changes in brain parenchyma due to plaque and tangle formation should translate into locally altered MRI relaxation times. High-field MRI has been used to investigate brain regional changes of MR relaxation times in two different murine AD models [76]. The transverse relaxation time T_2 was significantly reduced in various brain regions (hippocampus, cingulate, and retrosplenial cortex) of PSAPP mice [24] as compared to nontransgenic animals. No significant differences were observed between T_2-values measured in PS mice [23], which do not display deposition of solid Aβ-containing plaques, and control animals. These results indicate that T_2 might constitute a sensitive marker of parenchymal abnormalities due to massive deposition of insoluble Aβ. No significant changes have been found in the longitudinal relaxation time T_1.

A similar hypothesis has been pursuit by analyzing the water apparent diffusion coefficient (ADC) in brain parenchyma. Extracellular deposition of Aβ plaques impinges restrictions to interstitial fluid diffusion reflected by a reduction of the tissue ADC. In fact, in 24-month-old APP23 mice significantly decreased ADC values were observed in cortical regions that displayed high amounts of insoluble Aβ plaques as compared to wildtype animals. In 6-month-old animals, no difference was observed between transgenic and control mice [77].

Damage and dysfunction in AD is not only confined to gray matter but occurs also in white matter. White matter degeneration has been studied using diffusion-tensor (DT) MRI in APP overexpressing mice, in which APP was expressed under the control of the platelet-derived growth factor promoter (PDAPP line). Due to the fact that water diffusion is restricted by cellular membranes perpendicular to the fiber axis and is essentially free along the nerve fibers, high values of diffusion anisotropy reflect integrity of corresponding white matter tracts. DT anisotropy was significantly reduced in 15-month-old PDAPP mice with established pathology as compared to that of age-matched control mice, while no difference in DTI parameters was observed between the young, 3-month-old, PDAPP and control mice [78].

A final structural readout that has been proposed is the analysis of the cerebro-arterial systems. AD-related vasculopathy also affects lager vessels including the principal feeding arteries of the brain [79]. MR angiography (MRA) studies in APP23 mice confirmed this fact. Flow voids were detected at the internal carotid artery of 11-month-old APP23 mice. At the age of 20 months, more pronounced and additional flow disturbances were observed in large arteries at the Circle of Willis.

Vascular corrosion casts obtained from the same mice revealed that vessel elimination and/or deformation had taken place at the sites where flow voids were detected by MRA [80,81].

6.3.1.4 Assessment of the Neurochemical Profile Using MRS

MRS permits the quantification of metabolic biomarkers *in vivo* and *in vitro*, and has been used to characterize AD (for reviews see Ref. [82] and Chapter 7). The most consistent reported finding of 1H-MRS is a decrease in *N*-acetylaspartate (NAA), often considered as indicating neuronal number and health, even if the role of NAA in the brain is yet not fully understood. An increase of the signal from myo-inositol, which may either be a marker for osmotic stress or astrogliosis, has also been reported in AD patients. Thus, myo-inositol may be an earlier marker of pathological change in AD than NAA.

1H-MRS studies have also been carried out in Tg2576 [83] and in PS2APP mice [74]. *In vivo* 1H spectra of the frontal cortex of 19-month-old Tg2576 mice revealed significant decreases of NAA and increased levels of taurine compared to wildtype control mice. Subsequent *in vitro* MRS in corresponding areas of the cortex showed in addition decreased levels of glutamate and glutathione [83]. The decreased levels of NAA and the increased level of taurine are consistent with neuronal variability and increased glial volume, being equivalent to findings of decreased NAA and increased myo-inositol in human AD [82,84]. Taurine is much more concentrated in the rodent than in the human brain and may serve a similar role as myo-inositol in the human brain. Decreased NAA/creatine and glutamate/creatine ratios have been found in the frontal cortex of 24-month-old double-transgenic PS2APP mice compared to age-matched controls [74]. In a longitudinal study in the same model from age 4 to 24 months, the difference in the metabolic profile between mutant and wildtype animals became only significant at the age of 20 months. Thus, a reliable phenotyping using MRS readouts could only be undertaken at an age when Aβ deposits were widespread and pathophysiological changes had progressed to advanced stages. Nevertheless, the levels of NAA and glutamate were inversely correlated to the plaque load determined by histology, thus providing a valid biomarker to monitor the progression of the disease in this model.

6.3.1.5 From Structural to Functional Readouts

A common feature of various morphological and neurochemical phenotyping approaches, except the target-specific imaging methods probing the plaque load of the mice, is their lack of sensitivity. Reliable deviations from normal values (brain atrophy, changes in ADC, T_2, vascular defects, and neurochemical alterations) are only observed in advanced disease states (i.e., in old animals). This limits the value of these readouts for early diagnosis and as prognostic tools for monitoring disease evolution or therapeutic interventions.

In neurodegenerative diseases such as Alzheimer's disease (AD), early symptoms comprise functional (cognitive) deficits, which appear before gross morphological alterations of associated brain regions. This led to the hypothesis that functional neuroimaging that demonstrate physiological changes in the brain have the potential to identify subtle alterations of neuronal function before anatomical abnormalities become apparent in structural images. Therefore, functional readouts would be of high diagnostic relevance [85]. The various transgenic mouse models available today, which manifest characteristic neuropathological and behavioral features of AD, offer an attractive basis for the evaluation of this concept.

6.3.2 Functional MRI in Transgenic Models of AD

6.3.2.1 Introduction: Functional MRI in Mice

fMRI does not measure the neural activity *per se*, but rather the physiological consequences thereof, such as regional changes in cerebral blood volume (CBV) [86], cerebral blood flow (CBF) [87–89], and blood oxygenation [90]. Due to its noninvasiveness, it has become a very popular technique mapping human and animal brain function (Ref. [91]; see also Chapter 10 and Chapter 11). Moreover, fMRI methods have been applied to study neuronal function in rat models of brain disorders and can be regarded as an established tool in biomedical research. However, despite the proven utility of fMRI in preclinical studies, only a relatively small number of fMRI studies have focused on the mouse brain [92–98]. This is partly due to the small size of the mouse brain resulting in limited SNR. Moving towards a high-field system to improve SNR bears the problem of an increased susceptibility due to the large air-tissue interface of the small brain coupled with generally poorer shimming capabilities. Additionally, in mice, which are an order of magnitude smaller than rats, maintaining normal physiology (i.e., body temperature, blood-gas levels, and blood pressure), critical for eliciting robust functional responses, is challenging.

In animal fMRI studies performed under anesthesia, paradigms include sensory [99–101], pharmacological stimulation [102,103], or physiological stimulation [104]. Since some of the CNS active compounds used (e.g., bicuculline) produced large relative CBV changes of the order of 30 to 40% of baseline values [103], pharmacological stimulation was considered attractive to test the feasibility of fMRI studies in mice. In fact, intravenous infusion of bicuculline prompted region-specific increases in local relative CBV values, which were found to be dose-dependent [96] and comparable to the activation pattern observed in fMRI studies in the rat [103]. Similarly, robust CBV responses have been obtained in the respective cortical region of isoflurane-anesthetized and mechanically ventilated mice during unilateral electrical stimulation of the hind paw [94]. These feasibility studies show that with adequate temporal and spatial resolution CBV-based noninvasive fMRI is feasible in such small structures as the murine brain and open the way to a broad range of applications in genetically engineered mouse models of CNS disorders.

6.3.2.2 Functional MRI Readouts in Transgenic Mouse Models of AD

To investigate the potential of such functional readouts to phenotype transgenic models of AD, fMRI was applied to the APP23 line [20] of various ages (Figure 6.1). The CBV response in 6-, 13–15- and 25-month-old mutant mice to a standardized challenge was analyzed and compared to age-matched control littermates. The stimuli applied were those previously described [94–96], i.e., pharmacological stimulation using the $GABA_A$ receptor antagonist bicuculline, physiological stimulation by inducing hypercapnia using the carbonic anhydrase inhibitor acetazolamide, and peripheral sensory activation using electrical stimulation of the hind paws. All three stimulation paradigms evoked CBV responses in 13–15- and 25-month-old APP23 mice that were significantly smaller when compared to age-matched, control littermates [94,95]. In young animals of 6 months of age, there was no difference between the transgenic and wildtype group. The acetazolamide experiments indicated that the reduced response to the different stimuli might be due to a compromised vascular reserve capacity caused by the severe CAA found in this model [29,30,80]. Perivascular Aβ deposits impair the ability of the cerebral arteriolar and/or capillary compartments to effectively regulate CBF. As fMRI probes the hemodynamic changes associated with brain activity and not the neuronal activation *per se*, it is currently unclear to what extent the reduced response to the $GABA_A$ receptor inhibition and the sensory input is caused by impaired neural excitability or by the lack of cerebrovascular reactivity.

Assuming that the impaired vascular reactivity reflects CAA-related vasculopathy, the acetazolamide challenge might detect early phases of CAA, which involve focal discontinuities of the smooth muscle cell (SMC) layer that progresses later to a dramatic loss of SMCs in the tunica media of amyloid-loaded vessels. CAA has not been observed in young mice of 8 months of age [30]; in the framework of this hypothesis the normal response observed in 6-month-old APP23 mice as compared to controls might be explained by the absence of CAA at this age. Hence, fMRI data in this mouse model yield valuable information for the evaluation of the role of CAA in AD-related pathology. In APP23 mice, parenchymal Aβ levels have been reported to be increased already in

6-month-old mice [105]. Thus, the fMRI response observed in the mice correlates rather with CAA than with parenchymal Aβ levels. Furthermore, these studies in APP23 mice reveal that fMRI is an attractive tool for phenotyping of genetically engineered mice modeling human neuropathologies. Due to its noninvasive nature, functional consequences of disease progression can be investigated in longitudinal studies providing information on disease evolution in the individual that can be combined with more traditional readouts (i.e., behavioral assessments). The experimental procedures for our fMRI studies have been designed to allow repetitive measurement with a throughput as high as possible. Inhalatory anesthesia (isoflurane) has been chosen due to the ease of its administration and relative safety. Induction of anesthesia is fast and its maintenance easily performed. Recovery from inhalation anesthesia is fast. Mechanical ventilation using endotracheal intubation combined with a muscle relaxant provides stable values that can be maintained in the normal physiological range by adaptation of both the ventilation rate and volume based on continuous determination of blood-gas levels using a transcutaneous monitoring device. Further studies investigating the potential of fMRI readouts in genetically engineered mouse models of CNS disorders to characterize the disease phenotype and to assess the efficacy of a therapeutic intervention are therefore warranted.

6.4 CONCLUSION

MRI theoretically provides the spatial resolution needed to resolve neuritic plaques and the detection of Aβ plaques has been reported in postmortem human brain tissue [49]. Subsequent studies investigated the feasibility of visualizing Aβ deposits in brain tissue specimen of AD transgenic and in the intact animal either directly or following injection of targeted MR contrast agents possibly invasive after opening the blood–brain barrier [51–57]. Although measurement time recently approached a range acceptable to *in vivo* imaging [55], the sensitivity of this MR readout has to be further validated and evaluated in comparison with other imaging modalities (e.g., PET). Additional MRI readouts which have been used *in vivo* to successfully phenotype transgenic models of AD include volumetric measurements of brain atrophy [73,74], changes in MR relaxation times (T_2) [76], and in the proton diffusion properties of the brain parenchyma (ADC and DTI) [77, 78]. All these readouts could only detect reliable deviations from normal tissue in advanced disease stage. Similarly, the altered metabolic profile (i.e., NAA, glutamate, taurine) which has been detected in Tg2576 [83] and PS2APP [74] occur only in aged animals reflecting secondary pathophysiological changes, which are not specific for AD pathology. This limits the value of these readouts for early diagnosis and as prognostic tools for monitoring disease evolution or therapeutic interventions in preclinical studies.

The first clinical manifestation of AD is cognitive impairment such as degradation of short-term memory. fMRI has been shown to be an attractive tool for quantitative assessment of brain function in response to defined pharmacological or peripheral sensory stimulation also in mice [96]. Analyzing the CBV response in APP23 mice at various ages using a variety of stimuli (bicuculline, acetazolamide, and electrical stimulation of the hind paws), a reduced CBV response compared to control wildtype mice could be detected in 13 to 15-month-old transgenic animals [94,95]. The acetazolamide experiments indicate that this reduced response is due to a compromised vascular reserve capacity caused by the severe CAA. In fact, changes reflecting cerebrovascular abnormalities could be detected at an early time-point using time-of-flight angiography [80]. fMRI readouts probing the brain functional architecture complements more conventional morphological phenotyping and, at least in APP23 mice, display a high sensitivity to pathophysiological alterations and are superior in detecting early pathological alterations. Since the various AD mouse models are based on different APP cDNAs, FAD mutations, promoters and/ or genetic backgrounds, the appropriate MR readout for successful phenotyping may vary from line to line. Similarities and differences in the pathology of these various mouse models are being currently investigated. An important aspect is to differentiate transgenic "artifacts" from true disease-related changes. Therefore, measuring very young transgenic and their age-matched, wildtype littermates, and following age-related changes preferentially in a longitudinal approach is essential.

REFERENCES

1. Selkoe, D. J., Alzheimer's disease: genes, proteins, and therapy, *Physiol. Rev.*, 81, 741, 2001.
2. Hampel, H. et al., Biological marker candidates of Alzheimer's disease — perspectives for diagnosis, prediction of outcome and reflection of biological activity, *J. Neural. Transm.*, 111, 247, 2004.
3. Nestor, P. J., Scheltens, P., and Hodges, J. R., Advances in the early detection of Alzheimer's disease, *Nat. Rev. Neurosci.*, 5, S34, 2004.
4. Higgins, G. A. and Jacobsen, H., Transgenic mouse models of Alzheimer's disease: phenotype and application, *Behav. Pharmacol.*, 14, 419, 2003.
5. Phinney, A. L. et al., Mouse models of Alzheimer's disease: the long and filamentous road, *Neurol. Res.*, 25, 590, 2003.
6. Scorer, C. A., Preclinical and clinical challenges in the development of disease-modifying therapies for Alzheimer's disease, *Drug Discovery Today*, 6, 1207, 2001.
7. Nordberg, A., Towards an early diagnosis and treatment of Alzheimer's disease, *Int. Psychogeriatr.*, 15, 223, 2003.
8. Citron, M., Strategies for disease modification in Alzheimer's disease, *Nat. Rev. Neurosci.*, 5, 677, 2004.
9. Van Dam, D. et al., Symptomatic effect of donepezil, rivastigmine, galantamine and memantine on cognitive deficits in the APP23 model, *Psychopharmacology*, 180, 177, 2005.
10. Alzheimer, A., Ueber eine eigenartige Erkrankung der Hirnrinde, *Allg. Z. Psychiat. Psych.-Gericht. Med.*, 64, 146, 1907.
11. Graeber, M. B. et al., Histopathology and APOE genotype of the first Alzheimer disease patient, Auguste D, *Neurogenetics*, 1, 223, 1998.
12. Brion, J. et al., Mise en evidence immunologique de la protein tau au niveau des lesions de degenerescence neurofibrillaire de la maladie D'Alzheimer, *Arch. Biol.*, 95, 229, 1985.
13. Selkoe, D. J., The molecular pathology of Alzheimer's disease, *Neuron*, 6, 487, 1991.
14. Jarrett, J. T., Berger, E. P., and Lansbury, P. T. J., The carboxy terminus of the beta amyloid protein is critical for the seeding of amyloid formation: implications for the pathogenesis of Alzheimer's disease, *Biochemistry*, 32, 4693, 1993.
15. Masliah, E. and Rockenstein, E., Genetically altered transgenic models of Alzheimer's disease, *J. Neural. Transm.*, 59, 175, 2000.
16. Hock, B. J. J. and Lamb, B. T., Transgenic mouse models of Alzheimer's disease, *Trends Genet.*, 17, S7, 2001.
17. German, D. C. and Eisch, A. J., Mouse models of Alzheimer's disease: insight into treatment, *Rev. Neurosci.*, 15, 353, 2004.
18. Games, D. et al., Alzheimer-type neuropathology in transgenic mice over-expressing V717F beta-amyloid precursor protein, *Nature*, 373, 523, 1995.
19. Hsiao, K. et al., Correlative memory deficits, Abeta elevation, and amyloid plaques in transgenic mice, *Science*, 274, 99, 1996.
20. Sturchler-Pierrat, C. et al., Two amyloid precursor protein transgenic mouse models with Alzheimer disease-like pathology, *Proc. Natl. Acad. Sci. USA*, 94, 13287, 1997.
21. Chen, K. S. et al., Neurodegenerative Alzheimer-like pathology in PDAPP 717V− > F transgenic mice, *Prog. Brain Res.*, 117, 327, 1998.
22. Staufenbiel, M. and Sommer, B., Transgenic animal models in the development of therapeutic strategies for Alzheimer's Disease, In *Molecular Biology of Alzheimer's Disease: Genes and Mechanisms Involved in Amyloid Generation*, Haass, C., Ed., Harwood Academic Publishers, Amsterdam, pp. 309–326, 1998.
23. Duff, K. et al., Increased amyloid-beta42(43) in brains of mice expressing mutant presenilin 1, *Nature*, 383, 710, 1996.

24. Holcomb, L. et al., Accelerated Alzheimer-type phenotype in transgenic mice carrying both mutant amyloid precursor protein and presenilin 1 transgenes, *Nat. Med.*, 4, 97, 1998.
25. Richards, J. G. et al., PS2APP transgenic mice, coexpressing hPS2mut and hAPPswe, show age-related cognitive deficits associated with discrete brain amyloid deposition and inflammation, *J. Neurosci.*, 23, 8989, 2003.
26. Calhoun, M. E. et al., Neuron loss in APP transgenic mice, *Nature*, 395, 755, 1998.
27. Calhoun, M. E. et al., Neuronal overexpression of mutant amyloid precursor protein results in prominent deposition of cerebrovascular amyloid, *Proc. Natl. Acad. Sci. USA*, 96, 14088, 1999.
28. Phinney, A. L. et al., Cerebral amyloid induces aberrant axonal sprouting and ectopic terminal formation in amyloid precursor protein transgenic mice, *J. Neurosci.*, 19, 8552, 1999.
29. Burgermeister, P. et al., Mechanisms of cerebrovascular amyloid deposition. Lessons from mouse models, *Ann. N.Y. Acad. Sci.*, 903, 307, 2000.
30. Winkler, D. T. et al., Spontaneous hemorrhagic stroke in a mouse model of cerebral amyloid angiopathy, *J. Neurosci.*, 21, 1619, 2001.
31. Moechars, D. et al., Early phenotypic changes in transgenic mice that overexpress different mutants of amyloid precursor protein in brain, *J. Biol. Chem.*, 274, 6483, 1999.
32. Dodart, J. C. et al., Behavioral disturbances in transgenic mice overexpressing the V717F beta-amyloid precursor protein, *Behav. Neurosci.*, 113, 982, 1999.
33. Arendash, G. W. et al., Behavioral assessment of Alzheimer's transgenic mice following long-term Abeta vaccination: task specificity and correlations between Abeta deposition and spatial memory, *DNA Cell Biol.*, 20, 737, 2001.
34. Christie, R. et al., Structural and functional disruption of vascular smooth muscle cells in a transgenic mouse model of amyloid angiopathy, *Am. J. Pathol.*, 158, 1065, 2001.
35. Kelly, P. H. et al., Progressive age-related impairment of cognitive behavior in APP23 transgenic mice, *Neurobiol. Aging*, 24, 365, 2003.
36. Van Dam, D. et al., Age-dependent cognitive decline in the APP23 model precedes amyloid deposition, *Eur. J. Neurosci.*, 17, 388, 2003.
37. Chapman, P. F. et al., Impaired synaptic plasticity and learning in aged amyloid precursor protein transgenic mice, *Nat. Neurosci.*, 2, 271, 1999.
38. Hsia, A. Y. et al., Plaque-independent disruption of neural circuits in Alzheimer's disease mouse models, *Proc. Natl. Acad. Sci. USA*, 96, 3228, 1999.
39. Walsh, D. M. and Selkoe, D. J., Oligomers on the brain: the emerging role of soluble protein aggregates in neurodegeneration, *Protein Pept. Lett.*, 11, 213, 2004.
40. Cummings, B. J. and Cotman, C. W., Image analysis of beta-amyloid load in Alzheimer's disease and relation to dementia severity, *Lancet*, 346, 1524, 1995.
41. Morris, J. C. and Price, A. L., Pathologic correlates of nondemented aging, mild cognitive impairment, and early-stage Alzheimer's disease, *J. Mol. Neurosci.*, 17, 101, 2001.
42. Parvathy, S. et al., Correlation between Abetax-40-, Abetax-42-, and Abetax-43-containing amyloid plaques and cognitive decline, *Arch. Neurol.*, 58, 2025, 2001.
43. Kuo, Y. M. et al., Comparative analysis of amyloid-beta chemical structure and amyloid plaque morphology of transgenic mouse and Alzheimer's disease brains, *J. Biol. Chem.*, 276, 12991, 2001.
44. Gordon, M. N. et al., Time course of the development of Alzheimer-like pathology in the doubly transgenic PS1_APP mouse, *Exp. Neurol.*, 173, 183, 2002.
45. Brun, A., An overview of light and electron microscopic changes, In *Alzheimer's Disease: The Standard Reference Book*, Reisberg, B., Ed., The Free Press, New York, pp. 37–47, 1983.
46. Wisniewski, H. M., Neuritic (senile) and amyloid plaques, In *Alzheimer's Disease: The Standard Reference Book*, Reisberg, B., Ed., The Free Press, New York, pp. 57–61, 1983.
47. Huesgen, C. T. et al., In vitro MR microscopy of the hippocampus in Alzheimer's disease, *Neurology*, 43, 145, 1993.
48. Grundke-Iqbal, I. et al., Ferritin is a component of the neuritic (senile) plaque in Alzheimer dementia, *Acta Neuropathol*, 81, 105, 1990.
49. Benveniste, H. et al., Detection of neuritic plaques in Alzheimer's disease by magnetic resonance microscopy, *Proc. Natl. Acad. Sci. USA*, 96, 14079, 1999.
50. Dhenain, M. et al., Senile plaques do not induce susceptibility effects in T_2^*-weighted MR microscopic images, *NMR Biomed.*, 15, 197, 2002.

51. Rudin, M. et al., Characterization of CNS disorders and evaluation of therapy using structural and functional MRI, *Anal. Bioanal. Chem.*, 377, 973, 2003.
52. Lee, S. P. et al., Visualization of beta-amyloid plaques in a transgenic mouse model of Alzheimer's disease using MR microscopy without contrast reagents, *Magn. Reson. Med.*, 52, 538, 2004.
53. Zhang, J. et al., Detection of amyloid plaques in mouse models of Alzheimer's disease by magnetic resonance imaging, *Magn. Reson. Med.*, 51, 452, 2004.
54. Vanhoutte, G. et al., *In vivo* MRI can discern amyloid plaques in the Alzheimer APP[V717I] mouse model, *Proceedings of the International Society for Magnetic Resonance in Medicine, 10th Scientific Meeting Honolulu*, 2002, p. 1205.
55. Jack, C. R. Jr et al., In vivo visualization of Alzheimer's amyloid plaques by magnetic resonance imaging in transgenic mice without a contrast agent, *Magn. Reson. Med.*, 52, 1263, 2004.
56. Poduslo, J. F. et al., Molecular targeting of Alzheimer's amyloid plaques for contrast-enhanced magnetic resonance imaging, *Neurobiol. Dis.*, 11, 315, 2002.
57. Wadghiri, Y. Z. et al., Detection of Alzheimer's amyloid in transgenic mice using magnetic resonance microimaging, *Magn. Reson. Med.*, 50, 293, 2003.
58. Nordberg, A., PET imaging of amyloid in Alzheimer's disease, *Lancet Neurol.*, 3, 519, 2004.
59. Klunk, W. E. et al., Imaging the pathology of Alzheimer's disease: amyloid-imaging with positron emission tomography, *Neuroimaging Clin. N. Am.*, 13, 781, 2003, ix.
60. Klunk, W. E. et al., Imaging brain amyloid in Alzheimer's disease with Pittsburgh Compound-B, *Ann. Neurol.*, 55, 306, 2004.
61. Bacskai, B. J. et al., Four-dimensional multiphoton imaging of brain entry, amyloid binding, and clearance of an amyloid-beta ligand in transgenic mice, *Proc. Natl. Acad. Sci. USA*, 100, 12462, 2003.
62. Hintersteiner, M. et al., *In vivo* detection of amyloid-beta deposits by near-infrared imaging using an oxazine-derivative probe, *Nat. Biotechnol.*, 23, 577, 2005.
63. Sato, K. et al., Fluoro-substituted and 13C labeled styrylbenzene derivates for detecting brain amyloid plaques, *Eur. J. Med. Chem.*, 39, 573–578, 2004.
64. Higuchi, M. et al., 19F and 1H MRI detection of amyloid b plaques in vivo, *Nat. Neurosci.*, 8, 527, 2005.
65. Scheltens, P. et al., Structural magnetic resonance imaging in the practical assessment of dementia: beyond exclusion, *Lancet Neurol.*, 1, 13, 2002.
66. Knopman, D. S. et al., Practice parameter: diagnosis of dementia (an evidence-based review). Report of the Quality Standards Subcommittee of the American Academy of Neurology, *Neurology*, 56, 1143, 2001.
67. Frisoni, G. B. et al., Neuroimaging tools to rate regional atrophy, subcortical cerebrovascular disease, and regional cerebral blood flow and metabolism: consensus paper of the EADC, *J. Neurol. Neurosurg. Psychiat.*, 74, 1371, 2003.
68. Chetelat, G. and Baron, J. C., Early diagnosis of Alzheimer's disease: contribution of structural neuroimaging, *Neuroimage*, 18, 525, 2003.
69. Petrella, J. R., Coleman, R. E., and Doraiswamy, P. M., Neuroimaging and early diagnosis of Alzheimer disease: a look to the future, *Radiology*, 226, 315, 2003.
70. de Leon, M. J. et al., MRI and CSF studies in the early diagnosis of Alzheimer's disease, *J. Intern. Med.*, 256, 205, 2004.
71. Kantarci, K. and Jack, C. R. Jr., Neuroimaging in Alzheimer disease: an evidence-based review, *Neuroimaging Clin. N. Am.*, 13, 197, 2003.
72. Jack, C. R. Jr. et al., Comparison of different MRI brain atrophy rate measures with clinical disease progression in AD, *Neurology*, 62, 591, 2004.
73. Mueggler, T., Functional Magnetic Resonance Imaging of the Murine Brain: Application to a Transgenic Model of Alzheimer's Disease, Ph.D. thesis, University of Basel, 2002.
74. von Kienlin, M. et al., Altered metabolic profile in the frontal cortex of PS2APP transgenic mice, monitored throughout their life span, *Neurobiol. Dis.*, 18, 32, 2005.
75. Redwine, J. M. et al., Dentate gyrus volume is reduced before onset of plaque formation in PDAPP mice: A magnetic resonance microscopy and stereologic analysis, *Proc. Natl. Acad. Sci. USA*, 100, 1381, 2003.
76. Helpern, J. A. et al., MRI assessment of neuropathology in a transgenic mouse model of Alzheimer's disease, *Magn. Reson. Med.*, 51, 794, 2004.

77. Mueggler, T. et al., Restricted diffusion in the brain of transgenic mice with cerebral amyloidosis, *Eur. J. Neurosci.*, 20, 811, 2004.
78. Song, S. K. et al., Diffusion tensor imaging detects age-dependent white matter changes in a transgenic mouse model with amyloid deposition, *Neurobiol. Dis.*, 15, 640, 2004.
79. Gilbert, J. J. and Vinters, H. V., Cerebral amyloid angiopathy: incidence and complications in the aging brain. I. Cerebral hemorrhage, *Stroke*, 14, 915, 1983.
80. Beckmann, N. et al., Age-dependent cerebrovascular abnormalities and blood flow disturbances in APP23 mice modeling Alzheimer's disease, *J. Neurosci.*, 23, 8453, 2003.
81. Krucker, T. et al., Magnetic resonance angiography and vascular corrosion casting as tools in biomedical research: application to transgenic mice modeling Alzheimer's disease, *Neurol. Res.*, 26, 507, 2004.
82. Kantarci, K. et al., 1H MR spectroscopy in common dementias, *Neurology*, 63, 1393, 2004.
83. Dedeoglu, A. et al., Magnetic resonance spectroscopic analysis of Alzheimer's disease mouse brain that express mutant human APP shows altered neurochemical profile, *Brain Res.*, 1012, 60, 2004.
84. Block, W. et al., In-vivo proton MR-spectroscopy of the human brain: assessment of *N*-acetylaspartate (NAA) reduction as a marker for neurodegeneration, *Amino Acids*, 23, 317, 2002.
85. Small, S. A., Measuring correlates of brain metabolism with high-resolution MRI: a promising approach for diagnosing Alzheimer Disease and mapping its course, *Alzheimer Dis. Assoc. Disord.*, 17, 154, 2003.
86. Belliveau, J. W. et al., Functional cerebral imaging by susceptibility-contrast NMR, *Magn. Reson. Med.*, 14, 538, 1990.
87. Detre, J. A. et al., Perfusion imaging, *Magn. Reson. Med.*, 23, 37, 1992.
88. Kwong, K. K. et al., Dynamic magnetic resonance imaging of human brain activity during primary sensory stimulation, *Proc. Natl. Acad. Sci. USA*, 89, 5675, 1992.
89. Williams, D. S. et al., Fast serial MRI of perfusion in the rat brain using spin inversion of arterial water, *Bull. Magn. Reson.*, 15, 60, 1993.
90. Ogawa, S. et al., Brain magnetic resonance imaging with contrast dependent on blood oxygenation, *Proc. Natl. Acad. Sci. USA*, 87, 9868, 1990.
91. Buxton, R. B., *Introduction to Functional Magnetic Resonance Imaging: Principles and Techniques*, Cambridge University Press, Cambridge, 2002.
92. Nair, G. and Duong, T. Q., Echo-planar BOLD fMRI of mice on a narrow-bore 9.4 T magnet, *Magn. Reson. Med.*, 52, 430, 2004.
93. Kuriwaki, J. et al., Comparison of brain activity between dopamine D2 receptor-knockout and wild mice in response to dopamine agonist and antagonist assessed by fMRI, *Neurosignals*, 13, 227, 2004.
94. Mueggler, T. et al., Age-dependent impairment of somatosensory response in the amyloid precursor protein 23 transgenic mouse model of Alzheimer's disease, *J. Neurosci.*, 23, 8231, 2003.
95. Mueggler, T. et al., Compromised hemodynamic response in amyloid precursor protein transgenic mice, *J. Neurosci.*, 22, 7218, 2002.
96. Mueggler, T. et al., Bicuculline-induced brain activation in mice detected by functional magnetic resonance imaging, *Magn. Reson. Med.*, 46, 292, 2001.
97. Ahrens, E. T. and Dubowitz, D. J., Peripheral somatosensory fMRI in mouse at 11.7 T, *NMR Biomed.*, 14, 318, 2001.
98. Huang, W. et al., Magnetic resonance imaging (MRI) detection of the murine brain response to light: temporal differentiation and negative functional MRI changes, *Proc. Natl. Acad. Sci. USA*, 93, 6037, 1996.
99. Hyder, F. et al., Dynamic magnetic resonance imaging of the rat brain during forepaw stimulation, *J. Cereb. Blood Flow Metab.*, 14, 649, 1994.
100. Mandeville, J. B. et al., Dynamic functional imaging of relative cerebral blood volume during rat forepaw stimulation, *Magn. Reson. Med.*, 39, 615, 1998.
101. Reese, T. et al., Cytoprotection does not preserve brain functionality in rats during the acute post-stroke phase despite evidence of non-infarction provided by MRI, *NMR Biomed.*, 13, 361, 2000.
102. Chen, Y. C. et al., Detection of dopaminergic neurotransmitter activity using pharmacologic MRI: correlation with PET, microdialysis, and behavioral data, *Magn. Reson. Med.*, 38, 389, 1997.

103. Reese, T. et al., Regional brain activation by bicuculline visualized by functional magnetic resonance imaging. Time-resolved assessment of bicuculline-induced changes in local cerebral blood volume using an intravascular contrast agent, *NMR Biomed.*, 13, 43, 2000.
104. Graham, G. D. et al., BOLD MRI monitoring of changes in cerebral perfusion induced by acetazolamide and hypercarbia in the rat, *Magn. Reson. Med.*, 31, 557, 1994.
105. Sommer, B. et al., Transgenic approaches to model Alzheimer's disease, *Rev. Neurosci.*, 11, 47, 2000.

7 Imaging Alzheimer's Disease with MRI

Scott A. Small

CONTENTS

7.1 INTRODUCTION

Historical progress in medicine can be charted along the lines of technical innovations that have visualized the invisible. In this regard, the end of the 19th century was a landmark period. At around the same time that staining techniques were developed that visualized the histology of normal and diseased brains, Wilhelm Roentgen introduced the x-ray that visualized normal and abnormal internal structures in living people. In 1906, a few years after Roentgen received the first Noble prize in physics for his achievement, Alois Alzheimer first visualized amyloid plaques and neurofibrillary tangles — key features of his eponymonous disease — by looking at dead brains under the microscope. Now, almost a century later, these separate achievements are converging with the development of imaging techniques that visualize Alzheimer's disease among the living.

Alzheimer's disease (AD), one of the most common disorders of the brain, begins as mild forgetfulness by targeting the hippocampal formation, ultimately sweeping throughout the cortical surface and devastating most cognitive abilities in its wake. Almost a 100 years since Alzheimer first described his disease, we still do not have effective drugs to treat this ravaging disorder. Nevertheless, remarkable strides have been made during the last decade uncovering some, though not all, of the molecular mechanisms contributing to AD. With these advances, there is now justifiable optimism that we have entered a new pharmacological era in which treatment for AD will soon be available.

Magnetic resonance imaging (MRI)-based imaging techniques have the potential to impact this new era in two fundamental ways: First, MRI can be used to test the efficacy of new drugs, and second, MRI can be used to diagnose AD, preferably in its earliest stages.

In the long and often treacherous course of drug development, many compounds that work *in vitro* need to be tested *in vivo*. Although ameliorating cognitive deficits are the ultimate goal of any treatment, relying solely on neuropsychological testing to assess drug efficacy is problematic.

Longitudinal testing is the ideal experimental design for drug testing, in which an outcome measure is tested repeatedly before and multiple time points after drug delivery. Unfortunately, cognitive testing suffers from the test-retest artifact. Because of repeated exposure, subjects simply perform better by improving their test-taking skills, masking the true cognitive metric under investigation. Resorting to cross-sectional designs is possible — comparing separate groups on and off drug — but then a large number of subjects is needed to control against the long list of demographic confounds that notoriously affect neuropsychological performance.

Aside from the parametric artifacts associated with experimental design, neuropsychological testing has to contend with a number of theoretical concerns as well. The hippocampal formation is in fact a complex circuit made up of interconnecting subregions. The entorhinal cortex is the hippocampal subregion most vulnerable to AD, manifesting as relatively subtle synaptic dysfunction. Because of compensatory mechanisms that are known to exist within the hippocampal circuit, these earliest changes may not be readily apparent at the behavioral level. Even when they do become apparent, early deficits on tests of hippocampal-dependent memory may not distinguish early AD from other entities that target the hippocampus. For example, normal aging itself also affects hippocampal function, cognitively overlapping with the earliest stages of AD, although aging interrupts the hippocampal circuit by targeting subregions other than the entorhinal cortex. Thus, neuropsychological tests may be insensitive at the earliest stages of AD, and even when early AD is behaviorally detectable, hippocampal-dependent memory tests are currently not specific enough to reliably diagnosis AD.

Despite these concerns, there is no question that behavioral testing must be included during the final stages of drug development. In fact, through complex experimental design and more detailed longitudinal studies, both the practical and theoretical concerns of neuropsychological testing can be addressed. Nevertheless, an imaging technique that can visualize the pathological changes associated with AD holds great promise as a tool that can significantly enhance our precision in determining the true utility of any drug.

Diagnostics is the second utility for which MRI holds great promise. As drugs do become available, the issue of early diagnosis will become a matter of great urgency. For obvious reasons, drugs will more likely achieve the therapeutic goal of arresting disease progression when applied to the earliest stage of disease. Currently, the greatest diagnostic challenge is for detecting AD in its earliest stages, when it cognitively overlaps with normal aging.

In this chapter, the anatomy and pathophysiology of AD will first be reviewed, serving as a guiding post for how best to translate the remarkable power of MRI into a clinically useful tool. Then, different MRI approaches will be reviewed that, in principle, can visualize the separate pathological stages through which AD progresses. Separate sections will cover different general approaches, and each section will end with a summary of strengths and weaknesses. The section on functional MRI requires the most discussion, since this MRI approach is in many ways the most varied, both in meaning and in practical implementation (see also Chapter 11, Section 11.4.1). Although a potentially important technique, because of its limited spatial resolution, MRS will not be covered in this chapter. Finally, the different MRI approaches will be compared in terms of their ability to diagnose and detect drug efficacy in AD.

7.2 THE ANATOMY AND PATHOPHYSIOLOGY OF ALZHEIMER'S DISEASE

Prospective neuropsychological studies have made the fundamental observation that AD begins in the hippocampal formation [1,2]. The hippocampus itself is made up of anatomically distinct subregions (Figure 7.1) and recent microarray studies have shown that each hippocampal subregion expresses a unique molecular profile [3]. Although over time most subregions manifest AD pathology, these molecular observations underlie the assumption that early on AD targets the hippocampus with regional selectivity [4].

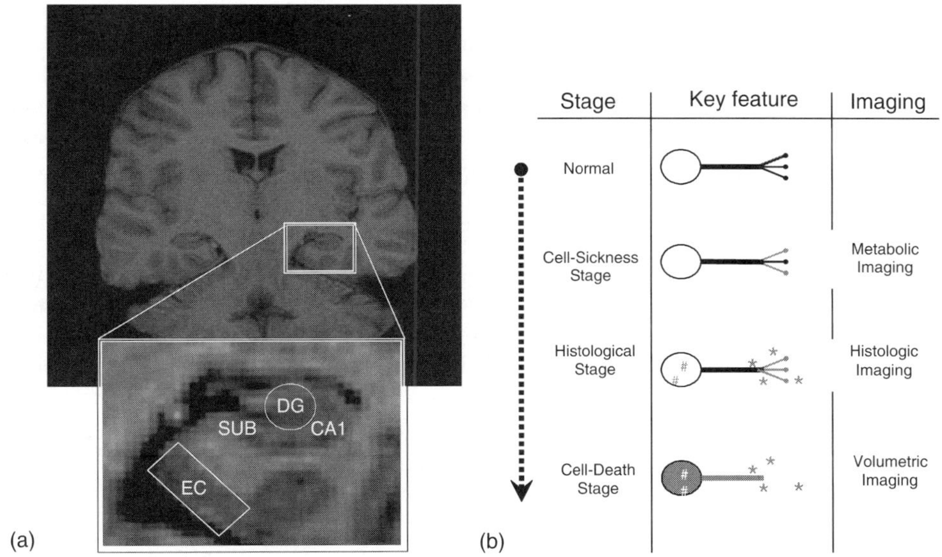

FIGURE 7.1 The anatomy and pathophysiology of Alzheimer's disease (AD) (a) The anatomy of AD. Cognitive studies have identified the hippocampal formation as the brain structure where Alzheimer's begins. *Post-mortem* and imaging studies have pinpointed the entorhinal cortex (EC) as the subregion within the hippocampal formation that is most vulnerable to AD. The dentate gyrus (DG) is the hippocampal subregion most resistant to dysfunction and cell death. The subiculum (SUB) forms the most inferior portion of the hippocampus and controls most of the entorhinal-hippocampal output. (b) The pathophysiology of AD. Recent studies in humans and mouse models of disease suggests that AD progresses through the following pathological stages. During the first cell-sickness stage, AD causes neurons to malfunction, manifesting as synaptic or metabolic failure; during the second histological stage, AD causes insoluble protein aggregation, typified by amyloid plaques and neurofibrillary tangles; and finally, during the cell-death stage, Alzheimer's begins killing off neurons, resulting in neuronal and volumetric loss.

In vitro markers of AD pathology — such as amyloid plaques, neurofibrillary tangles, or cell loss — applied to *post-mortem* tissue can be used to test this assumption. With notable exceptions [5], *post-mortem* studies suggest that either the entorhinal cortex [6–11] or the CA1 subfield [6–8, 12,13] are candidate sites of primary vulnerability. In many of these studies, the entorhinal cortex and the CA1 were not assessed simultaneously, accounting in part for the reported inconsistencies. More generally, however, isolating the hippocampal subregion most vulnerable to AD may be challenging relying on *post-mortem* studies alone. Not only are *post-mortem* series biased against the earliest and most discriminatory stages of disease, but synaptic dysfunction is an early defect that can occur independently of amyloid plaques, neurofibrillary tangles, and cell loss [14].

In this regard, functional imaging techniques that assess synaptic dysfunction in all hippocampal subregions have nicely complemented *in vitro* studies [15]. These studies have pinpointed the entorhinal cortex as the single hippocampal subregion most vulnerable to AD (Figure 7.1). Furthermore, in agreement with histological findings, imaging studies have also showed that the dentate gyrus is the hippocampal subregion most resistant to AD [16].

The entorhinal cortex, therefore, appears to be the nidus in which AD begins and from where AD progresses anatomically, ultimately involving other hippocampal subregions and sweeping throughout the temporal, parietal, and frontal lobes. Thus, the anatomy of AD suggests that an imaging technique that can visualize the entorhinal cortex is ideally suited for detecting and mapping the clinical course of disease. Among all imaging techniques, MRI possesses the best spatial resolution, and high resolution is required to reliably visualize the diminutive entorhinal cortex.

AD does not only progress anatomically, but within each region, AD progresses pathophysiologically as well. Human studies and, in particular, studies investigating mouse models of disease (see Chapter 6) have suggested different stages through which Alzheimer's disease progresses (Figure 7.1). During the first cell-sickness stage, AD causes neurons to malfunction, manifesting as synaptic or metabolic failure. During the second histological stage, AD causes insoluble protein aggregation, typified by amyloid plaques and neurofibrillary tangles. Finally, during the cell-death stage, Alzheimer's begins killing off neurons, resulting in neuronal and volumetric loss.

It is important to emphasize that these stages are not categorically exclusive, and at this point this pattern of progression serves only as a working model. Only by perfecting imaging techniques sensitive to each pathological feature and following a group of subjects over time, will the true pathological progression of the disease be established. In any case, our current understanding of the pathological progression of AD — even if only a working model — provides the backbone upon which imaging techniques can be organized. In the next three sections, we will review how MRI can, in principle, capture each of these pathological stages of AD.

7.3 IMAGING THE CELL-SICKNESS STAGE OF AD WITH FUNCTIONAL MRI

It is important to maintain a precise definition of the function in functional imaging, so as not to misinterpret its meaning or utility. Over the 50 years that the field has evolved, since the seminal work by Kety and Schmidt [17], functional brain imaging has come to imply a method that detects regional energy metabolism. Energy metabolism is best defined as the rate with which cells produce ATP, which in neurons — obligate aerobes who do not store glucose — requires the consumption of oxygen and glucose from the bloodstream. Visualizing ATP directly is challenging, but imaging techniques have been developed that can visualize correlates of oxygen and glucose consumption. With the use of radiolabeled glucose, positron emission tomography (PET) can quantify the regional rates of glucose uptake, which under certain assumptions corresponds to energy metabolism.

In contrast, MRI-based techniques have typically relied on the second ingredient of ATP production, oxygen consumption, to visualize correlates of energy metabolism. As in any organ, an increase in oxygen consumption is accompanied by an increase in oxygen delivery, i.e., accelerated blood flow. In the brain, this relationship is governed intrinsically and with regional specificity, although the biochemical mechanisms for this regional regulation remain poorly understood. Arterial spin labeling (ASL), a technique introduced by Alsop and Detre [18], is the only MRI approach that can directly and absolutely quantify regional cerebral blood flow (CBF).

Because postcapillary venules are low resistant vessels, pressure shifts caused by changes in CBF lead to concomitant changes in regional cerebral blood volume (CBV). Predictably, CBV turns out to be another hemodynamic variable that corresponds to oxygen consumption and that correlates with energy metabolism. In fact, metabolic-induced changes in CBV is what Roy and Sherrington measured in their historic studies over a century ago — not CBF as commonly and mistakenly thought [19]. Belliveau et al. introduced the first MRI-based technique, which relies on intravascular contrast agents like gadolinium to estimate regional CBV [20]. Note, that in the clinical setting this technique is often called perfusion MRI, because CBV maps can be converted to CBF maps by making certain assumptions about mean transit time and arterial input functions. One limitation of this approach for the purposes of diagnostics is that it only generates a relative estimate of CBV, not an absolute quantification measure. Lin et al. introduced a modification of this approach [21], in which a contrast agent is injected but the signal changes are measured in the steady state, not in the dynamic state. This approach offers the advantage of more precise quantification of CBV and greater spatial resolution [21].

Finally, deoxyhemoglobin content is the third hemodynamic variable that correlates with oxygen consumption and energy metabolism, and which can be visualized with MRI. By having rodents breath different concentrations of oxygen, Ogawa and colleagues were the first to show that regional differences in basal levels of deoxyhemoglobin can be visualized with MRI [22]. By using drugs to alter basal brain metabolism [23] and then by using behavioral task to alter metabolism more acutely [24], subsequent studies have documented that the correlation between deoxyhemoglobin content and energy metabolism is inverted: an increase in energy metabolism will lead to a decrease in deoxyhemoglobin content.

This somewhat counterintuitive inversion can be understood by examining the formulae with which deoxyhemoglobin content is derived:

$$\text{deoxyhemoglobin content} = \text{deoxyhemoglobin concentration} \times \text{CBV} \tag{7.1}$$

Based on Fick's principle,

$$\text{deoxyhemoglobin concentration} = \text{oxygen consumption}/\text{CBF} \tag{7.2}$$

so that

$$\text{deoxyhemoglobin content} = (\text{oxygen consumption}/\text{CBF}) \times \text{CBV} \tag{7.3}$$

A range of empirical studies have established that for every unit increase in oxygen consumption there is an approximately squared increase in CBF [25], and thus, according to the derivations above this will lead to a decrease in deoxyhemoglobin concentration. Note, also, that because it is based on a complex and conflicting interplay between CBF and CBV, deoxyhemoglobin content is the only MRI correlate of metabolism that is nonquantitative.

Now that function has been defined as a correlate of oxygen metabolism, metabolism itself needs to be linked to cell-sickness. Energy metabolism is by definition a dynamic process, constantly shifting its rates in response to internal or external stimuli. Thus, the term resting metabolism, which we and others have previously used [26], is in fact a misnomer; brain metabolism is never at rest. More accurately, a distinction should be made between internal or external stimuli that change metabolism acutely — over milliseconds or seconds — vs. stimuli that change metabolism over longer time periods, affecting basal metabolic rates. The distinction of acute vs. basal changes in metabolism layers on to the way in which investigators of metabolism have dichotomized the primary sources of neuronal energy production. Half of neuronal ATP production is dedicated to bioelectric processes [27], in particular any shift in the membrane potential. Note that a shift in postsynaptic potentials can occur with and without spike activity. The other 50% of ATP is dedicated to a long list of biochemical processes, which importantly includes protein synthesis, axonal transport, and synaptogenesis [28].

Finally, the distinction between bioelectric vs. biochemical sources of energy consumption layers on the two physiologic mechanisms with which neurons change function — either by changing synaptic activity or by changing synaptic strength (Figure 7.1). Long-term increases in synaptic strength occurs by increasing presynaptic neurotransmitter release, by increasing postsynaptic receptor density, or by synaptogenesis. In any case, the relatively long time courses of the biochemical mechanisms that govern these long-term effects will alter the basal metabolic rates of the neuron.

This scheme is helpful not only for understanding the different meanings of brain function viz-à-viz brain metabolism, but also for determining the type of function that is most informative for a particular question (Figure 7.2). Cognitively, one can ask which brain regions change synaptic activity in response to a brief external stimulus — i.e., mapping sensory representation — in which case an imaging technique is required to map acute changes in energy metabolism. In contrast,

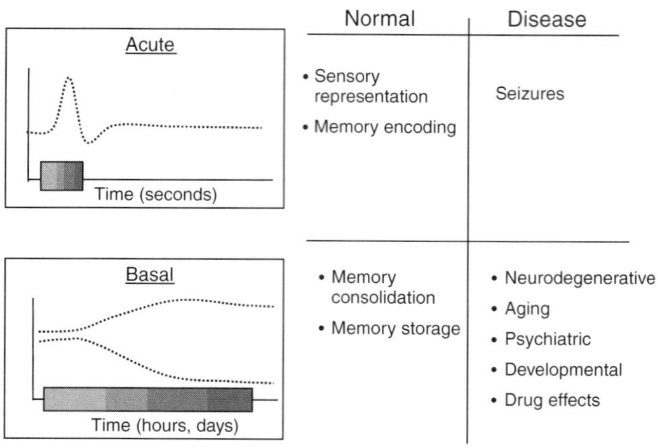

FIGURE 7.2 Functional MRI can be used to map normal brain function and brain disease. Normal brain function. Functional imaging can map changes in acute metabolism that occurs during sensory representation or memory encoding, or to map changes in basal metabolism that occurs during memory consolidation and memory storage. Abnormal brain function. Functional imaging can be used to map acute changes in metabolism that occur during seizure activity, or to map changes in basal metabolism that occur in most diseases of the brain, including AD.

asking which brain regions change synaptic strength in order to store the sensory representation in long-term memory is, metabolically speaking, a different question. Insofar that the biochemical mechanisms that govern synaptic strength — mechanisms that underlie long-term memory — require synaptogenesis, protein synthesis, and even axonal transport, than this change will be most evident in measures of basal metabolism (Figure 7.2).

Clinically, functional imaging is typically used to localize the lesion for diagnostic purposes, or for mapping the natural clinical course of disease or in response to therapeutic intervention. In the case of mapping seizures, the primary disorder is one of transient increase in synaptic activity and so a metabolic map should be sensitive to changes in bioelectricity. In contrast, the cell-sickness stage of AD, or cell-sickness that occurs in other physiological disorders, is characterized by a decrease in synaptic strength and not by a change in synaptic activity *per se* (Figure 7.2). This has been demonstrated in humans relying on molecular markers of synaptic function such as synaptophysin [28], and in mice relying on electrophysiological measures showing uniform deficits in basal synaptic transmission [29], or sometimes long-term potentiation. The primary change in synaptic strength accounts for why both *in vitro* and *in vivo* measures of basal metabolism uniformly detect focal deficits in these disorders, even when cell loss is not a factor.

In principle, of course, changes in basal metabolism might be difficult to detect and in this case using an external stimuli that acutely activates an affected brain area may further enhance lesion detection — akin to cardiac testing when a resting electrocardiogram is normal or ambiguous and a stress-test brings out the lesion. In fact, stimulus-induced changes in deoxyhemoglobin content, the so-called BOLD effect, has been used to map metabolic defects in AD [30–32].

Nevertheless, a number of advantages are gained if a lesion can be detected in its primary basal state. Because AD does have basal metabolic defects, the BOLD response is essentially an acute-on-chronic experiment, which is prone to misinterpretation. This point can be illustrated by considering the differences in the BOLD response between primary visual cortex and motor cortex. The basal metabolic state of the visual cortex is typically lower compared to the motor cortex [33], which is reflected by higher levels of basal deoxyhemoglobin [34]. Thus, when the visual cortex is stimulated there is more deoxyhemoglobin to be washed out, which will artificially amplify the BOLD response [34]. This wash-out effect has been invoked to account for why visual stimulation results in an artificially larger BOLD response compared to motor stimulation [34], even if the degree of neuronal stimulation is assumed equivalent. One might conclude that the motor cortex is dysfunctional compared to the visual cortex, but this would obviously be a mistake, and is simply caused by differences in the basal state. Thus, differences in basal metabolic rates act as a confound when comparing the acute BOLD response between separate brain regions. A similar acute-on-chronic problem exists when comparing the same brain regions in AD patients and controls, because AD reduces basal metabolic states.

A second advantage of relying of measurements of basal metabolism is the greater superior spatial resolution it affords. Higher temporal resolution is needed when setting out to measure a stimulus-induced change in acute metabolism. Like the logic of any camera, temporal resolution trades off with spatial resolution. Although this trade-off may be irrelevant when measuring acute metabolic changes in large cortical areas, the compromise in spatial resolution makes it more difficult to reliably visualize small brain regions, such as the entorhinal cortex. Because the entorhinal cortex is only a few millimeters in dimension, MRI pulse sequences with submillimeter resolution have been found preferable when investigating the entorhinal cortex. When optimized, BOLD scanning has been able to visualize the entorhinal cortex; however, because the resolution is supramillimeter only a few pixels can be sampled from the entorhinal cortex, and is therefore prone to error. In contrast, a submillimeter image — which is more easily achieved when investigating the basal metabolic state — provides dozens of entorhinal cortex pixels, yielding and, because of the high sampling, generating a more reliable metric.

To summarize, MRI can be made sensitive to three hemodynamic variables that correlate with neuronal energy metabolism and thus all can, in principle, detect the metabolic changes associated with AD-related cell-sickness. Nevertheless, important differences exist among the MRI measurements, as summarized in Figure 7.3, with a particular emphasis placed on two factors: The first is whether the measurement can be acquired with sufficient spatial resolution with which to generate multiple sample points from the diminutive entorhinal cortex; and the second is whether the measurement generates an absolute quantification of the hemodynamic correlate, a factor critical for diagnostics. For example, measurements of CBF using techniques like ASL, score high marks on quantification, but unfortunately cannot achieve the desired submillimeter resolution. In direct opposition, measurements sensitive to basal deoxyhemoglobin can be acquired with sufficient spatial resolution, but for the reasons listed above cannot be acquired quantitatively. Fortunately, measurements of CBV fulfill both requirements — submillimeter resolution and quantification — and therefore may turn out to be the best MRI metric with which to visualize cell-sickness in the entorhinal cortex of AD.

7.4 IMAGING THE HISTOLOGIC STAGE OF ALZHEIMER'S DISEASE WITH STRUCTURAL AND CONTRAST-ENHANCED MRI

Almost a century after Alzheimer himself visualized amyloid plaques and neurofibrillary tangles in dead brains, imaging techniques are being perfected allowing us to visualize this histological stage of AD in living brains. As mentioned earlier, the true pattern of histological progression — both spatially and temporally — is still a matter of debate for the very reason that, until recently, we did not have the opportunity to follow these histological changes in living subjects over time. For example, recent findings using PET radioligands, suggest that amyloid plaques may begin in the frontal lobes [35], which agrees with studies investigating transgenic mice who develop both plaques and tangles [36]. Whether this spatial mismatch between plaque burden and cognitive deficits, which show that frontal lobes deficits occur only later in the disease, is real or simply reflects the relatively coarse spatial resolution of PET remains to be determined.

Indeed, PET imaging struck first when it comes to visualizing amyloid plaques in living brains [10,35]. However, in the playing field of *in vivo* imaging there are those who maintain that anything

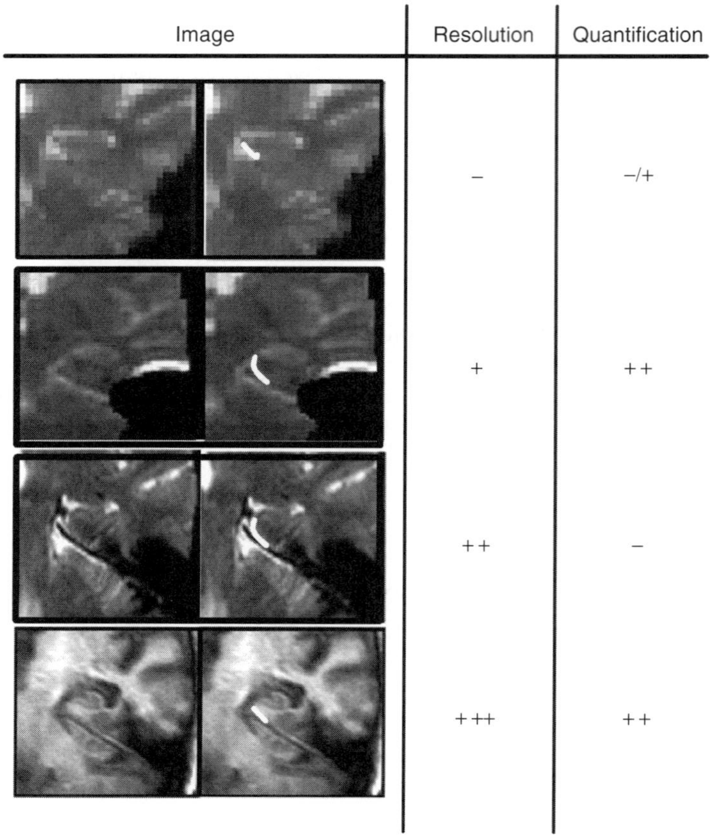

FIGURE 7.3 Detecting metabolic changes in the entorhinal cortex in Alzheimer's disease. MRI can visualize three correlates of oxygen metabolism: cerebral blood flow (CBF), cerebral blood volume (CBV), and deoxyhemoglobin (dHB) content. The left column shows the actual images acquired for assessing acute changes in dHB with BOLD (top panel), basal CBF with ASL (second panel), basal dHB (third panel), and basal CBV with a steady-state approach (bottom panel). The MRI techniques that assess these three correlates differ along two factors, spatial resolution and degree of quantification, as prioritized with +s or −s in the middle and right columns.

PET can do MRI can do better. MRI does in fact enjoy a number of theoretical and practical advantages over PET. Key among these is the superior spatial resolution afforded by MRI which can more reliably visualize the diminutive entorhinal cortex. From a practical point of view, MRI is safer than PET since it does not require the injection of radioactive material. MRI is also cheaper, typically costing a quarter of the price of a PET scan. Finally, because MRI technology is conventionally used in medicine, MRI scanners are more readily available. These practical advantages will play an increasing important role as these imaging techniques become clinically relevant.

For these reasons, a number of teams have been trying to develop MRI-based approaches to visualize amyloid plaques in living brains [37–39]. Two general approaches have been developed; however, to date they have only been tested in transgenic mice (see also Chapter 6). The first relies on the observation that amyloid plaques cause a loss of signal in T_2-weighed MRI scans, likely because of their high iron content. The second approach is conceptually similar to the PET scanning. By developing MRI-sensitive compounds that pass through the blood-brain barrier and bind to amyloid plaques *in vivo*, these approaches have visualized amyloid plaques in living brains.

A recent variation of this approach relies on plaque-binding compounds that are fluorinated with F19, thereby maximizing signal-to-noise [40].

Of course, visualizing AD in living patients, not in mice, is the ultimate goal of this technical development. In contrast to PET, all MRI-based approaches that visualize amyloid plaques have, to date, done so only in mice. Successfully translating these approaches to humans is the next important step — a step that is not trivial. The main hurdle is the long scanning time, typically hours in duration, used to visualize amyloid plaques in mice. In humans, particularly elderly patients, scan time must be drastically reduced to less than 60 min. Furthermore, mouse imaging is performed under anesthesia which artificially reduces head motion, and in high-field scanners that are not conventionally available for humans. Mice studies do, however, provide proof-of-principle, and there is reason to believe that the current technical limitations can be overcome, and that these techniques will, in the future, become applicable to humans.

Because they are intracellular, image-sensitive ligands directed against neurofibrillary tangles have the added challenge of penetrating the cell membrane, and as such are more likely to be toxic. Nevertheless, a prior PET study has reported visualizing neurofibrillary tangles [10].

7.5 IMAGING THE CELL-DEATH STAGE OF ALZHEIMER'S DISEASE WITH VOLUMETRIC MRI

A strikingly shriveled cortex is one of the most remarkable features of a brain removed from a patient who dies with many years of AD. Historically, this shrinkage was thought to be caused by the severe cell loss that characterizes late-stage AD under the microscope. Recent studies have demonstrated, however, that cortical thinning and volume loss can occur independently of cell loss [41], suggesting that other mechanisms contribute to brain shrinkage. Nevertheless, most experts in the field who use volumetric MRI to image AD maintain they are measuring cell death.

Almost as soon as imaging techniques began visualizing brain anatomy in living subjects, investigators applied the technique to search for anatomical correlates of brain disorders, including AD. By the late 1980s, a number of groups sprearheaded the effort to translate the exquisite anatomical detail provided by MRI into a clinically meaningful tool [42–45]. Since that time, additional groups have introduced protocols that are ideally suited to quantify the volume of the entorhinal cortex and the rest of the hippocampus [46–53]. Multiple studies have now applied these approaches, both cross-sectionally as well longitudinally, typically documenting entorhinal volume loss as the best indicator of disease.

Volume, by definition, is a measure that can be absolutely quantified. Although attempts can be made to quantify the measures generated by either metabolic MRI or histologic MRI (i.e., plaque detection), they will likely never reach the parametric purity of a simple volume. Thus, even though there are issues remaining about how best to outline structures, volumetric MRI scores the highest marks on parametric precision. Nevertheless, of all the MRI measures discussed the actual biologic underpinnings of brain volume are the least understood. Gaining this understanding is imperative, not only to fend off accusations of neophrenology but also to better interpret what volume loss means diagnostically and what kind of volume changes should be expected in association with treatment.

7.6 CONCLUSION

During the last decade important insights have been obtained about the molecular mechanisms underlying AD, and these insights have ushered in a new era of pharmacologic optimism. Accordingly, the ability to develop an imaging technique that can reliably detect the earliest stage of AD has become more important than ever. Not only would this technique be used to screen for efficacy among the growing numbers of candidate compounds designed to treat AD, but also once compounds are identified, it could be used to determine which subjects are truly harboring early, predementia, AD.

The progression of AD can be provisionally subdivided into different pathological stages, and, in principle, the pathological feature of each stage can be captured with different MRI-based approaches. Diagnostically, the greatest challenge is detecting AD in its earliest stages, when it causes only mild forgetfulness that overlaps with normal aging. Therefore, the ability to detect the first cell-sickness stage of AD may be the most promising approach. Of course, detecting soluble protein aggregation or volume loss with MRI will be helpful in diagnosing the later stages of disease. In terms of using imaging to screen for effective drugs, the proposed mechanism of a given drug will dictate which imaging tool is warranted. Thus, an imaging tool that visualizes amyloid plaques is ideally suited to test the effect of drugs designed to reduce plaque burden (the so called plaque busters), while volumetric MRI can test for drugs that prevent cell death, and metabolic techniques can test for drugs designed to stave off the earliest manifestations of disease.

The remarkable technical developments in MRI technology justify the excitement engendered by this latest era in the history of visualizing disease. Nevertheless, generating a picture is only the beginning. Let's not forget that it took x-ray technology many years before it was proven clinically useful, and, for example, the true utility of mammography is still debated. Indeed, not a single MRI technique discussed in this chapter has been validated, either diagnostically or as a tool for drug discovery.

Future studies must progress along two parallel lines of investigation. First, all MRI approaches need to be investigated in animal models of disease, so that the *in vivo* images can be correlated with gold standard *in vitro* measures of synaptic function, histological markers, or cell loss. Only by performing this due diligence will we avert misinterpretations, such as the false conclusion that spike activity must underlie the BOLD response, or that cell death must underlie volume loss. Second, all MRI approaches, no matter how conceptually sound, need to be tested in large-scale, epidemiologically rigorous, human studies. Only by imaging a large of group of healthy subjects and following them prospectively through dementia and until death will establish the true clinical utility of MRI as a tool to visualize AD.

ACKNOWLEDGMENTS

This work was supported in part by federal grants, AG07232, AG08702, AG025161; the Beeson Faculty Scholar Award from the American Federation of Aging; the McKnight Neuroscience of Brain Disorders Award; and The James S. McDonnell Foundation.

REFERENCES

1. Jacobs, D. M. et al., Neuropsychological detection and characterization of preclinical Alzheimer's disease, *Neurology*, 45, 957, 1995.
2. Masur, D. M. et al., Neuropsychological prediction of dementia and the absence of dementia in healthy elderly persons, *Neurology*, 44, 1427, 1994.
3. Zhao, X. et al., Transcriptional profiling reveals strict boundaries between hippocampal subregions, *J. Comp. Neurol.*, 441, 187, 2001.
4. Small, S. A., Age-related memory decline; current concepts and future directions, *Arch. Neurol.*, 58, 360, 2001.
5. Simic, G. et al., Volume and number of neurons of the human hippocampal formation in normal aging and Alzheimer's disease, *J. Comp. Neurol.*, 379, 482, 1997.
6. Price, J. L. et al., Neuron number in the entorhinal cortex and CA1 in preclinical Alzheimer disease, *Arch. Neurol.*, 58, 1395, 2001.

7. Fukutani, Y. et al., Neuronal loss and neurofibrillary degeneration in the hippocampal cortex in late-onset sporadic Alzheimer's disease, *Psychiatry Clin. Neurosci.*, 54, 523, 2000.
8. Giannakopoulos, P. et al., Tangle and neuron numbers, but not amyloid load, predict cognitive status in Alzheimer's disease, *Neurology*, 60, 1495, 2003.
9. Braak, H. and Braak, E., Evolution of the neuropathology of Alzheimer's disease, *Acta Neurol. Scand. Suppl.*, 165, 3, 1996.
10. Shoghi-Jadid, K. et al., Localization of neurofibrillary tangles and beta-amyloid plaques in the brains of living patients with Alzheimer disease, *Am. J. Geriatr. Psychiatry*, 10, 24, 2002.
11. Schonheit, B., Zarski, R., and Ohm, T. G., Spatial and temporal relationships between plaques and tangles in Alzheimer-pathology, *Neurobiol. Aging*, 25, 697, 2004.
12. West, M. J. et al., Hippocampal neurons in pre-clinical Alzheimer's disease, *Neurobiol. Aging*, 25, 1205, 2004.
13. West, M. J., Regionally specific loss of neurons in the aging human hippocampus, *Neurobiol. Aging*, 14, 287, 1993.
14. Selkoe, D. J., Alzheimer's disease is a synaptic failure, *Science*, 298, 789, 2002.
15. Small, S. A. et al., Evaluating the function of hippocampal subregions with high-resolution MRI in Alzheimer's disease and aging, *Microsc. Res. Tech.*, 51, 101, 2000.
16. Small, S. A. et al., Imaging hippocampal function across the human life span: is memory decline normal or not?, *Ann. Neurol.*, 51, 290, 2002.
17. Kety, S. S. and Schmidt, C. F., The nitrous oxide method for the quantitative determination of cerebral blood flow in man: theory, procedure and normal values, *J. Clin. Invest.*, 27, 476, 1948.
18. Alsop, D. C. and Detre, J. A., Reduced transit-time sensitivity in noninvasive magnetic resonance imaging of human cerebral blood flow, *J. Cereb. Blood Flow Metab.*, 16, 1236, 1996.
19. Small, S. A., Quantifying cerebral blood flow: regional regulation with global implications, *J. Clin. Invest.*, 114, 1046, 2004.
20. Belliveau, J. W. et al., Functional cerebral imaging by susceptibility-contrast NMR, *Magn. Reson. Med.*, 14, 538, 1990.
21. Lin, W., Celik, A., and Paczynski, R. P., Regional cerebral blood volume: a comparison of the dynamic imaging and the steady state methods, *J. Magn. Reson. Imaging*, 9, 44, 1999.
22. Ogawa, S. et al., Oxygenation-sensitive contrast in magnetic resonance image of rodent brain at high magnetic fields, *Magn. Reson. Med.*, 14, 68, 1990.
23. Ogawa, S. et al., Brain magnetic resonance imaging with contrast dependent on blood oxygenation, *Proc. Natl. Acad. Sci. USA*, 87, 9868, 1990.
24. Ogawa, S. et al., Intrinsic signal changes accompanying sensory stimulation: Functional brain mapping with magnetic resonance imaging, *Proc. Natl. Acad. Sci. USA*, 89, 5951, 1992.
25. van Zijl, P. C. et al., Quantitative assessment of blood flow, blood volume and blood oxygenation effects in functional magnetic resonance imaging, *Nat. Med.*, 4, 159, 1998.
26. Small, S. et al., Imaging physiologic dysfunction of individual hippocampal subregions in humans and genetically modified mice, *Neuron*, 653, 2000.
27. Erecinska, M. and Silver, I. A., ATP and brain function, *J. Cereb. Blood Flow Metab.*, 9, 2, 1989.
28. Masliah, E. et al., Synaptic and neuritic alterations during the progression of Alzheimer's disease, *Neurosci. Lett.*, 174, 67, 1994.
29. Mucke, L. et al., High-level neuronal expression of abeta 1-42 in wild-type human amyloid protein precursor transgenic mice: Synaptotoxicity without plaque formation, *J. Neurosci.*, 20, 4050, 2000.
30. Rombouts, S. A. et al., Functional MR imaging in Alzheimer's disease during memory encoding, *Am. J. Neuroradiol.*, 21, 2000, 1869.
31. Small, S. A. et al., Differential regional dysfunction of the hippocampal formation among elderly with memory decline and Alzheimer's disease, *Ann. Neurol.*, 45, 466, 1999.
32. Bondi, M. W. et al., fMRI evidence of compensatory mechanisms in older adults at genetic risk for Alzheimer disease, *Neurology*, 64, 501, 2005.
33. Raichle, M. E. et al., A default mode of brain function, *Proc. Natl. Acad. Sci. USA*, 98, 676, 2001.
34. Davis, T. L. et al., Calibrated functional MRI: mapping the dynamics of oxidative metabolism, *Proc. Natl. Acad. Sci. USA*, 95, 1834, 1998.
35. Klunk, W. E. et al., Imaging brain amyloid in Alzheimer's disease with Pittsburgh Compound-B, *Ann. Neurol.*, 55, 306, 2004.

36. Oddo, S. et al., Amyloid deposition precedes tangle formation in a triple transgenic model of Alzheimer's disease, *Neurobiol. Aging*, 24, 1063, 2003.
37. Jack, C. R. Jr. et al., *In vivo* visualization of Alzheimer's amyloid plaques by magnetic resonance imaging in transgenic mice without a contrast agent, *Magn. Reson. Med.*, 52, 1263, 2004.
38. Lee, S. P. et al., Visualization of beta-amyloid plaques in a transgenic mouse model of Alzheimer's disease using MR microscopy without contrast reagents, *Magn. Reson. Med.*, 52, 538, 2004.
39. Skovronsky, D. M. et al., *In vivo* detection of amyloid plaques in a mouse model of Alzheimer's disease, *Proc. Natl. Acad. Sci. USA*, 97, 7609, 2000.
40. Higuchi, M. et al., 19F and 1H MRI detection of amyloid bold beta plaques *in vivo*, *Nat. Neurosci.*, 8, 527, 2005.
41. Redwine, J. M. et al., Dentate gyrus volume is reduced before onset of plaque formation in PDAPP mice: a magnetic resonance microscopy and stereologic analysis, *Proc. Natl. Acad. Sci. USA*, 100, 1381, 2003.
42. Seab, J. P. et al., Quantitative NMR measurements of hippocampal atrophy in Alzheimer's disease, *Magn. Reson. Med.*, 8, 200, 1988.
43. de Leon, M. J. et al., Early marker for Alzheimer's disease: the atrophic hippocampus, *Lancet*, 2, 672, 1989.
44. Jack, C. R. Jr. et al., Anterior temporal lobes and hippocampal formations: normative volumetric measurements from MR images in young adults, *Radiology*, 172, 549, 1989.
45. Scheltens, P. et al., Atrophy of medial temporal lobes on MRI in probable Alzheimer's disease and normal ageing: diagnostic value and neuropsychological correlates, *J. Neurol. Neurosurg. Psychiatry*, 55, 967, 1992.
46. Killiany, R. J. et al., Temporal lobe regions on magnetic resonance imaging identify patients with early Alzheimer's disease, *Arch. Neurol.*, 50, 949, 1993.
47. Insausti, R. et al., MR volumetric analysis of the human entorhinal, perirhinal, and temporopolar cortices, *Am. J. Neuroradiol.*, 19, 659, 1998.
48. Insausti, R. et al., Human medial temporal lobe in aging: anatomical basis of memory preservation, *Microsc. Res. Tech.*, 43, 8, 1998.
49. Kaye, J. A. et al., Volume loss of the hippocampus and temporal lobe in healthy elderly persons destined to develop dementia, *Neurology*, 48, 1297, 1997.
50. Fox, N. C. et al., Presymptomatic hippocampal atrophy in Alzheimer's disease. a longitudinal MRI study, *Brain*, 119, 1996, 2001.
51. De Toledo-Morrell, L. et al., From healthy aging to early Alzheimer's disease: *in vivo* detection of entorhinal cortex atrophy, *Ann. N.Y. Acad. Sci.*, 911, 240, 2000.
52. Du, A. T. et al., Higher atrophy rate of entorhinal cortex than hippocampus in AD, *Neurology*, 62, 422, 2004.
53. Raz, N. et al., Differential aging of the medial temporal lobe: a study of a five-year change, *Neurology*, 62, 433, 2004.

8 MRI and MRS in Animal Models of Focal Cerebral Ischemia

Markus Rudin, Peter R. Allegrini, and Martin Rausch

CONTENTS

8.1 INTRODUCTION

Stroke is a leading cause of death in industrialized nations. The only treatment that is currently approved by the regulatory authorities is thrombolysis using recombinant tissue plasminogen activator (rtPA) when administered within 3 h following cerebral infarction [1–3]. Because of this time constraint, only a very small fraction of stroke patients of less than 5% are amenable to rtPA treatment.

This illustrates the strong medical need to develop novel pharmacological therapies to alleviate the disastrous consequences of a cerebral ischemic insult for the patients. While the pathophysiological cascade leading to reversible tissue necrosis in human embolic stroke is well understood [4,5], translation of this knowledge into efficacious clinical therapy concepts has not been successful up to now, despite many promising preclinical results. The reason for these failures are manifold, the discussion of which is beyond the scope of this chapter. Instead, we will focus on the role of magnetic resonance imaging (MRI) and spectroscopy (MRS) for the characterization of structural, functional and metabolic consequences of global and focal cerebral ischemia. MRI and MRS have been extensively used both in clinical settings (see Chapter 9) as well as for the analysis of preclinical models of stroke. We discuss the basic physiological and metabolic processes that are initiated following induction of ischemia, some frequently used rodent models of global and focal cerebral ischemia, the use of imaging readouts for disease phenotyping, pharmacological concepts that have been evaluated for treatment of acute and chronic stroke therapy, and the application of imaging methods to evaluate therapy response.

8.2 PATHOPHYSIOLOGY OF STROKE

Focal cerebral ischemia is caused by transient or permanent occlusion of a major cerebral artery. Cessation of local perfusion and thereby supply of oxygen and nutrients initiates a cascade of detrimental effects to the respective cerebral tissue, which leads to loss of function and ultimately to infarction [4,5].

Lack of oxygen and glucose results in energy failure within minutes due to the shut-down of cerebral aerobic ATP synthesis. Biochemical tissue analysis [6] and MRS studies [7–9] in models of global ischemia revealed that pools of high energy phosphates, such as phosphocreatine (PCr) and adenosine triphosphate (ATP) become depleted within 2 to 4 min following the complete cessation of perfusion. Moreover, due to the oxygen deficiency, energy metabolism switches to anaerobic ATP synthesis, which is ineffective with only 2 moles of ATP being synthesized per mole of glucose as compared to 34 for the oxidative pathway, leading to severe tissue acidosis due to excessive formation of lactate [10].

Calcium (Ca^{2+}), a crucial regulator of many physiological processes, acts as a second messenger (Figure 8.1). A variety of stimuli produces cellular effects by increasing the cytosolic

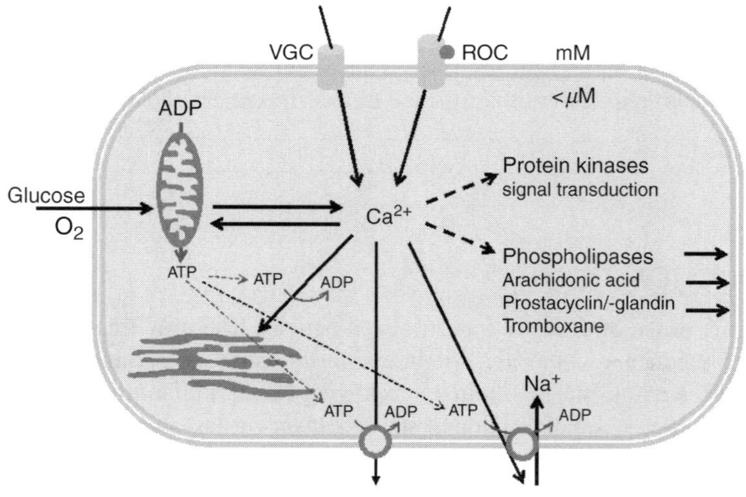

FIGURE 8.1 Ca^{2+} plays a central role in tissue ischemia. Due to its central role as second messenger tight regulation of intracellular Ca^{2+} levels, which are in the submicromolar range, is of vital importance. Cessation of perfusion will deprive tissue from nutrients and oxygen leading to failure of oxidative ATP synthesis in mitochondria and thus to energy failure. ATP-dependent regulation mechanisms will lead to excessive intracellular levels with detrimental consequences for the cell. Interaction with protein kinases compromises proper signal transduction within the cell and in-between cells, while activation of phospholipases will affect membrane integrity ultimately leading to cellular necrosis. VGC, voltage-gated Ca^{2+} channels; ROC, receptor-operated Ca^{2+} channels (e.g., NMDA receptor).

free Ca^{2+} concentration ($[Ca^{2+}]_i$). The increase in $[Ca^{2+}]_i$ can be achieved by Ca^{2+} entry from the extracellular space or from intracellular stores of calcium, predominantly from endoplasmic reticulum. The regulatory role of Ca^{2+} requires tight control of intracellular levels. Effective ion pumps are required to maintain the Ca^{2+}-concentration gradient between the extracellular compartment with millimolar and the intracellular compartment with submicromolar concentration. Energy depletion will affect all energy-dependent processes of the cell including membrane pumps required to maintain ion homeostasis and intracellular signaling cascades via ATP-dependent protein kinases. Failure of ATP-dependent membrane pumps will lead to a large excess of intracellular Ca^{2+} prompting a cascade of downstream events for the cell. In addition to the regulation of $[Ca^{2+}]_i$, the concentration gradients of Na^+ and K^+ will break down, leading to membrane depolarization. The altered ion distribution changes the cellular osmolality leading to a massive inflow of water into the cells (cytotoxic edema).

Consequences of elevated levels of intracellular Ca^{2+} are excessive activation of phospholipases, which play a central role in membrane turnover. Elevated activity of phospholipases will cause excessive degradation of phospholipids resulting in membrane breakdown. In addition, hydrolysis of phosphatidylinositol-biposphate releases the signaling molecule inositol-1,4,5-trisphosphate (IP_3), which will interact with its receptor (IP_3R) at the membrane of intracellular in Ca^{2+} stores, which operate as ligand gated channels. Activation of IP_3R will further increase $[Ca^{2+}]_i$ [11]. Loss of $[Ca^{2+}]_i$ regulation will ultimately lead to cell death.

Additional relevant factors ultimately leading to tissue necrosis are excitatory neurotransmitters, such as glutamate. Glutamate interacts with two types of receptors: ionotropic receptors such as the kainate, the *N*-methyl-D-aspartate (NMDA), or the alpha-amino-3-hydroxy-5-methyl-isoxazole-4-propionate (AMPA) receptor, and metabotropic receptors [12]. NMDA receptors are permeable to both Ca^{2+} and Na^+, while AMPA and kainate receptors are only permeable to Na^+ions [13]. Inactivation of glutamate via glial and neuronal uptake is energy-dependent; hence, during energy failure glutamate accumulates leading to exhaustive neuronal stimulation (convulsions, seizures). Elevated glutamate levels cause opening of receptor-operated Ca^{2+}-channels (NMDA receptors) and correspondingly increased Ca^{2+} influx with the consequences already discussed. In addition, glutamate interaction with metabotropic glutamate receptors (mGluRs) activates second-messenger-mediated signal transduction processes via guanosine triphosphate (GTP) binding proteins. There are three main classes of mGluRs: one class is related to phosphatidyl-inositol hydrolysis and the other two classes are negatively coupled to the cyclic-AMP formation via adenylate cyclase [14]. Regulation of the levels of second messenger pools is energy-dependent; hence, energy failure will lead to excessive cellular stimulation via second messenger pathways.

Glutamate-induced spreading depressions are believed to play a relevant role with regard to infarct growth. Excessive excitotoxic stimulation by the receptor agonist glutamate has been shown to induce waves of electrical depolarization that propagate from the infarct core into the ischemic penumbra at a speed of 3 to 4 mm/min [15,16]. Glutamergic stimulation increases focal energy consumption, which in a tissue area with compromised energy supply might cause energy failure. In fact, in focal cerebral ischemia the transient changes in the apparent diffusion coefficient (ADC) of water observed during spreading depression do not fully recover leading to an overall growth of the ischemic lesion [16].

Unless blood flow is restored within a short period, irreversible tissue necrosis will occur; hence, in order to protect tissue from becoming infarcted restoration of blood flow and correspondingly supply of oxygen and nutrients is mandatory. Although there is substantial evidence that reperfusion is beneficial when performed in due time, restoration of blood flow has also been demonstrated to cause additional tissue damage. Several mechanisms might account for this, in particular elevated levels of oxygen free radicals might induce a cascade of deleterious events including lipid peroxidation and membrane damage. High levels of free radicals during reperfusion have been demonstrated in the perfused isolated rat heart using electron spin resonance techniques [17]. Reperfusion damage is also associated with the infiltration of inflammatory cells, in particular neutrophils [18], and microvascular plugging [19,20].

It is well known that lesion volumes increase 24 and 48 h postinfarction due to recruitment of penumbra regions. This delayed loss of neurons encompasses apoptosis [21], which is commonly associated with neuro-inflammation due to the proximity of apoptotic neurons and immune-competent cells [22]. Increases in the activity of the effector caspase-3, which plays a central role in the apoptotic cascade, occur within hours after infarction [23,24]. Other caspases, both pro-inflammatory and apoptotic, are upregulated as well. The relevance of caspase inhibition has been demonstrated using oxamyl dipeptide caspase inhibitors [25] and genetically modified animals: caspase-3-deficient mice showed significantly reduced infarct volume when subjected to focal cerebral ischemia [26].

A second factor causing delayed tissue damage is neuro-inflammation. Expression of pro-inflammatory mediators such as chemokines and cytokines has been observed both in human stroke and in animal models thereof [27]. For example, early induction of the chemokine monocyte chemoattractant protein-1 (MCP-1) has been reported after focal cerebral ischemia in rats and mice [28,29]. MCP-1 plays a crucial role in monocyte recruitment in several neuro-inflammatory models. In addition, MCP-1 acts as regulatory chemokine inducing the expression of interleukins 1β and 6, which seem to be important mediators of brain damage following focal ischemia [30]. MCP-1-deficient mice (MCP-$1^{-/-}$) displayed resistance to experimental autoimmune encephalomyelitis with drastically reduced recruitment of macrophages to the central nervous system [31]. When subjecting MCP-1($^{-/-}$) mice to focal cerebral ischemia, infarct volumes determined 24 h following vascular occlusion were found to be significantly smaller (−30%) as compared to wildtype animals [32]. Immunostaining carried out at 2 weeks showed a significant reduction of tissue macrophages in MCP-1($^{-/-}$) mice both in the infarct core and in the periphery. Nevertheless, the acute protective effect of MCP-1 deficiency is not attributed to a reduced monocyte recruitment, which is commonly observed days after stroke onset, but rather to a significantly weaker early-ischemia induced cytokine response, potentially leading to a reduced activation of brain resident microglia. These and related studies indicate an important role of chemokines following ischemic brain injury with implications for therapy strategies (see Section 8.5.5).

8.3 ANIMAL MODELS OF STROKE

Although various global and focal cerebral ischemia models have been developed, we will limit the discussion to only a few rodent models widely used by the scientific community.

8.3.1 Global Cerebral Ischemia Models in Rodents

Studies of tissue metabolism have been largely carried out using global ischemia models such as cardiac arrest in rats and mice by intravenous administration of magnesium chloride [9] or the four-vessel occlusion model in rats [33]. The advantage of the first model is its simplicity and the high degree of reproducibility. However, relevant aspects of ischemic stroke, such as effects due to spontaneous or induced reperfusion, cannot be studied. Some of these deficiencies are addressed in the second model, which consists of the permanent occlusion of the two vertebrate arteries via electrocauterization through the foramen ovale of the first cervical vertebra and transient occlusion of the two common carotid arteries using removable clips. Occlusion of all four principal feeding arteries of the brain induces an almost complete global ischemia, while removal of the carotid clips provides reperfusion to all brain areas via blood supply through the Circle of Willis. High energy phosphate (HEP) levels are depleted within minutes following onset of ischemia and do rapidly recover during reperfusion episodes (Figure 8.2).

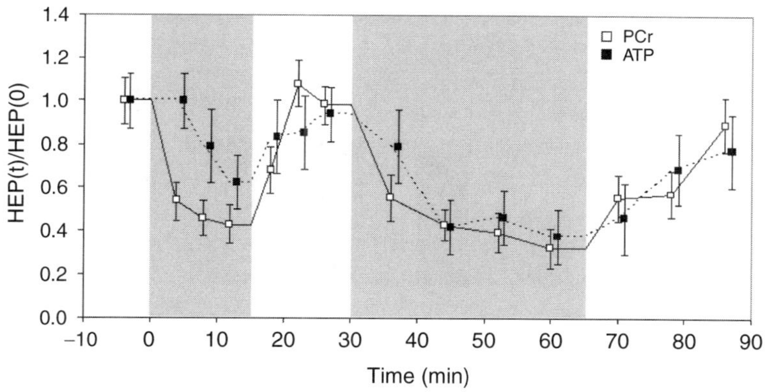

FIGURE 8.2 Relative levels of high energy phosphates (HEPs) PCr and ATP, measured noninvasively using ^{31}P MRS, as a function time during ischemia/reperfusion in the rat four-vessel occlusion model. Ischemic periods are indicated as gray areas. (Sauter, A. and Rudin, M., unpublished.)

Global ischemia models mimic the cerebral consequences of cardiac arrest in humans and may be used to study mechanistic aspects associated with cerebral ischemia. However, human embolic stroke is a focal event with different brain regions being affected to a different degree, aspects that are not reproduced by these simple models. Obviously, experimental studies of human embolic stroke require focal ischemia models.

8.3.2 Focal Cerebral Ischemia Models in Rodents

Mongolian gerbils have an incomplete Circle of Willis, therefore unilateral occlusion of the common carotid artery causes cerebral infarction in the ipsilateral hemisphere in approximately 30% of the animals [34].

The most frequently used focal ischemia model is the permanent or transient occlusion of the middle cerebral artery (MCA) in the rat. In the permanent occlusion model the MCA is exposed through a craniectomy approximately 1 mm superior to the foramen ovale at the inferotemporal fossa. After opening of the dura the MCA is occluded by electrocoagulation at a proximal location close to the Circle of Willis [35,36]. This leads to a significant infarction that invariably comprises the caudate putamen and neighboring areas of parietal and temporal cortex depending on the rat strain used. Differences in total infarct volumes are largely due to variability of cortical infarction: while cortical infarction is almost absent in Wistar-Kyoto rats, the genetically closely related spontaneously hypertensive (SH) rats display massive cortical lesions involving large portions of frontal, parietal, and occipital cortex. Infarct volumes for Wistar, Sprague-Dawley, and Fischer F344 rats are in-between (Figure 8.3) [37]. The reasons for these differences are not completely understood, but a significant factor is the strain-specific cerebral vascular anatomy with varying numbers of arterial branchings, anastomoses, and collaterals [37–39]. Measurement of cortical cerebral blood flow (CBF) supported this interpretation: the reduction of the ipsilateral cortical CBF during MCA occlusion was significantly smaller in Wistar-Kyoto than in SH rats and not sufficient to induce tissue necrosis [37].

An alternative permanent focal ischemia model in the rat is based on photothrombotic lesioning [40]. It combines the infusion of a photosensitive dye such as Rose Bengal with focal irradiation, for example, of the motor cortex area through the exposed skull using a halogen lamp inducing photothrombosis of cortical microvessels. This leads to a half-sphere-shaped lesion, which comprises cortical structures only.

While the permanent MCAO model has been widely used to study the pathophysiology of focal cerebral ischemia, it lacks an important feature of human stroke: potential reperfusion. To address

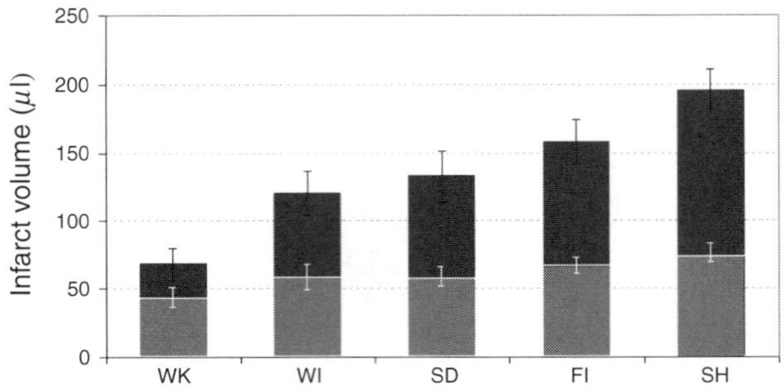

FIGURE 8.3 Strain-dependent infarct volumes following unilateral permanent occlusion of the rat MCA. Quantitative analysis was carried out 48 h following electrocauterization. While striatal lesions are essentially constant for the different rat strains (light gray), cortical infarction displays significant strain-dependence (dark gray). Values are given as mean ± s.e.m. WK, Wistar—Kyoto; Wi, Wistar; SD, Sprague-Dawley; Fi, Fischer F344; SH, spontaneously hypertensive rats. (Adapted from Sauter, A. and Rudin, M., *J. Pharmacol. Exp. Ther.*, 274, 1008, 1995.)

this aspect of the disease transient MCA occlusion models have been developed [41]. A monofilament thread with a rounded tip is introduced into the internal carotid artery through the external carotid artery and is gently advanced to the site where the MCA branches off the Circle of Willis (in rats, approximately 18 mm from the carotid bifurcation). The thread is then left in this position for the duration of the ischemia and then moved back to allow for reperfusion of the ischemic territory. The success of the intervention can be monitored using perfusion-weighted MRI [42] or simply by analysis of the infarct volume. A modification of the thread model includes the placement of blood clots in the Circle of Willis at the site of the MCA origin. Recirculation is achieved by clot lysis by infusion of rtPA [43]. Alternatively, transient focal ischemia is induced by local administration of endothelin-1 [44]. For both models, accurate control of the ischemia duration is difficult.

Essentially all models described here have been translated to the mouse. Murine models are becoming increasingly attractive, as the availability of genetically modified strains allows the evaluation of novel hypothesis relating to the pathophysiology of stroke and of potential therapeutic concepts.

8.3.3 Mechanism-Specific Neurotoxic/Excitotoxic Lesion Models in Rats

Quinolinic acid, an endogenous metabolite of L-tryptophan and NMDA receptor agonist, was found to accumulate in cortical areas of a traumatized rat hemisphere [45] or in traumatized guinea pig spinal cord [46], implicating a role in the evolving neuronal damage. Quinolinic acid is a so-called "excitotoxin," i.e., it belongs to a family of acidic amino acids which are neuroexcitants. These compounds produce a characteristic type of axon-sparing neuronal lesions reflecting characteristics of human neurodegenerative disorders. Intracerebral (commonly intrastriatal) infusions of members of this family, such as quinolinates, kainates, NMDA agonists, malonates, or ibotenates, which interact with specific receptors/receptor subtypes in the mammalian central nervous system, result in focal tissue damage at the injection site, the severity of which depends on the dose administered and the age of the animals [47–50]. While such excitotoxicity models address rather specific aspects of the pathophysiology of cerebral ischemia, pharmacological blockade of excitotoxicity as such constitutes an attractive strategy for cytoprotectiv therapy. Focal excitotoxin lesion models are of some value for evaluating antiexcitotoxic therapies that might be relevant for a variety of neurological indications including stroke [51,52]. Nevertheless, when targeting human embolic stroke as clinical indication, final compound evaluation should be based on focal cerebral ischemia models.

8.4 EXPERIMENTAL STROKE: DISEASE PHENOTYPING USING MRI/MRS

Due to the vital role of energy metabolism for proper tissue function, noninvasive ^{31}P MRS has been applied to monitor levels of HEP such as ATP and PCr, characterizing the metabolic state of tissue (Figure 8.2). Cerebral HEP synthesis not matching HEP consumption will ultimately lead to energy failure, to brain dysfunction, and ultimately to brain death. This is the case, e.g., for *status epilepticus*, during which energy consumption is dramatically increased. Prolonged seizures have been shown to compromise tissue levels of PCr and later of ATP with a concomitant increase of intracellular pH reflecting anaerobic glucose metabolism [7]. Brain ischemia has analogous metabolic consequences: during global cerebral ischemia, PCr levels disappear within 2 min following cessation of blood flow, while ATP reservoirs are depleted within typically 4 min following cardiac arrest [9]. Intracellular pH values drop from a normal value of 7.2 to values around 6.5, depending on the resting blood glucose levels [7–9]. Additional ^{1}H-MRS investigations demonstrated that energy failure is accompanied by massive build-up of intracellular lactate levels due to anaerobic glycolysis [53,54].

HEP levels as indicator of tissue state have been shown to be of limited value: due to highly efficient regulatory mechanisms only severe metabolic stress will lead to observable changes of HEP steady-state levels. As long as their synthesis rate accounts for the energy consumption, HEP levels will remain unchanged. HEP turnover, on the other hand, has to match the demands of tissue function; thus, a direct assessment of turnover rates provides superior information. This has been demonstrated in normal rat brain exposed to various "workloads." while cerebral steady-state ATP levels were not different for pentobarbital and isoflurane anesthetized rats and animals with mild epileptic seizures following administration of the γ-butyric amino acid A ($GABA_A$) receptor antagonist bicuculline, there was a high correlation between the forward rate constant, k_f, for the creatine kinase reaction

$$\mathrm{PCr} + \mathrm{ADP} + \mathrm{H}^+ \xrightarrow{k_f} \mathrm{ATP} + \mathrm{Cr} \tag{8.1}$$

as a measure for ATP turnover, and the cerebral energy consumption as reflected by the integrated electrical activity [55]. A similar correlation has been observed for the glucose perfused rat heart [56]. Kinetic information was derived from so-called magnetization transfer experiments, in which the transfer of a magnetic label between two reaction partners (in the case of the creatine kinase reaction PCr and ATP) was monitored [56–59].

MRS studies, while providing valuable mechanistic information, are limited (1) by the lack of sensitivity; (2) by a small dynamic range (it is difficult to detect drug effects of less than 20 to 30%); and (3) by poor spatial resolution, Therefore, MRS has played a minor role in the management of stroke patients and for the development of novel antiischemic therapies. In contrast, MRI methods emerged as an indispensable tool to identify and stage cerebral ischemic tissue (see also Chapter 9).

The classical MRI method for assessment of cerebral infarction is based on T_2 contrast: accumulation of water in the infarcted brain area (vasogenic edema) leads to significantly elevated T_2 values providing a good demarcation between ischemic and intact tissue. The contrast-to-noise ratio is high enough to allow for application of tissue segmentation algorithms based on intensity thresholding and the method has been extensively applied to quantitative assessments of drug effects on infarct volume in animal models of focal cerebral ischemia [36,60]. There is an excellent correlation between infarct volumes determined *in vivo* using T_2-weighted MRI and lesion volumes derived from histology [61].

Tissue areas displaying increased T_2 values are already irreversibly damaged; thus, earlier indicators that provide a significant contrast for tissue that is still salvageable would be highly relevant. Cerebral ischemia is caused by occlusion of a major brain artery, therefore assessment of CBF should immediately reflect hypoperfused brain regions. A number of MRI methods to assess local CBF has been developed [62–64] and applied to studies of stroke patients [65] or in animal models of stroke. In rat focal cerebral ischemia models, perfusion deficits have been visualized within seconds after occlusion of a major brain artery such as the MCA [42,66]. Relative perfusion values as compared to normally perfused brain regions can be obtained in a straightforward manner, but the determination of absolute values in ml/g tissue/min remains difficult. Yet, assessment of absolute values would be essential as reduced values of tissue perfusion do not necessarily imply tissue necrosis, and there are region-specific perfusion thresholds for neuronal function and neuronal survival [67].

As pointed out in Section 8.2, a consequence of cellular energy failure is the loss of ion homeostasis; the altered cellular osmolality leads to a massive influx of water and, hence, to cell swelling. This cytotoxic edema is reflected by a decrease of the water ADC value. The ADC measured in a voxel is the weighted average of the intra- and extracellular contributions. Since the extracellular diffusion coefficient is larger than the intracellular one, an increase in the intracellular volume fraction will lead to a decrease of the ADC. The correlation of cerebral ADC values with measurements of electrical conductivity in brain parenchyma in a neurotoxic lesion model supported this interpretation [68]. Nevertheless, this view is an oversimplification; additional factors to be considered are changes of diffusion constants within the individual tissue compartments [69,70]. Indeed, ADC reduction of the intracellular metabolites after global ischemia or cytotoxic lesions were observed [71].

Decreases in cerebral ADC values occur within minutes after onset of ischemia [72], i.e., diffusion-weighted MRI detects early microstructural changes following an ischemic insult. More importantly even, it has been demonstrated at least in animal models of global [73] and focal ischemia [74] that ADC changes are reversible: in both cases tissue reperfusion led to normalization of ADC values that were decreased during the ischemic episode. Similarly, it has been demonstrated that pharmacological interventions in NMDA-induced neurotoxicity normalized ADC values in newborn rats [68]. The evolution of the water ADC in ischemic tissue shows a characteristic profile both in stroke patients [75] and in animals models of focal cerebral ischemia [76]. The initial drop to 60% of the baseline values is followed by a pseudonormalization, which is commonly observed between 4 to 8 days after the insult.

The combination of the various MR readouts (T_2, T_1, CBF, CBV, ADC) provides a comprehensive characterization of the ischemic brain parenchyma (see also Chapter 9, Section 9.2.3). As the temporal evolution following infarction is different for the various parameters, a combination of them may provide a fingerprint regarding the state of the infarcted tissue (Figure 8.4). For instance, decreased CBF and ADC but still normal T_2 values indicate brain regions with reversible tissue damage that might be potentially saved by pharmacological treatment, while areas with decreased CBF, ADC and increased T_2 values are destined to becoming necrotic. Hence, the tissue stroke signature [76,77] might be used to predict the eventual final outcome of the infarction and to identify the brain region that might be responsive to a therapeutic intervention. Unfortunately, applications of such concepts were of limited success up to now [78].

Pathological brain regions are characterized by deviations of MRI parameters from "normality." Needless to say, that this procedure is to some extent arbitrary. How much must T_2 values deviate from normality to be identified as abnormal? This depends on a variety of factors such as the general signal-to-noise ratio of the image and the morphological heterogeneity of the corresponding brain area. Moreover, clinical stroke is highly heterogeneous, spontaneous recanalization may occur with profound influence on the evolution of the MRI parameters and thus to their prognostic quality. In animal models, rather homogeneous conditions can be achieved. For instance, in the rat unilateral permanent MCAO model, it has been found that the extent of the lesion derived from CBF maps recorded 1 h postinfarction (based on relative CBF values in the ischemic region that were significantly smaller than contralateral values) predicted the outcome at 48 h with good accuracy in untreated animals [76]. In contrast, the ischemic regions as derived from ADC and T_2 maps at 1 h were significantly smaller than those determined at 48 h, i.e., there was significant growth of the lesion area both in ADC- and T_2-weighted images. Hence, the prognostic

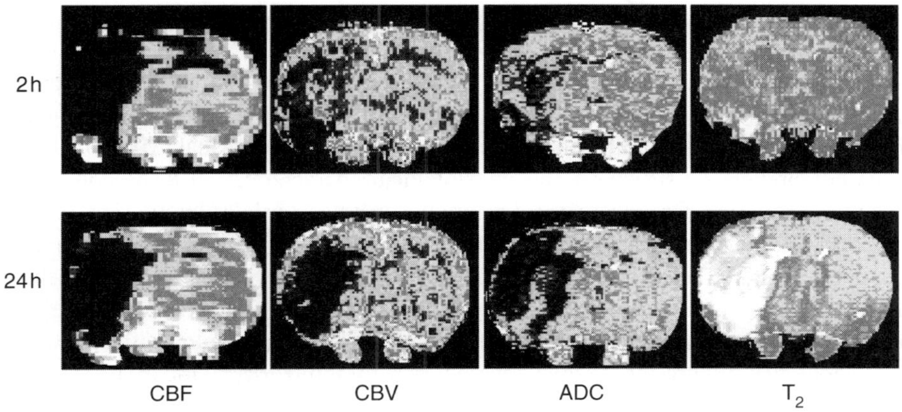

FIGURE 8.4 Characteristic tissue signatures based on MRI parameters for rat permanent MCA occlusion. At 2 h after occlusion CBF, CBV, and ADC are decreased in the infarcted area (left side) as compared to the healthy control side, while T_2 maps display no left/right asymmetry yet. At 24 h, CBF, CBV, and ADC remain decreased in the lesion area, while T_2 now is clearly elevated due to the formation of a vasogenic edema. The temporal evolution of the various MRI parameters allows staging of tissue and potentially the prediction whether a specific region might by salvagable by a therapeutic intervention. (Adapted from Rudin, M. et al., *Exp. Neurol.*, 169, 56, 2001. With permission.)

value of CBF measurements was found to be superior to that of ADC and T_2 values. This has also been reported in clinical stroke (see also Chapter 9, Section 9.2.1): a significant perfusion/diffusion mismatch, with the "perfusion lesion" being larger than that derived from ADC maps, implied significant growth of the ADC lesion [79].

Over many years, research in stroke was focused on the acute phase, i.e., the first 48 h following infarction. The therapy objective was to protect tissue from becoming infarcted by intervening at the early steps in the pathophysiological cascade. However, therapy successes achieved in animal models of focal cerebral ischemia could not be translated into the clinics due to a variety of reasons. A critical factor is the short time window available for successful cytoprotective interventions, probably of only a few hours, which is a severe hurdle for clinical drug development. In recent years, focus in stroke research was shifted to later phases of the pathology, in particular the inflammatory component of the disease has been addressed. Correspondingly, MRI methods to assess these aspects of cerebral ischemia have been developed.

Inflammation is characterized by massive infiltration of immune-competent cells, predominantly blood-borne monocytes that infiltrate tissue by transcytosis to become activated macrophages. These cells of the monocyte phagocytotic system (MPS) are often found at the border of ischemic/necrotic tissue. Ultrasmall particles of iron-oxide (USPIO) have been developed as contrast agents for visualization of structures with phagocytotic function, such as the spleen or lymph nodes [80]. These nanoparticles are efficiently internalized by monocytes/macrophages via absorptive endocytosis and, hence, can be used to track such cells. Feasibility of USPIO-based macrophage imaging in the brain has been demonstrated in the rat experimental autoimmune encephalomyelitis model of multiple sclerosis [81,82] (see also Chapter 12). In these studies, focal areas characterized by shortening of T_2 and T_2^* have been observed 24 h following the systemic administration of USPIOs. Histological analysis confirmed the presence of USPIO-labeled macrophages in the inflamed tissue regions. Application of the same approach to models of permanent [83] and transient MCAO in rats [18] displayed massive macrophage infiltration in focal ischemia. During the first 2 days after vessel occlusion USPIO accumulation was predominantly observed in patches in the core lesion comprising the caudate putamen and at the periphery of the infarction. At later time points, maximal label accumulation was observed at the boundary of the lesion. USPIO loaded macrophages could be monitored up to 7 days following systemic administration of the contrast agent.

MRI can be applied to visualize different phases of the pathophysiological cascade of stroke, from the initial vascular occlusion visualized by MR angiography [84,85] to the chronic phase with neuro-inflammatory and apoptotic processes. Application of functional MRI (fMRI) methods allows this comprehensive structural and physiological characterization to be complemented by readouts of CNS function. Obviously, focal cerebral ischemia translates into loss of functionality in the affected brain areas. In the rat permanent MCA occlusion model sensory stimulation of the forepaw contralateral to the infarction side did not evoke a hemodynamic response in the infarcted somatosensory cortex [86,87]. Similarly, global stimulation using bicuculline identified significant functional dropouts in the infarcted territory [86]. Functional deficits could be identified in transient MCA occlusion of short duration, despite apparent structural integrity of the tissue [88]. Functional readouts are particularly attractive when studying functional recovery, e.g., following cytoprotective therapy (see Section 8.6.3).

8.5 THERAPY CONCEPTS

Potential antiischemic therapies have been developed for various processes and targets throughout the ischemic cascade. Again, a comprehensive discussion of the various concepts pursuit is beyond the scope of this chapter and we will highlight some specific approaches.

8.5.1 RECANALIZATION

Long-term tissue survival can only be achieved by restoring blood supply to the ischemic lesion. Therefore, one therapy concept targets the initial cause of infarction trying to dissolve the blood clot responsible for vessel occlusion. Recanalization by administration of rtPA is currently the only approved treatment for acute stroke, provided it can be applied within 3 h following stroke onset [1–3] (see also Chapter 9, Section 9.2). There are two issues with rtPA treatment: hemorrhages must be absolutely excluded as potential source of stroke symptoms (see also Chapter 9, Section 9.2). Administration of rtPA to a hemorrhagic patient would be fatal. Secondly, it has been found in animal models of focal cerebral ischemia that the lesion area was significantly larger in cases in which reperfusion was initiated later than 2 h following infarction as compared to the permanent occlusion situation, due to the reperfusion damage.

8.5.2 MAINTENANCE OF LOW INTRACELLULAR CA^{2+} LEVELS

Due to the critical role of the tight control of intracellular Ca^{2+} levels for proper cell function, a number of strategies to reduce/inhibit Ca^{2+} influx into the cell has been developed. Blockade of voltage-gated channels using, for example, dihydropyridine Ca^{2+} antagonists has been successfully applied as antihypertensive therapy, and several compounds also showed promising efficacy in animal models of global [9] and focal cerebral ischemia [36,60]. Significant reduction of the infarct volume could be achieved when administering isradipine immediately after stroke onset. Similarly, posttreatment efficacy, which is critical with regard to clinical application in acute stroke, could be demonstrated: significant drug effects have been reported when the compound was administered up to 4 h post infarction [54]. Other compounds of the same structure type, such as nimodipine, showed similar efficacy [89]. Despite these promising preclinical data, clinical trials could not confirm efficacy in acute stroke trials.

An alternative strategy to control intacellular Ca^{2+} levels is the inhibition of Ca^{2+} influx via receptor-operated channels such as the NMDA receptor. The NMDA receptor has been shown to contain several ligand-binding sites that constitute targets for therapeutic interventions: the

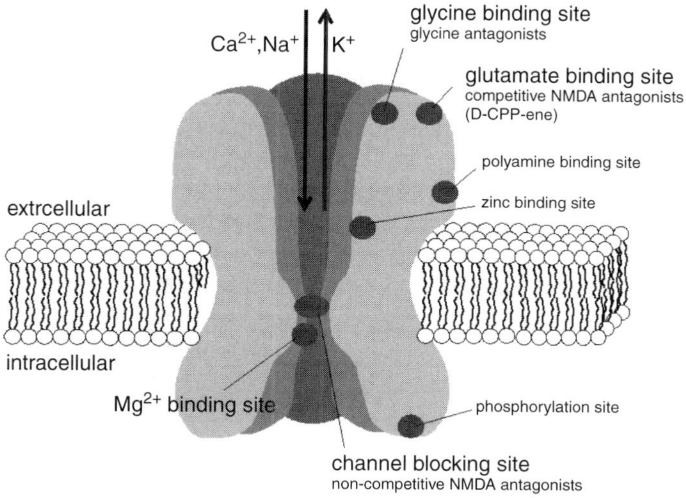

FIGURE 8.5 Schematic representation of an ionotropic NMDA receptor, which is a membrane spanning ion channel regulating the entry of Ca^{2+} and Na^+ consisting of five subunits. The receptor comprises a number of agonist binding sites. The glutamate binding site is the target for competitive NMDA antagonists (D-CPP-ene, selfotel). The interaction site for noncompetitive antagonsists (dizolcipine, phencyclidene) sits in the channel. The glycine binding site is close to the glutamate site, glycine acting as co-agonist. (Adapted from Tranquillini, M. E. and Reggiani, A., *Exp. Opin. Invest. Drugs*, 8, 1837, 1999.)

glutamate recognition site, a binding site associated with noncompetitive channel blockers, such as dizolcipine or phencyclidine, and a glycine binding site (Figure 8.5). NMDA activation strongly depends on the presence of glycine as co-agonist [12]. Inhibition of agonist binding to the glutamate site using noncompetitive NMDA antagonists such as selfotel [90,91] or SDZ 220–581 [92] has led to significant neuroprotective effects in rodent focal cerebral ischemia models. Similarly, noncompetitive blockage of the receptor channel using, for example, dizolcipine was shown to reduce the infarct volume in the rat MCA occlusion model [37]. Alternative strategies aimed at suppressing NMDA channel function by inhibiting the binding of the co-agonist glycine showed remarkable efficacy in animal models [93,94]. However, similar to the situation with dihydropyridine Ca^{2+} antagonists, preclinical efficacy achieved with the various approaches of NMDA inhibition could not be confirmed in clinical trials of acute stroke, at least not up to now. In addition to the lack of efficacy under posttreatment conditions, adverse side-effects such as the occurrence of hallucinations have been observed [92].

Glutamergic activity through AMPA receptors is a critical feature of the excitotoxic damage associated with ischemia. Therefore, inhibition of AMPA receptors has also been identified as an attractive strategy to reduce ischemia-induced necrosis with considerable preclinical success [95,96]. Nevertheless, also inhibition of AMPA receptors could not be translated into a clinically effective stroke therapy.

8.5.3 Free Radical Scavengers

Significant lesion growth has been observed following successful reperfusion of the ischemic territory. Reperfusion damage is largely attributed to the high levels of oxygen free radicals, probably due to the fact that radical trapping mechanisms, for example, via superoxide dismutase activity have been downregulated during the ischemic episode. Administration of radical scavenging compounds (e.g., ascorbic acid) should lower the levels of reactive oxygen radicals and thereby the disastrous consequences thereof. In fact, administration of the free radical scavenger U74389, a so-called lazaroid, significantly reduced the infarct volume in the rat MCA occlusion model as derived from diffusion-weighted MRI [97]. Yet, again the clinical drug evaluation did not confirm the preclinical results.

8.5.4 Antiapoptotic Therapy Using Inhibitors of Death Proteases

The clinical failure of cytoprotective therapy concepts for the treatment of acute stroke shifted interest to the chronic phase of the pathophysiological cascade. There is evidence of lesion growth due to apoptosis of neurons and glial cells at the periphery of the necrotic core [98]. Key enzymes in the apoptotic cascade are the members of the caspase family (death proteases). Inhibition of caspase activity thereby constitutes an attractive therapeutic strategy. Proof-of-concept was established by demonstrating reduced infarct volume in caspase-3-deficient mice subjected to focal cerebral ischemia [26]. Several irreversible caspase inhibitors were shown to be efficacious in transient and permanent focal cerebral ischemia models when administered directly into the cerebral ventricles [99,100]. Also, inhibition of multiple caspases using brain penetrable peptidomimetic has been shown to significantly reduce infarct volumes following MCA occlusion in the rat [101].

8.5.5 Antiinflammatory Therapy

The immunosuppressive drugs cyclosporin A and FK506, which are currently used in organ transplantation to prevent allograft rejection, have been shown to be neuroprotective in models of global cerebral ischemia [102,103] and in rat focal cerebral ischemia following MCA occlusion [104,105]. The specific mechanisms involved are not fully understood: cyclosporin A and FK506 bind to endogenous receptors termed immunophilins, which are prominent in the mammalian brain [106]. A major hypothesis is that these immune-suppressive drugs inhibit the Ca^{2+}-calmodulin-dependent phosphatase (calcineurin) [107]. Calcineurin inhibition causes deactivation of nitric oxide synthase and correspondingly reduces the nitric oxide synthesis rate and the associated production of free oxygen radicals, and has been shown to protect cultured neurons against glutamate toxicity. The interaction between the ligand-immunophilin complex and calcineurin has been shown to be essential for neuroprotection: binding of rapamycin to FK-binding protein (FKBP12), which prevents the interaction to calcineurin, blocks the neuroprotective efficacy of FK506.

Other potential therapeutic targets are chemokines such as MCP-1, which have been shown to play a crucial role in the activation of brain resident macrophages and the recruitment of blood-borne monocytes. MCP-1 also has regulatory activity inducing, for example, the expression of interleukins or adhesion molecules [108]. Inhibition of MCP-1 activity using low molecular weight inhibitors that are brain penetrable constitutes therefore an attractive therapeutic concept.

Expression of adhesion molecules by activated endothelium is an important early step for the extravasation of leukocytes and monocytes. Correspondingly, inhibition of the adhesion of these inflammatory cells to the endothelial cell, for example, by administration of antiadhesion molecule antibodies, should reduce the severity of an inflammatory response. This could be demonstrated by treatment of rats that underwent experimental stroke with antibodies directed against adhesion molecules, such as an antileukocyte adhesion antibody anti-CD18 or an anti-P-selectin antibody. This intervention reduced ischemic cell damage and improved the neurological and physiological outcome following transient focal cerebral ischemia [109,110]. While administration of anti-CD18 alone was not protective, the combination of antiadhesion therapy with thrombolysis using rtPA administered 2 and 4 h after stroke yielded superior treatment efficacy than rtPA alone [111].

8.5.6 Regeneration/Stem Cell Therapy

In the chronic phase of stroke with persistent tissue damage being fully established, potential therapeutic strategies aim at improving functional performance by either enhancing brain plasticity or by inducing neuroregeneration, e.g., by cellular transplants (see Chapter 25 for more details).

Early attempts of stem cell therapy in Parkinson's patients have been reported in the early 1990s. Intrastiatal implantation of fetal dopaminergic cells led to remarkable improvements of motor function [112,113]. Similarly, experimental studies in rat focal cerebral ischemia resulted in a significantly improved outcome following treatment with stem cells [114] or fetal neural grafts [115,116]. The development of imaging methods that allow the monitoring of cell migration in the intact organism and potentially also provides information on the viability of these cells would be of outmost importance for the evaluation of cell transplantion therapy. Migration of USPIO-labeled neuronal stem cells can be monitored with high temporal and spatial resolution in the rat MCA occlusion model [117]: labeled cells injected into the contralateral hemisphere were shown to migrate along the corpus callosum to the ischemic necrotic area probably following a chemotactic signal. The migration occurred over a period of 8 to 10 days.

Alternatively, stem cells can be labeled using a reporter gene. For instance, neuronal progenitor cells C17.2, which are known to differentiate into mature neuronal and glial cells, have been stably transfected to express firefly luciferase, an oxygenase that processes the substrate D-luciferin. Following administration of D-luciferin, luciferase expressing cells within the intact animal yield a bioluminescent signal that can be detected noninvasively using a CCD camera [118]. Implantation of labeled cells contralateral to the ischemic hemisphere in a murine MCA occlusion model revealed migration of the cells to the infarcted area within 7 to 14 days. While the spatial resolution of the bioluminescence readout is by far inferior to MRI, the reporter gene assay yields direct information on cell viability. Only viable cells will express the luciferase and, thus, yield a detectable bioluminescent signal [119].

One of the most potent inhibitors of neurite growth inhibitors and thus a hurdle for neuronal repair is the membrane protein Nogo-A [120]. Recently, attempts were made to enhance neuronal plasticity by infusion of anti-Nogo antibodies at a late time point after onset of cerebral ischemia, when the lesion had reached its final extent. Significant improvements in forepaw function without effect on infarct size as measured by MRI was found in rat stroke models [121].

8.6 NONINVASIVE ASSESSMENT OF THERAPY RESPONSE USING MR TECHNIQUES

In vivo MRS and MRI have been extensively used to assess the response to therapeutic interventions. The suitability of an *in vivo* parameter as efficacy biomarker is given by the ratio of its dynamic range $|\mu_{\text{drug}} - \mu_{\text{placebo}}|$, where μ_{drug} and μ_{placebo} are the expected drug and placebo effects, and the total variability of the measurement σ, which is composed of the error of the measurement method σ_{method}, the variability of the model σ_{model}, and the variability in the drug effect σ_{drug}, which we assume to be independent from each other, hence

$$\frac{|\mu_{\text{drug}} - \mu_{\text{placebo}}|}{\sigma} \approx \frac{|\mu_{\text{drug}} - \mu_{\text{placebo}}|}{\sqrt{\sigma^2_{\text{method}} + \sigma^2_{\text{model}} + \sigma^2_{\text{drug}}}} \tag{8.2}$$

Ideally this expression should be maximized in a pharmacological experiment. In this section, we will discuss some specific parameters used for the evaluation of the cytoprotective efficacy of drug candidates in global and focal ischemia models.

8.6.1 Effect of Cytoprotective Drugs on Cerebral Energy Metabolism

Energy failure due to lack of supply by nutrients and oxygen is the primary cause of tissue damage in ischemia. Hence, drug interventions that improve the energy charge of the cell (the ratio of HEPs divided by the total amount of phosphate containing metabolites) are potentially cytoprotective. Evaluation of drug effects on the energy charge requires accurate determination of HEP metabolite concentrations ([ATP], [PCr]) from ^{31}P MR spectra. This implies a high signal-to-noise ratio (SNR), fully relaxed (T_1) spectra or correction for relaxation effects provided that the T_1 values for each metabolite are known, and deconvolution of spectra in case of overlapping resonance lines. In addition, for determination of absolute concentrations, the distribution of the metabolites within the various compartments in the region-of-interest (intra- vs. extracellular) has to be known. However, in most cases, relative concentrations with respect to the initial state or with respect to a reference signal would be sufficient to assess drug efficacy. For example, using steady-state ^{31}P MRS it has been shown that the depletion of HEP levels following global cerebral ischemia is delayed by the administration of dihydropyridine Ca^{2+} antagonists [9]. Limitations of MRS is poor spatial resolution, which is a significant drawback when studying models of focal ischemia, and a poor SNR, which under typical experimental conditions (0.5 ml sampling volume, 1 min acquisition time) hardly exceeds a value of 5 to 10.

An additional limitation of steady-state measurements is the fact that changes in energy turnover will not be reflected by changes in substrate levels as long as the energy production matches the consumption. Therefore, direct measurements of energy turnover using magnetization transfer techniques have been suggested [54,56,57]. Drug effects are then assessed via the determination of a reaction flux of a metabolite X, v_X, which by itself is given by the product of the reaction rate constant k_X for the conversion of the metabolite and its concentration [X],

$$v_X = k_X[X] \tag{8.3}$$

We have assumed that the metabolite X is only participating in one reaction, which is governed by first-order kinetics [59]. This is, for example, the case for PCr, which is substrate for the creatine kinase reaction only. The pseudo-first-order forward rate constant k_f can be derived from a MRS saturation transfer experiment according to Ref. [59]

$$\frac{S_{PCr}(t)}{S_{PCr}} = \frac{T_{1,PCr}}{(1+k_f)T_{1,PCr}}\left\{\frac{1}{T_{1,PCr}} + k_f \exp\left[-\left(k_f + \frac{1}{T_{1,PCr}}\right)t\right]\right\} \tag{8.4}$$

with $S_{PCr}(t)$ and $S_{PCr}(0)$ being the PCr signal at time t and at baseline, respectively, and $T_{1,PCr}$ being the longitudinal relaxation time for PCr in the absence of the saturating pulse used to magnetically label the signal of the exchange partner (ATP). A frequency-selective saturation pulse (saturating the γ-phosphate resonance of ATP when analyzing the creatine kinase forward reaction rate) is applied during the transfer time t. Measurement of $S_{PCr}(t)$ at various transfer times allows the accurate determination of the rate constant and of $T_{1,PCr}$, the relaxation time employed in the conventional regression analysis. With this approach, it could be demonstrated that the dihydropyridine Ca^{2+} antagonist isradipine dose-dependently reduced the flux through the creatine kinase reaction in the normoxic rat brain [54]. The result indicated that the dihydropyridine Ca^{2+} antagonist rather reduced the energy consumption than enhanced the energy production. The accuracy of the approach is comparable to the measurement of steady-state HEP levels and, therefore, suffers from the same limitations.

8.6.2 Structural Changes Following Focal Cerebral Ischemia

Most of the preclinical studies evaluating drug efficacy were based on morphometric readouts in focal cerebral ischemia models. The underlying assumption was that a reduction of the structural damage, i.e., a reduction of the infarct volume, would necessarily translate into an improved behavioral or correspondingly clinical outcome. In other words, infarct volume served as an efficacy biomarker.

Accurate volume determinations depend on a high contrast-to-noise ratio between infarcted and healthy brain parenchyma; this is commonly provided by T_2-weighted images recorded 24 or 48 h following infarction. In fact, an excellent correlation has been found between infarct volumes determined *in vivo* using T_2-weighted MRI and those derived from histological analysis [61]. A significant number of drug candidates have been evaluated using this approach [60]. Alternatively, contrast based on other MRI parameters (ADC, CBF) has been used for the identification of the ischemic territory. In this case estimates for the final infarction might be obtained at an earlier time point, presumably prior to the onset of drug treatment.

A potential structural readout is the hemispheric swelling $\Delta H(\%)$, which is a measure for the vasogenic edema formation. It might be defined as [76]

$$\Delta H(\%) = 100\frac{H_{\text{ipsi}} - H_{\text{contra}}}{H_{\text{ipsi}} + H_{\text{contra}}} \tag{8.5}$$

with H_{ipsi} and H_{contra} being the ipsi- and contralateral hemispheric volumes. For example, it has been reported for SH rats that underwent unilateral MCA occlusion that the dihydropyridine Ca^{2+} antagonists, isradipine and nimodipine, significantly reduced hemispheric swelling to $2.3 \pm 1.5\%$, as compared to $6.6 \pm 1.9\%$ for placebo-treated animals [36]. In this study, hemispheric swelling was determined from *postmortem* hemispheric weights and not from *in vivo* MRI measurements. Values for hemispheric swelling might be used to correct infarct volumes for the different hemispheric volumes [76]. Two issues associated to *in vivo* determinations of $\Delta H(\%)$ are the low dynamic range and potential problems in determining the brain midline from MR images.

Drug-induced changes in tissue parameters *per se* were hardly used for assessment of therapeutic efficacy. Yet, demonstration that a pharmacological intervention, e.g., raised CBF values in the penumbral region of the infarction from 0.4 ml/g tissue/min to 0.6 ml/g tissue/min, would be highly relevant, as it might implicate the difference between tissue necrosis and survival. Such readouts should be envisaged in future studies.

8.6.3 Assessment of Drug Efficacy Using Functional Readouts

It should not be forgotten that the objective of stroke therapy is not to reduce infarct volume but to improve the clinical outcome of the patient, i.e., to preserve/restore brain functionality. Many experimental stroke studies have therefore used functional readouts to assess therapy, subjecting experimental animals to a battery of behavioral tests. In fact, rats with focal cerebral ischemia display an astonishing functional plasticity, and lost functions are recovered within relatively short periods of time. Therapeutic interventions may accelerate functional recovery significantly [122]. Yet it is not clear whether this is due to enhanced plasticity or whether the brain regions that have been spared from becoming infarcted are in fact functional. Functional reorganization (plasticity) of the brain is certainly a major factor leading to functional recovery. This has been demonstrated both in stroke patients [123] and in experimental animals [124]. In both cases, sensory/motor input following stimulation of fingers (or paws) contralateral to the infarction site was rerouted, in part, to the contralateral healthy somatosensory cortex.

Cytoprotective therapy using a variety of pharmacological strategies has been demonstrated to reduce the volume of infarction in animal models of focal cerebral ischemia. Demonstration that these regions are functional would be evidence that the assessment of the infarct volume is a valid efficacy biomarker for antiischemic therapy. Studies in rats that underwent permanent MCA occlusion and that were treated with isradipine confirmed this hypothesis only in part [86,87]. Albeit isradipine led to a significant reduction of the infarct volume, and in particular spared the somato-sensory cortex from becoming necrotic, electrical stimulation of the forepaws revealed no fMRI response in the corresponding cytoprotected cortical region during the first 48 h following MCA occlusion. The relative CBV response (determined using a blood–pool contrast agent) in the somato-sensory cortex was derived as

$$\frac{\Delta \mathrm{CBV}(t)}{\mathrm{CBV}_0} = \frac{\ln\{S(t)\} - \ln\{S(0)\}}{\ln\{S(0)\} - \ln\{S_0\}} \tag{8.6}$$

with S_0 and $S(0)$ being the signal intensities prior and 10 min after the administration of the intravascular contrast agent, and $S(t)$ the corresponding value at time t, e.g., during stimulation. At days 5 to 12 after vascular occlusion, some recovery of the function was observed; yet, only a fraction of the animals showed a fully recovered fMRI response, while the remaining animals of the drug-treated group displayed no CBV response whatsoever (Figure 8.6). In all animals, the corresponding fMRI signal in the healthy hemisphere was used as a reference [86,87]. Obviously, structural integrity is a necessary yet not sufficient prerequisite for functional integrity. The different responses were attributed to differences in CBF values in the cytoprotected territory [87]. CBF was sufficient to ensure survival of cells, but not sufficient in all cases to ensure proper functionality. This stresses the importance of accurate measurements of absolute perfusion rates.

8.6.4 Cell Tracking to Assess the Efficacy of Cell-based Therapies

Two factors contribute to the attractiveness of using MRI techniques for cell tracking studies: (1) the high temporospatial resolution provided by MRI and (2) the potentially high payloads of labels that can be achieved for a cell without affecting its vital functions (see Chapter 25 for more details). This overcomes in part the inherent sensitivity issues associated with MRI. Cell trafficking studies can be applied to qualitatively monitor the migration of cells within the intact organism. This has been discussed in the previous section with regard to the evaluation of stem cell therapies in stroke. Alternatively, quantitative assessments are feasible by either measuring the volume occupied by the labeled cells [82] or by estimating local cell densities via quantitative analyses of relaxation effects.

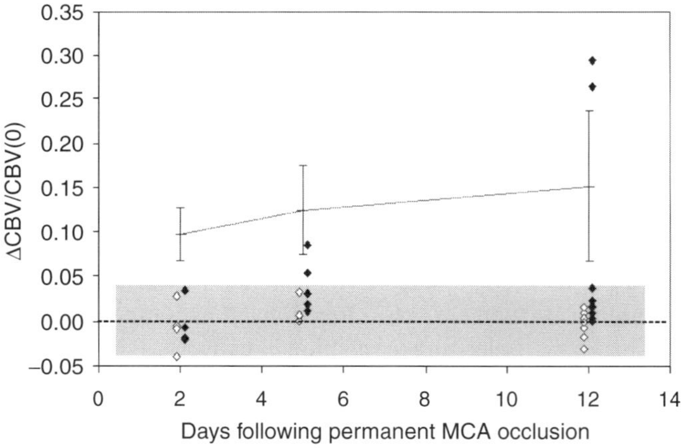

FIGURE 8.6 Functional recovery in cytoprotected cortex in rat permanent MCA occlusion model. Treatment with the Ca^{2+} antagonist isradipine spared the ipsilateral somatosensory cortex from becoming infarcted. Functional integrity was probed using electrical stimulation of the contralateral forepaw. The fMRI response in the cortical S1 area was analyzed at days 2, 5, and 12 following infarction. Signals from individual rats receiving isradipine (filled symbols) or vehicle (open symbols) are shown. The dashed line with error bars (standard deviation) represents the response measured on the contralateral intact hemisphere when stimulating the forepaw ipsilateral to the MCA occlusion site. Only a fraction of the animals displayed recovery of functionality in the cytoprotected area despite the fact that structural imaging revealed morphological integrity. (Adapted from Sauter, A. et al., *Magn. Reson. Med.*, 47, 759, 2002.)

The concentration of contrast agents can be estimated based on their effects on tissue relaxation rates according to

$$c(t) = \frac{T_{i0} - T_i(t)}{r_i T_{i0} T_i} \tag{8.7}$$

with T_i and T_{i0} ($i = 1,2$) being the tissue relaxation times measured prior to and after administration of the contrast agent, while r_i is the molar relaxivity of the contrast agent. The same approach can be extended in a straightforward manner to estimate local concentration of magnetically labeled cells [83], provided the corresponding r_i value for the chosen labeling conditions is known. Even if this is not the case, accurate measurement of relaxation times would allow one to estimate relative cell concentrations, which might be sufficient for drug studies.

8.7 CONCLUSION

A large variety of animal models of human embolic stroke has been developed and widely used for the evaluation of potential therapeutic intervention. Over decades, pharmacological research has largely focused on cytoprotective approaches, i.e., intervention in the acute phase of cerebral infarction. Strategies comprised rapid tissue reperfusion via thrombolysis, alleviating the detrimental consequences of energy failure by lowering intracellular levels of Ca^{2+}, or reducing exhaustive neuronal stimulation by excitatory amino acids such as glutamate, to name a few. Yet, despite impressive results in preclinical models, none of these approaches, with the exception of thrombolysis using rtPA, could be successfully translated into the clinics. The reasons are manifold and a discussion is beyond the scope of this article. Factors of relevance are the time window following infarction: drug administration has to occur within the first few hours following infarction in order to be successful. The patient population is much less homogeneous than the respective animal models used, i.e., large groups are required to demonstrate efficacy. Last but not least, the prognostic value of the animal models may be limited: a vascular occlusion in a healthy young animal does not necessarily correspond to the situation in an elderly patient, potentially with a prolonged history of hypertension and/or atherosclerotic disease. More realistic models are feasible, e.g., when using SH stroke-prone rats [125], which spontaneously develop infarction. Such models, however, are less practicable for drug testing on a large scale.

The value of imaging, and in particular MRI, in stroke research is manifold. The MRI signal is governed by a multitude of parameters, which allow the investigation of various aspects of the pathophysiological cascade of cerebral infarction. The characteristic fingerprint of MRI parameters has been suggested as tissue signature suitable for staging cerebral tissue [76,77]. Moreover, some of the readouts are of prognostic value: the lesion volume as derived from CBF maps measured within hours after infarction seems to provide a good estimate for the "final" infarct size in the absence of treatment. This would enable use of a patient as their own control, i.e., assessment of the treatment efficacy with respect to a hypothetical untreated lesion volume. Yet, this concept is highly speculative and extensive studies are still required for validation of the approach (see Chapter 9, Section 9.2.3).

MRI methods allow a direct correlation of structural measures (infarct location and volume) with functional readouts (behavior or brain activity measures). Experimental evidence suggests that both are required for a comprehensive characterization of drug efficacy. The paradigm that reduced infarct volumes will translate into improved functional outcome seems not always to be true [86,87]. Finally, the lack of success of treatment strategies for acute stroke has shifted the interest to the chronic phase addressing aspects such as inflammation and eventually neuroregeneration. Imaging approaches also provide solutions to monitor these processes; for instance, inflammation can be tracked by monitoring the migration of immune-competent cells, such as macrophages, labeled *in vivo* using contrast agents composed of iron-containing nanoparticles [18,83]. Analogous methods have been applied to visualize the migration of stem cell therapy [117]. Similar to the situation described for cytoprotective treatment, functional readouts have to be used to assess the functionality of neuronal stem cell grafts.

In conclusion, MRI methods enable a comprehensive characterization of both the pathophysiology of cerebral infarction and therapeutic interventions providing quantitative structural and functional readouts. As such, MRI has become an indispensable tool in the development of novel therapies of human embolic stroke, as will be discussed in the next chapter.

REFERENCES

1. Hacke, W. et al., Thrombolysis in acute ischemic stroke: controlled trials and clinical experience, *Neurology*, 53(Suppl. 4), S3, 1999.
2. Leira, E. C. and Adams, H. P., Management of acute ischemic stroke, *Clin. Geriatr. Med.*, 15, 701, 1999.
3. Schellinger, P. D. and Warach, S., Therapeutic time window of thrombolytic therapy following stroke, *Curr. Atheroscler. Rep.*, 6, 288, 2004.
4. Siesjö, B. K., *Brain Energy Metabolism*, John Wiley & Sons, New York, 1978.
5. Hossmann, K. A., Treatment of experimental cerebral ischemia, *J. Cereb. Blood Flow Metab.*, 2, 275, 1982.
6. Siesjö, B. K. and Wieloch, T., Cerebral metabolism in ischemia: neurochemical basis for therapy, *Brit. J. Anaesth.*, 57, 47, 1985.
7. Delpy, D. T. et al., Noninvasive investigation of cerebral ischemia by phosphorus magnetic resonance, *Pediatrics*, 70, 310, 1982.
8. Prichard, J. W. et al., Cerebral metabolic studies in vivo by ^{31}P NMR, *Proc. Natl. Acad. Sci. U.S.A*, 80, 2748, 1983.
9. Sauter, A. and Rudin, M., Effects of calcium antagonists on high-energy phosphates in ischemic rat brain measured by ^{31}P NMR spectroscopy, *Magn. Reson. Med.*, 4, 1, 1987.
10. Rehncrona, S., Rosen, I., and Siesjö, B. K., Brain lactic acidosis and ischemic cell damage. 1. Biochemistry and neurophysiology, *J. Cereb. Blood Flow Metab.*, 2, 297, 1981.
11. Dutta, D., Mechanism of store-operated calcium entry, *J. Biosci.*, 25, 397, 2000.
12. Tranquillini, M. E. and Reggiani, A., Glycine-site antagonists and stroke, *Exp. Opin. Invest. Drugs*, 8, 1837, 1999.
13. Schneggenburger, R. et al., Fractional contribution of calcium to the cation current through glutmate receptor channels, *Neuron*, 11, 133, 1993.
14. Henrich-Noack, P. et al., Distinct influence of the group III metabotropic glutamate receptor agonist (R,S)-4-phosphonophenylglycine [(R,S)-PPG] on different forms of neuronal damage, *Neuropharmacology*, 39, 911, 2000.
15. Rother, J. et al., MR detection of cortical spreading depression immediately after focal ischemia in the rat, *J. Cereb. Blood Flow Metab.*, 16, 214, 1996.
16. Busch, E. et al., Potassium-induced spreading depressions during focal cerebral ischemia in rats: contribution to lesion growth assessed by diffusion-weighted NMR and biochemical imaging, *J. Cereb. Blood Flow Metab.*, 16, 1090, 1996.
17. Pietri, S., Culcasi, M., and Cozzone, P. J., Real-time continuous-flow spin trapping of hydroxyl free radical in the ischemic and post-ischemic myocardium, *Eur. J. Biochem.*, 186, 163, 1989.
18. Rausch, M. et al., In-vivo visualization of phagocytotic cells in rat brains after transient ischemia by USPIO, *NMR Biomed.*, 15, 278, 2002.
19. Zhang, R. L. et al., Temporal profile of ischemic tissue damage, neutrophil response, and vascular plugging following permanent and transient (2h) middle cerebral artery occlusion in the rat, *J. Neurol. Sci.*, 125, 3, 1994.
20. Matsuo, Y. et al., Role of neutrophils in radical production during ischemia and reperfusion of the rat brain: effects of neutrophil depletion and extracellular ascorbyl radical formation, *J. Cereb. Blood Flow Metab.*, 15, 941, 1995.
21. Banasiak, K. J., Xia, Y., and Haddad, G. G., Mechanisms underlying hypoxia-induced neuronal apoptosis, *Prog. Neurobiol.*, 16, 202, 2000.

22. Del Zoppo, G. J. et al., Infalmmation in stroke: putative role of cytokines, adhesion molecules and iNOS in brain response to ischemia, *Brain Pathol.*, 10, 95, 2000.
23. Fink, K. et al., Prolonged therapeutic window for ischemic brain damage caused by delayed caspase activation, *J. Cereb. Blood Flow Metab.*, 18, 1071, 1998.
24. Namura, S. et al., Activation and cleavage of caspase-3 in apoptosis induced by experimental cerebral ischemia, *J. Neurosci.*, 18, 3659, 1998.
25. Linton, S. D. et al., Oxamyl dipeptide caspase inhibitors developed for the treatment of stroke, *Bioorg. Med. Chem. Lett.*, 14, 2685, 2004.
26. Wu, Y. et al., Caspase-7 activation after ischemia in caspase-3 deficient mice, *Soc. Neurosci. Abstr.*, 26, 245, 2000.
27. Stoll, G., Jander, S., and Schroeter, M., Inflammation and glial responses in ischemic brain lesions, *Prog. Neurobiol.*, 56, 149, 1998.
28. Wang, X. et al., Monocyte chemoattractant protein-1 messenger RNA expression in rat ischemic cortex, *Stroke*, 26, 661, 1995.
29. Kim, J. S. et al., Expression of monocyte chemoattractant protein-1 and macrophage inflammatory protein-1 after focal cerebral ischemia in the rat, *J. Neuroimmunol.*, 56, 127, 1995.
30. Rothwell, N. J. and Lusheshi, G. N., Interleukin-1 in the brain: biology, pathology, and therapeutic target, *Trend Neurosci.*, 23, 618, 2000.
31. Huang, D. R. et al., Absence of chemoattractant protein-1 in mice leads to decreased local macrophage recruitment and antigen-specific T helper cell type 1 immune response in experimental autoimmune encephalomyelitis, *J. Exp. Med.*, 193, 713, 2001.
32. Hughes, P. M. et al., Monocyte chemoattractant protein-1 deficiency is protective in a murine stroke model, *J. Cereb. Blood Flow Metab.*, 22, 308, 2002.
33. Pulsinelli, W. A. and Brieley, J. B., A new model of bilateral hemispheric ischemia in the unanaesthetized rat, *Stroke*, 10, 267, 1979.
34. Ito, U. et al., Experimental cerebral ischemia in Mongolioan gerbils: I. Light microscopic observations, *Acta Neuropathol. (Berl.)*, 32, 209, 1975.
35. Tamura, A. et al., Focal cerebral ischemia in the rat: 1. Description of techniques and early neuropathological consequences following middle cerebral artery occlusion, *J. Cereb. Blood Flow Metab.*, 1, 53, 1981.
36. Sauter, A. and Rudin, M., Calcium antagonists reduce the extent of infarction in rat middle cerebral artery occlusion model as determined by quantitative magnetic resonance imaging, *Stroke*, 17, 1228, 1986.
37. Sauter, A. and Rudin, M., Strain-dependent drug effects in rat middle cerebral artery occlusion model of stroke, *J. Pharmacol. Exp. Ther.*, 274, 1008, 1995.
38. Coyle, P., Spatial relations of dorsal anastomoses and lesion border after middle cerebral artery occlusion, *Stroke*, 18, 1133, 1987.
39. Duverger, D. and McKenzie, E. T., The quantification of cerebral infarction following focal ischemia in the rat: influence of strain, arterial pressure, blood glucose concentration, and age, *J. Cereb. Blood Flow Metab.*, 8, 449, 1988.
40. Grome, J. J. et al., Quantitation of photochemically induced focal cerebral ischemia in the rat, *J. Cereb. Blood Flow Metab.*, 8, 89, 1988.
41. Koizumi, J. et al., Experimental model of ischemic brain edema. 1. A new experimental model of cerebral embolism in rats in which recirculation can be introduced in the ischemic area, *Jpn. J. Stroke*, 8, 1, 1986.
42. van Dorsten, F. A. et al., Diffusion- and perfusion-weighted MR imaging of transient focal cerebral ischaemia in mice, *NMR Biomed.*, 12, 525, 1999.
43. Jiang, Q. et al., Diffusion-, T_2-, and perfusion-weighted nuclear magnetic resonance imaging of middle cerebral artery embolic stroke and recombinant tissue plasminogen activator intervention in the rat, *J. Cereb. Blood Flow Metab.*, 18, 758, 1998.
44. Sharkey, J., Ritchie, I. M., and Kelly, P. A., Perivascular microapplication of endothelin-1: a new model of focal cerebral ischaemia in the rat, *J. Cereb. Blood Flow Metab.*, 13, 865, 1993.
45. Faden, A. I. et al., The role of excitatory amino acids and NMDA receptors in traumatic brain injury, *Science*, 244, 798, 1989.

46. Blight, A. R., Saito, K., and Heyes, M. P., Increased levels of the excitotoxin quinolinic acid in spinal cord following contusion injury, *Brain Res.*, 632, 314, 1993.
47. Schwarcz, R. et al., Excitotoxic models for neurodegenerative disorders, *Life Sci.*, 35, 19, 1984.
48. Pappius, H. M., Neurochemical approaches to the amelioration of brain injury, *J. Neural Transm. Supp.*, 29, 49, 1990.
49. Winn, P. et al., A comparison of excitotoxic lesions of the basal forebrain by kainate, quinolinate, ibotenate, *N*-methyl-D-aspartate or quisqualate, and the effects on toxicity of 2-amino-5-phosphonovaleric acid and kynurenic acid in the rat, *Br. J. Pharmacol.*, 102, 904, 1991.
50. Henshaw, R. et al., Malonate produces striatal lesions by indirect NMDA receptor activation, *Brain Res.*, 647, 161, 1994.
51. van Lookeren-Campagne, M. et al., Early evolution and recovery from excitotoxic injury in the neonatal rat brain: a study combining magnetic resonance imaging, electrical impedance, and histology, *J. Cereb. Blood Flow Metab.*, 14, 1011, 1994.
52. Laurent, D. et al., Reduction of excitotoxicity-induced brain damage by the competitive NMDA antagonist CGP 40116: a longitudinal study using diffusion-weighted imaging, *Neurosci. Lett.*, 213, 209, 1996.
53. Williams, S. R., Gadian, D. G., and Proctor, E., A method for lactate detection in-vivo by spectral editing without the need for double irradiation, *J. Magn. Reson.*, 66, 562, 1986.
54. Rudin, M. and Sauter, A., Dihydropyridine calcium antagonists reduce the consumption of high-energy phosphates in the rat brain. A study using combine $^{31}P/^{1}H$ magnetic resonance spectroscopy and ^{31}P saturation transfer, *J. Pharmacol. Exp. Ther.*, 251, 700, 1989.
55. Sauter, A. and Rudin, M., Determination of creatine kinase kinetic parameters in rat brain by NMR magnetization transfer: correlation with brain function, *J. Biol. Chem.*, 268, 13166, 1993.
56. Bittl, J. A. and Ingwall, J. S., Reaction rates of creatine kinases and ATP synthesis in the isolated rat heart, *J. Biol. Chem.*, 26, 3512, 1985.
57. Forsen, S. and Hoffman, R. A., Study of moderately rapid chemical exchange reaction by means of nuclear magnetic double resonance, *J. Chem. Phys.*, 40, 1189, 1963.
58. Koretsky, A. P. et al., ^{31}P NMR saturation transfer measurements of phosphorus exchange reactions in rat heart and kidney in situ, *Biochemistry*, 25, 77, 1986.
59. Rudin, M. and Sauter, A., Measurement of reaction rates in vivo using magnetization transfer techniques, In *NMR: Basic Principles and Progress*, Vol. 27, Diehl, P., Ed., Springer, Heidelberg, p. 257, 1992.
60. Rudin, M. et al., In vivo magnetic resonance in pharmaceutical research: current status and perspectives, *NMR Biomed.*, 12, 69, 1999.
61. Allegrini, P. R. and Sauer, D., Application of magnetic resonance imaging to the measurement of neurodegeneration in rat brain: MRI data correlate strongly with histology and enzymatic analysis, *Magn. Reson. Imaging*, 10, 773, 1992.
62. Villringer, A. et al., Dynamic imaging with lanthanide chelates in normal brain: contrast due to magnetic susceptibility effects, *Magn. Reson. Med.*, 6, 164, 1988.
63. Rudin, M. and Sauter, A., Noninvasive determination of regional cerebral blood flow in rats using dynamic imaging with Gd(DTPA), *Magn. Reson. Med.*, 22, 32, 1991.
64. Detre, J. A. et al., Perfusion imaging, *Magn. Reson. Med.*, 23, 37, 1992.
65. Warach, S., Dashe, J. F., and Edelman, R. R., Clinical outcome in ischemic stroke predicted by early diffusion-weighted and perfusion magnetic resonance imaging: a preliminary analysis, *J. Cereb. Blood Flow Metab.*, 16, 53, 1996.
66. Busch, E. et al., Reperfusion after thrombolytic therapy of embolic stroke in the rat — magnetic resonance and biochemical imaging, *J. Cereb. Blood Flow Metab.*, 18, 407, 1998.
67. Astrup, J., Siesjö, B. K., and Symon, L., Thresholds in cerebral ischemia — the ischemic penumbra, *Stroke*, 12, 723, 1981.
68. Verheul, H. B. et al., Comparison of diffusion-weighted MRI with changes in cell volume in a rat model of brain injury, *NMR Biomed.*, 7, 96, 1994.
69. Norris, D. G., The effects of microscopic tissue parameters on the diffusion weighted magnetic resonance imaging experiment, *NMR Biomed.*, 14, 77, 2001.
70. Vorisek, I. et al., Water ADC, extracellular space volume, and tortuosity in the rat cortex after traumatic injury, *Magn. Reson. Med.*, 48, 994, 2002.

71. Dijkhuizen, R. M. et al., Changes in the diffusion of water and intracellular metabolites after excitotoxic injury and global ischemia in neonatal rat brain, *J. Cereb. Blood Flow Metab.*, 19, 341, 1999.
72. van der Toorn, A. et al., Dynamic changes in water ADC, energy metabolism, extracellular space volume, and tortuosity in neonatal rat brain during global ischemia, *Magn. Reson. Med.*, 36, 52, 1996.
73. Davis, M. et al., The effect of age on cerebral oedema, cerebral infarction and neuroprotective potential in experimental occlusive stroke, *Acta Neurochir. (Wien)*, 60(Suppl.), 282, 1994.
74. Hasegawa, Y. et al., MRI diffusion mapping of reversible and irreversible ischemic injury in focal brain ischemia, *Neurology*, 44, 1484, 1994.
75. Schlaug, G. et al., Time course of the apparent diffusion coefficient (ADC) abnormality in human stroke, *Neurology*, 49, 113, 1997.
76. Rudin, M. et al., MRI analysis of the changes in apparanet water diffusion coefficient, T_2 relaxation time, and cerebral blood flow and volume in the temporal evolution of cerebral infarction following permanent middle cerebral artery occlusion in rats, *Exp. Neurol.*, 169, 56, 2001.
77. Jiang, Q. et al., The temporal evolution of MRI tissue signatures after transient middle cerebral artery occlusion in rat, *J. Neurol. Sci.*, 145, 15, 1997.
78. Warach, S., Measurement of the ischemic penumbra with MRI: it's about time, *Stroke*, 34, 2533, 2003.
79. Neumann-Haefelin, T. et al., Diffusion- and perfusion-weighted MRI: the DWI/PWI mismatch region in acute stroke, *Stroke*, 30, 1591, 1999.
80. Weissleder, R. et al., Ultrasmall superparamagnetic iron oxide: an intravenous contrast agent for assessing lymph nodes with MR imaging, *Radiology*, 175, 494, 1990.
81. Dousset, V. et al., Comparison of ultrasmall particles of iron oxide (USPIO)-enhanced T_2-weighted, conventional T_2-weighted, and gadolinium-enhanced T_1-weighted MR images in rats with experimental autoimmune encephalomyelitis, *Am. J. Neuroradiol.*, 20, 223, 1999.
82. Rausch, M. et al., MRI-based monitoring of inflammation and tissue damage in acute and chronic relapsing EAE, *Magn. Reson. Med.*, 50, 309, 2003.
83. Rausch, M. et al., Dynamic pattern of USPIO enhancement can be observed in macrophages after ischemic brain damage, *Magn. Reson. Med.*, 46, 1018, 2001.
84. Reese, T. et al., Magnetic resonance angiography of the rat cerebrovascular system without the use of contrast agents, *NMR Biomed.*, 12, 189, 1999.
85. Beckmann, N., Stirnimann, R., and Bochelen, D., High-resolution magnetic resonance angiography of the mouse brain: application to murine focal cerebral ischemia models, *J. Magn. Reson.*, 140, 442, 1999.
86. Reese, T. et al., Cytoprotection does not preserve brain functionality in rats during acute post-stroke phase despite evidence of non-infarction provided by MRI, *NMR Biomed.*, 13, 361, 2000.
87. Sauter, A. et al., Recovery of function in cytoprotected cerebral cortex in rat stroke model assessed by functional MRI, *Magn. Reson. Med.*, 47, 759, 2002.
88. Reese, T. et al., Impaired functionality of reperfused brain tissue following short transient focal ischemia in rats, *Magn. Reson. Imaging*, 20, 447, 2002.
89. Germano, I. M. et al., Magnetic resonance imaging in the evaluation of nimodipine-treated acute experimental focal cerebral ischemia, *Acta Radiol.*, 369(Suppl.), 49, 1986.
90. Sauer, D. et al., Differing effects of alpha-difluormethylornithin and CGP40116 on polyamine levels and infarct volume in a rat model of focal cerebral ischemia, *Neurosci. Lett.*, 141, 131, 1992.
91. Sauer, D. et al., The competitive NMD antagonist CGP 40116 permanently reduces brain damage after middle cerebral artery occlusion in rats, *J. Cereb. Blood Flow Metab.*, 15, 602, 1995.
92. Urwyler, S. et al., Biphenyl-derivatives of 2-amino-7-phophono-heptanoic acid, a novel class of potent competitive *N*-methyl-D-aspartate receptor antagonists. II. Pharmacological characterization in vivo, *Neuropharmacology*, 35, 655, 1996.
93. Qiu, H. et al., Progression of a focal ischemic lesion in rat brain during treatment with a novel glycine/NMDA antagonist: an in vivo three-dimensional diffusion-weighted MR microscopy study, *J. Magn. Reson. Imaging*, 7, 739, 1997.
94. Petty, M. A. et al., In vivo neuroprotective effects of ACEA 1021 confirmed by magnetic resonance imaging in ischemic stroke, *Eur. J. Pharmacol.*, 474, 53, 2003.
95. Buchan, A. M. et al., Blockade of AMPA receptors prevents CA1 hippocampal injury following severe but transient forebrain ischemia in adult rats, *Neurosci. Lett.*, 132, 1358, 1991.

96. Nellgard, B. and Wieloch, T., Postischemic blockade of AMPA but not NMDA receptors mitigates neuronal damage in the rat brain following transient severe cerebral ischemia, *J. Cereb. Blood Flow Metab.*, 12, 2, 1992.
97. Muller, T. B. et al., Perfusion and diffusion-weighted MR imaging for in vivo evaluation of treatment with U74389G in a rat stroke model, *Stroke*, 26, 1453, 1995.
98. Mattson, M. P., Culmsee, C., and Yu, Z. F., Apoptotic and antiapoptotic mechanisms in stroke, *Cell Tissue Res.*, 301, 173, 2000.
99. Loddick, S. A., McKenzie, A., and Rothwell, N. J., An ICE inhibitor, z-VAD-DCB attenuates ischemic brain damage in the rat, *Neuroreport*, 7, 1465, 1996.
100. Wiessner, C. et al., Protective effects of caspase inhibitors in models for cerebral ischemia in vitro and in vivo, *Cell. Mol. Biol.*, 46, 53, 2000.
101. Deckwerth, T. L. et al., Longterm protection of brain tissue from cerebral ischemia by peripherally administered peptidomimetic caspase inhibitors, *Drug Dev. Res.*, 52, 579, 2001.
102. Uchino, H., Ishii, N., and Shibasaki, F., Calcineurin and cyclophilin D are differential targets of neuroprotection by immunosuppressants CsA and FK506 in ischemic brain damage, *Acta Neurochir*, 86(Suppl.), 105, 2003.
103. Li, P. A. et al., Amelioration by cyclosorine A of brain damage following 5 or 10 min of ischemia in rats subjected to preischemic hyperglycemia, *Brain Res.*, 753, 133, 1997.
104. Sharkey, J. et al., Tacrolimus (FK506) ameliorates skilled motor deficits produced by middle cerebral artery occlusion in trats, *Stroke*, 27, 2282, 1996.
105. Bochelen, D., Rudin, M., and Sauter, A., Calcineurin inhibitors FK506 and SDY ASM 981 alleviate the outcome of focal cerebral ischemic/reperfusion injury, *J. Pharmacol. Exp. Ther.*, 288, 653, 1999.
106. Pong, K. and Zaleska, M. M., Therapeutic implications for immunophilin ligands in the treatment of neurodegenerative diseases, *Curr. Drug Targets CNS Neurol. Disord.*, 2, 349, 2003.
107. Bram, R. J. et al., Identification of the immunophilins capable of mediating inhibition of signal transductionby cyclosporine A and FK506: roles of calcineurin binding and cellular binding cellular location, *Mol. Cell. Biol.*, 13, 4760, 1993.
108. Jiang, Y. et al., Monocyte chemoattractant protein-1 regulates adhesion molecule expression and cytokine production in human monocytes, *J. Immunol.*, 148, 2423, 1992.
109. Chopp, M. et al., Post ischemic administration of an anti-MAC-1 antibody reduces ischemic cell damage after transient middle cerebral artery occlusion in the rat, *Stroke*, 25, 869, 1994.
110. Goussev, A. V. et al., P-selectin antibody reduces hemorrhage and infarct volume resulting from MCA occlusion in the rat, *J. Neurol. Sci.*, 161, 16, 1999.
111. Zhang, R. L., Zhang, Z. G., and Chopp, M., Increased therapeutic efficacy with rt-PA and anti-CD18 antibody treatment of stroke in the rat, *Neurology*, 52, 273, 1999.
112. Freed, C. R. et al., Transplantation of human fetal dopamine cells for Parkinson's disease. Results at 1 year, *Arch. Neurol.*, 47, 505, 1990.
113. Lindvall, O. et al., Grafts of fetal dopamine neurons survive and improve motor function in Parkinson's disease, *Science*, 247, 574, 1990.
114. Modo, M. et al., Effects of implantation site of stem cell grafts on behavioral recovery from stroke damage, *Stroke*, 33, 2270, 2002.
115. Mattsson, B. et al., Neuronal grafting to experimental neocortical infarcts improves behavioral outcome and reduces thalamic atrophy in rats housed in enriched but not in standard environments, *Stroke*, 28, 1225, 1997.
116. Kelly, S. et al., Transplanted human fetal neural stem cells survive, migrate, and differentiate in ischemic rat cerebral cortex, *Proc. Nati. Acad. Sci. U.S.A*, 101, 11839, 2004.
117. Hoehn, M. et al., Monitoring of implanted stem cell migration in vivo: a highly resolved in vivo magnetic resonance imaging investigation of experimental stroke in rat, *Proc. Nati. Acad. Sci. U.S.A*, 99, 16267, 2002.
118. Contag, C. H. et al., Visualizing gene expression in living mammals using a bioluminescent reporter, *Photochem. Photobiol.*, 523, 1997.
119. Kim, D. E. et al., Imaging of stem cell recruitment to ischemic infarcts in a murine model, *Stroke*, 35, 952, 2004.
120. Schwab, M. E., Nogo and axon regeneration, *Curr. Opin. Neurobiol.*, 14, 118, 2004.

121. Wiessner, C. et al., Anti-Nogo-A antibody infusion 24 hours after experimental stroke improved behavioral outcome and corticospinal plasticity in normotensive and spontaneously hypertensive rats, *J. Cereb. Blood Flow Metab.*, 23, 154, 2003.
122. van der Staay, F. J., Augstein, K. H., and Horvath, E., Sensorimotor impairments in Wistar Kyoto rats with cerebral infarction, induced by unilateral occlusion of the middle cerebral artery: recovery of function, *Brain Res.*, 715, 180, 1996.
123. Cramer, S. C., Functional imaging in stroke recovery, *Stroke*, 35, 2695, 2004.
124. Dijkhuizen, R. M. et al., Correlation between brain reorganization, ischemic damage, and neurologic status after transient focal cerebral ischemia in rats: a functional magnetic resonance imaging study, *J. Neurosci.*, 23, 510, 2003.
125. Yamori, Y., Importance of genetic factors in stroke: an evidence obtained by selective breeding of stroke-prone and -resistant SHR, *Jpn. Circ. J.*, 38, 1095, 1974.

9 MRI in Clinical Studies of Stroke

Eric Juettler, Jochen B. Fiebach, and Peter D. Schellinger

CONTENTS

9.1 INTRODUCTION

This chapter presents an overview of magnetic resonance imaging (MRI) as a diagnostic approach to stroke management. Over the last decade there have been major breakthroughs in stroke research and the understanding of the pathophysiology of ischemic stroke has grown considerably. Consequently, there have been numerous drug trials of acute stroke trying to take benefit from our knowledge of the regulation of brain circulation and metabolism, glutamate excitotoxicity, peri-infarct depolarization, free radicals, apoptosis, and inflammation. Yet, so far all of these efforts using antiinflammatory and antiapoptotic drugs, growth factors, and gene therapy, to name but a few, have shown disappointing results in clinical trials and thrombolysis is still the treatment of choice for acute stroke within the first few hours after symptom onset. One reason for the failure of these new therapies is that they usually affect only one aspect of stroke pathophysiology. Stroke, however, is a heterogeneous disorder encompassing several etiologies with different pathobiological mechanisms often co-existing in one patient. All of these may need a different therapeutic approach and may be useful only in a distinct time window so that a specific treatment option may be beneficial in one patient but of no benefit or even detrimental in another. Therefore, it seems reasonable to apply improved selection criteria that allow categorization of those patients who have a relevant indication for a given therapy from those who do not.

New MRI techniques have revolutionized diagnostic imaging in stroke. MRI is a powerful tool that allows not only quick definition of the state of stroke and the time window for thrombolysis and other therapies, but is also capable of differentiating several etiologies, underlying causes and co-existing disorders and therefore to individualize patient management based on pathophysiological reasoning and not on rigid time windows. MRI to date is therefore the most promising diagnostic tool to translate preclinical developments to the bedside.

This chapter concentrates in the first part on giving the reader an integrated knowledge of the current status of the use of MRI in the diagnosis of stroke based on the definition of the underlying etiology, as well as in stroke therapy based on pathophysiological information rendered by a multiparametric stroke-MRI protocol. This will be compared to other imaging techniques with a special focus on computerized tomography (CT). The second part gives an overview of current or upcoming stroke trials that use MRI as a selection criteria to include patients. Finally, in the third part we review new MR imaging techniques and novel sequences that will provide further information and may be used in the diagnosis of stroke in the future.

9.2 CURRENT STATUS OF THE USE OF MRI IN THE DIAGNOSIS AND THERAPY OF STROKE

Up to 85% of all strokes are of ischemic origin and mostly due to blockage of a cerebral artery by a blood clot [1]. The target for most therapeutic interventions for focal ischemia is ischemic tissue that can respond to treatment and is not irreversibly injured. Such tissue must be distinguished from nonsalvageable ischemic tissue, which has evolved to a state, in which recovery is no longer possible. The characterization of potentially reversible vs. irreversible loss of function is based on the concept of the ischemic penumbra [2]. Until recently only PET and SPECT imaging could approximately define ischemia and penumbra thresholds. This is, however, not feasible for caregivers in a broad population, where diagnostic imaging in an acute setting is confined to CT and MRI imaging.

In the acute phase of ischemic stroke, the penumbra is defined as hypoperfused but still viable brain tissue. The underlying pathophysiological concept is that of neuronal damage caused by reduced cerebral blood flow (CBF). CBF values normally range from 60 to 70 ml/100 g/min in gray and 20 to 30 ml/100 g/min in white matter. A reduction of CBF to 10–20 ml/100 g/min results in a loss of neuronal function but preserved brain structure. This area is the so-called ischemic penumbra (semishadow, twilight zone). Below a threshold of 10–12 ml/100 g/min absolute ischemia is present, which immediately after onset leads to loss of neuronal function and within minutes to neuronal structural damage with irreversible ischemic infarction. The area thus affected is the so-called ischemic core. With time, the size of the ischemic penumbra diminishes and the infarct core progressively grows. If CBF is restored in time, the ischemic damage in the penumbra is reversible, and in most instances there is no manifest ischemic stroke. Therefore, the lysis of the thrombus with subsequent reestablishment of cerebral blood flow by cerebrovascular recanalization is the most promising therapy in this state of stroke [3].

Four large trials (NINDS, ECASS I and II, and ATLANTIS studies) investigated the use of recombinant tissue plasminogen activator (rtPA) for intravenous thrombolysis. These trials randomized a total of 2775 patients to treatment with placebo ($n = 1384$ patients) or intravenous rtPA ($n = 1391$ patients) within 0 to 3 h (NINDS), 3 to 5 h (ATLANTIS), or 0 to 6 h (ECASS I and II) after symptom onset. Meta-analyses of these studies [4–6] underlined the crucial meaning of the time window for treatment showing a significant correlation of outcome with time from symptom onset to start of treatment. Within the first 3 h, there were significant changes in outcome even at 10-min increments. The two clinical trials for intraarterial thrombolytic therapy (PROACT I and II) [7,8] used pro-urokinase for acute middle cerebral artery occlusion and showed significant improvement in outcome if administered within 3 to 6 h after stroke onset [8]. These clinical trials clearly demonstrated a negative correlation between the time to re-establish cerebral blood flow and the clinical outcome. They supported the pathophysiological concept of hypoperfusion as a main treatment target and established the therapeutic principle of Time is Brain in the early phase of stroke.

To identify patients who most likely benefit from thrombolytic therapy in the acute phase of cerebral ischemia, the diagnostic technique of choice should therefore be capable to (1) be performed as quickly as possible; (2) exclude other causes of stroke symptoms, the most common being intracerebral hemorrhage and epileptic seizures; (3) detect the ischemic tissue and the duration of ischemia; (4) distinguish between irreversibly damaged tissue and hypoperfused, but potentially salvageable tissue, i.e., tissue at risk; (5) identify risk factors and identify patients to whom treatment may be harmful; and (6) provide further information about the underlying etiology of the stroke, i.e., show any vessel occlusion and its location.

9.2.1 Diagnosis and Treatment of Acute Stroke and Underlying Etiology Based on MRI

A stroke-MRI protocol consists at least of standard MR sequences such as T_2-weighted imaging (T_2-WI), FLAIR, and MR Angiography (MRA).

On T_2-WI, ischemic infarction appears as a hyperintense lesion. Definite signal changes, however, are at the earliest seen 2 h after stroke onset in animal experiments and 6 to 8 h after stroke onset in human stroke [9]. Neither a diagnosis of parenchymal ischemia nor the differentiation of ischemic core from penumbral tissue is possible with T_2-WI. On the other hand, T_2-WI provides a good anatomical definition of the brain, and depicts microangiopathic changes, edema, old infarcts, or other pathologies [10] (Figure 9.1). FLAIR demonstrates hyperintense vessel sign [11] (Figure 9.2). MRA demonstrates vessel occlusion or patency [12] (Figure 9.3). T_2^*-WI (e.g., source images from PWI) shows the presence or absence of acute and chronic intracranial hemorrhages.

The advent of perfusion-(PWI) and diffusion-(DWI) weighted imaging in the early 1990s has added another dimension to diagnostic imaging in stroke [13–15]. During the last years a growing body of evidence has accumulated, documenting the usefulness of this methodology in the clinical setting of acute ischemic stroke including the differentiation of infarct patterns in hyperacute stroke and the prediction of clinical outcome, which may allow a more rational selection of therapeutic strategies based on the presence or absence of a tissue at risk [16–21].

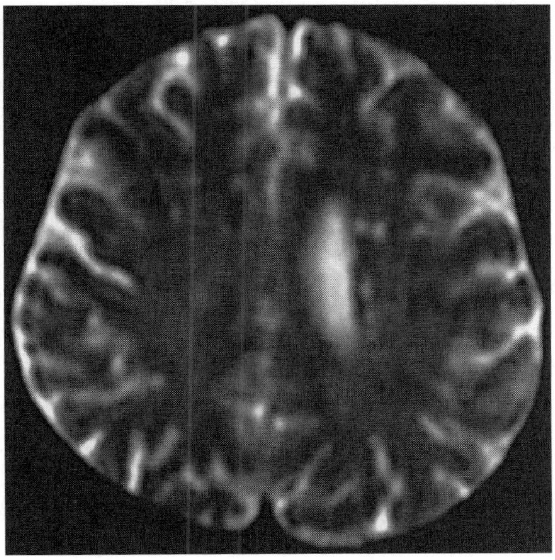

FIGURE 9.1 Acute MCA infarction 2 h after symptom onset. T_2-WI, axial, TR 3800 msec, TE 22 msec flip angle 180°, slice thickness 5 mm, FOV (mm) 240, acquisition matrix 128 × 256, acquisition time 1 min 42 sec.

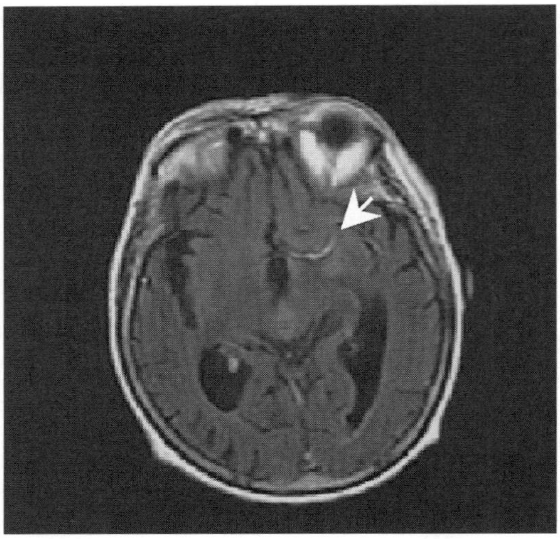

FIGURE 9.2 Acute MCA infarction 2 h after symptom onset. FLAIR, axial, TR 4500 msec, TE 105 msec, TI 1870 msec, flip angle 90°, slice thickness 5 mm, FOV (mm) 230, acquisition matrix 224 × 256, acquisition time 3 min 22 sec.

Diffusion-weighted imaging (DWI) exploits the net movement of water in tissue due to random (Brownian) molecular motion as a contrast mechanism. It is based on a methodology described in 1965 [22] and was incorporated 20 years later into MRI sequences [23]. In tissue, the free movement of water is limited by physical and chemical interactions, thus leading to an apparent diffusion coefficient (ADC) (see also Chapter 8, Section 8.2 and Section 8.4). DWI, earlier than any other imaging modality, allows demonstratation of ischemic tissue changes within minutes after vessel occlusion with a reduction of the ADC [23]. A net shift of extracellular water into the intracellular compartment (cytotoxic edema) with a consecutive reduction of free water diffusion is the main underlying mechanism for ADC change [24]. First, it has to be stressed that decreases in the ADC and increased signal on DWI represent tissue bioenergetic compromise, and not necessarily irreversible ischemia. Secondly, in order to interpret changes on DWI correctly, a variety of artifacts must be known and identified, i.e., anisotropy (physical effects, like diffusion of molecules in the brain, depending on the direction in space are called anisotropic) and T_2-shine through.

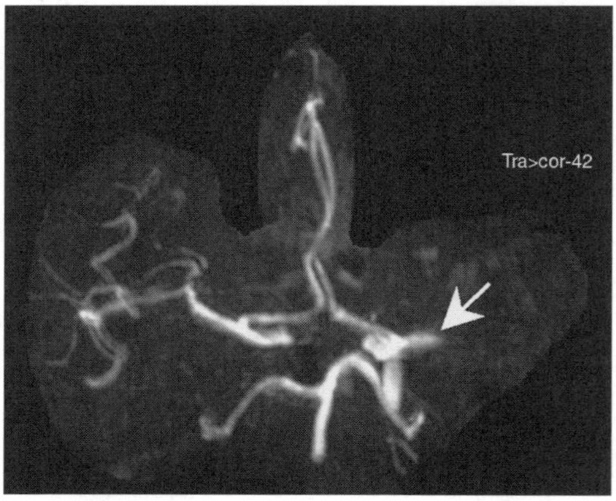

FIGURE 9.3 Acute MCA infarction 2 h after symptom onset. MRA (3D TOF), axial, TR 35 msec, TE 6.4 min flip angle 20°, slice thickness 319 mm, gap −0.38 mm, FOV (mm) 240, acquisition matrix 160 × 512, acquisition time 6 min 14 sec.

In the clinical setting of a hyperacute stroke, a lesion on strongly isotropic DWI (indicating acute cellular edema) and a normal T_2-WI (indicating that the hyperintense area on DWI is not older than 6 to 8 h) favor an acute lesion. The maximum information can be obtained when isotropic ADC maps are calculated, in addition to DWI and T_2-WI. Whereas DWI provides only part of the information on cellular necrosis, ADC provides in addition dynamic information about cerebrovascular hemodynamics [25] (Figure 9.4).

A review of the current literature reveals that more than 1000 patients have been imaged with DWI for acute stroke within 12 h. In 93% of them was capable to demonstrate areas of acute ischemia. When individuals without stroke were included, DWI was negative (i.e., did not show ischemia) in all of them (100% specificity) [26], while in transient ischemic attacks (TIAs), where symptoms resolved within 24 h, DWI was positive in only 21% of the patients.

Perfusion-weighted MR imaging (PWI) allows the measurement of capillary perfusion with the dynamic susceptibility contrast-enhanced technique. Paramagnetic contrast agent is injected as an intravenous bolus and the signal change is tracked by ultrafast MR sequences in the area of interest (Figure 9.5). Cerebrovascular hemodynamic parameters, such as relative cerebral blood volume (CBV), mean transit time (MTT), time-to-peak (TTP), and cerebral blood flow (CBF) can be estimated from the MR-derived contrast-bolus over the time curve in a semiquantitative fashion. In ischemic brain tissue with reduced perfusion or zero perfusion less (or no) contrast agent is present and T_2^*-WI thus do remain hyperintense, respectively, keep their high signal [27]. It is not yet clear, which PWI parameter gives the optimum approximation to critical hypoperfusion and allows to differentiate infarct core from penumbra and penumbra from oligemia. Most authors, however, agree that in clinical practice the MTT or the TTP give the best prognostic information [29]. Determination of the absolute CBF requires knowledge of the arterial input function, which in clinical practice is estimated from a major artery, such as the middle cerebral artery (MCA) or the internal carotid artery.

The attempt to differentiate potentially salvageable ischemic tissue, or tissue at risk, and nonsalvageable ischemia, that has reached a status in which recovery is no longer possible, by imaging techniques was made possible by introducing DWI and PWI into the clinical setting. In a simplified approach it has been hypothesized that DWI more or less reflects the irreversibly damaged infarct core and PWI the complete area of hypoperfusion [28]. The difference

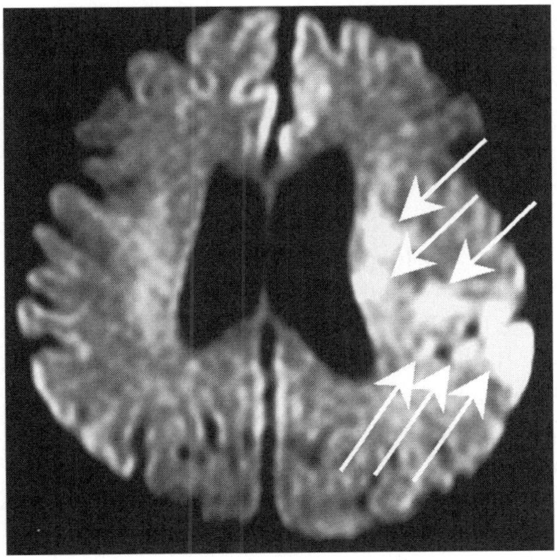

FIGURE 9.4 Acute MCA infarction 2 h after symptom onset. DWI, axial, TR 6000 msec, TE 114 msec flip angle, slice thickness 5 mm, FOV (mm) 240, acquisition matrix 98 × 128, $b = 0$ and $b = 1000$ sec/mm^2 (directions), acquisition time 23 sec.

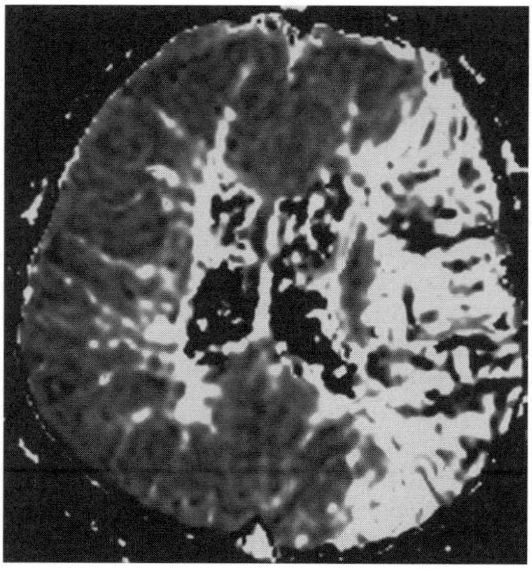

FIGURE 9.5 Acute MCA infarction 2 h after symptom onset. PWI, axial, TR 0.8 msec, TE 47 msec flip angle 60°, slice thickness 7 mm, FOV (mm) 240, acquisition matrix 96 × 128, 40 phases, acquisition time 40 sec.

(or sometimes also the ratio) between the lesion volumes assessed by PWI and DWI, also termed PWI–DWI-mismatch, would therefore be a measure of the tissue at risk of infarction or the stroke-MRI correlate of the ischemic penumbra. On the other hand, if there is no difference in PWI and DWI volumes (PWI–DWI-match) or even a negative difference (negative PWI–DWI-mismatch), according to this model the patient is expected to have no penumbral tissue because of normalization of prior hypoperfusion or due to completion of infarction leading to total loss of the penumbra [15,29]. It may be criticized that this model does not take into account that the PWI lesion also encompasses areas of oligemia which are not in danger and that DWI abnormalities do not necessarily turn into infarction [30–33]. In other words, neither DWI nor PWI presently allows to completely and reliably differentiate ischemic core from critical hypoperfusion [30]. Also the assessment of mismatch as a percentage may be less reliable than previously thought [34]. Overall and besides these questions, however, the model of PWI–DWI-mismatch is attractive due to its simplicity; it seems to have a tolerable accuracy in most acute stroke patients and its findings seem to be consistent with our current pathophysiological understanding [15,29].

The hope prevails that by using the mismatch concept patients can be categorized into two groups: those that may profit from a specific therapy to salvage the penumbra and those where no ischemic tissue at risk is present any longer. Indeed, several smaller case series reported excellent correlations between findings on DWI and PWI with baseline and outcome clinical scores as well as with follow-up stroke volume [16,35]. Two large studies found that a combination of the baseline National Institute of Health Stroke Scale (NIHSS) score, the estimated time interval from stroke onset to the MRI examination, and the baseline stroke volume on DWI gave the best prediction of stroke recovery with a 77% sensitivity and 88% specificity. DWI volume was an independent predictor of outcome, together with age and NIHSS score [18,36]. Four other studies found significant positive correlations between the baseline lesion volumes assessed by PWI and DWI, and the outcome lesion volumes [5,37–39]. Yet, these studies were either retrospective, not blinded, or imaging was not performed within the relevant time window. There are only two studies that investigated the correlation of baseline DWI and PWI volumes with baseline stroke severity and clinical outcome in a blinded and independent fashion [17,40] and showed a good correlation with follow-up lesion volume acute and chronic NIHSS score. However, multiple linear regression analysis revealed a significantly lower acute NIHSS score on the right compared with the left side when adjusted for stroke volume on T_2 imaging performed in the chronic phase. There are differences in NIHSS scores when the left hemisphere is affected, because usually the areas for speech are in the left hemisphere and patients with aphasia have a much higher NIHSS score [41]. In addition, it has also been reported that in the very early time window after symptom onset these correlations are substantially lower as DWI and PWI may reflect a best and worst case scenario at these time points [29]. Taken together, due to the heterogeneity of the present literature and the lack of truly randomized class I trials, it is still difficult to analyze the prognostic value of PWI–DWI-mismatch in MRI-based therapeutic trials.

9.2.2 Comparison of MRI with Other Imaging Techniques

Six years ago there were only five centers worldwide, which could perform stroke-MRI on a routine basis around the clock. Currently the number is estimated to exceed 500 centers and substantially more that have part-time access to stroke-MRI capabilities. Acute stroke is not only treated at specialized academic medical centers; indeed, the majority of patients initially seek help in local hospitals that usually have no MRI facilities [42]. The main advantage of CT is its widespread availability in many hospitals 24 h a day. CT scanners of the third, fourth, or even fifth generation (volume scanners) are less expensive as compared to MRI scanners, being available even in smaller community hospitals, where they are mostly used for extracranial scanning. Furthermore, substantial doubts remain regarding the feasibility and practicality as well as the validity of stroke MRI in the clinical setting [31,33], although it has been shown that logistic obstacles can be overcome [3,18].

9.2.2.1 Time Needed for Imaging and Availability of Imaging Techniques

A dedicated stroke service with multimodal imaging availability around the clock (CT, MRI, digital subtraction angiography, DSA) requires a sufficiently large staff, infrastructure such as a stroke service, stroke or neurocritical care unit, and small distances between emergency room, stroke unit, and imaging facilities to save time. Practice and experience with stroke-MRI in a dedicated team significantly reduces the time effort for a complete protocol that need not exceed 15 min including patient transfer and positioning and thus facilitates a 24 h availability [43]. There is no doubt that noncontrast CT scan can be done in approximately one third of the time. Yet, the amount of information obtained through noncontrast CT scanning is limited. When new CT imaging techniques are used to obtain additional information, the time needed for imaging gets close to the time needed for stroke-MRI [44].

9.2.2.2 Exclusion of Other Causes of Acute Stroke Symptoms

Nontraumatic intracranial hemorrhage (ICH) accounts for 10 to 15% of all strokes and up to 25% of more severe strokes [45,46]. Hyperacute stroke does not only demand an all-round diagnostic work-up, with which all the important pathophysiologic aspects can be investigated, but also the differentiation between ischemic stroke and ICH by the radiologist, which is impossible to achieve by clinical means only. Although early deterioration of vigilance, vomiting in anterior circulation as opposed to posterior circulation syndrome, coumadine therapy, or hypertensive crisis may hint towards ICH, these symptoms can also be seen in ischemic stroke.

Noncontrast CT imaging is still the current diagnostic standard for imaging of acute stroke mainly due to its close to 100% sensitivity to confirm or exclude ICH [15,42,47]. Until recently, MRI was considered to be of little value for the diagnosis of ICH or subarachnoid hemorrhage (SAH). As opposed to CT, due to the complexity of the ICH appearance in different MR sequences at different stages, there is a considerable amount of disagreement among clinicians and radiologists as to the role of MRI in the evaluation of hyperacute stroke. Many authors even claim that the sensitivity of MRI for detecting hyperacute ICH is poor [48–51]. The appearance of intracranial hemorrhage in MR images depends primarily on the age of the hematoma and the type of MR contrast (i.e., T_1- or T_2-weighting).

While hyperacute ICH is hyperdense on CT scans acquired during the acute phase, there is a loss of density with time and hematoma degradation and the ICH may appear isodense or hypodense. The typical appearance of ICH on the MRI images is a heterogeneous focus of high and low signal intensities [52–54]. Acute hematomas are characterized by an unspecific central hyperintensity on T_2-WI, whereas they appear isointense on conventional T_1-WI and therefore cannot be seen unless there is a substantial mass effect. The key substrate for early MRI visualization of acute hemorrhage is deoxyhemoglobin, a blood degradation product with paramagnetic properties due to unpaired electrons. Sequences which are susceptible to paramagnetic effects of deoxyhemoglobin may detect hyperacute ICH. For instance, T_2^*-WI shows no or few areas of hyperintensity, or merely a faint ring around a central core of signal loss. In the very first minutes after symptom onset, the center of the lesion appears heterogeneous on T_2-WI, T_2^*-WI, and T_1-WI, which is due to a local predominance of oxyhemoglobin. The periphery of the hematoma is more hypointense on susceptibility-weighted images than on T_2-WI and shows a progressive enlargement over the next minutes and first hours. This is due to a progressive centripetal increase in concentration of deoxyhemoglobin. There is a surrounding rim, which appears hyperintense on T_2-WI and T_2^*-WI, but hypointense on T_1-WI and represents perifocal vasogenic edema [52]. Methemoglobin formation in the subacute stage leads to a T_1-shortening and therefore to centripetal hyperintensity on T_1-WI after 3 days, which is also taking effect on T_2-WI causing a hyperintense signal. In late subacute and chronic ICH, a hypointense rim caused by the paramagnetic effect of ferritin and hemosiderin demarcates the border zone of the hematoma, which is better seen on T_2-WI than on T_1-WI. This may allow approximate classification of the stage and thus age of the ICH [55].

There are only few publications which report a high diagnostic accuracy of MRI for ICH within a time window of 6 h or less after symptom onset [52–56]. In the hyperacute and acute stage a sensitivity of 46% is reported for MRI, when T_2-WI and T1-WI are employed (93% for CT). However, in the subacute and chronic stages of ICH the sensitivity of MRI increases to 97 and 93%, respectively, (for CT, it decreases dramatically to 58 and 17%, respectively) [57]. Patel et al. [53] were the first to demonstrate early changes in susceptibility-weighted T_2^*-WI in acute ICH. Stroke-MRI allows a definitive diagnosis of ICH within the first hours of stroke on susceptibility-weighted T_2^*-sequences due to a profound signal loss caused by paramagnetic effects of deoxyhemoglobin, even when only present in traces [52,54,58] (Figure 9.6). Comparison of CT and stroke MRI findings in patients with acute ICH (CT, DWI, PWI with T_2^*-W source images, T_2-WI, FLAIR images, MRA) [54] showed that ICH was unambiguously identified on the basis of all stroke MRI sequences and volumetric analysis showed a good correlation of hematoma volumes in all MRI images compared to CT. Images obtained with sequences with a high sensitivity for susceptibility effects (T_2^*-WI, FLAIR) generally overestimate the actual hematoma size in comparison to the lesion volume assessed on CT [59], whereas conventional T_2-WI substantially underestimates hematoma size. Hematoma volumes on DWI followed by FLAIR corresponded best with lesion size on CT.

In a randomized, blinded prospective multicenter trial, the role of stroke-MRI in ICH was investigated by sets of diffusion-, T_2-, and T_2^*-weighted images [58]. Experienced readers, who were unaware of clinical details, identified ICH with a 100% sensitivity (confidence interval, 97 to 100%) and a 100% overall accuracy. The authors concluded that hyperacute ICH is detectable in MRI with excellent accuracy and that there is no need to perform CT for exclusion of ICH in addition to stroke MRI, which would be time-consuming (time is brain), medicoeconomically questionable, and also unpractical. Since small amounts of deoxyhemoglobin present within the very first minutes after onset of ICH are detectable by susceptibility-weighted MRI sequences, T_2^*-WI are suited best for the diagnosis of ICH, which also holds true for the qualitative detection of

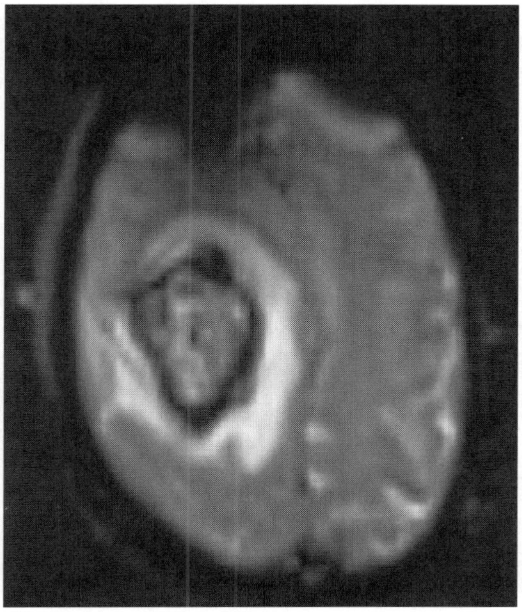

FIGURE 9.6 Acute ICH infarction 1.5 h after symptom onset. T_2^*-WI, axial, TR 800 msec, TE 26 msec flip angle 20°, slice thickness 5 mm, FOV (mm) 240, asymmetric matrix 256, acquisition time 6 min.

relatively small hematomas without mass effect. Further information such as the presence of space occupying edema, midline shift, and ventricular hemorrhage is best derived from conventional T_2-WI. Detection of old as well as new microbleeds and early hemorrhagic infarction by T_2^*-WI may allow the exclusion of patients from thrombolysis, who have an excessive bleeding risk [60, 61]. Beside the differentiation between ischemia and hemorrhage, MRI may provide information with regard to the etiology of ICH (Figure 9.7). Basal ganglia hemorrhage in combination with older microbleeds or vascular leukencephalopathy implies a hypertensive etiology of ICH as do lobar hematomas in the elderly [62]. Multiple cortical ICH in the elderly may hint towards an amyloid angiopathy [63] and postcontrast T1-WI scans may be obtained after PWI if another primary disease is suspected (e.g., hemorrhage in glioma or metastases). In young patients, additional information from MRA may detect aneurysms, arteriovenous malformations, vasculitis-like changes, such as multiple intracranial stenoses, or cerebral venous thrombosis and thus may make an invasive conventional angiography unnecessary [50,59]. Taking all of this into consideration MRI is far superior to CT in the subacute and chronic stages especially with regard to concomitant or underlying pathology [57,64].

In the acute phase, CT is the imaging standard for the diagnosis of SAH [65,66], with a sensitivity of 85 to 100%. Nevertheless, the diagnosis of SAH by CT may be difficult in the posterior fossa due to bone artifacts, as well as with small amounts of blood. Furthermore, in the subacute stage, the sensitivity of CT for SAH diminishes substantially with sensitivities of 50% after 1 week, 30% after 2 weeks, and approximately 0% at 3 weeks [66]. At the latter time point, lumbar puncture, the diagnostic gold standard for detecting SAH, must be carried out. Currently there is only scarce information about the sensitivity of stroke MRI for SAH (Figure 9.8). Yet, MRI techniques such as MRA, DWI, and PWI may be useful to detect early complications of SAH such as vasospasm and spreading depression [67]. MRA and DSA provide complementary information with regard to aneurysm detection [68]; however, when SAH is diagnosed, DSA is still the diagnostic and in certain instances, when immediate coiling is performed at the same time, it is the therapeutic method of choice.

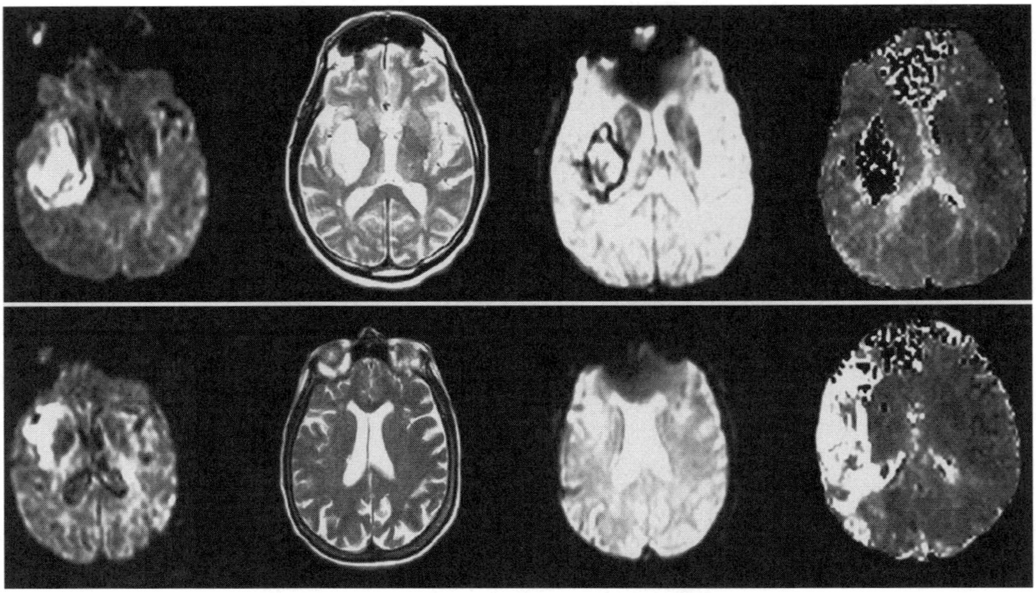

FIGURE 9.7 Comparison of acute ICH (upper row) and ischemia using MRI. From left to right: DWI, T_2-WI, T_2^*-WI, PWI.

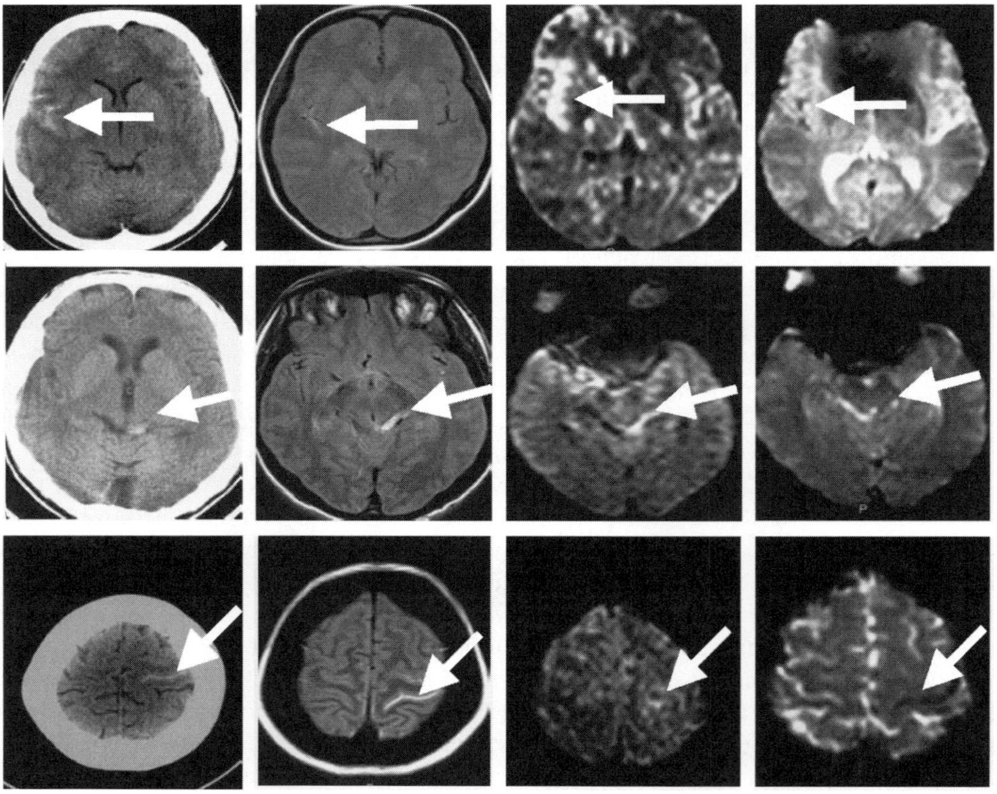

FIGURE 9.8 CT and MRI in the diagnosis of SAH. From left to right: CT, T_1-WI, DWI, T_2^*-WI.

9.2.2.3 Detection of Ischemic Tissue

During the last years it has been generally accepted by the neuroradiological community that CT can demonstrate early infarct signs within the first 6 h after stroke. With the availability of high-quality CT scanners, more and more investigators reported their positive CT findings in early ischemic stroke [69–71]. However, the sensitivity of noncontrast CT to detect early signs of infarct is still a matter of debate as these signs may often be subtle and require a high level of experience for detection and interpretation. The use of CT angiography source images may further increase the sensitivity for early ischemic changes missed on noncontrast scans [72,73].

There has been cumulating evidence of the superiority of MRI over CT in the diagnosis of hyperacute ischemic stroke [14,15,74,75]. In the earlier years of DWI, case series and small comparative studies with CT suggested a 100% sensitivity for DWI in the hyperacute stage of stroke [13,76,77]. With an increasing frequency, however, cases of stroke lesions not detected by DWI have been reported especially in patients with early arterial recanalization or transient ischemic attacks (TIAs), where symptoms resolved within 24 h [78,79]. Despite an inference among stroke physicians that DWI has the highest diagnostic accuracy for the diagnosis of ischemic stroke among all imaging modalities applied in the acute setting, there remains a lack of methodologically pristine studies to assess its diagnostic strength accurately and beyond doubt [79]. When DWI is performed after conventional imaging (i.e., CT), the likelihood is high that more lesions are shown [80]. However, up to now in only one study the order in which DWI and CT were performed was actually randomized [81]; in another study, the time interval between both imaging modalities was reduced by having some patients studied with DWI first [82].

In the acute phase, the overall sensitivity of DWI is between 91 and 100%, while that reported for CT is between 42 and 77% [75–77,81,82]. The specificity and accuracy of lesion detection by DWI are, respectively, 100 and 91% (respectively, 56 to 100 and 47% for CT). According to the literature, acute DWI lesions are present in up to 50% of patients with the clinical diagnosis of a TIA, a finding which correlates with symptom duration [79]. Compared to FLAIR, DWI more than triples the likelihood of detecting ischemic stroke [11]. These studies establish DWI as the superior imaging modality and therefore optimum imaging standard of care [76,80,81]. It has to be stressed that one study compared novices with experts and that the novices achieved a high diagnostic accuracy in DWI imaging [81]. This is of clinical significance since usually novices rather than an international expert panel are on routine calls and treat the majority of stroke patients. Therefore, a stroke-MRI protocol with DWI, if available, should be used instead of CT as the modality of choice in acute stroke patients.

Determination of the diagnostic accuracy of PWI for acute stroke has not yet been the objective of any trial published to date. This is especially notable considering its suggested importance for decision-making in acute stroke [15,30,83]. An analysis of the role of vascular imaging, as well as the importance of the combined information provided by a multiparametric stroke-MRI protocol, exceeds the scope of this chapter but is stressed at this point.

9.2.2.4 Distinction between Irreversibly Damaged Tissue and Tissue at Risk

PWI has to meet the critique that it renders only a qualitative (at best semiquantitative) index of tissue perfusion [84], whereas other methods such as SPECT und PET, neither of which have become a standard for patient management, may offer accurate quantitative regional CBF measurements [31]. The evaluation of perfusion status and identification of a tissue at risk by Xenon CT, SPECT, or PET, however, are not practical for routine use [15]. While it is not clinically feasible yet to obtain quantitative PWI-parameters that differentiate oligemia from relevant hypoperfusion and infarct core, relative MTT (or TTP) parameter maps may be used to guide clinical management in patients with acute ischemic stroke [85].

Several studies compared the sensitivity and specificity of PWI for the diagnosis of acute ischemia with other physiologic techniques (SPECT, PET, Xenon-CT) [86–89]. In 91% of the patients examined, PWI was positive. None of these trials included patients without stroke or TIA and the lesions not detected by PWI were mostly lacunar lesions and anterior choroideal artery territory infarctions. In addition, none of them compared the diagnostic accuracy of PWI to other perfusion techniques. The absence of a perfusion defect at the time of imaging may be due to spontaneous recanalization and therefore a negative study in this setting is appropriate. Furthermore, there is no study that addressed quantitative perfusion imaging in humans with MR techniques compared to Xenon CT or PET. This is likely due to the inherent difficulties of having access to all these techniques in the clinical setting of acute stroke and remains therefore an important topic for ongoing clinical research.

Dynamic perfusion CT results in images, that can be used to generate functional maps of CBV, CBF, or time-to-peak enhancement. Areas with reduced CBF can be shown immediately after vessel occlusion with high contrast to areas with normal perfusion providing information about cerebrovascular parameters and their changes in acute stroke patients [88,90,91]. However, the necessary perfusion software is not yet available on many CT scanners serving emergency units.

Electron beam CT is also capable of performing multislice dynamic CT with calculation of absolute CBV and CBF. A disadvantage is the high image noise, limiting the demarcation of ischemic tissue [92]. In addition, ischemia may be located outside the scanning level of perfusion CT and could therefore be missed, because with each bolus injection only one brain section (multislice CT provides a maximum of two 1-cm-thick slices) can be evaluated and the maximum brain area that can be imaged is a 2-cm wide slab at the base of the brain, thus apical infarctions in the upper MCA and ACA territory may not be detected. This disadvantage may eventually be overcome with the next generation of CT scanners with larger detector rows [93].

9.2.2.5 Identification of Patients Who May Profit from Thrombolytic Treatment

The question that arises is whether patients that would seem to be the ideal candidates for thrombolytic therapy can be really characterized by the stroke-MRI concept, i.e., vessel occlusion and PWI–DWI-mismatch. In a prospective, open-label, nonrandomized multicenter trial patients with acute ischemic stroke were examined using a multiparametric stroke-MRI protocol within 6 h after symptom onset and at follow-up [94]. Patients were divided into two therapeutic groups: a no-thombolysis group with conservative treatment and a group with thrombolytic therapy. A relevant PWI–DWI-mismatch ratio >1.2 was present in 120 of 139 patients. MRA demonstrated a vessel occlusion in 90% of the patients. The mismatch ratio did not differ between the two groups, whereas the mismatch volume (i.e., the difference between the lesion volumes assessed by PWI and DWI) was smaller in the no-thrombolysis group. The final lesion volume (T_2-WI on day 7) was smaller in the thrombolysis group with 35 vs. 73 ml. rtPA had a strong effect on recanalization rates (see also Chapter 8, Section 8.3.2 and Section 8.5). This suggests that stroke MRI is a selection tool that allows substantially widening of the time window for treating stroke with thrombolytic therapy and can yield even better results than compared to historical studies. As there is a still growing body of evidence in favor of the recommended procedures, these recommendations may be seen as an expert consensus and form the basis for inclusion of patients in future stroke trials.

CT-angiography (CTA) with spiral CT is today a widely available tool to evaluate the Circle of Willis. It can provide accurate information on stenoses or occlusions in the basal arteries of the brain and can also reliably detect emboli and aneurysms of a moderate to large size [95,96]. Furthermore, CTA is superior to Doppler ultrasound in the assessment of the basilar artery patency in patients with the syndrome of an acute basilar artery ischemia, particularly in patients with distal basilar artery occlusion [97]. The method is noninvasive and comparatively safe. In a large series of stroke patients none had any immediate adverse reactions after administration of the intravenous nonionic iodinated contrast material [96]. Newer generations of CT scanners allow for lower contrast doses. While older studies reported an increase of the infarct size after administration of ionic contrast material, an experimental study clearly showed that bolus injection of nonionic contrast material does not affect infarct volume or worsen the symptoms of cerebral ischemia [98], although this should be more firmly established. In addition to the assessment of a major vessel occlusion, CTA has the potential to deliver information about the quality of the collateral circulation. In patients with good leptomeningeal collaterals contrast enhancement occurs in arterial branches beyond the occlusion site. This degree of enhancement can be taken as an estimate of the collateral blood flow [73,95]. Although CTA may have limitations in being less reliable in showing branch occlusions of the middle cerebral artery or other smaller vessels distal to the Circle of Willis [96], many experts suggest that it may be superior to fast MRA techniques and can easily be performed directly after noncontrast CT.

Analysis of CTA source images (CTA-SI) must be clearly differentiated from perfusion CT [91]. CTA-SI analysis is a strong predictor of clinical outcome and may predict final infarct volume. Patients with recanalization do not experience infarct growth, whereas those without complete recanalization do [99]. A comparison of acute stroke patients imaged with CT followed by MRI showed that all vessel occlusions detected on CTA were seen on MRA at the same location [100]. Neither in patients with poor collaterals nor in patients with good collaterals did lesion volumes at baseline assessed from CTA-SI differ significantly from those determined by DWI. In patients with poor collateral vessel status, initial CTA-SI lesion volumes differed significantly from T_2-WI lesion volumes on day 5, whereas in patients with good collaterals no significant difference was found. In all patients, the lesion volume measured in CTA-SI significantly correlated with the initial lesion volumes on DWI and with the outcome lesion volume determined on day 5 using T_2-WI [100].

As the substrate for thrombolytic therapy is an obliterating thromboembolus, the ability of CTA to detect intracranial vessel occlusion suggests that it is a useful screening tool for identifying patients in whom intravenous or intraarterial thrombolysis is appropriate [52]. In patients with a poor collateral vessel status, CTA-SI may provide information similar to that of the PWI–DWI-mismatch concept. One might ask if standard postcontrast CT should not suffice to visualize the extent of ischemic tissue. However, in comparison to postcontrast CT, CTA has the advantage of showing the leptomeningeal collaterals surrounding the lesion of reduced parenchymal enhancement which can be seen with both methods. The volume of the affected brain area that has inadequate blood supply can be estimated by the difference between the CTA-SI lesion volumes and the brain area supplied by the occluded artery, taking the qualitative assessment of the collateral status into account. The patients with poor collaterals seem to represent those who may have a PWI–DWI-mismatch revealed by stroke-MRI, whereas the patients with good collaterals probably have no tissue at risk (i.e., small stroke, lacunar stroke, or tissue at risk already completely infarcted).

Compared to MRA, CTA is at least as reliable in demonstrating a vessel occlusion. The combination of CT and CTA may also be more cost-effective than stroke-MRI. The main disadvantages are the additional amount of time needed for imaging. Furthermore, the use of contrast medium is required. Although rarely seen, problems may arise in some patients with renal failure or allergic reactions. With regard to clinical trials, there is also the risk that contrast medium may interfere with the use of new pharmacological therapies.

9.2.2.6 Identification of Patients to Whom Thrombolytic Treatment Is Harmful

The clinical studies ECASS I and II showed that rtPA had no benefit but increased the risk for a fatal brain hemorrhage in patients with a large area of hypoattenuation ($>33\%$ of the MCA-territory) [47]. Furthermore, several studies demonstrated that physicians including general radiologists and neurologists do not uniformly achieve a sufficient level of sensitivity for identification of CT-contraindications for thrombolytic therapy (i.e., intracerebral hemorrhage or early signs of ischemia) [101]. History of a previous ICH is in general considered to be a contraindication for thrombolytic therapy [102].

Another potential use of stroke-MRI could be the identification of those patients who carry a high risk of subsequent symptomatic ICH after treatment with rtPA. The association of old microbleeds with risk for secondary ICH after thrombolytic therapy was investigated in two studies [60,61]. In one study major symptomatic ICH occurred in 20% of patients with 11% of patients without microbleeds undergoing intraarterial thrombolysis. The other study revealed that 20% of patients with acute stroke had microbleeds according to T_2^*-WI and 26% of patients had secondary hemorrhagic conversion or symptomatic ICH. Both suggest that microbleeds represent the presence of vascular vulnerability that contributes to an excessive risk of spontaneous ICH after ischemic stroke [61] and, even more, predisposes the patient to a therapy-associated hemorrhagic complication [60]. Detection of old as well as new microbleeds and early hemorrhagic infarction by T_2^*-WI may allow exclusion from thrombolysis patients who have an excessive bleeding risk [60, 61,63,103]. However, in a retrospective analysis in stroke patients with a small number of microbleeds revealed by MRI before treatment, Derex et al. [104] showed that thrombolysis did not significantly increase the frequency of symptomatic intracerebral hemorrhage. Larger prospective studies are needed to address the predictive value of microbleeds detected by MRI as a risk factor for tPA-induced ICH.

9.2.3 Stroke Treatment Based on a Multiparametric Stroke-MRI Protocol

At this point we would like to summarize the above comments by proposing a multiparametric stroke-MRI protocol which would currently best address the relevant questions in acute ischemic stroke patients. Such a protocol, which should not take longer than 15 min, would consist of:

1. MRA to demonstrate vessel occlusion or patency
2. T_2^*-WI (e.g., source images from PWI) to show the presence of or to exclude intracranial hemorrhage
3. DWI to show the infarct core and infarct age (ADC-maps)
4. T_2-WI to give a more anatomical image of the brain in stroke patients and depict microangiopathic changes, edema, old infarcts, other pathologies
5. PWI to show the complete area of hypoperfusion and derive the tissue at risk by comparing the results with the findings on DWI

Three distinct categories of patients considered for thrombolytic therapy could be selected by applying this protocol:

1. Patients with large infarctions exceeding 50% of the MCA territory according to DWI should not be treated with thrombolysis but are good targets for other upcoming therapies.
2. (a) Patients without PWI–DWI-mismatch but with vessel occlusion, patients with PWI–DWI-mismatch but without (identifiable) vessel occlusion (e.g., distal MCA branch); (b) patients without proof of vessel occlusion and without mismatch (e.g., lacunar stroke); and (c) individual patients with PWI–DWI-mismatch, vessel occlusion, and DWI lesion volume between 33 and 50% of the MCA territory. The use of thrombolysis in these patients is still a matter of debate which makes them good targets for either thrombolytic therapy with individual study protocols to select those who profit from thrombolysis, as well as other alternative (future) therapies or both.
3. Intravenous and/or intraarterial thrombolysis are indicated and essential in patients with MCA occlusions distal to the lenticulostriate branches and with presence of a PWI–DWI-mismatch and in patients with distal internal carotid artery or proximal MCA occlusions and presence of a PWI–DWI-mismatch, which makes them targets only for studies where new therapies are investigated in addition to thrombolysis.

The earlier the time point of imaging, the lower the correlation between DWI and PWI volumes with neurological baseline and outcome scores [29]. The more subacutely stroke-MRI is performed, the more likely that DWI and PWI findings approximate the final infarct size and thus correlate with clinical outcome [16,20,35] which is consistent with older CT and MRI data [29,71,105]. Thus, the baseline lesion sizes determined by DWI and PWI neither reflect the clinical degree of severity at baseline nor at outcome, but rather illustrate the potential best- and worse-case scenarios. The clinical and morphological course of hyperacute ischemic infarction is completely open and may thus be influenced by therapy. Therefore, the PWI–DWI-mismatch and the evaluation of best or worse outcome should be used to differentiate which patients are at high risk and which are not. Stroke-MRI findings are far more reliable in predicting what fate the patient may face if not treated (final stroke size $\approx$ PWI size) or effectively treated (final stroke size $\approx$ DWI size). Also, there is a highly significant association of vessel occlusion and presence of a PWI–DWI-mismatch (98%) and vessel patency and PWI–DWI-match in the first hours after stroke. Patients with vessel occlusion and PWI–DWI-match in the first hours probably have infarcted their tissue at risk due to poor collaterals or profound drops in blood pressure or oxygenation. Early recanalization as shown by resolution of a PWI–DWI-mismatch, however, leads to smaller infarcts, improved (restituted) perfusion, and a significantly better clinical outcome [29,106]. In patients with proximal vessel occlusions, a larger area of tissue is at risk, the recanalization rate is lower, and outcome is worse. Therefore, vessel patency should be achieved by all means in this patient group.

9.3 THE USE OF MRI IN CURRENT AND UPCOMING STROKE TRIALS

Stroke-MRI protocols will play a major role in stroke trial design in the future [54,83,107]. To demonstrate efficacy in a clinical trial with a treatment time window beyond 3 h, several features of the trial design need to be optimized, and proof of pharmacological activity in phase II is needed before lengthy, expensive, labor-intensive and potentially risky phase III clinical trials are undertaken. The requirement of proof of concept phase II studies will prevent the wastefulness of phase III trials that are doomed to fail. MRI-guided phase II studies may answer the question of biological activity in fewer than 200 patients, the typical sample size in phase II trials.

Trends toward benefit using clinical scales at phase II have been notoriously poor predictors of clinical outcomes in phase III trials on much larger samples. It would be unthinkable for clinical trials in cardiology or oncology to enrol patients by bedside clinical impression alone, without objective evidence from diagnostic testing confirming the pathology before inclusion of a patient. Yet this has been the traditional standard by which clinical trials for ischemic stroke have been conducted, because until recently there has been no practical alternative. Stroke-MRI parameters, such as lesion growth or tissue saved have been and are currently used as surrogate markers for drug efficacy [83,108] in acute stroke studies. The goal of image-based patient selection is to narrow the range of patient characteristics, leading to a more homogeneous sample, reducing group variance, and increasing the statistical power (lowering sample size requirement) of the experimental design to demonstrate efficacy. Open clinical trials such as those presented by Röther et al. [94] provide an idea about sample sizes needed when homogeneous patient groups are selected and monitored by stroke-MRI. The sample size of approximately 800 patients required in trials based on clinical outcome can be easily reduced to 150 individuals when MRI is included as a readout.

Several planned or ongoing trials using stroke-MRI for the inclusion of patients can be named (a list of ongoing acute stroke trials adopting MRI as readout can be found in Ref. [109]). A phase I study with the thrombolytic drug tenecteplase has been concluded, the results however have not yet been published. In DIAS (desmoplase in acute ischemic stroke), a stroke-MRI based study on the efficacy of recombinant desmoteplase (derived from the saliva of the vampire bat *Desmodus rotundus*) for treatment of stroke in the 3 to 9-h time window, all dose-finding tiers have been completed. The start of the phase III of the DIAS trial is planned for the end of 2004. DEFUSE (in the USA) and EPITHET (in Australia) are two studies that perform MRI-based thrombolysis with rtPA in the 3–6-h time window.

The benefits of arterial recanalization may be supplemented by neuronal protection (a first protocol draft including MRI in the clinical trial is underway), particularly when the two strategies are used simultaneously, and if they can be used very early following symptom onset. A further very interesting approach being tested in the clinic is ultrasound-enhanced recanalization in stroke patients under treatment with rtPA. Ultrasound can be applied via intravascular devices (EKOS, EPAR, Angiojet), or clot lysis facilitation with transcranial ultrasound is another option. Two trials examining these possibilities are underway: TRUMBI is an international trial, while CLOTBUST is an oligocentric trial headed by the university medical center at Houston, Texas. Preliminary data from CLOTBUST (Alexandrov and Grotta, unpublished data) showed a significantly higher rate of early recanalization in patients treated with rtPA and ultrasound as opposed to rtPA alone. Further data are pending. Also, protocols combining fibrinolytics with GPIIb/IIIa antagonists (ROSIE 1: Retavase + Abciximab; ROSIE 2: rtPA + Eptifibatide, SATIS: rtPA + Tirofiban) have started recruiting patients. Another study (PROACT III) examining the efficacy of intraarterial pro-urokinase for acute stroke within 6 h is planned, but due to funding problems is still a matter of debate.

9.4 CONCLUSIONS

At present, thrombolytic therapy is still underutilized. A major problem of the approach is that relatively few candidates meet the clinical and time criteria. Educating the general public to regard stroke as a treatable emergency and training emergency caregivers in the use of thrombolysis can decrease these problems but demands a continuous effort. Healthcare institutions should be made aware of the potential in long-term cost savings, once stroke management is optimized and thrombolysis is more widely available. Patients and their relatives should be informed not only about the hazards of thrombolytic therapy, but also about its potential benefits and thus the risks of not adopting it.

At the same time, numerous new stroke therapies find their way from the laboratories into clinical studies including neuroprotection, antiinflammation, antioxidative therapy, and the use of growth factors, to name but a few. However, not every subtype of stroke may be a good target for an individual therapy, thus emphasizing the role of selection tools that allow identification of the subgroups of stroke patients. Since stroke therapy seems to be most effective in the first few hours after symptom onset, the selection tools should be able to be performed quickly and in a standardized way. To date stroke-MRI is the only tool to meet these criteria. The combined information provided by DWI, PWI, MRA, T_2-WI, and PWI/DWI-mismatch allows the early identification of those patients whose outcome and final infarct size, ultimately the patients' fate, have not yet been determined. With an increasing distribution and availability of stroke-MRI protocols, the identification of patients suitable for thrombolytic therapy, and those who are not, will lead to an increased benefit and a reduction of complications [15]. Furthermore, the rather strictly defined therapeutic window may be qualified and individualized according to the findings in each patient.

The idea that quantitative perfusion imaging is required for stroke assessment is derived from concepts of ischemic thresholds and ischemic penumbra, the premise being that if CBF could be accurately quantified then the tissue could be characterized as normal, reversibly ischemic, or irreversibly damaged. Unfortunately, a variety of factors noted above make this unlikely to be the case in human patients. First, the duration as well as extent of ischemia must be known, and such information is not available from a single examination performed at the time of presentation. Secondly, human stroke typically involves both gray and white matter, whereas threshold data apply primarily to gray matter. Thirdly, while some human strokes such as those caused by thromboembolism in atrial fibrillation consist of a solitary MCA occlusion, many human strokes are multifocal or are caused by partial occlusions and in these cases a complex topological relationship is likely to occur between core and penumbra including variations between cortical laminae. Finally, it is now recognized that delayed cell death occurs as a result of ischemia (apoptosis) and also that recurrent sublethal ischemia can make the brain less sensitive to subsequent ischemic events (ischemic conditioning) [110].

Thus, while hypoperfusion remains a key pathophysiological mechanism in stroke it is no longer clear that absolute quantification of CBF at any time point is sufficient or even necessary for predicting tissue outcome. More practically, the ischemic penumbra may be operationally defined as those brain regions which are at risk of infarction but remain salvageable based on any criteria, namely the target of stroke therapy. Over the past decade, a variety of potential imaging markers have been identified, with MRI-based DWI and PWI being among the most widely available. Multiparametric hemodynamic information, pertaining both to the extent of hypoperfusion and to the existence and viability of collateral flow sources, derived using PWI remains likely to contribute to tissue assessment, along with direct measures of tissue injury (diffusion tensor imaging, magnetization transfer ratio, ^{23}Na MRI). Assuming the predictive value of such hemodynamic measures can be validated in clinical trials, it will be more critical that the measurements can be performed reliably and reproducibly than that they correspond to classical CBF measurements using ^{15}O-PET scanning or other diffusible tracer techniques.

Larger studies of DWI and PWI are needed, with clear patient and clinical details (inclusions, exclusions, and failures), blinding of analyses, valid clinical outcome measures, and comparison with routine imaging, such as CT, so that an assessment of added clinical value of the combined multiparametric stroke-MRI protocol including presence or absence of arterial occlusion can be made. Therefore, research should focus on the utility of MRA along with DWI and PWI in predicting outcome. The imaging results of randomized trials of new or existing acute stroke treatments, where patients with suspected stroke receive a screening MRI, are a potential source of class I evidence (provided by one or more prospective, randomized controlled trials). These data, however, are not yet available. Further improvement of these imaging techniques to reliably differentiate the irreversibly damaged ischemic infarct core from the critically ischemic but salvageable tissue and the noncritically hypoperfused oligemic brain tissue, e.g., by establishing and developing quantitative PWI techniques, is an important objective for ongoing and future research.

Newer MRI approaches are being developed that do not require the use of exogenous contrast media [111]. These techniques tag or label the spins in the arterial blood flowing into the brain and are broadly termed arterial spin labeling techniques. These methods have the advantage of precluding the administration of a contrast agent, being therefore easily repeatable. Furthermore, in theory, these methods could produce absolute quantification of flow. Enthusiasm for these techniques has been tempered by their ongoing and rapid evolution and subsequent lack of standardization, and also the relatively low signal to noise ratio of the images even with a long ($\sim$5 min) imaging time. However, these approaches are promising and may resolve both the quantitation issues and allow for noncontrast measurement. As noted above, the technical issues must play a secondary role since the relationship between blood flow abnormalities (no matter how expertly calculated) and tissue and clinical outcome remains to be established. This will require controlled multicenter clinical studies.

REFERENCES

1. WHO Task Force Stroke, Recommendations on stroke prevention, diagnosis, and therapy. Report of the WHO Task Force on Stroke and other Cerebrovascular Disorders, *Stroke*, 20, 1407, 1989.
2. Astrup, J., Siesjö, B., and Symon, L., Thresholds in cerebral ischemia — the ischemic penumbra, *Stroke*, 12, 723, 1981.

3. Schellinger, P. D. et al., Thrombolytic therapy for ischemic stroke — a review. Part I, intravenous thrombolysis, *Crit. Care Med.*, 29, 1812, 2001.
4. Brott, T. G., *A Combined Metaanalysis of NINDS, ECASS I and II, ATLANTIS, International Stroke Conference, San Antonio, TX, USA. February 7–9th*, 2002.
5. Hacke, W. et al., Thrombolysis in acute ischemic stroke: controlled trials and clinical experience, *Neurology*, 53, S3, 1999.
6. Wardlaw, J. M., del Zoppo, G., and Yamaguchi, T., Thrombolysis for acute ischaemic stroke, *Cochrane Database Syst. Rev.*, 2, CD000213, 2000.
7. del Zoppo, G. J. et al., PROACT: a phase II randomized trial of recombinant pro-urokinase by direct arterial delivery in acute middle cerebral artery stroke, *Stroke*, 29, 4, 1998.
8. Furlan, A. et al., Intra-arterial prourokinase for acute ischemic stroke. The PROACT II study: a randomized controlled trial. Prolyse in acute cerebral thromboembolism, *JAMA*, 282, 2003, 1999.
9. Lev, M. H. et al., Utility of perfusion-weighted CT imaging in acute middle cerebral artery stroke treated with intra-arterial thrombolysis: prediction of final infarct volume and clinical outcome, *Stroke*, 32, 2021, 2001.
10. Gilman, S., Imaging the brain. First of two parts, *N. Engl. J. Med.*, 338, 812, 1998.
11. Perkins, C. J. et al., Fluid-attenuated inversion recovery and diffusion- and perfusion-weighted MRI abnormalities in 117 consecutive patients with stroke symptoms, *Stroke*, 32, 2774, 2001.
12. Yang, J. J. et al., Comparison of pre- and postcontrast 3D time-of-flight MR angiography for the evaluation of distal intracranial branch occlusions in acute ischemic stroke, *Am. J. Neuroradiol.*, 23, 557, 2002.
13. Fisher, M. and Albers, G. W., Applications of diffusion–perfusion magnetic resonance imaging in acute ischemic stroke, *Neurology*, 52, 1750, 1999.
14. Hacke, W. and Warach, S., Diffusion-weighted MRI as an evolving standard of care in acute stroke, *Neurology*, 54, 1548, 2000.
15. Schellinger, P. D., Fiebach, J. B., and Hacke, W., Imaging-based decision making in thrombolytic therapy for ischemic stroke: present status, *Stroke*, 34, 575, 2003.
16. Barber, P. A. et al., Prediction of stroke outcome with echoplanar perfusion- and diffusion-weighted MRI, *Neurology*, 51, 418, 1998.
17. Lovblad, K. O. et al., Ischemic lesion volumes in acute stroke by diffusion-weighted magnetic resonance imaging correlate with clinical outcome, *Ann. Neurol.*, 42, 164, 1997.
18. Thijs, V. N. et al., Is early ischemic lesion volume on diffusion-weighted imaging an independent predictor of stroke outcome? A multivariable analysis, *Stroke*, 31, 2597, 2000.
19. Tong, D. C. et al., Correlation of perfusion- and diffusion-weighted MRI with NIHSS score in acute (<6.5 hour) ischemic stroke, *Neurology*, 50, 864, 1998.
20. Warach, S., Dashe, J. F., and Edelman, R. R., Clinical outcome in ischemic stroke predicted by early diffusion-weighted and perfusion magnetic resonance imaging: a preliminary analysis, *J. Cereb. Blood Flow Metab.*, 16, 53, 1996.
21. Warach, S., Boska, M., and Welch, K. M., Pitfalls and potential of clinical diffusion-weighted MR imaging in acute stroke, *Stroke*, 28, 481, 1997.
22. Stejskal, E. O. and Tanner, J. E., Spin diffusion measurements: spin echoes in the presence of a time-dependent field gradient, *J. Chem. Phys.*, 42, 288, 1965.
23. Le Bihan, D. et al., MR imaging of intravoxel incoherent motions: application to diffusion and perfusion in neurologic disorders, *Radiology*, 161, 401, 1986.
24. Röther, J., Gass, A., and Busch, E., Diffusion- and perfusion-weighted MRI in cerebral ischaemia — part 1: results of animal experiments, *Akt. Neurol.*, 26, 300, 1999.
25. Taleb, M. et al., Reperfusion demonstrated by ADC mapping after local intra-arterial thrombolysis for human ischemic stroke, *Neuroradiology*, 43, 591, 2001.
26. Grandin, C. B. et al., Usefulness of magnetic resonance-derived quantitative measurements of cerebral blood flow and volume in prediction of infarct growth in hyperacute stroke, *Stroke*, 32, 1147, 2001.
27. Fiebach, J. B. and Schellinger, P. D., Modern magnetic resonance techniques for stroke, *Nervenarzt*, 73, 104, 2002.
28. Jansen, O. et al., Early recanalization in acute ischemic stroke saves tissue at risk defined by MRI, *Lancet*, 353, 2036, 1999.

29. Schellinger, P. D. et al., Stroke magnetic resonance imaging within 6 hours after onset of hyperacute cerebral ischemia, *Ann. Neurol.*, 49, 460, 2001.
30. Kidwell, C. S., Alger, J. R., and Saver, J. L., Beyond mismatch: evolving paradigms in imaging the ischemic penumbra with multimodal magnetic resonance imaging, *Stroke*, 34, 2729, 2003.
31. Powers, W. J. and Zivin, J., Magnetic resonance imaging in acute stroke: not ready for prime time, *Neurology*, 50, 842, 1998.
32. Powers, W. J., Testing a test: a report card for DWI in acute stroke, *Neurology*, 54, 1549, 2000.
33. Zivin, J. A. and Holloway, R. G., Weighing the evidence on DWI: caveat emptor, *Neurology*, 54, 1552, 2000.
34. Coutts, S. B. et al., Reliability of assessing percentage of diffusion–perfusion mismatch, *Stroke*, 34, 1681, 2003.
35. Beaulieu, C. et al., Longitudinal magnetic resonance imaging study of perfusion and diffusion in stroke: evolution of lesion volume and correlation with clinical outcome, *Ann. Neurol.*, 46, 568, 1999.
36. Baird, A. E. et al., A three-item scale for the early prediction of stroke recovery, *Lancet*, 357, 2095, 2001.
37. Keir, S. L. and Wardlaw, J. M., Systematic review of diffusion and perfusion imaging in acute ischemic stroke, *Stroke*, 31, 2723, 2000.
38. Schaefer, P. W. et al., Predicting cerebral ischemic infarct volume with diffusion and perfusion MR imaging, *Am. J. Neuroradiol.*, 23, 1785, 2002.
39. Wittsack, H. J. et al., MR imaging in acute stroke: diffusion-weighted and perfusion imaging parameters for predicting infarct size, *Radiology*, 222, 397, 2002.
40. Warach, S. et al., Effect of citicoline on ischemic lesions as measured by diffusion-weighted magnetic resonance imaging. Citicoline 010 investigators, *Ann. Neurol.*, 48, 713, 2000.
41. Spilker, J. et al., Using the NIH stroke scale to assess stroke patients. The NINDS rt-PA stroke study group, *J. Neurosci. Nurs.*, 29, 384, 1997.
42. Handschu, R. et al., Acute stroke management in the local general hospital, *Stroke*, 32, 866, 2001.
43. Schellinger, P. D. et al., Feasibility and practicality of MR imaging of stroke in the management of hyperacute cerebral ischemia, *Am. J. Neuroradiol.*, 21, 1184, 2000.
44. Chalela, J. A. et al., Hemorrhage and early MRI evaluation from emergency room (HEME-ER): a prospective, single center comparison of MRI to CT for the emergency diagnosis of intracranial hemorrhage in patients with suspected acute cerebrovascular disease, *Stroke*, 34, 239, 2003.
45. Jorgensen, H. S. et al., Intracerebral hemorrhage versus infarction: stroke severity, risk factors, and prognosis, *Ann. Neurol.*, 38, 45, 1995.
46. Qureshi, A. I. et al., Spontaneous intracranial hemorrhage, *N. Engl. J. Med.*, 344, 1450, 2001.
47. von Kummer, R. et al., Acute stroke: usefulness of early CT findings before thrombolytic therapy, *Radiology*, 205, 327, 1997.
48. Bradley, W. G. Jr., MR appearance of hemorrhage in the brain, *Radiology*, 189, 15, 1993.
49. Hayman, L. A. et al., Mechanisms of MR signal alteration by acute intracerebral blood: old concepts and new theories, *Am. J. Neuroradiol.*, 12, 899, 1991.
50. Jäger, H. R. et al., MRA versus digital subtraction angiography in acute subarachnoid haemorrhage: a blinded multireader study of prospectively recruited patients, *Neuroradiology*, 42, 313, 2000.
51. Weingarten, K. et al., Detection of acute intracerebral hemorrhage on MR imaging: ineffectiveness of prolonged interecho interval pulse sequences, *Am. J. Neuroradiol.*, 12, 475, 1991.
52. Linfante, I. et al., MRI features of intracerebral hemorrhage within 2 hours from symptom onset, *Stroke*, 30, 2263, 1999.
53. Patel, M. R., Edelman, R. R., and Warach, S., Detection of hyperacute primary intraparenchymal hemorrhage by magnetic resonance imaging, *Stroke*, 27, 2321, 1996.
54. Schellinger, P. D. et al., A standardized MRI stroke protocol: comparison with CT in hyperacute intracerebral hemorrhage, *Stroke*, 30, 765, 1999.
55. Allkemper, T. et al., Acute and subacute intracerebral hemorrhages: comparison of MR imaging at 1.5 and 3.0 T — initial experience, *Radiology*, 232, 874, 2004.
56. Ebisu, T. et al., Hemorrhagic and nonhemorrhagic stroke: diagnosis with diffusion-weighted and T_2-weighted echo-planar MR imaging, *Radiology*, 203, 823, 1997.

57. Steinbrich, W. et al., Intracranial hemorrhages in the magnetic resonance tomogram. Studies on sensitivity, on the development of hematomas and on the determination of the cause of the hemorrhage, *Rofo Fortschr. Geb. Rontgenstr. Neuen Bildgeb. Verfahr.*, 152, 534, 1990.
58. Fiebach, J. B. et al., Stroke magnetic resonance imaging is accurate in hyperacute intracerebral hemorrhage. A multicenter study on the validity of stroke imaging, *Stroke*, 35, 502, 2004.
59. Ruiz-Sandoval, J. L., Cantu, C., and Barinagarrementeria, F., Intracerebral hemorrhage in young people: analysis of risk factors, location, causes, and prognosis, *Stroke*, 30, 537, 1999.
60. Kidwell, C. S. et al., Magnetic resonance imaging detection of microbleeds before thrombolysis: an emerging application, *Stroke*, 33, 95, 2002.
61. Nighoghossian, N. et al., Old microbleeds are a potential risk factor for cerebral bleeding after ischemic stroke: a gradient-echo T_2^*-weighted brain MRI study, *Stroke*, 33, 735, 2002.
62. Fazekas, F. et al., Histopathologic analysis of foci of signal loss on gradient-echo T_2*-weighted MR images in patients with spontaneous intracerebral hemorrhage: evidence of microangiopathy-related microbleeds, *Am. J. Neuroradiol.*, 20, 637, 1999.
63. Hagen, T., Intracerebral hemorrhage in the context of amyloid angiopathy, *Radiologe*, 39, 847, 1999.
64. Felber, S. et al., MRI characteristics of spontaneous intracerebral hemorrhage, *Radiologe*, 39, 838, 1999.
65. Scotti, G. et al., Computed tomography in the evaluation of intracranial aneurysms and subarachnoid hemorrhage, *Radiology*, 123, 85, 1977.
66. van Gijn, J. and van Dongen, K. J., The time course of aneurysmal haemorrhage on computed tomograms, *Neuroradiology*, 23, 153, 1982.
67. Busch, E. et al., Diffusion MR imaging during acute subarachnoid hemorrhage in rats, *Stroke*, 29, 2155, 1998.
68. Jansen, O., Knauth, M., and Sartor, K., Advances in clinical neuroradiology, *Akt. Neurol.*, 26, 1, 1999.
69. Barber, P. A. et al., Validity and reliability of a quantitative computed tomography score in predicting outcome of hyperacute stroke before thrombolytic therapy. ASPECTS study group. Alberta stroke programme early CT score, *Lancet*, 355, 1670, 2000.
70. Pexman, J. H. et al., Use of the alberta stroke program early CT score (ASPECTS) for assessing CT scans in patients with acute stroke, *Am. J. Neuroradiol.*, 22, 1534, 2001.
71. von Kummer, R. et al., Early prediction of irreversible brain damage after ischemic stroke at CT, *Radiology*, 219, 95, 2001.
72. Koenig, M. et al., Quantitative assessment of the ischemic brain by means of perfusion-related parameters derived from perfusion CT, *Stroke*, 32, 431, 2001.
73. Wildermuth, S. et al., Role of CT angiography in patient selection for thrombolytic therapy in acute hemispheric stroke, *Stroke*, 29, 935, 1998.
74. Baird, A. E. and Warach, S., Magnetic resonance imaging of acute stroke, *J. Cereb. Blood Flow Metab.*, 18, 583, 1999.
75. Barber, P. A. et al., Identification of major ischemic change — diffusion-weighted imaging versus computed tomography, *Stroke*, 30, 2059, 1999.
76. Fiebach, J. B. et al., Comparison of CT with diffusion-weighted MRI in patients with hyperacute stroke, *Neuroradiology*, 43, 628, 2001.
77. Lansberg, M. G. et al., Comparison of diffusion-weighted MRI and CT in acute stroke, *Neurology*, 54, 1557, 2000.
78. Ay, H. et al., Normal diffusion-weighted MRI during stroke-like deficits, *Neurology*, 52, 1784, 1999.
79. Kidwell, C. S. et al., Diffusion MRI in patients with transient ischemic attacks, *Stroke*, 30, 1174, 1999.
80. Buckley, B. T. et al., Audit of a policy of magnetic resonance imaging with diffusion-weighted imaging as first-line neuroimaging for in-patients with clinically suspected acute stroke, *Clin. Radiol.*, 58, 234, 2003.
81. Fiebach, J. B. et al., CT and diffusion-weighted MR-imaging in randomized order: DWI results in higher accuracy and lower interrater variability in the diagnosis of hyperacute ischemic stroke, *Stroke*, 33, 2206, 2002.

82. Saur, D. et al., Sensitivity and interrater agreement of CT and diffusion-weighted MR imaging in hyperacute stroke, *Am. J. Neuroradiol.*, 24, 878, 2003.
83. Warach, S., Stroke neuroimaging, *Stroke*, 34, 345, 2003.
84. Yamada, K. et al., Magnetic resonance perfusion-weighted imaging of acute cerebral infarction: effect of the calculation methods and underlying vasculopathy, *Stroke*, 33, 87, 2002.
85. Parsons, M. W. et al., Perfusion magnetic resonance imaging maps in hyperacute stroke. Relative cerebral blood flow most accurately identifies tissue destined to infarct, *Stroke*, 32, 1581, 2001.
86. Jäger, H. R., Diagnosis of stroke with advanced CT and MR imaging, *Br. Med. Bull.*, 56, 318, 2000.
87. Karonen, J. O. et al., Diffusion and perfusion MR imaging in acute ischemic stroke: a comparison to SPECT, *Comput. Methods Programs Biomed.*, 66, 125, 2001.
88. Kim, J. H. et al., Comparative evaluation of cerebral blood volume and cerebral blood flow in acute ischenic stroke using perfuaion-weighted MR imaging and SPECT, *Acta Radiol.*, 43, 365, 2002.
89. Sobesky, J. et al., Which time-to-peak threshold best identifies penumbral flow?. A comparison of perfusion-weighted magnetic resonance imaging and positron emission tomography in acute ischemic stroke, *Stroke*, 35, 2843, 2004.
90. Hamberg, L. M. et al., Measurement of cerebral blood volume with subtraction three-dimensional functional CT, *Am. J. Neuroradiol.*, 17, 1861, 1996.
91. Koenig, M. et al., CT perfusion imaging in acute ischemic cerebral infarct: comparison of cerebral perfusion maps and conventional CT findings, *Röfo Fortschr. Geb. Röntgenstr. Neuen Bildgeb. Verfahr.*, 172, 219, 2000.
92. Bruning, R. et al., Calculation of absolute cerebral blood volume and cerebral blood flow by means of electron-beam computed tomography (EBT) in acute ischemia, *Radiologe*, 38, 1054, 1998.
93. Röther, J. et al., Hemodynamic assessment of acute stroke using dynamic single-slice computed tomographic perfusion imaging, *Arch. Neurol.*, 57, 1161, 2000.
94. Röther, J. et al., Effect of thrombolysis on MRI parameters and functional outcome in acute stroke <6 h, *Stroke*, 33, 2438, 2002.
95. Knauth, M. et al., Potential of CT angiography in acute ischemic stroke, *Am. J. Neuroradiol.*, 18, 1001, 1997.
96. Shrier, D. A. et al., CT angiography in the evaluation of acute stroke, *Am. J. Neuroradiol.*, 18, 1011, 1997.
97. Brandt, T. et al., CT angiography and doppler sonography for emergency assessment in acute basilar artery ischemia, *Stroke*, 30, 606, 1999.
98. Doerfler, A. et al., Are iodinated contrast agents detrimental in acute cerebral ischemia? An experimental study in rats, *Radiology*, 206, 211, 1998.
99. Koenig, M. et al., Perfusion CT of the brain: diagnostic approach for early detection of ischemic stroke, *Radiology*, 209, 85, 1998.
100. Schramm, P. et al., Comparison of CT and CT angiography source images with diffusion-weighted imaging in patients with acute stroke within 6 hours after onset, *Stroke*, 33, 2426, 2002.
101. Schriger, D. L. et al., Cranial computed tomography interpretation in acute stroke: physician accuracy in determining eligibility for thrombolytic therapy, *JAMA*, 279, 1293, 1998.
102. The European Stroke Initiative, Recommendations for stroke management, *Cerebrovasc. Dis.*, 10(Suppl. 3), 1, 2000.
103. Kidwell, C. S. et al., Predictors of hemorrhagic transformation in patients receiving intra-arterial thrombolysis, *Stroke*, 33, 717, 2002.
104. Derex, L. et al., Thrombolysis for ischemic stroke in patients with old microbleeds on pretreatment MRI, *Cerebrovasc. Dis.*, 17, 238, 2004.
105. Saver, J. L. et al., Infarct volume as a surrogate or auxiliary outcome measure in ischemic stroke clinical trials, *Stroke*, 30, 293, 1999.
106. Kidwell, C. S. et al., Thrombolytic reversal of acute human cerebral ischemic injury shown by diffusion/perfusion magnetic resonance imaging, *Ann. Neurol.*, 47, 462, 2000.
107. Warach, S., Tissue viability thresholds in acute stroke: the 4-factor model, *Stroke*, 32, 2460, 2001.

108. Warach, S., Kaste, M., and Fisher, M., The effect of GV150526 on ischemic lesion volume: the GAIN Americas and GAIN international MRI substudy, *Neurology*, 54, A87, 2000.
109. Major ongoing stroke trials, *Stroke*, 36(6), e59, 2005.
110. Wegener, S. et al., Transient ischemic attacks before ischemic stroke: preconditioning the human brain? A multicenter magnetic resonance imaging study, *Stroke*, 35, 616, 2004.
111. Alsop, D. C. and Detre, J. A., Reduced transit-time sensitivity in noninvasive magnetic resonance imaging of human cerebral blood flow, *J. Cereb. Blood Flow Metab.*, 16, 1236, 1996.

Editorial Comments

Functional magnetic resonance imaging (fMRI) has the capacity to provide data with spatial and temporal resolutions exceeding those achieved by other currently available methods of noninvasive investigation of brain function. This fact coupled with the ability of the technique to perform serial studies makes fMRI an attractive tool for investigating the effects of pharmacological agents in the animal and human brain, as extensively discussed in Chapter 10 and Chapter 11. However, there are various associated complications to be taken into account, such as the different means by which drugs may interfere with the mechanisms that give rise to the pharmacologically induced fMRI signal, and local or global cardiovascular changes that might produce functional responses unrelated to neural activity. Furthermore, in animals, there is the complicating effect of anesthesia. Proper consideration of these concerns, along with careful attention to experimental details and verification procedures, are fundamental in this context.

The designation pharmacologic magnetic resonance imaging (phMRI) has been introduced in the literature to mean the application of fMRI to monitor drug-induced changes in brain activity [1–4]. Unfortunately, it turns out that this nomenclature may be too restrictive. As the many chapters of this book illustrate, MRI techniques can be sensibly used to perform pharmacological studies addressing various disease areas besides neurological disorders. In addition, MRI is being successful in deriving functional information not only from the brain, but also from other organs, for instance the heart, the lungs, the kidneys, and even the joints. A more appropriate terminology to designate the use of fMRI to follow drug-induced changes in the brain may thus be, for instance, pharmacological functional MRI (phfMRI) of the brain.

REFERENCES

1. Chen, Y. I. et al. Detection of dopaminergic neurotransmitter activity using pharmacologic MRI: correlation with PET, microdialysis, and behavioral data, *Magn. Reson. Med.*, 38, 389, 1997.
2. Chen, Y. I. et al. Detection of dopaminergic cell loss and neural transplantation using pharmacological MRI, PET and behavioural assessment, *NeuroReport*, 10, 2881, 1999.
3. Nguyen, T. V. et al. Detection of the effects of dopamine supersensitivity using pharmacological MRI and correlations with PET, *Synapse*, 36, 57, 2000.
4. Leslie, R. A. and James, M. F., Pharmacological magnetic resonance imaging: a new application for functional MRI, *Trends Pharmacol. Sci.*, 21, 314, 2000.

10 Pharmacologic Magnetic Resonance Imaging (phMRI)

Bruce G. Jenkins, Ji-Kyung Choi, Joseph B. Mandeville, and Yin-Ching Iris Chen

CONTENTS

10.1 INTRODUCTION

10.1.1 IMAGING TECHNIQUES FOR STUDYING NEURONAL ACTIVITY

The technique of functional magnetic resonance imaging (fMRI) using either relative cerebral blood volume (rCBV), blood oxygenation level dependent (BOLD) or T_1-based cerebral blood flow (CBF) techniques has led to a revolution in brain mapping [1–3]. This is largely due to the fact that the advent of a noninvasive tool with reasonable contrast to noise, spatial, and temporal resolution, allows for studies to be conducted more easily than the prior positron emission tomography (PET) studies of brain activation. Both fMRI and PET studies of brain activation are based upon the coupling between neuronal activity, metabolism, and hemodynamics (see also Chapter 11, Section 2). The possibility that fMRI may help understand the organization and flow of information in the brain has led to an explosion in the number of centers dedicated to performing the technique. In addition to the interest in fMRI by the neuroscience community, a number of clinical conditions has the potential to benefit from the development of fMRI techniques, such as perfusion studies of stroke, presurgical planning for conservation of eloquent cortex during brain surgery, and investigation of motor systems in movement disorders. Most fMRI studies have used task activation, such as photic stimulation or finger movements, or a cognitive challenge to induce neuronal activity. However, it is also possible to elicit neuronal activity using pharmacologic ligands. This approach has the potential to generate maps of the metabolic consequences of receptor stimulation of relevance to a large number of cerebral disorders. Studies of receptor binding can be performed *in vivo* using PET imaging, or *post mortem* with autoradiography. These techniques allow one to use direct agonists or antagonists to map out the receptor binding parameters or the density of these sites in the brain. Such studies are of diagnostic value for the examination of dopamine receptor depletion in Parkinson's disease (PD) and have great potential for study of conditions such as drug abuse and schizophrenia.

Autoradiographic and PET studies have also examined metabolic changes (both blood flow and glucose utilization) after neurotransmitter stimulation using, for example, amphetamine [4]. While PET is the gold standard tool for measurement of regional changes in glucose utilization *in vivo*, the same cannot be said for PET studies of metabolic activation using CBF. A number of studies used PET to assess changes in CBF after drug stimulation. These studies suffer from the fact that, with PET, CBF is usually only measured once after administration of the drug whereas with MRI one can obtain the entire hemodynamic time course with temporal resolution on the order of 1 sec. The technique of fMRI is well suited to study these metabolic changes [5]. Several reports using MRI to study the acute effects of amphetamine [5–7], cocaine or cocaine analogs [5,8–10], apomorphine or *L*-dopa [11–13], nicotine [14], heroin [15], and serotonin ligands [16] have appeared. Nonetheless, there is a number of issues that render interpretation of the signal changes induced more difficult than in conventional task-related fMRI. Since drugs are used as the stimuli of interest, and because drugs can have effects very different from functional activation tasks, we have coined the term pharmacologic MRI (phMRI) to describe these experiments [5].

Unlike in conventional task-related fMRI studies where the time courses of the stimuli can be controlled at will, in phMRI the time course is determined by the pharmacodynamic profile of the drug administered to induce the signal changes. Since most drugs can be anticipated to have long time courses compared with task-related stimuli (tens of minutes or more compared with seconds for conventional fMRI), data collection and analysis schemes become important for accurate determination of metabolically induced signal changes after pharmacologic stimulus. A number of approaches to this problem will be discussed in Section 10.2.

There are generally two flavors of what might be considered pharmacologic MRI. The first is what has been discussed in the papers referenced above. This paradigm is most often run in the form of a drug challenge study in which MR signal changes are monitored after the acute administration of the drug of interest. Clearly, there are many permutations on this basic model, such as antagonism of the effects of one drug with another, or examining perhaps the acute effects of one drug upon the chronic effects of another (useful perhaps for studying cocaine addiction). The second flavor of what might be considered phMRI is the observation of the modulatory effects of a pharmaceutical upon a conventional task-related fMRI study, such as the effects of dopaminergic and glutamatergic drugs upon cognitive tasks [17,18]. Since this chapter is primarily concerned with animal studies such approaches will not be discussed further; however, the review by Honey and Bullmore provides an excellent summary of the work to date in humans [17] (see also Chapter 11, Section 11.3 and Section 11.4). The effects of such a drug administration during a cognitive task however, must be kept in mind when interpreting the hemodynamic changes — as the drug itself may have modulatory effects upon the hemodynamics. With this as a general background we proceed to compare the possibilities of studying neuroreceptors using MRI techniques with the more traditional techniques, such as PET and autoradiography.

10.1.2 Pharmacologic MRI Compared with PET and Autoradiography. How Well Do Hemodynamic Changes Reflect Receptor Distributions?

The ability of both PET and autoradiography to measure direct binding of drugs to neuroreceptors would, at first glance, render the possibility of measuring specific receptor parameters based upon simple hemodynamic changes seem rather remote. At best, one might hope to verify the assumption that the hemodynamic changes observed after administration of a particular drug correlate with the activation of the receptor systems targeted by the drug. In this manner one would hope that there is a pharmacologically induced metabolic coupling entirely analogous to the metabolic coupling usually assumed in standard fMRI studies. Such correlations can be established empirically using techniques capable of measuring receptor binding, receptor distribution, and the attendant metabolic circuitry. These parameters in turn can be correlated with electrophysiologic data and companion metabolic studies. Such correlations might entail measuring BOLD signal changes and correlating these with changes in the cerebral metabolic rate of glucose consumption (CMRglc) as well as evoked potentials and perhaps even EEG or magnetoencephalography data. In such a manner it is possible to painstakingly verify which correlations characterize the BOLD signal and to stand on firmer ground when trying to interpret BOLD signal changes. Recently, such studies have become quite popular, and are underway in many different laboratories around the world.

Monitoring hemodynamic changes after administration of a drug will lead to three obvious general outcomes. First, one may obtain no response or correlation whatsoever with other measured parameters. In such an instance the only conclusion to be drawn is that a drug targeted towards a specific receptor has no hemodynamic effect. This does not mean that it has no behavioral effect or even that it has no metabolic effect, since for instance the vasodilatory and vasoconstrictive properties of the drug may cancel one another. The second outcome one might envisage is that there is a hemodynamic effect that is measurable, but that it does not correlate with any obvious pattern of receptors, or that the targeted receptors have such a widespread distribution that distinguishing nonspecific from specific effects is quite difficult. We have observed just such effects with caffeine and theophylline where activation (more precisely, negative rCBV changes) is seen over almost the entire brain, mirroring the distribution of adenosine A1 receptors, but also being indistinguishable from global vasoconstrictive changes. Another twist on this basic scenario is that the hemodynamic effects resulting from administration of the drug are sufficiently complicated that specific correlation with a receptor system is not possible. In this regard, the phMRI study can be anticipated to mirror a PET measurement of glucose utilization or CBF. This, by the way, is the situation encountered in almost every fMRI study. In these cases the neurovascular coupling is considered as a black box and the interpretation of the hemodynamic patterns are anatomic or contextual in nature. The third and most copacetic possibility is that a very good correlation exists between the hemodynamic changes induced by the drug and a given receptor distribution. This situation is most likely to occur when the administered drug causes release of a vasoactive molecule reflective of the targeted receptor system or when the pattern of vascular targets is reflective of the receptor targets in the brain tissue.

Shown in Table 10.1 is a comparison of PET and MRI with the relative advantages and disadvantages of each considering the types of information that can be obtained by the techniques and issues related to the data collection. PET can examine both the metabolic response to neuronal stimulation (usually performed using measures of glucose accumulation with ^{18}F-fluorodeoxyglucose or CBF using ^{15}O-labeled water) as well as the direct binding of the compound to its targets. PET has the added advantage of utilizing either tracer-level doses of the ligand or to examine the metabolic coupling evoked by behaviorally relevant doses as MRI can. MRI is better, in general, at examining the hemodynamic changes possessing superior temporal and spatial resolution if one considers the BOLD effect (the relative advantages of CBF measurements are more murky given the relatively low sensitivity of arterial spin-labeling). MRI is also better at examining changes in rCBV. PET is obviously superior at determining changes in glucose utilization, although this can be examined using MR spectroscopy (both ^{13}C and proton spectroscopy of the glucose peak at 5.23 ppm) with inferior spatial and temporal resolution compared with PET. The superior temporal sampling characteristics of MR in general, make examination of drug time courses more flexible than with PET, although both techniques are clearly useful.

Utilization of PET imaging to examine receptor populations requires administration of drugs that bind specifically to a given receptor population. The data interpretation is not quite as straightforward as might be anticipated. A complicated multicompartmental model is derived with compartments for the free, specifically bound, nonspecifically bound, and plasma components with transfer coefficients for the compartments, as shown in Figure 10.1. To render so many parameters experimentally tractable, a number of assumptions are made. For instance, in the case of dopamine receptors, it is usually assumed that the cerebellar time activity curves represent only the nonspecifically bound compound and that the specifically bound curve in other brain regions, such as

TABLE 10.1
Comparisons of phMRI and PET for Measurement of Neuroreceptors

	phMRI	PET
In plane spatial resolution	0.1–3 mm	1.5–12 mm
Direct drug binding	No	Yes
Metabolic coupling (Indirect (I) Direct (D))	$rCMRO_2$ (I), rCBV (D), CBF (D), BOLD (I)	rCMRglc (D/I), $rCMRO_2$ (D/I), CBF (D)
Drug time course (hemodynamic)	Yes	No
Drug time course (binding)	Maybe	Yes
Multiple studies	Yes	Sometimes
Tracer level doses	No	Yes
Behaviorally relevant doses	Yes	Yes

Direct means the parameter is derived from data with minimal modeling. Indirect means the parameter requires either extensive models or no direct relation to a metabolic/physiologic parameter. D/I suggests elements of both direct and indirect.

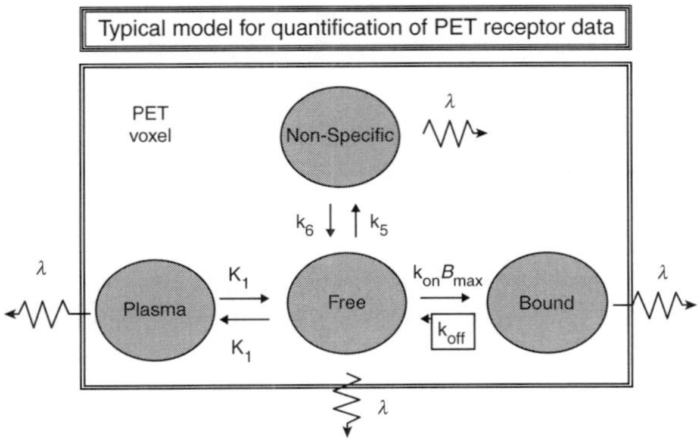

FIGURE 10.1 Schematic for the data obtained in a PET study. The rate constants are determined from fitting time activity curves corrected for both the arterial input function and the radioactive decay (λ). The cerebellum is often used as a brain region that provides a measure of the nonspecific binding parameters for study of dopaminergic drugs. B_{max} is the total number of receptors, the other ks are transfer coefficients and rate constants for binding to the receptor.

in the striatum, can be fit using parameters for the plasma, transfer coefficients, and nonspecifically bound compartment derived from the cerebellar curves. A further problem for PET imaging is that a radiolabeled ligand is required for each target. Development of new ligands is laborious, especially when compared with MRI where standard nonradiolabeled ligands can be used.

The obvious advantages of no requirement for radioactivity (or the presence of a cyclotron and PET scanner which are much rarer than MR machines), means that multiple repeated studies in the same subject are more feasible using MR. Nonetheless, it is better to characterize the relationship between PET and MR as complementary techniques that have much to offer in the study of pharmaceutical interactions.

Autoradiographic techniques have the obvious disadvantage of being terminal. There is also the issue of tissue fixation and preparation, which may affect some of the parameters. However, autoradiography can measure nearly the full complement of parameters measurable by PET, and can also examine mRNA expression levels, receptor protein levels as well as the direct ligand binding to the receptors. The large array of parameters that can be examined using autoradiography makes it an attractive complement to PET or phMRI. Unfortunately, for the purposes of validation, there is often not a direct relationship between the regional mRNA expression levels, ligand binding, or even protein expression levels [19–21] for a given receptor system. This means that selection of a gold standard for comparison of an phMRI or PET activation pattern can be problematic. Secondly, the empirical determination of what patterns of activity can be observed after administration of various drugs is also very much a work in progress, and will probably be very different for different classes of drugs targeted towards the various neurotransmitter systems. We will consider in more detail later specific correlations between receptor densities measured with PET or autoradiography and those determined using phMRI. However, as a way of introducing the concept let us examine a hypothetical phMRI examination. In this case we may have injected drug X which was targeted towards the dopaminergic system, for instance. Obviously, the first step would be to determine the regional pattern of hemodynamic changes elicited by the chosen drug. In the case of the dopaminergic system, for instance, the drug might be an agonist or antagonist of a specific dopamine receptor subtype, or it might be a compound targeted towards the dopamine transporter. If the drug had a hemodynamic consequence (not a foregone conclusion) then the spatial pattern of hemodynamic changes induced by the drug can be compared with a number of different autoradiographic parameters. Is the pattern similar to that of the receptor mRNA expression levels? Is the pattern similar to the pattern of drug binding measured autoradiographically? Is the pattern similar to the immunohistochemical distribution of the receptor proteins? Lastly, is the pattern induced similar to the pattern of CMRglc induced around the brain? All of these are good questions, and in an ideal study they would be addressed in animals (clearly, it is not as easy to perform such studies on post-mortem human tissue — but one can examine PET data for both the CMRglc as well as the direct drug binding). It must be said that at this point in time, no one has performed such a study. The histologic/autoradiographic studies have exquisite spatial resolution, however, the quantitative measurements of mRNA expression and protein levels can be problematic. Those studies such as CBF using iodoantipyrene, and CMRglc, which are quantitative, have the problem of trying to catch a metabolic snapshot by allowing enough time for accumulation of labeled compound (such as glucose, for which it can be 45 min) in a system where the metabolic parameters may be changing dynamically. This factor may account for the differences which may be observed between phMRI and autoradiographic measurements of CMRglc. In Section 10.3 of this chapter we will examine in detail some of the correlations observed between PET, autoradiographic, and phMRI studies in selected model systems.

As an example we compare the distribution of adenosine A2a receptors, as measured using autoradiography, with that of a phMRI study using the selective A2a antagonist DMPX (3,7-dimethyl-1-propargylaxanthine) (Figure 10.2). There is a close relationship between the rCBV changes and the distribution of A2a receptors in the brain. Such a close relationship is what makes the possibilities of the MRI technique so tantalizing for drug studies.

10.1.3 Neurovascular Coupling: Many Neurotransmitters Are Vasoactive

Changes in neuronal activity have long been known to lead to changes in metabolic activity. Both the mechanisms of the coupling between the metabolic and hemodynamic changes as well as the location of where these changes occur is still a subject of intense research activity. Most of the data and models that exist have been developed to describe changes that take place for cortical glutamatergic neuronal systems. As such, we will review these, however, we believe that many of the unifying principles that exist for the glutamatergic system may not be universal across neurotransmitter systems. One particular example of this is that the reuptake of glutamate released during firing occurs through astrocytes. In the dopaminergic system, most of the reuptake occurs at the presynaptic neuron. Thus, the coupling mechanisms of these two systems may well be different.

The origins of the concept of increases in neuronal activity coupling to increased metabolic and hemodynamic changes go back over 100 years to the pioneering work of Roy and Sherrington, who postulated coupling between brain activity and blood flow. More recently, much work has gone into

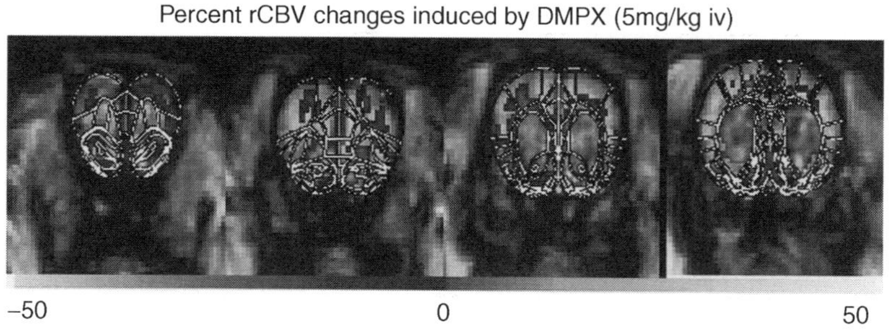

FIGURE 10.2 (See color insert following page 328.) Illustrative map of rCBV changes induced in the rat brain by the A2a antagonist DMPX. The rCBV changes induced by this drug are negative. The rCBV map is shown overlaid on a gradient-echo image. Also overlaid on the image is a coregistered rat anatomic template demonstrating that the rCBV changes induced by DMPX are almost exclusively found in the caudate/putamen and nucleus accumbens consistent with the distribution of A2a receptors in the brain.

developing models of what happens during firing of a glutamatergic neuron. The majority of this work has addressed what happens to glucose metabolism as a surrogate marker for neuronal activity. Early work investigated the subcellular distribution of glycolytic enzymes and led to the conclusion that much of the glycolytic apparatus is localized in the nerve terminals rather than in the cell bodies [22–24]. This work was followed by a series of experiments by Sokoloff and others showing that the localization of increased glucose utilization during neuronal activity was in the terminal regions rather than in the perikarya [25–27].

These early experiments have led to the paradigm, elegantly articulated by Magistretti and Pellerin [28–30], and supported by others [31], in which a cycle of glutamate release from the presynaptic terminal is followed by reuptake of the synaptic glutamate by the astrocyte. The glutamate is then converted into glutamine and lactate may also be produced for transport back to the neuron to use as a fuel, although whether the lactate is used routinely as a fuel is controversial [32]. This model makes two important predictions: first, since transport of glutamate (along with Na^+) into the glia is fueled by Na^+K^+ATPase and the neurons consume lactate, then most of the glucose utilization that occurs must happen in the glial cells and not the neurons. Second, this model predicts, consistent with the experimental data, that most of the increased glucose utilization is happening at the synaptic level. Clearly, however, much of the increased glucose utilization cannot be defined as either pre- or postsynaptic given that it is occurring in the glia. The simple fact to emerge from these results is that increased metabolic response is happening at the level of the synapse rather than at the cell bodies. The question of how the increased glucose consumption at the astrocyte is coupled to an increase in CBF is still unknown. Uptake of glutamate through astrocytes has been shown, *in vitro*, to be coupled to release of a number of vasoactive molecules, such as arachidonic acid or vasoactive intestinal peptide [33,34], thus providing possible coupling mechanisms. What actually happens *in vivo* is not known.

This fact will not necessarily generalize to the other neurotransmitter systems, such as the dopaminergic system, for the simple reason that in the case of dopamine most of the reuptake occurs on the presynaptic side of the dopamine neuron via the dopamine transporter (DAT) protein. This system is reviewed by Cooper et al. [35]. Second, dopamine synthesis and uptake are, to a large degree, controlled by presynaptic D2 autoreceptors that are more sensitive than postsynaptic dopamine receptors to the effects of dopamine or apomorphine. These data seem to suggest that the metabolic changes would be mediated via the presynaptic dopamine neurons. It was with this thought in mind that we investigated this hypothesis using unilateral lesioning of the nigrostriatal dopamine tracts using 6-hydroxydopamine [5]. These experiments showed that the hemodynamic changes induced by either amphetamine or 2β-carbomethoxy-3β-(4-fluorophenyl)tropane (CFT) were ablated by the presynaptic lesioning, and this was consistent with PET data obtained in the same animals. These data were also consistent with prior 2-deoxyglucose autoradiographic measurements of glucose utilization rates after stimulation with either amphetamine or cocaine in the same lesion model [36,37]. Nonetheless, these experiments do not prove that the hemodynamic response is being driven presynaptically, as one has also destroyed the neuron's ability to synthesize dopamine. Irrespective of whether or not the metabolic changes are induced at the level of the presynaptic neuron or whether they derive from the astrocytes, the million dollar question when it comes to understanding neurovascular coupling in a quantitative manner, is which molecules actually mediate the coupling between neurotransmitter reuptake, a metabolic change, and a change in hemodynamics.

One confound to dissecting completely the neurovascular coupling is that most neurotransmitters are also vasoactive, and indeed, many of the neurotransmitters have receptors on the vasculature. Several different brain neurotransmitters have now been identified as having axonal projections to the microcirculature in many brain regions. Many of the amino acid neurotransmitters, in particular glutamate, appear to couple to changes in blood flow via nitric oxide (NO) [38–40]. As discussed above, this coupling is thought to arise at the level of the astrocytes. Serotonin took its name from the fact that it was a potent vasoconstrictor — this was discovered before its role as a neurotransmitter was known (see review in [41]). Acetylcholine also has vasoactive properties [42]. A coupling of cholinergic M5 receptors on the vasculature apposed to NO neurons (which are vasodilatory) in the basal forebrain has been worked out to provide control of cerebral microcirculation [43,44]. Confounding the neurovascular coupling is the fact that cholinergic activation of the substantia innominata leads to increased CBF in the absence of increases in glucose utilization [45]. Strong histological evidence accrued over the past 20 years indicates that dopamine neurons are intimately associated with microvasculature in brain parenchyma [46,47]. It has, recently, even been suggested that much of the hemodynamic change observed in neuronal activation may be dopaminergic in origin [48]. This latter study by Krimer et al. showed direct immunocytochemical evidence for termination of central dopaminergic neurons on penetrating arterioles and the pericytes of capillaries. The pericytes are the contractile motors regulating capillary flow. The highest density of dopaminergic innervation of these microvessels was in areas of cortex known to be high in dopaminergic innervation in the parenchyma such as the frontal cortex. Thus, control of microvascular flow via dopamine release is certainly one important factor in regulating changes induced by dopaminergic drugs. It is, of course, well known that dopamine is a vasoactive substance in many other areas of the body.

Adenosine is another neurotransmitter whose vasoactive properties are well known — especially in the heart. Adenosine antagonists, such as caffeine and theophylline, have the interesting property of increasing energy metabolism and at the same time decreasing CBF [49]. The list of vasoactive molecules in the brain also includes many of the important neuropeptides [50].

A list of neurotransmitter systems amenable to analysis using phMRI based upon their known activation of CBF, as well as common drugs that might be studied and disease states relevant to those molecules, are provided in Table 10.2. It is clear that a wide array of molecules may be amenable to analysis. This does not, however, guarantee that all molecules targeted towards a given neurotransmitter system may have vasoactive properties. Isolating the neurovascular coupling interactions in the face of such a daunting array of vasoactive molecules can be quite complicated. In the case of stimuli that may ultimately drive many different brain regions, it is more than likely that numerous neurotransmitters may be involved in coupling metabolic changes to increases in CBF. Pharmacologic MRI may well be one very good way to isolate some of these interactions and coupling relationships.

Our laboratory has collected a great deal of data on the dopaminergic system that may be of interest to consider since it is quite different from the cortical glutamatergic and GABAergic systems usually considered in most fMRI studies. It has long been known that dopaminergic ligands are capable of increasing CBF. Measurement of CBF using autoradiography after amphetamine stimulus showed, over 20 years ago, regionally specific increases in dopamine-rich brain areas [4].

TABLE 10.2
Neurotransmitter Systems, Clinical Targets, and Ligands

System	Clinical Targets	Common Drugs with phMRI Potential
Glutamatergic	Drug Abuse, Schizophrenia	Ketamine, phencyclidine (PCP)
Dopaminergic	Drug Abuse, Schizophrenia, Parkinson's Disease	Cocaine, amphetamine, L-DOPA apomorphine, haldol
Cholinergic	Alzheimer's disease, cigarette addiction	Nicotine, scopolamine, tacrine
Opioid	Drug Abuse, Pain Research	Fentanyl, morphine
GABAergic	Epilepsy, Anxiety	Vigabatrin, flumazenil, diazepam
Serontinergic	Drug abuse, sleep disorders	Prozac, fenfluramine, MDMA (ecstasy)
Adenosinergic	Neurodegeneration, Coffee and Tea consumption	Caffeine, theophylline

Increases in cerebral glucose utilization rates after dopaminergic stimulus are also found in similar brain regions [4,51–53]. Thus, it is not surprising that MRI techniques sensitive to hemodynamics can measure changes due to stimulation with either amphetamine or cocaine. One question that naturally arises is, what agents and synaptic activities actually mediate the coupling between the receptor activation and blood flow? Obviously, this is a complicated question that has not been completely answered for any of the various phenomena that can modulate cerebral hemodynamics, such as hypercapnia, hypoxia, or neuronal activation. Nonetheless, great strides have been made in this direction.

Let us first look at the events that may occur after stimulation of the dopaminergic system using a drug such as amphetamine or cocaine. Amphetamine's main mechanism appears to be twofold. First, it may reverse the dopamine transporter protein to provide reverse transport of the dopamine from the presynaptic neuron to the synaptic cleft [54]. Second, it can apparently render the vesicular environment alkaline to enhance vesicular release of dopamine and reverse transport [55]. Cocaine is a member of a family of drugs (including nomifensene and methylphenidate) that blocks the DAT, thus blocking reuptake of dopamine. The end result of these two mechanisms is an increase in synaptic dopamine concentrations (one has to keep in mind that there are other targets as well — cocaine also binds to the serotonin transporter). As its concentration increases, dopamine diffuses both across the synapse and away from the synapse. Since there is good evidence for dopamine receptors on the vasculature, it is reasonable to assume that some of the dopamine will directly affect the vessels. In addition, there will be stimulation of the postsynaptic dopamine neurons. These neurons in turn control afferent output via the striatum and globus pallidus to the thalamus and hence to the cortex. Thus, in addition to the effects of any dopamine released directly upon the vasculature there is the potential for downstream effects in areas metabolically activated by dopamine. Since reuptake of dopamine, similar to that of glutamate, is coupled to energy demands mediated by Na^+K^+ATPase, changes in metabolism may also lead to further hemodynamic changes at the level of the presynaptic dopamine neuron. Changes in hemodynamics elicited in the downstream areas are likely to be coupled via other vasoactive substances. These two perspectives are illustrated as follows:

$$\text{Mechanism I : Drug} \rightarrow \Delta\text{DA} \rightarrow \Delta\text{CBV} \tag{10.1a}$$

$$\text{Mechanism II : Drug} \rightarrow \Delta\text{DA} \rightarrow \Delta\text{metabolism} \rightarrow \Delta\text{substance[s]X} \rightarrow \Delta\text{CBV} \tag{10.1b}$$

It is probable that in any stimulation a combination of these two mechanisms is operative with a relative weighting determined by the brain region and local conditions. Vascular and metabolic effects may be usefully compared using phMRI to obtain the hemodynamic effects and PET or autoradiography of glucose utilization to determine the metabolic changes. However, such comparisons, as mentioned above, may be difficult to make based upon the different time courses of the techniques.

A simple schematic diagram illustrating the perspective that we believe is a reasonable one to take with regards to regulation of blood flow or volume in the brain is shown in Figure 10.3. This diagram indicates that a drug can cause a metabolic change after which vasocactive molecules will be released (referred to as the indirect pathway). Alternatively, or more probably in addition, the drug may cause an increase in the concentration of a molecule such as dopamine that will in turn lead to a direct increase in CBF or CBV. This direct pathway is further schematized as a baseline state in which the vascular volume and flow are under the control of any number of vasoactive molecules (some vasoconstrictive, other vasodilatory). After administration of a drug such as amphetamine, the dopamine concentration becomes so large that it is the biggest hammer which drives a vasodilatory response thereby increasing CBV, CBF, and the BOLD effect. Interestingly, this type of model allows for the fact that other substances might actually antagonize the CBV effects of amphetamine, without actually changing the dopaminergic neurotransmission. We hypothesized previously that dopamine

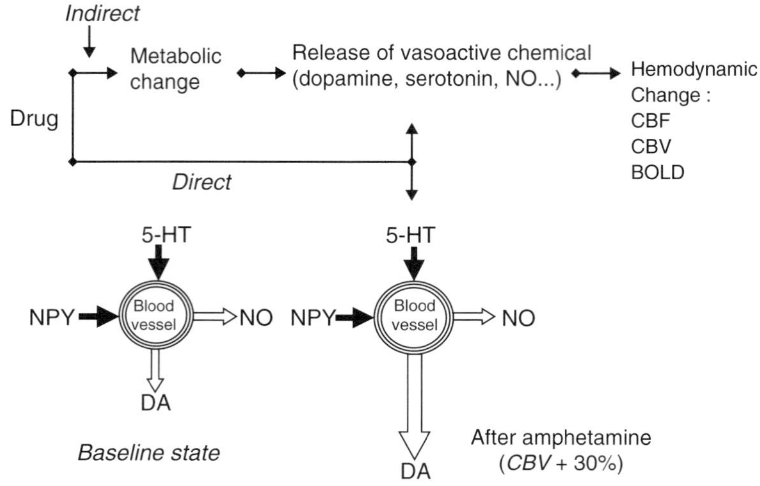

FIGURE 10.3 Schematic illustrating a plausible situation for hemodynamic changes. The top of the figure shows two pathways for driving the hemodynamic changes. The indirect pathway is that most familiar to all fMRI studies where metabolic changes induced by a drug lead to release of vasoactive substances and a resultant hemodynamic (or BOLD) change. Also shown is a direct pathway whereby the drug can directly cause release of a vasoactive substance. In this model many vasoactive substances control the baseline flow. A large increase in one of the molecules (in this case dopamine) may be responsible for driving the hemodynamic change due to administration of a drug such as amphetamine. NO is nitric oxide, NPY is neuropeptide Y, and 5-HT is 5-hydroxytryptamine.

may actually drive the hemodynamic changes, based upon the strong temporal correlation between the time course of the dopamine release measured by microdialysis and the changes in either BOLD or rCBV. Such a correlation is presented in Figure 10.4 where we show the time course of dopamine release in the nucleus accumbens after 2 mg/kg amphetamine in eight animals with and without pretreatment with the D2 antagonist eticlopride [56]. The eticlopride acts to increase dopamine release (by antagonism of autoreceptors) and increases rCBV proportionately. The time courses and relative changes in the amplitude of the rCBV and dopamine release are well correlated ($R > 0.9$ for a linear correlation $p < 0.01$).

Detailed study of stimulation of neurotransmission, however, quickly leads one to the conclusion that no single neurotransmitter is an island. That is, there is a coupling between the many neurotransmitters in a given brain region such that increasing the level of one leads to reciprocal changes in coupled systems to maintain homeostasis. As an example, we will examine the interactions between the dopaminergic and adenosinergic system in the brain. It should be pointed out that a large body of literature also exists on interactions between dopamine and glutamate, dopamine and serotonin, and dopamine and GABA!

Dopamine release and function are strongly affected by adenosine A2a receptors in the basal ganglia and nucleus accumbens (see reviews in Ref. [57–59]). In particular, administration of A2a receptor antagonists such as DMPX or 3-(3-hydroxypropyl)-8-(m-methoxystyryl)-7-methyl-1-propargylxanthine (MSX-3) reduces dopamine release induced by electrical stimulation [60]. We used amphetamine as a means of increasing dopamine release and tried to antagonize it using the selective A2a antagonist DMPX [61]. DMPX induced a large reduction in the amphetamine-induced rCBV changes in brain regions with high densities of A2a receptors — as well as in downstream circuits such as the thalamus. These results are consistent with a decrease in amphetamine-induced dopamine release evoked by administration of DMPX, and this was demonstrated by the companion microdialysis results in the caudate/putamen. The decrease in rCBV induced by DMPX alone can be interpreted as being due to decreased basal dopamine levels,

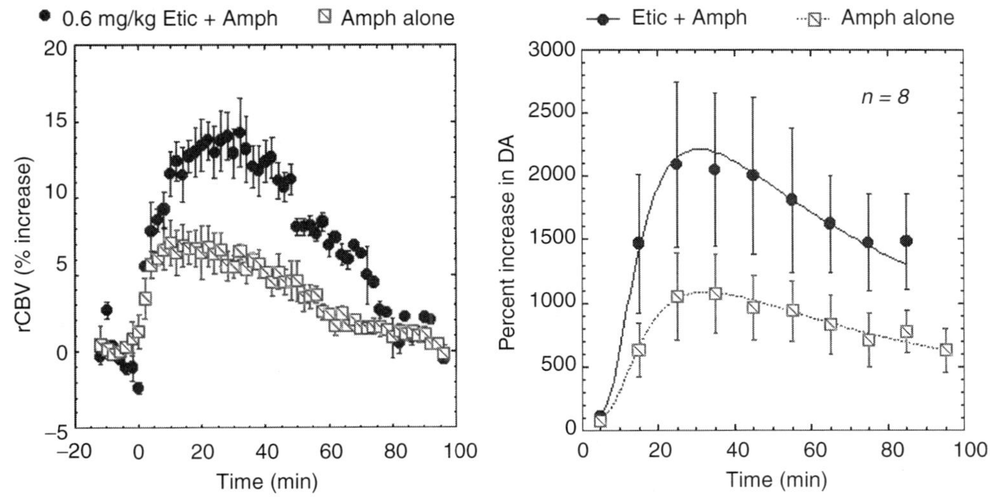

FIGURE 10.4 Comparison of microdialysis data of dopamine release and rCBV data from nucleus accumbens in rats. Two sets of curves are shown. On the left is the increase in rCBV over time with amphetamine alone or with pretreatment with the D2 antagonist eticlopride. It is seen that blocking D2/D3 receptors leads to an increase in the rCBV induced by amphetamine. This increase in rCBV is paralleled by an increase in dopamine release by an almost identical percent. The time courses for the rCBV and dopamine release data match quite closely. Both data sets were collected under 1.5% halothane anesthesia.

as well as from hemodynamic consequences of A2a antagonism that may be independent of dopamine. These data accord with behavioral studies and appear to be modulated via the opposing effects of D2 and A2a receptors upon stimulation evoked GABA release by striatal neurons [62].

The purpose of the discourse above is not to bore the reader with the gory details of the interaction between adenosine and dopamine, but rather to point to the fact that such a story is likely to be found in many brain regions for many different neurotransmitters. Thus, administration of a given pharmacologic agent may often need to be considered in light of interactions with multiple neurotransmitter systems. Indeed, many of the most behaviorally efficacious drugs — whether a drug of abuse such as cocaine, or an antipsychotic such as clozapine — target multiple neurotransmitter systems. Cocaine clearly blocks the serotonin as well as the dopamine transporter, whereas clozapine may be one of the dirtiest drugs ever studied, having activity at multiple serotonin receptors, dopamine D4 receptors, and adrenergic receptors. In light of this fact, one must consider potential phMRI data with an eye towards parsimonious interpretation of the data. This problem is especially acute in human studies where separation of all the competing hemodynamic interactions is probably not possible. In animal studies there is no excuse for such a lack of thoroughness.

10.2 METHODOLOGIES

10.2.1 Magnetic Resonance Techniques Used for Collecting Hemodynamic Data

The contrast-to-noise ratio (CNR) is a logical way to describe the relative merits/demerits of both functional and pharmacological MRI due to the relatively low sensitivity of these techniques in general. Thus, sensitivity becomes a logical criterion with which to arrange the various techniques. What follows are brief descriptions of the major MR methods, arranged in the order of increasing CNR, that have been used to follow changes in brain activity as a result of task or pharmacologic stimulation. These techniques are all based upon hemodynamic metrics.

10.2.1.1 The Original Technique: First Pass Bolus Mapping of Changes in rCBV

The first functional MR images were collected by Belliveau and colleagues at the Massachusetts General Hospital (MGH) around 1989 and 1990 and published in 1991 [1]. The technique these investigators chose to use was one that had also been pioneered at the MGH (no accident) [63] using intravenous administration of a bolus of paramagnetically labeled salt, $Gd(DTPA)^{2-}$. This technique allows the measurement of relative cerebral blood volume based upon the fact that the contrast agent remains in the intravascular space. Since the contrast agent is chosen to have a high magnetic susceptibility a large gradient is induced between the blood and the brain tissue. These gradients, which spread out far beyond the actual spatial volume distribution of the blood vessels, decrease in turn the T_2^* relaxation rates of the water spins that diffuse through the gradients thereby affecting a relatively large proportion of the total water signal (i.e., in excess of the actual CBV). This renders the technique more sensitive than it might otherwise be, but at a cost of only being able to measure the relative, rather than absolute, cerebral blood volume. At commonly used concentrations of agents and imaging parameters, the total signal loss observed as the bolus passes through the brain can be close to 100%. This signal rapidly returns to baseline. Then, standard tracer kinetic analyses can be applied to the signal to derive parameters related to cerebral hemodynamics. The area under the curve is roughly proportional to CBV, while the peak drop is roughly proportional to CBF.

The main limitations of this technique are twofold. First, there is the requirement of injection of at least two doses of contrast agent (before and after the stimulus). Even though $Gd(DTPA)^{2-}$ is extremely nontoxic there is still a minimal risk associated with its use. Second, in order to collect multiple time points one must perform multiple injections. This quickly becomes prohibitive, and dramatically limits the statistical power of the technique. Since this technique is no longer used for functional imaging-type experiments we will not consider it further. Interested readers can obtain further details from some of the original reports [1,64]. It should be pointed out, however, that this technique is still widely used for measuring hemodynamic parameters in a clinical setting for many types of cerebral pathologies, such as strokes and tumors. Its direct descendent is, however, being used more frequently, as described below.

10.2.1.2 CBF-Based Techniques

The original brain functional imaging experiments using PET/SPECT methodologies were based upon increases in either CBF [65] or glucose utilization [66–68]. CMRglc is likely to be a more direct marker for synaptic activity than measures of hemodynamics. Nonetheless, a number of studies have indicated a relatively tight coupling between increases in CMRglc and CBF during neuronal activation [69–72]. Thus, CBF would appear to be a logical choice for MR studies of brain function given the limitations of measuring glucose utilization with MR. A number of techniques have been developed to measure changes in either absolute or relative CBF. These techniques, which evolved into a veritable alphabet soup of acronyms, rely upon the fact that blood spins flowing into a voxel will change the apparent longitudinal relaxation time (T_1), based upon the fact that they attain a different saturation level compared with the intravoxel spins. In principle, all these methods are similar to tracer kinetic methodologies that have evolved over the years with the difference that instead of the diffusion of a labeled substance, such as iodoantipyrene used in autoradiographic measurements of CBF, one uses water as a freely (or close to freely) diffusible tracer. The origins of the approach go back many years to studies of flow using MR spectroscopy [73], and the physics are similar to those used in time-of-flight MR angiography methods [74]. The first practical demonstration of this approach in the brain was by Detre and Koretsky et al. [75], and the first demonstration of the effect for functional brain imaging was by Kwong et al. [2], in the same paper where BOLD imaging was demonstrated.

The approach was also used in one of the first phMRI studies ever of increased CBF caused by administration of 20 mg/kg amphetamine (a nearly lethal dose) in rats [6]. As mentioned, numerous variations on these techniques have evolved, and we will not spend time here covering all the permutations, largely because they have lower CNRs than other methodologies, such as BOLD and increased relaxation with iron oxide nanoparticles (IRON), and hence are not likely to prove as useful. Nonetheless, the ability to measure absolute flow with these methods makes it worth discussing them in some detail.

We will discuss the general principles behind arterial spin labeling. As mentioned, flowing spins will alter the effective T_1 within a voxel. It can be assumed that the flow of spins in and out of a voxel alters the magnetization in the following manner (we follow the approach outlined in [75]):

$$\frac{dM_z(t)}{dt} = \frac{M_0 - M_z(t)}{T_1} + \frac{f}{\lambda}M_a(t) - \frac{f}{\lambda}M_z(t) \tag{10.2}$$

where f is the perfusion (in ml/g/min), λ is the tissue:blood partition coefficient (ml/g — usual brain value of 0.88), M_a is the arterial magnetization, M_0 is the equilibrium longitudinal magnetization, and $M_z(t)$ is the longitudinal magnetization at time t. The incoming spins to a voxel can be altered either by saturation ($M_a(t) = 0$) or by inversion ($M_a(t) = -M_0$). One assumption of this approach is that water is a freely diffusible tracer, such that the incoming spins are effectively incorporated into the voxel, and the outgoing spins come from the voxel. This assumption has been tested to be reasonable under all but very high flow conditions. If one applies a long period of labeling, a steady-state is attained such that

$$\frac{dM_z(t)}{dt} = \frac{M_0 - M_z(t)}{T_1} + \frac{f}{\lambda}M_a(t) - \frac{f}{\lambda}M_z(t) = 0 \tag{10.3}$$

Solving and rearranging with the appropriate boundary conditions leads to

$$f = \frac{\lambda(M_{ss} - M_0)}{T_1(M_a - M_{ss})} \tag{10.4}$$

where M_{ss} is the apparent steady-state magnetization in the presence of continuous arterial spin labeling. The time to reach steady state is on the order of 5 sec at most field strengths. The amount of perturbation of inflowing spins is defined as

$$\alpha = \frac{M_0 - M_a}{2M_0} \tag{10.5}$$

where perfect inversion would mean $\alpha = 1$. Typically, efficiencies of $\alpha = 0.7 - 1$ can be achieved using a single surface coil on the neck for inversion (the longer the transit time from the labeling site to the voxel of interest the smaller α becomes — thus spin labeling the neck in a giraffe would likely result in a very small labeling in a brain voxel of interest). The true α is

$$\alpha_{voxel} = \alpha_{label}\exp(-\Delta t/T_{1_{blood}}) \tag{10.6}$$

In practice this is not a problem except in regions of very low flow. Combining the two previous equations leads to

$$f = \frac{\lambda(M_{ss,control} - M_{ss,label})}{T_1(M_{ss,label} + (2\alpha - 1)M_{ss,control})} \tag{10.7}$$

where $M_{ss,label}$ and $M_{ss,control}$ are respectively the steady-state magnetization in the control and continuously labeled states. This equation allows for calculation of the absolute CBF on the condition that we measure α and we assume or measure λ.

The approach relies upon differences between labeled and unlabeled images to achieve CBF contrast. The typical signal differences are small, leading to rather low CNR. There is, however, a number of circumstances where one might wish to use this approach. First, as has been shown quite elegantly in a number of papers, interleaving BOLD and CBF imaging may allow one to measure (albeit indirectly) relative changes in relative cerebral oxygen consumption ($rCMRO_2$). Second, there is a number of situations where one might wish to determine the absolute flow change, in order to dissect out components of neurovascular coupling. This might occur in cases where there is a large increase in flow in the absence of a concomitant increase in glucose utilization. Such a situation may happen, for instance, in stimulation of the cholinergic neurons in the basal forebrain [45]. There are other situations where one might anticipate a change in glucose utilization in the absence of a flow change [49]. Measurement of absolute CBF can be of great value in dissecting these two phenomena. In most situations, however, a good coupling can be anticipated between glucose utilization and oxygen utilization. More importantly, in cases where chronic treatments with drugs may lead to alterations in resting regional metabolism, measurement of absolute CBF changes would greatly aid in determining whether the hemodynamic changes observed during an acute drug challenge are altered by changes in resting perfusion.

10.2.1.3 BOLD Techniques

BOLD contrast was named by Ogawa in 1990, when he used this technique at a high magnetic field (11 T) to detect the contrast in veins in rat brain due the intrinsic magnetic susceptibility of deoxyhemoglobin [76]. Hemoglobin is paramagnetic in the deoxy-state and diamagnetic in the oxy-state. The technique was subsequently employed by others to detect changes in brain parenchyma during perturbations such as hypoxia [76,77]. After the original fMRI paper by Belliveau and colleagues [1], a number of groups applied the BOLD technique to examine changes in brain activity as a result of photic or motor stimulation. In 1992, three papers by Bandettini et al. [78], Kwong et al. [2], and Ogawa et al. [3] appeared in quick succession. These publications created quite a stir, as now one could map brain activity by simple, noninvasive, gradient-echo MRI. Thus, the technique became the province of the masses. At any place where an MRI machine was present one could start carrying out functional brain imaging (although in truth the technique requires high speed imaging, such as echo planar imaging, to attain reasonable statistical power). Since this technique is well documented, we will not cover it in any detail here. Rather, we will discuss how one can potentially use BOLD imaging to determine $rCMRO_2$. While BOLD imaging has the advantage of ease of use it has the disadvantage that the main parameter measured (percent signal change — that can be converted to ΔR_2^*) has no direct physiologic relevance. Thus, interpretation of BOLD contrast is problematic. BOLD contrast most accurately reflects the tissue concentration of deoxyhemoglobin. In cases where increases in CBF outstrip increases in $CMRO_2$ the result will be increased signal on images sensitive to T_2^*.

A number of papers have appeared utilizing modeling approaches to use the relative balance between CBF and BOLD contrast to determine the $rCMRO_2$ changes induced by brain stimulation [79–81]. The principle of these approaches is quite simple. An outline of the method is indicated below, following the approaches taken in [79,81,82]. We can write the R_2^* changes induced by a stimulus as:

$$\Delta R^*_{2_{\mathrm{BOLD}}}(t) \propto \mathrm{VF}(t)\left(\frac{\mathrm{CMRO_2}(t)}{\mathrm{CBF}(t)}\right)^{\beta} - \mathrm{VF}(0)\left(\frac{\mathrm{CMRO_2}(0)}{\mathrm{CBF}(0)}\right)^{\beta} \tag{10.8}$$

where $R_2^*(t)$ is the BOLD R_2^* changes, VF is the blood volume fraction, CBF and $CMRO_2$ are the blood flow and oxygen consumption at times 0 and t. One first determines, in the same subject and brain region, the increase in CBF in a stimulus where no increase in $CMRO_2$ is expected. Such a stimulus is found in hypercapnia (increased CO_2 concentrations). This then determines the coupling of ΔR_2^* to a given increase in CBF under conditions of constant $CMRO_2$. In these experiments one uses interleaved CBF and BOLD imaging to determine the simultaneous response of the given brain tissue. Then, one determines the response to a neuronal stimulus where increases in $CMRO_2$ are expected. In this situation, the BOLD percent signal increases (and ΔR_2^*) will be less than those observed under conditions of the same CBF increase due to the increased tissue $CMRO_2$

$$\mathrm{rCMRO_2}(t) = \left(\frac{\mathrm{CBF}(t)}{\mathrm{CBF}(0)}\right)^{1-(\alpha/\beta)} \left(1 - \frac{B(t) - 1}{M}\right)^{1/\beta} \tag{10.9}$$

where $rCMRO_2$ is the relative $CMRO_2$, $B(t)$ is the fractional BOLD signal change, α is 0.38 determined from the Grubb relationship between CBV and CBF (i.e., $\mathrm{CBV} \approx \mathrm{CBF}^{\alpha}$), and M is the parameter that represents the maximal BOLD signal change from the baseline state determined from the changes induced via hypercapnia (i.e., when there is no change in $CMRO_2 = 0$)

$$M = \frac{B(t) - 1}{1 - \left(\dfrac{\mathrm{CBF}(t)}{\mathrm{CBF}(0)}\right)^{-(\beta-\alpha)}} \tag{10.10}$$

Such studies have produced a remarkable consistency in estimates of the $CMRO_2$ changes induced by either forepaw stimulation in rats [81] or photic stimulation in humans [79,80]. All these studies, and more recent ones, indicate that $CMRO_2$ increases about a factor of 2 less than CBF. In most of these experiments the increase in $CMRO_2$ was about 20%. This is in contrast to earlier PET studies where increases of about 5% were noted [83], although more recent studies show changes of about the same magnitude (25%) $CMRO_2$. These numbers are in conflict with ^{13}C MRS studies in rats where changes on the order of 300% were noted [84,85]. It should be noted that the $CMRO_2$ measurements using PET and ^{13}C are considerably less sensitive than BOLD imaging. Thus, the original PET observation determined correctly, that the increase in CBF was considerably greater than that in $CMRO_2$. The discrepancy with the ^{13}C data is harder to reconcile, however, recent ^{13}C data in humans have led to an upper limit for the increase in $CMRO_2$ of about 30% for photic stimulation [86]. This value is consistent with the other MRI studies.

The reason for discussing these issues is that BOLD imaging of a pharmacological stimulus may very well alter relative changes in CBF or $CMRO_2$ differently (we discussed above such a finding in the case of cholinergic stimuli). Thus, use of such techniques may allow for discrimination of the origins of the BOLD signal changes, and may allow for separation of pure vascular stimuli from stronger metabolic changes.

10.2.1.4 IRON CBV Mapping

This technique is a relatively recent entry to brain imaging, although its principles were first demonstrated in the 1980s using the exact same principles as those described above for mapping of rCBV [63]. The idea is very simple. One injects an intravascular contrast agent with high magnetic susceptibility to sensitize the images to relative CBV. Then, functional imaging is performed using either drugs or tasks to cause increases in CBF and CBV. The contrast agent is designed to have a long plasma half-life in order to provide the ability to collect large numbers of images over relatively long periods of time. The much higher magnetic susceptibility of the contrast agents compared with deoxyhemoglobin leads to a much greater effect than is seen with BOLD contrast.

There are two other major differences between this technique and BOLD. First, the very high magnetic susceptibility renders the T_2^* of the intravascular signal so short that the intravascular signal essentially disappears. This is in sharp contrast to BOLD imaging where the venous intravascular signal is an important confound of the signals observed. Second, the magnetic susceptibility of the contrast agent is constant whereas the magnetic susceptibility of deoxyhemoglobin is constantly changing due to variations in oxygen extraction in the tissue. This has the effect of rendering the BOLD contrast a mixed parameter with no unique physiologic signature. In contrast, the contrast agent allows continual monitoring of changes in rCBV. These, in summary, are the major features of IRON CBV mapping.

The contrast agents that have been used for this technique are primarily based upon iron oxide nanoparticles. Thus, we dubbed the technique increased relaxation with iron oxide nanoparticles or increased relaxation for optimized neuroimaging (IRON) to distinguish it from BOLD [87]. In 1998 the technique appeared essentially simultaneously in a number of laboratories [88–90]. Further explorations of the method have proved that it provides a huge increase in CNR compared with BOLD imaging at most field strengths [87,91]. Since the different CNRs achieved by the various techniques are so important we discuss these in some detail below (Section 10.2.3).

Before discussing the CNR a brief description of the IRON technique is outlined here. A typical experimental protocol consists in collecting a series of baseline images before injection of contrast agent. Depending upon the expected time course of the pharmacologic stimulus, one can tailor the imaging time accordingly, trading off temporal resolution for spatial resolution if the expected time course is long enough. This point cannot be emphasized strongly enough, and is one compelling reason for use of IRON mapping for pharmacologic stimulus over BOLD imaging. The reason for this is simple. Owing to the intrinsic CNR of the BOLD effect being rather small, achieving the requisite statistical power usually necessitates using a rapid technique such as echo planar imaging. A large number of images per unit time then provides the requisite increase in statistical power over a slower, higher spatial resolution technique. With IRON imaging the large increase in CNR means that one can use a slower, higher spatial resolution technique. Figure 10.5 shows a typical time course of an IRON protocol after injection of a hypothetical drug that induces a CBV increase. First a series of baseline images is acquired. Then, a new baseline is acquired where the signal changes observed are proportional to relative CBV, as originally outlined in [63]. One converts the signal decrease observed after injection of

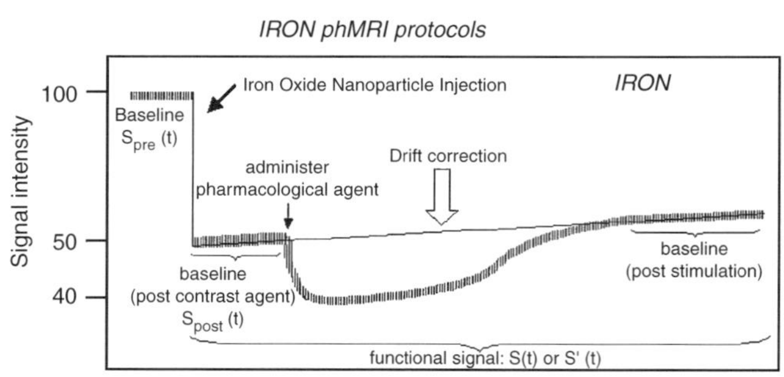

FIGURE 10.5 Typical protocols for an IRON phMRI experiment. IRON requires injection of a contrast agent with high magnetic susceptibility and long plasma half-life. This in turn renders the images sensitive to relative cerebral blood volume (rCBV). After a new steady-state baseline is reached, then drugs can be injected and any signal changes can be converted to changes in R_2^* that will be directly proportional to changes in rCBV. (From Villringer, A. et al., *Magn. Reson. Med.*, 6, 164, 1988; Mandeville, J. B. et al., *Magn. Reson. Med.*, 39, 615, 1998.)

iron oxide contrast agent to ΔR_2^* values as

$$\Delta R_2^* = -\ln(S/S_0)/\mathrm{TE} \tag{10.11}$$

and

$$\mathrm{rCBV} = K\Delta R_2^* \tag{10.12}$$

where K is a constant that scales the R_2^* values with the regional CBV. In cases where K might be known, it would be possible to calculate the absolute CBV. In practice, this is very difficult, however, numerous validation studies performed over the years have verified that the measures of relative CBV are consistent with what is expected. That being said, it is also true that no really good gold standard has evolved for the determination of absolute CBV. In a typical experiment one might use the following expression:

$$\frac{\Delta\mathrm{rCBV}(t)}{\mathrm{rCBV}_0} = \left(\frac{\Delta R_2^*(t)}{\Delta R_{2_0}^*}\right) - 1 \tag{10.13}$$

A number of different iron oxide agents has been used for this purpose (some of which are reviewed in [87]), having slightly different magnetic properties. Most of these agents are quite nontoxic and one of them is currently in human clinical trials as a method for coronary angiography [92] or liver imaging [93] at doses as high as 1.7 mg iron/kg. The typical doses in animal studies range from 4 to 10 mg/kg.

Our contention here is that use of intravascular contrast agents with high magnetic susceptibility, which allow mapping of rCBV, will greatly improve phMRI compared with BOLD imaging. Figure 10.6a shows two typical statistical maps of amphetamine activation in the striatal region using either IRON phMRI (top) or BOLD phMRI (bottom). These data were acquired at a magnetic field strength of 4.7 T, at which the BOLD effect is much stronger than at typical clinical magnetic fields such as 1.5 T. Nevertheless, it is clear that use of the contrast agents produced a functional map that is much cleaner due to greater statistical power. IRON phMRI increased CNR in the striatum relative to the BOLD method by a factor of about 3 for CFT and amphetamine. In order to produce a functional map of similar appearance to the map obtained in a single animal using the IRON method, BOLD data from about six rats would need to be averaged. Looking at the signal changes induced by amphetamine for the two methods (Figure 10.6b), it is apparent that the increase in CNR derives primarily from the much larger overall signal change using the IRON method (i.e., the area under the IRON curve is much larger than under the BOLD curve).

Another way to judge the relative statistical powers of these imaging methods is to compare volumes of striatum that exceed any statistical threshold for activation. Figure 10.6c compares the percent of activated striatum as a function of the statistical threshold (log of the p value) for BOLD and IRON phMRI. At a statistical threshold that selects almost 100% of the striatum using IRON phMRI, the BOLD method selects only about one third of the striatum. At a threshold such that less than 10% of the striatum is selected by the BOLD method, about one third of the striatum is shown to be activated using the IRON method.

It thus appears clear that following injection of CFT, IRON phMRI provides an increase of CNR in the striatum. These results lead us to make the following contentions, justified in Section 10.2.3, regarding comparisons between BOLD and IRON phMRI:

1. CNR should be increased everywhere in the brain for pharmacological stimuli.
2. The magnitude of the increase in CNR varies regionally, with subcortical structures generally benefiting from a larger increase in CNR than cortical structures.

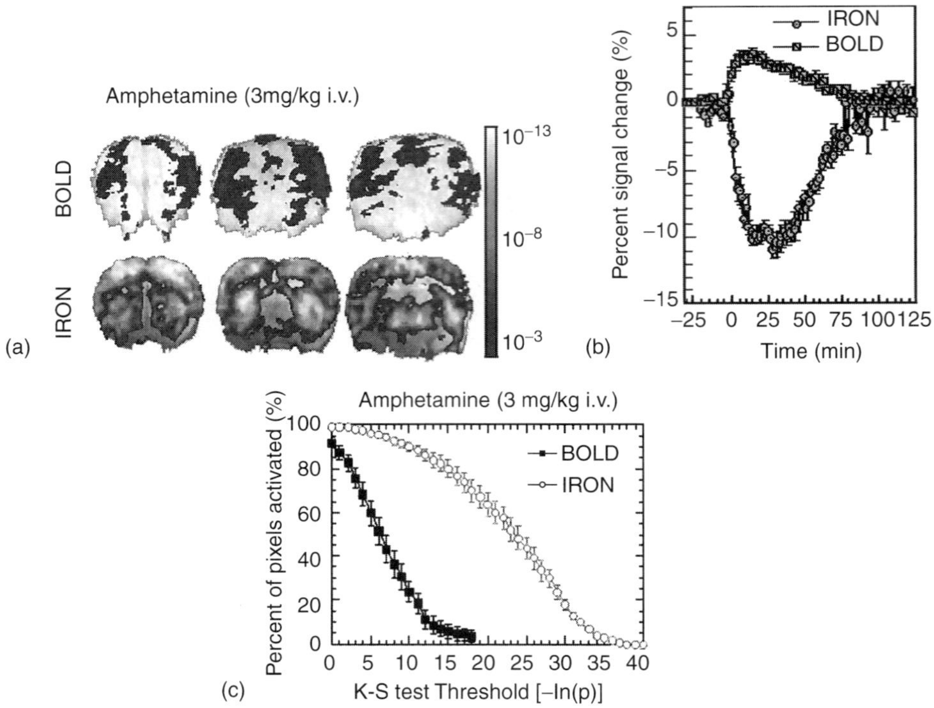

FIGURE 10.6 (See color insert for (a) following page 328.) (a) Comparison of BOLD and IRON images at 4.7 T at the same statistical threshold derived from a student's *t*-test after administration of 3 mg/kg amphetamine in a rat. Note the nearly ten orders of magnitude decrease in the *p*-value for the IRON technique compared with the BOLD technique (both data sets were collected with the same number of images and identical imaging parameters). (b) Plot of the percent signal changes induced by the same amphetamine stimulus for BOLD (top) or IRON (bottom). Note that the increased rCBV after amphetamine induces a negative percent signal change during IRON imaging. The large increase in the area under the curve for the IRON imaging is largely responsible for the increase in statistical power of this technique. (c) Plot of the percent of the striatum activated at a given statistical threshold for both a BOLD and IRON study of 3 mg/kg amphetamine stimulus in seven rats again illustrating the great increase in statistical power of the IRON technique at all statistical thresholds.

3. The percent change in CBV should correlate regionally with the percent change in the concentration of deoxyhemoglobin [dHb].
4. CNR in draining veins should be amplified by the BOLD method but attenuated by the IRON method.

10.2.2 Advantages and Disadvantages of MR Techniques: Brain–Vein Controversies Revisited

The BOLD technique is, by far, the most commonly employed method for both fMRI and phMRI studies. There are a number of reasons for this: it is the easiest to implement, provides higher contrast to noise than the CBF-based fMRI techniques, and requires no injection of contrast agents as do the CBV methodologies. Nonetheless, conventional BOLD techniques have many disadvantages, the principal one being that no direct physiologic parameter is measured. Aside from the obvious increase in CNR obtained using the contrast agents, IRON provides a number of other advantages. First, unlike with conventional BOLD imaging, one is able to obtain a direct measurement of a physiologically relevant parameter - CBV. A second quite distinct advantage is that the BOLD technique at field strengths such as 4.7 and 1.5 T shows a high degree of spatial weighting towards large veins. Mandeville et al. [91] showed that the BOLD technique is embedded with a vascular weighting factor and the activation map is shifted toward larger vessels than the brain tissue. Owing to the ring of arachnoid vessels surrounding the rat brain, the BOLD activation map, in general, tends to shift outwards towards the edge (compare the BOLD and IRON images in Figure 10.6a). The IRON technique, however, can be optimized to have the maximal sensitivity in tissue rather than in vessels and thus is able to show the location of neuronal activation more accurately. For the larger vessels the very short intravascular T_2^* leads to very little signal on the gradient-echo images, and hence less vascular weighting. For BOLD imaging such a feature may occur at very high magnetic field strengths, such as 9.4 T (or probably even higher). This latter point is quite important since many people (and especially many referees of submitted papers) are confused by the fact that a technique which produces maps of changes in relative CBV is insensitive to the intravascular signal. Relative comparisons of the BOLD and IRON techniques are outlined in Table 10.3 (the relative CNR comparisons are approximate only for field strengths between about 1.5 and 4.7 T). Previous work has shown that the CNR advantage of IRON over BOLD is about 8 at 2 T and about 3 at 4.7 T.

Recently, we also compared the BOLD and IRON techniques at higher magnetic field, 9.4 T, where BOLD CNR starts to match that attained by IRON [94]. Unfortunately, for BOLD to attain its maximal CNR the echo time must be equal to approximately T_2^*. Thus, at 9.4 T where the average brain T_2^* is about 20 msec the echo time should be about 20 msec. Such a long echo time will lead to GE images with unacceptably low quality, especially in regions where there are sinuses. Thus, the IRON technique allows one to use as short a TE as desired (the TE can be adjusted at will in tandem with the contrast agent concentration).

Clearly, the biggest disadvantage to the IRON technique is the large amount of iron that must be administered. Since the optimal signal changes and CNRs are attained when the signal loss is approximately 1/e [89] between 3 and 10 mg/kg of total iron per dose is typically injected, depending upon the agent and the echo time used. While iron is relatively nontoxic, such an increase in body iron load may represent an unwarranted cost for the relative benefit of the MR examination. In our studies we noted no toxicity with the relatively high doses that were used, and in this regard the SPBPA agent we used in some of our studies attains similar R_2^* changes with 4.5 mg/kg as MION does with 10 mg/kg [87]. In our previous studies in a rodent model of PD [12], we noted no toxicity due to the injection of the SPBPA agent, even after multiple studies in the same animals over the course of 1 year. This issue, however, will require further study for potential use in humans.

TABLE 10.3
Comparisons of Different MRI Hemodynamic-Based Techniques

	BOLD	IRON	FAIR	ASL
MR parameter	T_2^*	T_2^*	T_1	T_1
Physiologic parameter	None ($rCMRO_2$ can be modeled)	rCBV	rCBF	CBF
Spatial vascular weighting	High	Low	Low	Low
Relative CNR	1	5	≈0.25	≈0.5
Number of subjects to attain CNR at 3T	8–10	1	30	20
Temporal resolution	High	High	Low	Low

Relative CNR is approximate assuming a field strength of ca. 3 T. At higher fields this will be lower and at lower fields higher.

10.2.3 Theoretical Framework for Contrast-to-Noise Ratio

It is convenient to think of CNR at spatial location r and time t as the product of the signal-to-noise ratio (SNR), a vascular weighting function (W), and a term that depends upon functional changes (Φ) but is independent of baseline physiology:

$$\mathrm{CNR}(r,t) = \mathrm{SNR}(r)\, W(r)\, \Phi(r,t) \tag{10.14}$$

A theoretical framework for quantitatively comparing BOLD and CBV CNR can be developed by making simplifying assumptions. For CBV phMRI, these assumptions include: (1) changes in the transverse relaxation rate of MRI signal after injection of the contrast agent are linearly proportional to the blood volume fraction (V) at spatial location r and time t,

$$\Delta R_2^*(r,t) = KV(r,t) \tag{10.15}$$

where K depends upon the contrast agent dose; (2) noise does not depends upon contrast agent dose; (3) a sufficient amount of contrast agent is used so that BOLD contributions to relaxation rate changes during functional challenges can be neglected. For BOLD phMRI, assumptions include: (1) the transverse relaxation rate is a linear function of the voxel concentration of deoxygenated hemoglobin, $\Delta R_2 = K\ \Delta[\mathrm{dHb}]$; (2) the small arterial blood volume fraction (approximately 10 to 15%) can be neglected; (3) a tight linear regional relationship exists between resting state values of CBF and $\mathrm{CMRO_2}$, as consistently measured by PET studies. Under these assumptions, the expressions for the CNR of BOLD fMRI and CBV fMRI can be derived as follows:

$$W_{\mathrm{BOLD}}(r,t) \approx T_{\mathrm{E}} R_2^{*\mathrm{BOLD}}(r_0,0) v(r), \quad \Phi_{\mathrm{BOLD}}(r,t) \approx -\Delta[\mathrm{dHb}](r,t)/[\mathrm{dHb}](r,0) \tag{10.16a}$$

$$W_{\mathrm{CBV}}(r,t) \approx \mathrm{e}^{-v(r)} v(r), \quad \Phi_{\mathrm{CBV}}(r,t) \approx -\Delta V(r,t)/V(r,0) \tag{10.16b}$$

where $R_2^{*\mathrm{BOLD}}(\mathrm{r_0},0)$ is the BOLD part of the resting-state transverse relaxation rate at some location r_0, $\mathrm{T_E}$ is the gradient echo time of the BOLD imaging sequence, V is the blood volume fraction, and v is the resting state blood volume with respect to the point r_0

$$v(r) = V(r,0)/V(r_0,0) \tag{10.17}$$

In a comparison of the CNR of the two methods, a point r_0 must be selected such that injection of contrast agent drops the signal intensity to about e^{-1} of the preinjection value; this location depends upon both the contrast agent and the local blood volume fraction.

The forms of the weighting functions for these MRI methods differ due to injection of contrast agent, which reduces SNR proportional to a decreasing exponential of relative blood volume. Figure 10.7a graphically shows weighting functions vs. the negative log of the ratio of signal intensities before (S_{BOLD}) and after (S_{CBV}) injection of contrast agent; this quantity is proportional to the product of resting CBV and contrast agent dose. The dependence of CNR on the resting-state blood volume is expected to be much stronger for BOLD phMRI than for IRON phMRI, where CNR is insensitive to small changes in resting-state CBV about the point $v = 1$ and decreases when the magnitude of resting-state CBV deviates in either direction from this value. In contrast, BOLD CNR changes with a roughly linear dependence on the resting-state blood volume, exacerbating the brain vs. vein ambiguity due to CNR amplification in large veins. As seen from Figure 10.7a there is a much greater sensitivity to tissue with the IRON technique that falls away in the intravascular space because of the short blood T_2^* after contrast agent injection.

Equation 10.16a and Equation 10.16b suggest a way to compare CNR for the BOLD and IRON methods that will help illuminate functional couplings during an acute pharmacological challenge.

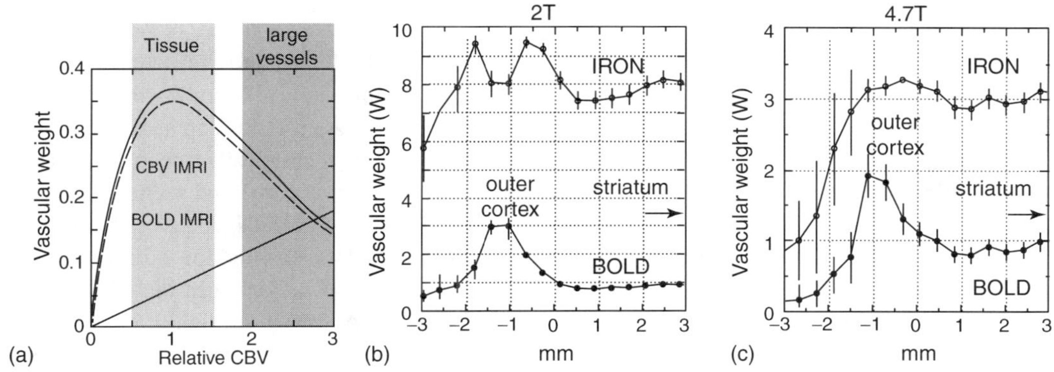

FIGURE 10.7 (a) Relative vascular weighting functions (proportional to CNR) for BOLD and IRON imaging at 2 T. The relevant equations describing the graph are shown in the text. BOLD imaging has its largest sensitivity in the large veins. IRON imaging has its greatest sensitivity in the tissue and little in the large veins. The dotted line in the curve for IRON indicates the decrease in weighting from signal increases due to the BOLD effect. The effects at 4.7 T can essentially be scaled by increasing the slope of the BOLD curve (4.7/2 = 2.35) and leaving the IRON curve unchanged. (b) Estimates of the relative CNR of BOLD phMRI and IRON phMRI at magnetic field strengths of 2 T (b) and 4.7 T (c) from the cortical rim towards the striatum. For equal percent changes in CBV, estimates are shown for the relative BOLD CNR normalized to 1 in striatum at each field strength. CNR is expected to increase in striatum by factors of about 8 and 3 at 2 and 4.7 T, respectively. The peaks seen at about -1 mm arise from the cortical rim of arachnoid vessels in the rat brain. The peaks are negative for the IRON technique due to the short T_2^* of the blood after injection of contrast agents.

By computing the CNR for BOLD and CBV phMRI separately (e.g., using a T statistic) and then dividing the two CNR maps, the result should be of the form

$$\mathrm{CNR_{BOLD}}/\mathrm{CNR_{CBV}} = K\mathrm{e}^{v(r)}\{\%\Delta[\mathrm{dHB}]/\%\Delta\mathrm{CBV}\} \tag{10.18}$$

If we assume that the percent change in [dHb] and the percent change in CBV scale together across different brain regions, then the ratio in Equation 10.18 should produce the appearance of a blood volume map, since $\mathrm{e}^{v(r)} \sim \mathrm{e}^1\ v(r)$ for a small change in CBV about the point r_0. By comparing this ratio with a blood volume map, created as $v = -\ln(S_{\mathrm{CBV}}/S_{\mathrm{BOLD}})$ following injection of the contrast agent, the hypothesis can be tested that the percent change in CBV and percent change in [dHb] scale regionally together.

Figure 10.7b and Figure 10.7c provide a theoretical estimate for the increase in CNR in the cortex and striatum at magnetic field strengths of 2 and 4.7 T. The vascular weights in these figures approximately represent the CNR values obtained for the two techniques. For them to represent the relative CNR magnitudes between the two methods properly, it must be assumed that the percent changes in CBV and [dHb] are approximately the same everywhere throughout the brain. For functional changes in rat somatosensory cortex due to forepaw stimulation, we have found that percent changes in these quantities are approximately equal [89]. The peak seen at approximately -1 mm comes from the ring of arachnoid vessels on the cortical rim in the rat. Figure 10.7c provides a similar plot for data at a field strength of 4.7 T. Note that there is a smaller difference between the BOLD and IRON techniques, however, there is still a substantial sensitivity gain. In both of these figures the relative CNR ratio can be determined from the relative vascular weight ratios.

10.2.4 Field Strength Dependencies of BOLD and IRON

An attractive feature of measurement of rCBV, as opposed to BOLD, is that rCBV changes should be independent of field strength, whereas BOLD signal changes are extremely field strength dependent. This means that drug-induced changes observed at different fields can be compared for IRON, but not for BOLD. We investigated whether or not such a contention was true, by comparing the activation due to two drugs targeting the dopamine transporter: cocaine and methylphenidate. We then compared the measured rCBV changes at 2 T, 4.7 T, and 9.4 T. As expected, the interanimal variability was much larger than the variation in rCBV as a function of field strength [94]. Both experimental data and simulations showed that the CNR advantages of IRON persist even at field strengths as high as 4.7 T by a factor of 3 [87,94]. At very high fields such as 9.4 T, BOLD CNR increases to the point where it is competitive with IRON. However, there are some additional considerations that render the IRON technique advantageous even at 9.4 T. For instance, echo times and iron oxide concentrations can be traded off. Long echo times can be traded off for less iron, conversely if one desires short echo times, then more iron can be used. The optimal CNR for BOLD comes when TE $\approx T_2^*$, however, at 9.4 T T_2^* in the brain is quite short being approximately 20 msec. Gradient-echo images collected with a T_2^* of 20 msec at 9.4 T will be of poor quality in many regions including those near sinuses. By using a higher concentration of iron oxide contrast agent, one can use ultrashort echo times and maintain constant CNR, at levels still higher than BOLD.

Since MRI in general, and functional or pharmacological MRI specifically, is almost always in need of more SNR as well as CNR (to push spatial and temporal resolution), we believe that the huge CNR increase of IRON over BOLD at most field strengths means that IRON is the technique of choice in animal models. In fact, at field strengths lower than 7 T one could even argue that the use of BOLD causes far more animals to be used than is necessary from a scientific and ethical point of view. Not to put a fine point on it, but at 4.7 T, BOLD imaging would require averaging data from about six animals to attain the same CNR as with a single drug challenge experiment using IRON. Thus, one could argue from the point of view of using the fewest animals with the least amount of suffering that BOLD experiments are unethical when the alternative to use IRON exists!

10.2.5 Nonhemodynamic MR Techniques of Potential Use for phMRI

Two other MR techniques have been used to investigate brain activation. We will briefly discuss them, not because they have proved very useful to date for examining pharmacologic stimuli, but rather because they have potential for the future to reveal alternative physiologic parameters than the simple hemodynamic metrics discussed above. The first of these techniques is magnetic resonance spectroscopy (MRS) and the other is T_1-weighted imaging of accumulation of manganese due to neuronal stimulation.

10.2.5.1 Magnetic Resonance Spectroscopy

This technique is widely used for research of various brain disorders, and clearly would have potential for study of pharmacologic challenges. However, even at high field strengths, such as 4.7 T, this technique has very poor spatial and temporal resolution (and these must be traded off starting from baselines that are already much lower than conventional MRI). This is due largely to the fact that water in the brain is present at 80 M in protons, whereas even the most abundant neurochemicals, such as *N*-acetylaspartate (NAA), are present at only about 25 mM in protons. If we compare the relative sensitivity of a T_2-weighted water image (assuming at 4.7 T a water T_2^* of 65 msec and a TE of 100 msec) and a short echo time NAA image (with a T_2 for NAA of 250 msec and a TE of 20 msec) we arrive at a relative sensitivity of NAA/H_2O of approximately

$$\frac{0.025\ \mathrm{M}^{*}\exp^{-(0.02/0.25)}}{80\ \mathrm{M}^{*}\exp^{-(0.1/0.065)}} = 0.0013 \tag{10.19}$$

where the longer T_2 of the NAA methyl group compared with that of water adds back (via $\exp[-TE/T_2]$) some of the signal lost due to the concentration difference. Nonetheless, this represents a factor of greater than 700 or an increase in averaging time of 500,000 for the equivalent signal to noise.

A number of studies have appeared examining photic stimulation using MRS. These studies have focused upon detection of increased lactate during photic stimulation [95], or on changes in glucose utilization [86,96,97]. These can be measured in two ways. Glucose resonances can be observed directly (optimally at 5.23 ppm [98]) and their decline assessed during photic stimulation [97]. This technique has the advantage of being a direct measure of glucose utilization, thus avoiding many of the modeling problems inherent to PET. The other method is to utilize ^{13}C-labeled glucose and observe its metabolic transformation through the TCA cycle to glutamate and other metabolites [86,96,99,100]. This technique has the advantage of providing incredible metabolic specificity, however, it also suffers from poor spatial and temporal resolution. Increases in both spatial and temporal resolution utilizing echo planar spectroscopy [101–103], especially at higher magnetic fields such as 7 or 9.4 T, and with phased array surface coils, may lead to more practical pharmacologic spectroscopy studies. At these high field strengths, with reasonable averaging times, we might hope to achieve spatial resolution on the order of a clinical PET scanner (about 3 to 4 mm in plane).

A number of studies examining the metabolic response to pharmacologic stimuli have appeared. The effects of the glutamate antagonist MK-801 were examined using proton and phosphorus spectroscopy [104]. The authors of this study showed increased lactate after MK-801 administration, indicative of nonoxidative glycolysis. Increased brain GABA concentrations were noted in occipital cortex after administration of vigabitrin (an inhibitor of GABA-transaminase) to epileptic patients [105]. We examined the effects of amphetamine stimulation on brain TCA cycle flux in the frontal cortex using ^{13}C MRS [106]. This study showed an increase in C2-glutamate labeling of about 34%, indicative of increased $CMRO_2$ of the same magnitude (interestingly, of C4-labeling, often taken as a surrogate marker for TCA cycle flux, was much faster). Nonetheless, these data were averages over about 90 min; it is unlikely that the metabolic profile was constant over this time period. Higher field strengths, as well as better carbon-edited proton observation techniques may improve the temporal and spatial resolution of these methods.

10.2.5.2 Manganese Enhanced MRI

The other nonhemodynamic technique, pioneered in the laboratory of Dr. Alan Koretsky, is the injection of paramagnetic manganese (after opening the blood–brain barrier with mannitol) to detect brain activity [107]. This technique relies upon the ability of manganese to substitute for calcium, and thus, cells which have increased uptake of calcium during brain stimulation will selectively accumulate manganese. This, in turn, leads to a decrease in T_1 that is readily detectable using conventional T_1-weighted imaging. In principle, this technique has high sensitivity and exquisite spatial resolution.

One study compared the focus of activation of BOLD fMRI to manganese enhanced MRI (MEMRI) at 9.4 T and showed the foci of the two techniques were within 200 μm of one another [108]. This lends credence to the utility of BOLD imaging.

The MEMRI technique suffers from a number of problems that render it less compelling than it might otherwise appear. First, the blood–brain barrier must be opened since Mn^{++} will not enter the brain otherwise. In our hands, opening the blood–brain barrier with mannitol often suffers from large interanimal variability. Another problem is that not all neurons accumulate Ca^{++} during stimulation. Reuptake of dopamine, for instance, on presynaptic neurons is not Ca^{++} dependent. Second, accumulation of Mn^{++} in the globus pallidus, and selectively in dopamine neurons [109], may confound results. Nevertheless, this technique shows great promise for animal models and has recently been applied to pharmacologic stimulation of the hippocampus [110]. The technique has the potential of very high spatial resolution, comparable to that attained in MR microscopy. This results from the fact that the stimulus can be performed outside the magnet where the manganese will accumulate at the active sites, and then the animal can be placed in the magnet for imaging. Since over a short time period images are not time dependent one can spend most of the imaging time averaging to obtain ultrahigh spatial resolution.

10.3 THE CONFOUNDS OF RESPIRATORY GASES AND ANESTHESIA

The great majority of phMRI studies is, and will continue to be, hemodynamic in nature. Thus, changes in respiratory gases during such a study can be a major confound when interpreting signal changes whether one is measuring CBF, rCBV, or BOLD. This, of course, is also true for all fMRI studies. Changes in breathing rate can readily and easily affect CO_2 levels in the blood. As an example of this we show the effects of increases and decreases in CO_2 and their relation to MRI signal changes. The reactivity curves for changes in CBF induced by changes in CO_2 are linear with similar slopes across species. Thus, a change in CO_2 from baseline (ca. 38 mmHg) to about 90 mmHg will produce an increase in CBF of approximately 350%. Increases in CBF produce increases in both T_2 and T_2^* signal intensity (BOLD effects) as well as in T_1 signal effects (CBF). This is shown in Figure 10.8a for a rat. Increases in CO_2 were induced by i.v. injections of acetozolamide, an inhibitor of carbonic anhydrase. The increases caused an increase in T_2-weighted (BOLD) signal intensity, due to the fact that increases in CO_2 increase CBF but do not increase

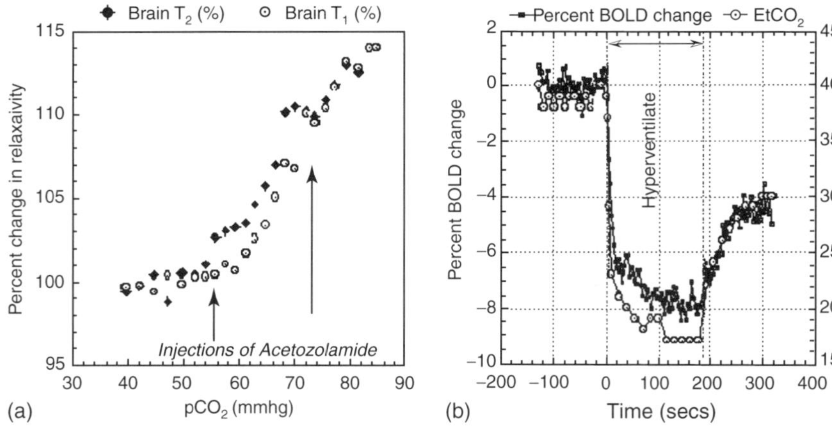

FIGURE 10.8 (a) Changes in either T_2-weighted (BOLD) or T_1-weighted (CBF) signal intensities in a rat as a function of increasing the CO_2 concentration via acetazolamined injections at 4.7 T. It is seen that increasing the pCO_2 to close to 90 mmHg only increases the signal by 10%. (b) Comparison of changes in BOLD signal (echo planar images; TR/TE 2500/45 msec; 1.5 T) from multiple gray matter regions in the cortex vs. the end tidal CO_2 ($EtCO_2$) measured simultaneously in a normal control human subject before, during, and after 3 min of hyperventilation. Note the tight correlation between the BOLD signal and $EtCO_2$. Note also the short time for the CO_2 to decrease and the much longer time to return to baseline. Such changes are critically important to measure during drug stimulation — for instance a short burst of hyperventilation can have a much longer-term effect on signal changes.

oxygen consumption. Likewise, an increase in T_1-weighted signal intensity is noted due to the increase in flow [2,75] as described above in Section 10.2.1.2. Increases in flow between 300 and 400% are about the largest that are possible in the brain. The data in Figure 10.8a show that even such large increases produce only a 10% change in BOLD signal intensity at this echo time (15 msec) and field strength. Larger changes than this must either come from large veins or movement, and papers claiming much larger changes (after adjusting for field strength and TE) almost certainly are quantifying artifacts such as motion.

Decreases in CO_2 will lead to decreases in CBV and decreased BOLD signal. For instance, hyperventilation will drop pCO_2 from about 38 to 20 mmHg in less than a minute. Shown in Figure 10.8b are studies where a human subject hyperventilated for 3 min. Changes in end tidal CO_2 ($EtCO_2$) and BOLD percent signal change are plotted. Note how rapidly the $EtCO_2$ changes — this is mirrored by a decrease in BOLD signal due to the decreased CBF. The $EtCO_2$ takes much longer to return to baseline (about 5 min). Such changes have been shown to alter the response of visual cortex to photic stimulation — paradoxically decreasing BOLD signal [111]. In situations where awake humans are being administered drugs such as cocaine or amphetamine, it is imperative to simultaneously measure $EtCO_2$ in order to determine the effects changes in this parameter might have. It has been reported that i.v. cocaine administration decreases $EtCO_2$ [112], probably due to hyperventilation. Changes in blood pressure can also have an effect upon hemodynamics, however, numerous studies of autoregulation suggest that maintenance of CBF in the face of decreased arterial pressure occurs over a fairly wide range of pressures. Simultaneous measurements of CBV and CBF using MRI suggest that between 65 and 140 mmHg pressure CBF and CBV are constant in rats [113]. Another study simultaneously monitored changes in BOLD contrast and blood pressure during a blood withdrawal protocol under varying anesthesia conditions [114]. Results suggested that there was a correlation between those two parameters that was regionally heterogeneous. Thus, once again, it is imperative to measure these parameters while imaging. Many drugs of interest can cause changes in mean arterial blood pressure.

The confounds of anesthesia are even more profound than those of changes in systemic physiologic variables. This is because the latter effects can be readily measured and potentially corrected for, whereas those of anesthesia often selectively affect different neurotransmitter systems. Furthermore, the goal of any good anesthetic is retention of systemic involuntary responses, such as respiration, while blunting cortical responsivity. This requirement is often in conflict with the goals of the functional or pharmacologic study. Many studies have investigated the effects of differing anesthetics on the coupling of cerebral metabolism and anesthetic dose [115,116]. These studies will not be reviewed here, except to say that for somatosensory stimuli different anesthetics can often lead to very large differences in CBF increases observed for the same stimulus [117]. In addition, the effects on basal metabolism for the various anesthetics are often quite different. However, the neurovascular coupling problem with respect to the differing neurotransmitter systems selectively affected by the various anesthetics has not yet been throughly examined. For a number of anesthetics, such as halothane or isoflurane, the exact mechanisms are not known, therefore it is difficult to predict a priori which receptor systems will be most affected. From studies on its mechanisms of action there is good evidence for an influence of halothane upon multiple systems including glutamate uptake, glucose utilization, phospholipid methylation, glycine receptor antagonism, decreased calcium channel binding sites, etc. Urethane, similar to the volatile anesthetics, is thought to target multiple neurotransmitter systems through potentiation and inhibition of neurotransmitter-gated ion channels [118]. For some anesthetics, however, the target neurotransmitter systems are known. Ketamine, a commonly used anesthetic for animal procedures, is a noncompetitive glutamate *N*-methyl-*D*-aspartate antagonist [119,120]. Ketamine can also potentiate dopamine release after administration of drugs such as amphetamine [121]. Similarly to MK-801, it can induce regionally selective changes in brain metabolism. Morphine sulfate is another anesthetic used for functional studies, and it obviously targets the opioid receptors. α-Chloralose is another common anesthetic for fMRI studies and has been shown to preserve the functional–metabolic coupling in the cortex [122]. Forepaw stimulation in α-chloralose anesthetized rats showed an increase of regional CMRglc (measured with autoradiography) [122] and an increase of CBF and CBV (measured by fMRI) in the forelimb area of the somatosensory cortex [89]. However, α-chloralose has also been shown to depress the activity of the dopaminergic neurons [123]. Halothane, in contrast to α-chloralose, attenuates the functional–metabolic coupling in the cortex [122] but preserves the dopamine activity in the striatum [123]. We showed that α-chloralose can turn off the effects of cocaine or amphetamine in the brain [124].

As an example of the effects of anesthetics on flow and metabolism coupling we show data from Maekawa et al. [125] examining the regional effects of isoflurane on CBF and CMRglc (Figure 10.9). Isoflurane decreases CMRglc compared with the awake state and at the same time increases CBF, thereby increasing the slope of the flow–metabolism coupling. This slope becomes even steeper at higher concentrations of isoflurane. Halothane has the same, but smaller, effect, while propofol dramatically decreases both glucose utilization as well as CBF. Thus, in picking an anesthetic it becomes imperative to understand not only the effects on the neurotransmitter system in question, but also how the flow–metabolism coupling curves may be affected.

Thus, it is clear that each neurotransmitter system one wishes to study must be carefully investigated — preferably with multiple anesthetics — before being confident of the results. In this manner the investigator can perform a differential diagnosis as to how the chosen anesthetic may be affecting the neurotransmitter system under study. A further, extremely important, point is that often the effects on metabolism by a given anesthetic are not regionally uniform, and may affect the very brain region in which the investigator is interested. The effects of anesthesia are not always a negative confound however. We previously showed that the phMRI response to the antipsychotic agent clozapine can be selectively modulated using different anesthetics. Use of α-chloralose allows one to turn off the dopamine-related components, whereas use of halothane retains them [124].

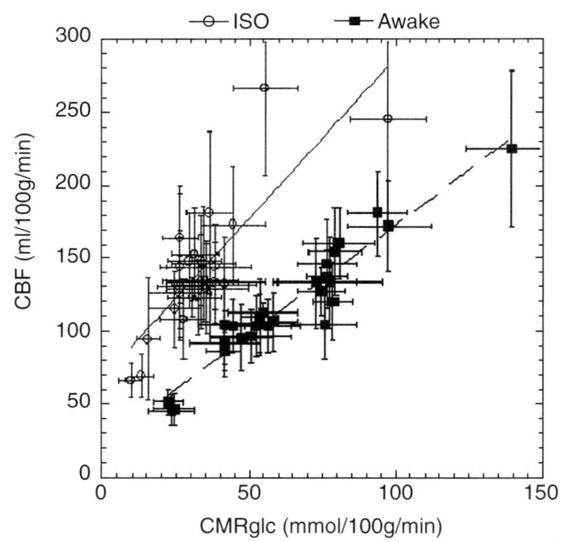

FIGURE 10.9 Changes in CBF vs. changes in CMRglc in rats in multiple brain regions in either the awake state or under isoflurane anesthesia (ca. 1% — MAC of 1). These data are taken from Maekawa et al. [125] and have been replotted. They indicate the profound decrease in CMRglc as well as the increase in CBF induced by isoflurane anesthesia. As shown in Table 10.4, these changes are more profound than those induced by halothane. The changes in CMRglc are similar to those induced by propofol, but propofol decreases CBF. The authors are grateful to Dr. John Marota for helpful discussions and pointers to the literature.

TABLE 10.4
Effects of Different Anesthetics on Neurotransmitter Systems and Metabolism

Anesthetic	Mechanism/Neurotransmitter Systems	Effect on Metabolism/CBF	References
α-Chloralose	Dopamine (?)	↑CMRglc, ↑CBF	[122,123]
Barbiturates	GABA	↓↓CMR, ↓↓CBF	[116,174]
Ketamine	Glutamate NMDA receptors	↑CMR, ↑CBF	[175–177]
Propofol	Multiple	↓$CMRO_2$, ↓CBF	[178,179]
Halothane	Multiple	↓$CMRO_2$, ↓CMRglc, ↑CBF	[125,180–182]
Isoflurane	Multiple	↓↓$CMRO_2$, ↓↓CMRglc, ↑CBF Burst — Suppression EEG pattern	[125,180,181,183,184]
Urethane	Multiple neurotransmitter system	↓CBF, ↓CMRglc	[118,185]

A comparison of the effects of different anesthetics is provided in Table 10.4 for the most commonly used anesthetics.

Comparisons of awake and anesthetized animals were made by Lahti et al. [126] using rats accustomed to a head-holder. Propofol anesthetized animals yielded BOLD signal changes of 1 to 6%. The awake animals yielded signal changes of up to 30%. Clearly, the latter change is too large to be credible at the field strength of that study (2 T) and most probably represents motion. Peters et al. [127] compared awake curarized (paralyzed animals) and animals under α-chloralose anesthesia using both fMRI and EEG analysis. The awake animals yielded activation patterns that were widespread and difficult to interpret. These authors concluded the paper with the following assertion "Definitely the problems and difficulties for interpretation that will be encountered using awake animals will mostly outweigh the advantages" [127]. As an editorial comment, we have yet to see convincing activation data from awake rats.

Conversely, in rhesus monkeys, a number of elegant fMRI studies have appeared in the awake state [13,128–131]. These studies, in contrast to the rat studies, show reproducible, readily interpretable patterns of activation. Unfortunately, in order to obtain reliable data, monkeys must be trained repeatedly over the course of about 2 years, and must continually enter the magnet (on a weekly basis) to maintain reliable task responsivity. These conditions severely limit the number of animals that can be scanned. Interestingly, it appears that rhesus monkeys are much easier to train for these studies than, say, cynomolgus macaques.

Clearly then, for any question it becomes an issue of the scientific problem to be addressed whether or not the awake animal is absolutely critical for answering the scientific question.

10.4 BASIC DRUG CHALLENGE DESIGNS

10.4.1 Acute Model

The most basic form of an phMRI experiment is to monitor signal changes (either BOLD or IRON) using a baseline condition followed by administration of the drug of interest (see also Chapter 11, Section 11.3). The relative nature of the signal changes measured by either BOLD or IRON CBV methods means that comparisons to absolute changes in metabolism are either difficult or impossible. The ability to measure an absolute metabolic parameter makes one capable of monitoring the chronic effects of a drug challenge. Such experiments have been performed, for instance, in PET studies concerning the effects of haloperidol (a rather dirty dopamine D2 antagonist).

These studies have shown decreases in glucose metabolism after chronic administration of the drug. Optimally, in such a case a technique is required that can measure absolute changes in the parameter of interest (CBV, CBF, CMRglc, etc.). The only MR technique that can be envisioned as of use for this purpose is that of arterial spin labeling which is capable of measuring absolute CBF. However, the low sensitivity of this technique has precluded its full exploration in such a context. In situations where one might expect the changes to be regional, it is possible that measurements of relative CBV might be of some value. Thus, while certainly feasible, most studies will probably continue to be performed as acute drug challenges. There is another point to be made with regard to the acute drug challenge model. Often, one is interested not in metabolic perturbations that may have resulted from administration of a drug, but in the pattern of receptor alterations that may have been induced by a drug. Our studies of the dopamine system have resulted in the conclusion that the dynamics and populations of the dopamine receptors have a major influence upon the metabolic changes induced by the acute administration of a dopaminergic drug such as amphetamine. Thus, one can interpret the acute administration of a drug as a means of indirectly probing the population and circuitry involved with a particular receptor population. Clearly, this type of interpretation has to be proved for each new ligand and receptor system. However, once such a conclusion can be made, the drug challenge becomes a means to probe such circuitry.

A schematic of data from an IRON experiment is depicted in Figure 10.5. In this experiment, baseline signal is measured in a number of images, then an iron oxide contrast agent is administered. Administration of this agent (as discussed above) leads to a loss of signal (an increase in R_2^*) proportional to the cerebral blood volume. Then, a drug such as amphetamine is injected, all the while imaging continuously. The signal changes are monitored for as long as one anticipates the drug of choice to have an effect. In instances where such a time period may be unknown, one might image as long as the animal remains physiologically stable. Increasing the number of images will obviously increase the statistical power of the experiment, assuming of course that everything is stable. In cases where there may be signal drift over a long period of time this must be accounted for (see also Chapter 11, Section 11.3).

In this regard it should be kept in mind that the pharmacodynamic profile of various drugs can often be very different even when targeted towards the same receptor system. For instance, cocaine and amphetamine have very similar effects upon the synaptic dopamine concentration, however, cocaine has a much shorter time course. In addition, cocaine has effects that are extremely sensitive to the method of administration. A similar effect upon synaptic dopamine changes and hemodynamic changes that occurs for cocaine at a dose of say 1 mg/kg i.v. requires about 10 mg/kg i.p. or p.o. For amphetamine, the relative difference for i.p. vs. i.v. challenge is about 30% less for the i.p. administration compared with the factor of 10 for cocaine. Thus, it cannot be stressed enough, to understand as much as possible about the pharmacodynamic profile of the drug of choice before performing the experiment. On the other hand, maybe phMRI will become a useful adjunct for performing such pharmacodynamic screening. Along these lines it is useful to note that the dissociation between direct vascular effects of the drug of choice and stimulation of the receptors must be examined. It is quite possible that the acute hemodynamics effects of a drug may be different from those that occur when, for instance, the drug reaches its peak concentration in brain tissue.

A permutation on the basic acute drug challenge is repeated administration of a drug with a relatively short time course. In this case, one can study, for instance, the effects of acute tolerance. Such experiments are feasible with drugs such as cocaine or nicotine, both of whose hemodynamic effects last for about 20 min. It is not necessarily feasible with drugs such as amphetamine that have very long time courses.

10.4.2 Antagonism and Agonism of Acute Drug Challenges

Many other permutations exist on the basic framework of the simple acute drug challenge study discussed above. One of the most basic and important, especially in initial phases of investigation of a new compound, is the antagonism and agonism of the drug effects. Examples of this type of experiment have been the use of D1 antagonists to turn off the effects of cocaine [10], the use of adenosine A2a antagonists to turn off the effects of amphetamine [61], the use of D2 agonists to turn off amphetamine-induced rCBV [56], and the use of D2 and D3 receptor antagonists to potentiate the effects of amphetamine [56,132].

There are a number of further permutations one can make. For instance, one could envision using repeated administrations of an agonist or antagonist to turn signal changes on and off. This type of format is mostly applicable when the time courses of the drugs of choice are relatively short, such as nicotine or D1 agonists. As alluded to above, the interpretation of these experiments can become extremely complicated in cases where the exact pharmacodynamics and brain distributions of the chemicals are not known. In such cases, alternative techniques must be employed to make such determinations to assist in the interpretation of the results. However, such studies should be performed anyway. Use of any technique by itself often results in the classic paradox of the blind men examining an elephant. The trap of approaching problems with the mindset of "to a man with a hammer every problem is a nail" is an occupational hazard in the MRI community. While this is a testimony to the breadth and depth of parameters that can be measured using MRI, it should never become a trap to application of an inappropriate technique.

10.4.3 The Acute Model for Examining the Effects of Chronic Drug Administration

At first glance it may appear as if the acute drug challenge model has severe limitations for examining the effects of chronic drug changes. Such changes are of crucial importance for understanding receptor dynamics in situations often encountered clinically. Two important examples stand out. The first is the effects of chronic administration of antipsychotic medications in schizophrenic populations. Drugs such as haloperidol, olanzapine, or clozapine often require a period of time before attaining full efficacy. A second salient example comes from the study of chronic abusers of drugs such as cocaine or ecstasy. It is well known that abusers often experience a tolerance to the effects of these drugs, implying changes in receptor populations that modulate the pharmacology of the drug of abuse. Thus, it would appear as if the acute drug challenge may not provide an adequate model for examining receptor dynamics. However, there are many ways to construe the acute drug challenge model. What we believe to be the most fruitful is to view such challenges as a means to probe a snapshot of a receptor population and its associated circuitry. Thus, one might wish to use a different ligand as the challenge agent if it has a more powerful effect upon the receptor system in question than the therapeutic agent. As an example, chronic cocaine abuse has been reported to lead to alterations in the populations of both dopamine transporters as well as dopamine D2 receptors [133,134]. One could thus plan an experiment to use a drug challenge to probe dopaminergic circuitry with more efficacy than cocaine (the short time course of cocaine's hemodynamic effects make it less than optimal). Such a drug might be amphetamine or apomorphine. In this case, one potential hypothesis might be that the decrease in dopamine transporter might lead to a much smaller effect of amphetamine than would be observed in a control population. This is because the effects of amphetamine are predicated upon reverse transport of the vesicular pool of dopamine via the dopamine transporter. Such an experiment might be tried to assay the effects of not only cocaine use, but also chronic haloperidol (schizophrenia) or methylphenidate (Ritalin) treatment (attention deficit hyperactivity disorder).

10.4.4 Pharmacodynamics

The above situations describe the basic drug challenge designs, but have elided over some major complications. In particular, the pharmacodynamics that underlie the brain metabolic response to a drug challenge needs to be addressed. Specifically, the question is, how well does the metabolic response to a drug reflect the time course of the drug in the brain? This question has not really been addressed by previous PET studies of the hemodynamic response to drug challenges, due to the limited temporal resolution of PET measurements. The exquisite temporal resolution of MRI lends itself well to study the brain pharmacodynamics. It is important to discriminate between three different phenomena:

1. The drug induces neuronal activity that diminishes with time in spite of the drug being present.
2. The drug induces a hemodynamic reponse that is proportional to the lifetime of the drug in the brain (the most favorable case).
3. The drug induces an indirect response that persists longer than the time course in the brain.

One of the first studies to address this issue was by Stein and colleagues [14,135], who set forth a kinetic model with which to interpret the phMRI data. The model included empirical terms for modeling the signal response including time to peak response, the peak response, the time to decay to 50% of peak, and the slope of the rising part of the curve. These parameters were then used to characterize the observed activation time–response curves in order to assess to what degree the brain hemodynamic response matched the plasma pharmacokinetics. A different approach was taken by Wise et al. [136,137] to stydy the modulation of pain-induced BOLD signal changes by remifentanil. These authors assumed a pharmacodynamic profile using a previously established three-compartment model for the effect site concentration. Then, the equilibration half-life and the washout half-life were characterized based upon the modulated BOLD signal due to a noxious (painful) stimulus. In this case it is not the drug-induced BOLD response, but the modulation of the BOLD response to another stimuli that is measured. Thus, this is tantamount to assuming the remifentanil will only modulate the signal as long as it is present at its effective site.

Both above studies examined the question and/or assumed that the BOLD response was proportional to the lifetime of the drug at its effective site (i.e., possibility (2) described above). In the first cited study, where the possibility was stated that the drug could persist in the brain for a time period longer than the hemodynamic effects. An instructive example of such a case is provided by the comparison of two different dopamine transporter blockers, cocaine and CFT. The latter has a much longer half-life at the dopamine transporter. PET imaging studies can provide excellent information on the time course for specific drug binding in the brain. Figure 10.10 shows data from PET studies on ^{11}C-CFT binding in the rat brain along with microdialysis measurements of dopamine release as well as changes in rCBV. It is clear that the specific binding in the striatum had an extremely long half-life (showing little decrease over at least) 2 h (Figure 10.10a), whereas both the rCBV changes induced by CFT as well as the increased synaptic dopamine had decreased to baseline by 2 h (Figure 10.10b). Thus, in this case, the hemodynamic time course reflected the extracellular dopamine concentration, and not the time course of the CFT in the brain. This is most probably explained by decreased dopamine release, possibly as a result of the blockade of the DAT leading to postsynaptic feedback inhibition of dopamine release [138].

Interestingly, this case is not necessarily representative of what happens with drugs targeting the DAT. Cocaine, similar to CFT, blocks the reuptake of dopamine through the DAT. Cocaine has a much shorter half-life (less than 20 min) in the brain than does CFT [139]. Cocaine's half-life is less than 20 min. This is quite consistent with the observed changes in rCBV measured using MRI [10,91]. Thus, in this case, the lifetime of the drug in the brain is nicely paralleled by the hemodynamic time course, and the approach of Stein et al. to modeling pharmacodynamic time courses is appropriate [14,135].

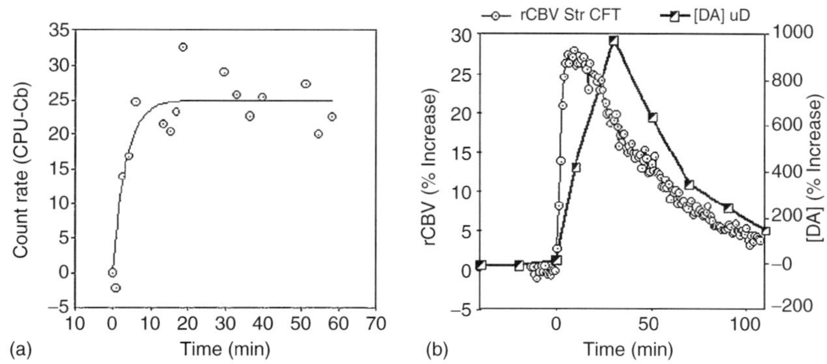

FIGURE 10.10 (a) ^{11}C-CFT study of the specific binding in the caudate/putamen of a rat. Note that the CFT has an extremely long time-constant for decline from the striatum (i.e., there is none detectable over 70 min). (b) Comparisons of the rCBV changes and increases in extracellular dopamine concentrations (measured from the caudate/putamen using microdialysis) after 0.75 mg/kg of CFT. Note the time course for rCBV parallels well that of the dopamine release. Both parameters decline, however, with much shorter time constants than that of the specific binding of CFT shown in (a). The PET data are from collaborative studies with Dr. Anna-Liisa Brownell.

10.4.5 Modeling CBV Changes Induced in the Brain Using a Pharmacologic Model

Data analysis of a PET pharmacologic study inherently includes all the different pharmacodynamic parameters of interest due to the fact that one is trying to determine either the concentration of a drug in the brain, or the kinetic parameters associated with its binding. No such analysis is usually attempted, perhaps wisely, for hemodynamic measures. The reasons for this were discussed in the first section of this chapter, i.e., that the total number of molecules responsible for the hemodynamic change is so large that any model is likely to have enough slop to make extraction of quantitative parameters difficult. Nevertheless, under favorable circumstances, there may be models of some use that can be derived. First, if the drug in question has a PET tracer analog then one could combine parameters derived from the PET model to extract the lifetime of the drug in the brain. Under such a circumstance, one could then postulate that the hemodynamic effects of the drug will be directly proportional to its concentration in the brain. Thus, such a model would be described as

$$\frac{\mathrm{dCBV}}{\mathrm{d}t} = K\frac{\mathrm{d[Drug]}}{\mathrm{d}t} \tag{10.20}$$

where the rate of change of CBV is proportional to the rate of change of the drug in the voxel of interest. If such a relationship can be validated then one might, under very controlled (blood gases, breathing rate, etc.) circumstances, extract the drug concentration or the relative drug concentration in the brain, after empirical estimates of K and determination of where such a relationship might break down. In the case of a drug such as amphetamine, which increases synaptic and extra synaptic dopamine concentrations, we can further predict that, at least in the striatum, the release of dopamine may directly lead to vasodilation (see Figure 10.3 above). In this case the equation above can be rewritten as

$$\mathrm{CBV}(t) = K^{*}C_{\mathrm{free}}^{\mathrm{DA}}(t) = R(t) - U(t) \tag{10.21}$$

where the instantaneous CBV at time t is CBV(t) and C_{free}^{DA} is the free dopamine concentration as a function of time that is the balance between release $R(t)$ and reuptake $U(t)$ — the latter is usually modeled as Michaelis-Menten kinetics for the dopamine transporter. The possibility of adding the phMRI and PET data together with microdialysis data is intriguing, and such attempts have been made using combinations of PET and microdialysis [140]. However, incorporating all the kinetic terms one might need even for the simplest description often produces solutions to differential equations which are the difference of two exponentials (characteristic of an phMRI time course). Fitting noisy BOLD data to such a model often leads to nonunique solutions at best, and nonsense at worst.

10.5 CURRENT APPLICATIONS OF phMRI TECHNIQUES

10.5.1 Criteria for Demonstration That the Hemodynamic Effects Are Due to the Neurotransmitter System in Question

As was discussed in the first section of this chapter, the coupling between pharmacologic stimulation, neural activity, and a hemodynamic change is a very complicated issue. Therefore, the first time one performs an phMRI experiment with a given drug or neurotransmitter system, great pains should be taken to determine that the hemodynamic changes observed are due to the neurotransmitter or receptor system in question. This should not be assumed as a foregone conclusion without proving it, otherwise, to paraphrase Lord Kelvin, one's ability to interpret the signal changes observed is of a meager and insubstantial nature. This is especially true in systems where the neurotransmitter may also be vasoactive. As discussed earlier, most neurotransmitters are indeed vasoactive.

In what follows we will outline some of the steps that can be taken to demonstrate that the hemodynamic changes observed are due to stimulation of the neurotransmitter system in question. It should be stated that this stimulation may activate not only the specific neuronal subtype targeted by the pharmacologic ligand, but may include as well the downstream circuitry that will probably encompass other neurotransmitter systems. With this in mind, we outline below some of the criteria that should be fulfilled. Many of these experiments by necessity have to be performed in animals, possibly in support of possible human studies.

Criteria for demonstration that hemodynamic changes induced by a given ligand are specific to neurotransmitter in question:

1. phMRI signal changes should not correlate with changes in systemic physiologic parameters (e.g., pCO_2, blood pressure).
2. phMRI signal changes should be correlated with the distribution of the neurotransmitter in question and/or the downstream circuitry measured using autoradiography or PET.
3. Selective lesioning of the receptor system in question should modulate phMRI signal changes in predictable ways.
4. Administration of agonists and antagonists of the receptor system should modulate the signal in a manner consistent with the proposed mechanisms of action of the agonists and antagonists.
5. phMRI signal changes should correlate with behavioral and/or neurotransmitter dynamics (the latter measured using, for instance, microdialysis).

Some of these may need to be explained in more detail. The first criterion may appear obvious, however, there are a number of circumstances where the relationship between regional changes in systemic parameters and specific activation of a given neurotransmitter may be correlated. For instance, administration of adenosine receptor agonists can produce decreases in blood pressure. If these drops are large enough, they may alter local tissue hemodynamic parameters, as discussed in Section 10.1.2. Such a drop may also be correlated with direct action of the ligand upon adenosine receptors. Since adenosine A1 receptors are found over almost the entire brain, disentangling these two phenomena may be impossible. In general then, if there are uniform changes that occur over the entire brain, and these correlate with changes in systemic physiologic variables, it will be difficult to determine which effects are specific to the neurotransmitter system in question in the absence of other information. To put a positive spin on this confound, one could also say that these types of data may be of some use in determining the hemodynamic effects of systemic changes in something like CO_2!

The second criterion can be considered as the *sine qua non* if phMRI is to be considered as a useful neuroreceptor mapping tool. As we discussed in Section 10.1, which of the various metrics might be chosen to correlate with the phMRI data is somewhat open to interpretation. However, the general distributions of most of the major neurotransmitters in the brain are known with some degree of specificity. The issue of the downstream circuitry is quite important and is the same problem encountered in all fMRI studies of task activation. That is, the metabolic effects of stimulation of a given set of neurons leads both to local changes as well as changes in the attendant circuitry. This question also needs to be reframed in light of the specific distribution of vascular receptors. In general, the distribution of vascular receptors is much less well known than the distribution of parenchymal receptors. Also, the spatial correlation between the vascular and parenchymal receptors is not well known. Thus, once again, disentangling the neurovascular coupling problem is a complicated conundrum. What can be stated with some certainty is that if, in general, the pattern of activation induced by a given drug is not consistent with any of the known receptor distributions of the drug administered, then the interpretation of the phMRI data is much less interesting than it would otherwise be. The likely place to look in such a situation is for specific vascular phenomena, for instance.

The third criterion is important, because it further helps to demonstrate that the phMRI activation observed is specific to the neurotransmitter system studied. If the lesion is made to ablate the neurotransmitter, for instance, then the response induced by a drug targeted towards that neuroreceptor system should also be reduced. This will be described in more detail below, where we discuss the criteria specifically for the dopamine system. The fourth criterion is important for much the same reasons. By examining the response to both agonists and antagonists of a given receptor system it is possible to have a much fuller understanding of the effects of the hemodynamic coupling. For instance, one could postulate that administration of a dopamine receptor D1 agonist might increase CBV (and this is indeed the case). Simple logic might suggest that administration of a dopamine D1 antagonist would decrease CBV (and this is also the case). Thus, one can immediately suggest that signal increases noted after administration of nonspecific ligands, such as amphetamine, are driven largely by D1 agonism! Such a criterion should always be attempted when performing animal studies.

Finally, the last criterion is important for a number of reasons. In PET imaging there is often interest in the regional binding of a tracer level of a given ligand. This provides information on the receptor distribution. In phMRI, in order to get a measurable response, one must typically inject a high enough dose that there are measurable systemic effects. Such doses are usually behaviorally active — hence the phMRI data should correlate, temporally and spatially, with behavioral data. In this context these studies can be considered to be similar to what is observed with task-activated fMRI studies where the behavioral response in general correlates spatial and temporally with the fMRI response (although in practice one is usually performing the inverse solution of manipulating a behavior and solving for the brain signal changes).

In order to make these criteria more concrete we will review the steps we took in animal studies of the dopamine system to establish that the hemodynamic changes observed after stimulation with dopaminergic drugs were truly due to stimulation of dopamine receptors. Luckily, in the case of the dopamine system, there was a large body of prior literature with which to compare in order to cross-validate the phMRI studies.

10.5.2 Application of the above Criteria to Study the Dopamine System

We investigated the application of the above criteria to the dopaminergic system in rats and to a less thorough degree in monkeys. We first chose to examine amphetamine, a drug that causes reverse transport of dopamine through the dopamine transporter as well as an increase of dopamine release from presynaptic vesicles [54]. The second drug we used was β-CFT (2β-carbomethoxy-3β-(4-fluorophenyl)tropane), which is a selective blocker of the dopamine transporter decreasing reuptake of presynaptic dopamine. In these studies we injected the drugs in an acute challenge design.

The first experiment one might perform in an animal is to inject a target drug and observe the hemodynamic changes. In the same animal one can simultaneously measure both mean arterial blood pressure (MABP) and pCO2, thereby assuring that any observed hemodynamic changes are not due to changes in systemic physiologic parameters. This is a necessary and good start, but it is hardly sufficient. We showed that injection of either amphetamine or β-CFT (a dopamine transporter blocker) led to systemic increases in MABP that were transient and much shorter than the BOLD or rCBV changes induced by these drugs [5], a fact that was already known for amphetamine [141]. The next step in such an experiment might be to compare how the spatial pattern of BOLD or rCBV changes compares to the known distributions of dopaminergic neurons. Dopamine D1 and D2 receptors have highest density of expression in the striatum, nucleus accumbens, substantia nigra, ventral tegmental area and prefrontal cortex [35]. In the rat, there is also an extremely high density in the large olfactory areas. Thus, the observed signal changes correlate, in general, with the known spatial pattern of dopamine receptors. Nevertheless, this correlation is not perfect. For instance, there is a very large induced phMRI signal change in the thalamus, an area not ordinarily considered to have high dopamine receptor density (except for D5 receptors). The thalamus is, however, the output circuit from the striatum to the cortex. Thus, it is not surprising that activation might be seen there.

In the dopamine system a number of well-described and specific lesion models exists for selective ablation of the nigral-striatal dopamine tracts using the toxin 6-hydroxydopamine [142]. These lesion models can be performed unilaterally as shown in Figure 10.11. The unlesioned side is essentially normal, and can be used as control. This then allows one to test that the signal changes are due to dopamine, as other related aminergic neurotransmitters such as norepinephrine and

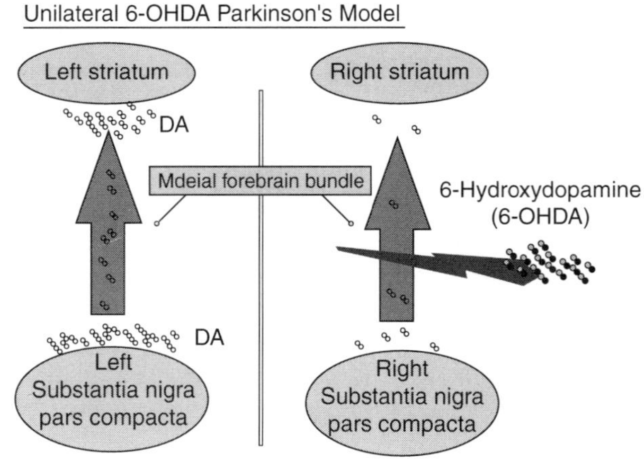

FIGURE 10.11 Schematic showing the unilateral destruction of the nigral-striatal dopamine tracts using the toxin 6-hydroxydopamine (6-OHDA). This well-characterized model provides a way of studying the effects of dopaminergic depletion while the other side is relatively normal. In this model the noradrenergic, serotonergic, and cholinergic neurons are spared.

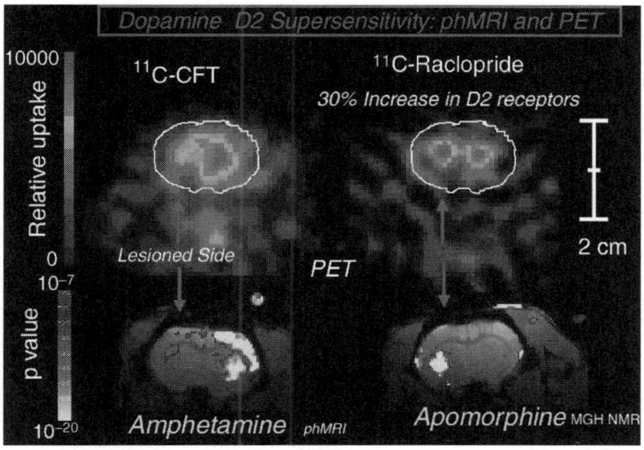

FIGURE 10.12 (See color insert following page 328.) Comparisons of PET and phMRI data of the same rat unilaterally lesioned with 6-OHDA scanned with four different drugs showing binding of ^{11}C-CFT to presynaptic DAT terminals (top left) or ^{11}C-raclopride to postsynaptic D2 receptors (top right). On the bottom is the rCBV response to amphetamine (left) or apomorphine (right). The loss of ^{11}C-CFT binding indicates loss of presynaptic DA terminals. Conversely, the ^{11}C-raclopride data indicate upregulation of postsynaptic D2 receptors. These findings correlate well with the amphetamine data where the lesioned side shows loss of presynaptic dopamine release. Apomorphine stimulation leads to increased rCBV on the lesion side only (apomorphine is an indirect dopamine agonist with lower affinity than dopamine, thus in the presence of the high levels of dopamine on the intact side apomorphine has little effect). These data indicate the sensitivity of phMRI to dopaminergic supersensitivity. (From Nguyen, T. V. et al., *Synapse*, 36, 57, 2000. With permission.)

noradrenaline can be spared. If one compares the BOLD or rCBV changes induced by amphetamine or CFT it can be seen that the signal changes are largely restricted to the intact side, and further, the intact side looks similar to a conventional amphetamine scan (Figure 10.12) [5,8,12]. In this lesion model a simple behavioral test correlates quite well with the degree of lesioning. In this test a dose of amphetamine is given to the rat, and a unilaterally lesioned animal will turn repeatedly to the contralateral side. The time course of the turning correlates well with the time course of the phMRI signal changes in the striatum. Not surprisingly, this time course parallels the release of dopamine induced by amphetamine. This time course is the same on both the intact side in a lesioned animal, and in a control animal [5,8,12].

One more experiment provides additional evidence that the phMRI signal changes are due to stimulation of dopamine neurons. Transplantation of fetal dopamine cells into the unilaterally lesioned striatum of a rat not only restores the behavioral profile (stopping the animal from rotating after injection with amphetamine) but it also restores binding of CFT as measured by PET as well as the phMRI response at the very same location where the graft is. This is readily verified using post-mortem histology on the same animal [8]. This may prove useful for studying fetal and stem cell grafting in PD [143]. This model is discussed in more detail in Section 10.5.4.

Proof: Hemodynamic changes induced by dopaminergic ligands are specific to dopamine in the striatum:

- phMRI signal changes do not correlate with pCO2 or BP changes
- phMRI signal changes are lost by destruction of dopaminergic fiber innervation (even when cholinergic, glutamatergic, adenosinergic, gabaergic, and adrenergic innervation is intact)

- the phMRI response is restored by transplantation of dopaminergic neurons
- the phMRI response correlates both spatially and temporally with dopamine efflux measured via microdialysis
- the phMRI response is strongest in areas with high dopamine innervation, as measured by PET or autoradiography
- the phMRI magnitude correlates with ability to release dopamine

10.5.3 phMRI Studies of Drug Abuse

Drugs of abuse such as nicotine, cocaine, and heroin are major problems plaguing the industrialized world. While each of the aforementioned drugs targets a different neurotransmitter system (cholinergic, dopaminergic, and opioid, respectively), there is a general consensus that much of the rewarding effects of the drugs act through the mesocortical limbic dopaminergic system including the sublenticular extended amygdala, hypothalamus, nucleus accumbens, striatum, and frontal cortex. This reward pathway is common to many other drugs of abuse, such as alcohol, as well as behaviors such as sex [144], video games [145], and even music [146]. Thus, there is a number of ways for investigating drugs of abuse using fMRI or phMRI. For instance, the effects of the drugs of abuse on cognitive or visual tasks targeting brain regions of interest can be studied. These effects can either be chronic or can be studied during administration of the drug of abuse [147–149]. In the latter case it is of paramount concern to understand the vascular effects of the drug in the absence of any cognitive challenge. Another potentially revealing approach is to study the effects of tasks targeting the reward circuitry in control and addicted populations [150,151]. Such studies may be of great use in understanding the imbalances in such circuitry that may precipitate or predispose individuals towards abuse. Attention must be paid to the potentially adaptive changes that may take place in, for instance, the dopaminergic system consequent to abuse of the drugs. It is the latter state that may be probed using the acute challenge methodology discussed in Section 10.4.1. In our conception, the acute challenge methodology is most sensitive to the basal state of the target receptors in the brain, and thus in some ways can be likened to a PET study of the receptor populations.

In what follows we will summarize some of the acute challenge phMRI literature that has been published concerning both animal and human studies. We will focus on what may be learned from such studies rather than to catalog the findings.

10.5.3.1 Dopaminergic Drugs

This category is, by far, the most studied using phMRI methods. Drugs such as cocaine, cocaine analogs, and amphetamine have been studied in both humans and animals. The animal data are reasonably consistent, in that increased CBV or BOLD signal is generally noted in the basal ganglia [5,7,10,152]. More or less cortical activation is seen with the different drugs in dopaminergically related brain areas, such as frontal and insular cortex, similar to prior studies using PET or autoradiography. Data on humans are more difficult to interpret. The reason for this is multifarious. In humans, we are restricted to using the BOLD effect (or the even less sensitive imaging of CBF by MRI). Signal changes due to primary sensory stimuli, such as photic stimulation, are often larger than those detected following cognitive stimuli, thus the cocaine-induced effects (given the relatively small doses used in human studies — usually around 0.5 mg/kg compared with the 1 mg/kg used in the rodent studies) are often rather small. In addition, work from Hans Breiter's laboratory has shown that expectancy is a severe confound of BOLD signal in, for instance, the nucleus accumbens, as it may determine the amplitude of the baseline BOLD signal [150]. A number of other confounds remain in the human data where acute administration of cocaine can lead to either vasoconstriction, and subsequent decreases in CBV or BOLD in many different brain regions [112,153], but also increased BOLD in limbic areas such as the nucleus accumbens [154].

The study by Kaufman et al. [153] is interesting in that there were significant differences in the rCBV induced after 0.4 mg/kg cocaine administration between both men and women, and between women as a function of the menstrual cycle. Some of these decreases in BOLD or rCBV may be related to hyperventilation. Following an infusion of cocaine under double-blind conditions, cocaine-dependent subjects demonstrated significant increases in heart rate and mean arterial blood pressure and decreases in $ETCO_2$ [154]. This latter study demonstrated that correlation maps of the signal changes induced by infusion of cocaine with behavioral measures of either euphoria or craving showed dramatic differences. Craving tended to be associated with activation in the nucleus accumbens and amygdala, while the rush or euphoria tended to correlate with activity in the anterior cingulate, basal forebrain and ventral tegmental area. Administration of cocaine in a double-blind fashion (where neither the subject nor investigator know whether the subject is receiving cocaine or placebo) is required to eliminate the possibility that cues as to the injection will change expectancy, and thereby modulate the signal.

A more recent study of cocaine identified brain regions associated with craving, rush, high, and anxiety during cocaine self-administration in the magnet [155]. The mesocortical limbic system is heavily involved in the high and craving. Numerous elements of the dopaminergic circuitry showed negative correlations of BOLD signal with the high and positive correlations in the same regions with craving. Interestingly, unlike in animal studies, many of these effects appear to be lateralized.

Other studies of brain regions involved in cocaine craving have examined the fMRI response to visual cues of cocaine use to stimulate craving [156,157]. Areas such as the anterior cingulate, dorsolateral prefrontal cortex, and caudate were significantly activated in cocaine-abusing subjects in response to visual cues. These studies do, however, point out that the response to a relatively small injection of cocaine will be a complicated effect of the multifarious cognitive and emotional responses to the drug, in addition to the direct pharmacologic and vasoactive effects.

Most of these studies have been successful in demonstrating the utility of phMRI for evaluating the effects of acute drug challenges to the dopaminergic reward circuitry. However, an assessment of changes in the dopamine system as a function of the addictive process, as well as withdrawal and therapy, has yet to be performed. Such a study could evaluate, for instance, the effects of addiction and withdrawal upon the D2 system, as decreases in D2 binding have been associated with increased cocaine craving and self-administration [158,159]. Such a study, might additionally evaluate changes associated in cocaine-induced activation by pretreatment with D2 agonists or antagonists. Another possibility is to examine changes that might occur in the dopamine transporter protein — the primary target of cocaine and amphetamine. Further correlation of the temporal changes in the acute challenge model (where one would plan to inject cocaine longitudinally in subjects) with the temporal changes in molecules such as CREB and Δ-FosB [160] would be invaluable in determining if those time courses were correlated. Such a study would have the capacity to associate potential changes in brain circuitry with molecular events known to correlate with behavioral profiles. For instance, increased CREB activity during the 25 days after cessation of cocaine has been shown to correlate with an acute withdrawal anhedonic effect. Buildup of Δ-FosB over later times correlated with potentiation of the abuse potential [160]. Such a study (of course in animals) would be of great value when examined concomitantly with behavioral and phMRI studies. Luckily, in humans, repeated injections of cocaine in the laboratory setting do not seem to influence future abuse of the drug [161].

We discussed above the correlations between extracellular dopamine and the phMRI signal changes. Interestingly, in rhesus monkeys there were no correlations of extracellular dopamine with drug-seeking activity in response to visual cues. There were, however, huge increases in extracellular dopamine induced by cocaine [162]. This is an important factor to keep in mind when trying to assess the origins of increased BOLD or CBF in the brain reward circuitry. Another very important confound is discussed below with respect to nicotine administration.

10.5.3.2 Nicotine

Likewise dopaminergics, nicotine can have specific vascular effects — most notably vasodilation. However, much of the observed vasodilatory effects appear to be mediated via NO [44]. Intravenous administration of nicotine to human subjects leads to increased BOLD signal in the nucleus accumbens, amygdala, cingulate, and frontal lobes, all areas associated with reward circuitry [14]. In addition, the primary sites of activation appear to correspond well with the distribution of nicotine cholinergic binding sites seen using ^{11}C-nicotine binding [163]. The highest concentration of sites are seen in the frontal, cingulate, and insular lobes of the cortex and in the thalamus and basal ganglia. These results are somewhat different from those obtained using PET measurements of changes in regional CBF. Nicotine reduced rCBF in the left anterior temporal cortex and in the right amygdala. Increases were noted in the right anterior thalamus [164,165]. In the case of the MRI study nicotine was administered i.v. whereas in the PET studies it was administered nasally. How these two administration routes may affect the observed signal changes is not known.

Separation of the activation components due to the reward circuitry vs. those caused by direct stimulation of the cholinergic receptors has not been attempted, nor has a systematic investigation of the effects of other cholinergic antagonists or agonists upon the nicotine-induced hemodynamic changes. A further confound related to activation of reward circuitry vs. the direct effects of the drug on its target receptors has been pointed out by Hans Breiter and colleagues in their studies of monetary reward [150]. In such studies one can obtain either positive or negative BOLD signal changes in the nucleus accumbens in response to the same stimulus depending upon what the expectation of the stimulus was. Thus, in cases where the drug is not administered in a double-blind fashion it is conceivable that the expectation of the subject may dramatically influence the activation seen in the accumbens! This is likely to be a confound in cases where the drug of interest, e.g., nicotine, does not produce a large change in dopamine release in the dopaminergic elements of the reward circuitry.

10.5.3.3 Heroin

A few studies have appeared examining the effects of heroin. One such study examined the effects of an acute heroin dose upon visual activation using fMRI. Not surprisingly, there was decreased activation after a heroin dose in all the subjects [148]. Another study followed visual drug cues in heroin users with an actual drug dose to evaluate different brain patterns associated with cues for use. The urge to use correlated strongly with increased regional CBF in the inferior frontal and orbitofrontal cortex regions implicated in conditioning and reward [166]. Autoradiographic studies of changes in blood flow in rats after acute doses of heroin showed increased CBF in many different brain regions that could be blocked by naloxone [167,168]. A phMRI study of heroin in rats showed that there was a large difference between spontaneously breathing and artificially ventilated rats with the former showing widespread decreases in BOLD [15]. In the latter case there were systematic increases in BOLD signal regions consistent with the distribution of opiate mu-receptors in rat brain. These increases were blocked by naloxone. These same authors also showed that heroin self-administration in rats led to a decreased number of activated voxels in a number of brain regions, including the nucleus accumbens [169].

The confounds of changes in respiratory gases is pointed out by a number of the studies discussed above. It is clear that simultaneous measurement of blood gases is critical in such studies. However, this introduces the interesting point that changes in global hemodynamic states induced by changes in blood gases may be overridden in selected brain regions by direct action of other vasoactive neurotransmitters. Such a complicated state of affairs means that simple corrections of drift in phMRI signals may not always be a useful, or even feasible proposition.

The use of phMRI for investigations of conditions and systems related to drug abuse can only be described as in its infancy. Nevertheless, MRI lends itself well to multiple longitudinal studies, which will be of great value for studying the effects of withdrawal and therapy. In addition, the high temporal and spatial resolution of MRI may well allow for more fine discrimination of subtle pharmacodynamic effects than is possible with other techniques.

10.5.4 phMRI Studies of Neurodegeneration

Neurodegenerative disorders such as Alzheimer's and Parkinson's disease (AD and PD) are devastating progressive illnesses for which much is known about the pathology, and much less about the etiology. Many of these diseases either target specific neurotransmitter systems or selectively damage specific regions in the brain. For instance, cholinergic neurons seem to be selectively vulnerable in AD whereas dopamine neurons are the primary target in PD. This selectivity with respect to neuronal populations makes the use of phMRI a potentially valuable adjunct for addressing questions of etiology, natural history, and progression. Numerous PET studies have investigated many of the same metabolic and neurotransmitter questions one would like to address with phMRI in various neurodegenerative conditions. These studies often show decreased glucose utilization in the parts of the brain undergoing selective degeneration. In addition, degeneration of dopamine neurons in PD and cholinergic neurons in AD can be shown using ligands selective for those neurotransmitter systems. We will not review this literature here, but instead, will discuss what has been performed using phMRI studies of the dopaminergic system in Parkinson's disease models.

Unlike the situation for many neurodegenerative conditions, good animal models for PD have existed for many years. With the advent of transgenic mouse models more neurodegenerative diseases will be able to avail themselves of the opportunity for good animal studies. In the case of PD, the models developed were based upon neurotoxins that are selective for dopamine neurons. The first model is based upon 6-hydroxydopamine. This compound is selectively taken up by dopamine neurons where it generates toxic hydroxyl radicals. Direct injection of 6-OHDA into the substantia nigra or medial forebrain bundle to destroy the nigrostriatal or nigrofrontal dopaminergic projections has been used for many years in rats. The nice feature of this model is that one can perform unilateral lesions and thereby keep one side of the animal relatively intact as a control. Such lesions generate a characteristic behavioral profile where injections of amphetamine cause rotations of the animal due to the dopamine released on the intact side. This behavior has been very well characterized over the years, and the amount of dopamine cell loss is quantitatively related to the number of rotations over a threshold value [170]. Another permutation of this model is to inject 6-OHDA into the striatum and follow the retrograde transport into, and subsequent degeneration of, the substantia nigra. Yet another toxin is capable of producing selective destruction of dopamine neurons which is the hallmark of PD. This molecule was originally discovered in humans when a bad batch of synthetic heroin led to a number of 20-year-old individuals with symptoms almost entirely reminiscent of idiopathic PD. It was subsequently discovered that the contaminant was a compound known as MPTP (*N*-methy-4-phenyl-1,2,3,6-tetrahydropyridine). This compound is converted via monoamine oxidase-B (MAO-B) into *N*-methyl-4-phenylpyridinium (MPP^+) [171]. The latter compound is an extremely selective inhibitor of complex I in the electron transport chain — thus inhibiting ATP production. Its selectivity for the dopaminergic system is thought to arise from selective uptake of MPTP via the dopamine transporter. This model has been most often studied in primates where it has the advantage of being capable of generating the PD model with systemic injections. Rats have very little MAO-B and so convert very little of the MPTP into MPP^+ thus suffering very little dopamine cell loss. We will cover these two PD models in both rats and monkeys. As above, we will try to cover what aspects of the pathology and therapy can be discovered using phMRI rather than perform a literature review.

10.5.4.1 Rat and Monkey Models of Parkinson's Disease

We have extensively studied the 6-OHDA rat PD model using phMRI [5,8,12]. A schematic of such a model was shown in Figure 10.11. Our studies have been geared towards multiple objectives. First, we wished to show that the hemodynamic effects of amphetamine or β-CFT (a selective dopamine transporter blocker similar to cocaine or methylphenidate) were due to dopamine release itself, and not some other neurotransmitter. This aspect of the experiment was discussed above in the beginning of Section 10.5. Careful lesioning leads to selective dopamine cell loss, whereas cholinergic, serotonergic, and noradrenergic neurons are preserved. Thus, we showed that there was loss of the hemodynamic response on the lesioned side, whereas the phMRI response was preserved on the intact side [5,8]. This effect is shown in Figure 10.12. In this figure there is a loss of response to amphetamine on the lesioned side. Conversely, there is an increased response to apomorphine. Second, we showed that the profile of the rotational behavior after administration of amphetamine correlated well with the phMRI time course. This lends credence to the utility of the technique for assessment of the behavioral consequences of the disease model. Such a phenomenon helps provide evidence that phMRI could be a useful marker for following potential therapies. We showed such a possibility where recovery of the dopaminergic response occurs after transplantation with fetal dopamine cells in the striatum (see also Chapter 25, Section 25.2 and Section 25.6). This recovery of the phMRI correlated with both the temporal pattern of the rotational behavior and with the spatial distribution of ^{11}C-CFT binding (a ligand selective for the DAT), as well as subsequent histology [8]. These experiments were conducted using BOLD phMRI. Newer experiments show that the IRON phMRI experiments (as expected) are even more sensitive and can show recovery of poststriatal cortical circuitry after the stem cell graft is able to successfully innervate the host [143].

A third issue we wished to investigate was the effect of receptor supersensitivity. It is well known that after unilateral lesioning with 6-OHDA, there is postsynaptic upregulation of dopamine receptors. This is referred to as supersensitivity, because it leads to unusual behavioral sensitivity to the effects of dopamine (this phenomenon has also been shown for other neurotransmitter systems). We showed that injection of amphetamine in unilaterally lesioned animals led to the expected loss of phMRI response on the lesioned side. Injection of apomorphine, a nonselective dopamine agonist, led to increased rCBV on the lesioned side only, and very little on the intact side [12]. This finding correlated well with PET measurements, in the same animals, of upregulation in D2 receptors postsynaptically (Figure 10.12). These studies, therefore, lend great credence to the belief that phMRI may be of considerable use for investigating dopamine receptor dynamics in PD models, and in PD itself. These studies amply demonstrate that phMRI is a useful tool for following dopamine cell loss, dopamine cell recovery using fetal and stem cell transplantation, and also show that receptor supersensitivity can be measured. The primate studies discussed below lead to further evidence that this is the case.

We also studied primates given chronic, low-dose MPTP to replicate the symptoms of PD. These animals showed many of the same behavioral and histopathological hallmarks of PD. We studied the response to amphetamine injection before and after MPTP had induced stable Parkinsonian symptoms. These studies, similar to the rat models, showed a loss of response to amphetamine, with preservation of the signal in the accumbens. The latter feature mirrors the well-known preservation of the A10 neurons innervating the accumbens in both PD as well as MPTP models [172]. An illustration of the exquisite spatial resolution of the IRON technique is shown in Figure 10.13. This figure demonstrates the loss of amphetamine-induced activation in the substantia nigra and caudate/putamen, while the response to amphetamine is preserved in the accumbens.

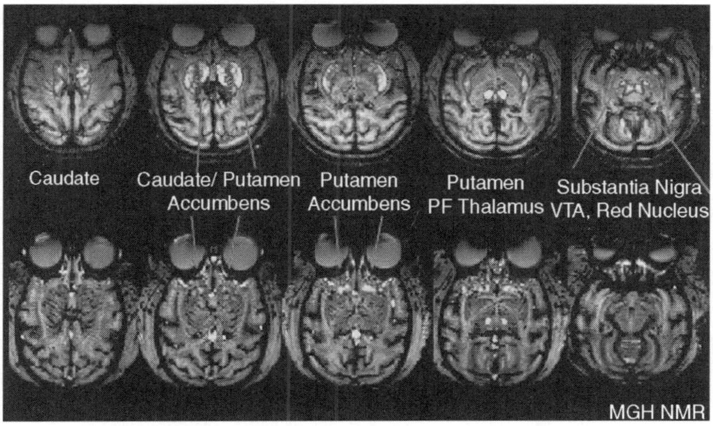

FIGURE 10.13 (See color insert following page 328.) Maps of amphetamine stimulation in cynomolgus macaques. The response to 2.5 mg/kg amphetamine is shown on the top. Note the large increases in rCBV in the dopaminergic circuitry including the caudate, putamen, nucleus accumbens, parafascicular thalamus, substantia nigra, and ventral tegmental area. The bottom of the figure shows the response to amphetamine after long-term chronic treatment with low-dose MPTP. Note the response to amphetamine is lost in most regions except for the nucleus accumbens and the parafascicular thalamus. The data were acquired at 3 T using the IRON technique and spatial resolution of 0.7 mm in plane with 1.5 mm slices.

One question that remains at the end of this section is the comparison with PET. The hemodynamic measurements made using phMRI are indirect, while PET can directly measure dopamine receptor binding, as well as dopamine metabolism using ^{18}F-labeled dopa. We will address the above issues comparing the PET and phMRI for measuring dopamine cell loss, dopamine cell recovery, and receptor supersensitivity. A snapshot of the comparisons of the parameters measured using either PET or phMRI to study dopamine cell loss in PD is presented in Table 10.5. PET measurements of dopamine cell loss seem to be best reflected in ligands specific for the DAT [173]. These ligands provide a marker for presynaptic dopamine terminals that are depleted in PD. By comparison, amphetamine stimulus, for example, reflects the amount of dopamine that can be released. Therefore, loss of the dopamine transporter will lead to a loss of an effect after either amphetamine stimulus or stimulation with a DAT blocker such as β-CFT. The lack of an effect from an amphetamine stimulus arises because not only are dopamine concentrations depleted (meaning less for release) but the reverse transport of dopamine into the synaptic cleft induced by amphetamine requires invagination of the DAT. Compounds such as

TABLE 10.5
Dopaminergic Decline in PD as Assessed Using PET or phMRI

Physical Effect or Symptom	Receptor Parameter	PET Marker	phMRI Marker
Loss of presynaptic DA terminals	Loss of DAT	^{11}C-CFT binding decreased	Amphetamine or Cocaine phMRI response decreased
Loss of DA synthesis	Loss of DA cell bodies	Decreased ^{18}F-Dopa uptake	Decreased response to amphetamine ?
Supersensitivity or Dyskinesias	Upregulation of postsynaptic D2 receptors	Increased binding potential of ^{11}C-raclopride	Large phMRI response to apomorphine or *L*-dopa

β-CFT are also ineffective at evoking an increase in the dopamine levels due to the lack of the target DAT. We showed a good correlation between PET measures of decreased CFT binding in unilaterally lesioned rats with both amphetamine and CFT-induced phMRI changes [5,152]. A comparison between CFT binding and amphetamine-induced rCBV changes in monkeys showed a weak, but statistically significant correlation between the two parameters. This reflects the fact that phMRI after amphetamine probably represents the remaining capacity to release dopamine, whereas CFT binding assessed by PET represents the remaining DAT. These two parameters are not necessarily correlated in a one-to-one fashion.

Another parameter of interest is that of supersensitivity caused by upregulation of postsynaptic dopamine receptors. In this instance, one can inject the nonspecific dopamine agonist apomorphine to elicit a large response on the lesioned side, while the intact side shows no response. In this case, the endogenous dopamine competes with apomorphine for binding to receptors on the intact side, whereas this is not possible on the lesioned side, therefore there is a large increase in the CBV after apomorphine injection. We showed this was a very sensitive marker for supersensitivity [12]. Other studies have shown decreases in R_2^* after administration of *L*-dopa in an MPTP-lesioned primate model [11]. This effect is similar to that noted with apomorphine, although the changes are smaller due to the relatively low increases in synaptic dopamine levels caused by *L*-dopa.

These results clearly indicate the utility of phMRI to assess various components of dopaminergic function. Separating some of these effects into their components may be difficult, but carefully designed experiments in the animal models may well do this. For instance, deciding whether there is loss of DAT or just loss of presynaptic dopamine stores is made by considering the differences between CFT and amphetamine. If both compounds cannot produce a signal increase in the lesioned brain then that must mean DAT targets are depleted, however, the sum of those experiments does not indicate whether or not the synthesis and presynaptic dopamine stores are intact (although in these models we know they are not). The use of *L*-dopa as a challenge may prove to be quantitatively related to the amount of presynaptic dopamine that can be released. In order to potentiate the effects of *L*-dopa it could be administered in conjunction with a DAT blocker such as cocaine or CFT.

PhMRI also makes a good tool for following therapeutic interventions in lesion models. We showed a good recovery of dopamine cell loss following transplantation of fetal dopamine cells or even stem cells [8,143]. The size of the grafts were shown by the phMRI to be consistent with the grafts seen in PET scans as well as subsequent histology. This has the potential to turn into a useful clinical tool when, and if, such therapies prove to be generally efficacious in PD.

ACKNOWLEDGMENTS

We would like to acknowledge the contributions of our many colleagues to this work, but especially: M. Flint Beal, Hans Breiter, Anna-Liisa Brownell, Anthony J-W. Chen, Keith Chiappa, Ole Isacson, Ekkehard Kuestermann, Joe B. Mandeville, John Marota, John B. Moore, T. Van Nguyen, and Bruce R. Rosen.

REFERENCES

1. Belliveau, J. W. et al., Functional mapping of the human visual cortex by magnetic resonance imaging, *Science*, 254, 716, 1991.
2. Kwong, K. K. et al., Dynamic magnetic resonance imaging of human brain activity during primary sensory stimulation, *Proc. Natl. Acad. Sci. U.S.A*, 89, 5675, 1992.

3. Ogawa, S. et al., Intrinsic signal changes accompanying sensory stimulation: functional brain mapping with magnetic resonance imaging, *Proc. Natl. Acad. Sci. U.S.A*, 89, 5951, 1992.
4. Carlsson, C., Hagerdal, M., and Siesjo, B. K., Influence of amphetamine sulfate on cerebral blood flow and metabolism, *Acta Physiol. Scand.*, 94, 128, 1975.
5. Chen, Y. I. et al., Detection of dopaminergic neurotransmitter activity using pharmacologic MRI: correlation with PET, microdialysis, and behavioral data, *Magn. Reson. Med.*, 38, 389, 1997.
6. Silva, A. C. et al., Multislice MRI of rat brain during amphetamine stimulation using arterial spin labelling, *Magn. Reson. Med.*, 33, 209, 1995.
7. Zhang, Z. et al., Pharmacological MRI mapping of age-associated changes in basal ganglia circuitry of awake rhesus monkeys, *Neuroimage*, 14, 1159, 2001.
8. Chen, Y. I. et al., Detection of dopaminergic cell loss and neural transplantation using pharmacological MRI, PET and behavioral assessment, *Neuroreport*, 10, 2881, 1999.
9. Febo, M. et al., The neural consequences of repeated cocaine exposure revealed by functional MRI in awake rats, *Neuropsychopharmacology*, 30, 936, 2005.
10. Marota, J. J. et al., Cocaine activation discriminates dopaminergic projections by temporal response: an fMRI study in rat, *Neuroimage*, 11, 13, 2000.
11. Chen, Q. et al., Mapping drug-induced changes in cerebral R_2^* by multiple gradient recalled echo functional MRI, *Magn. Reson. Imaging*, 14, 469, 1996.
12. Nguyen, T. V. et al., Detection of the effects of dopamine receptor supersensitivity using pharmacological MRI and correlations with PET, *Synapse*, 36, 57, 2000.
13. Zhang, Z. et al., Functional MRI of apomorphine activation of the basal ganglia in awake rhesus monkeys, *Brain Res.*, 852, 290, 2000.
14. Stein, E. A. et al., Nicotine-induced limbic cortical activation in the human brain: a functional MRI study, *Am. J. Psychiatry*, 155, 1009, 1998.
15. Xu, H. et al., Heroin-induced neuronal activation in rat brain assessed by functional MRI, *Neuroreport*, 11, 1085, 2000.
16. Scanley, B. E., Kennan, R. P., and Gore, J. C., Changes in rat cerebral blood volume due to modulation of the 5-HT(1A) receptor measured with susceptibility enhanced contrast MRI, *Brain Res.*, 913, 149, 2001.
17. Honey, G. and Bullmore, E., Human pharmacological MRI, *Trends Pharmacol. Sci.*, 25, 366, 2004.
18. Kimberg, D. Y. et al., Cortical effects of bromocriptine, a D-2 dopamine receptor agonist, in human subjects, revealed by fMRI, *Hum. Brain Mapp.*, 12, 246, 2001.
19. Palacios, J. M. et al., Recent trends in receptor analysis techniques and instrumentation, *J. Chem. Neuroanat.*, 4, 343, 1991.
20. Pompeiano, M., Palacios, J. M., and Mengod, G., Distribution and cellular localization of mRNA coding for 5-HT1A receptor in the rat brain: correlation with receptor binding, *J. Neurosci.*, 12, 440, 1992.
21. Schalling, M. et al., Comparison of gene expression of the dopamine D-2 receptor and DARPP-32 in rat brain, pituitary and adrenal gland, *Eur. J. Pharmacol.*, 188, 277, 1990.
22. Knull, H. and Minton, A. P., Structure within eukaryotic cytoplasm and its relationship to glycolytic metabolism, *Cell. Biochem. Funct.*, 14, 237, 1996.
23. Knull, H. R., Association of glycolytic enzymes with particulate fractions from nerve endings, *Biochim. Biophys. Acta*, 522, 1, 1978.
24. Knull, H. R. and Fillmore, S. J., Glycolytic enzyme levels in synaptosomes, *Comp. Biochem. Physiol. [B]*, 81, 349, 1985.
25. Kadekaro, M., Crane, A. M., and Sokoloff, L., Differential effects of electrical stimulation of sciatic nerve on metabolic activity in spinal cord and dorsal root ganglion in the rat, *Proc. Natl. Acad. Sci. U.S.A*, 82, 6010, 1985.
26. Sokoloff, L., Measurement of local cerebral glucose utilization and its relation to local functional activity in the brain, *Adv. Exp. Med. Biol.*, 291, 21, 1991.
27. Sokoloff, L., Sites and mechanisms of function-related changes in energy metabolism in the nervous system, *Dev. Neurosci.*, 15, 194, 1993.
28. Magistretti, P. J., Cellular bases of functional brain imaging: insights from neuron-glia metabolic coupling, *Brain Res.*, 886, 108, 2000.

29. Pellerin, L. and Magistretti, P. J., Glutamate uptake into astrocytes stimulates aerobic glycolysis: a mechanism coupling neuronal activity to glucose utilization, *Proc. Natl. Acad. Sci. U.S.A*, 91, 10625, 1994.
30. Pellerin, L. and Magistretti, P. J., Excitatory amino acids stimulate aerobic glycolysis in astrocytes via an activation of the Na + /K + ATPase, *Dev. Neurosci.*, 18, 336, 1996.
31. Sokoloff, L. et al., Contribution of astroglia to functionally activated energy metabolism, *Dev. Neurosci.*, 18, 344, 1996.
32. Chih, C. P., Lipton, P., and Roberts, E. L. Jr., Do active cerebral neurons really use lactate rather than glucose?, *Trends Neurosci.*, 24, 573, 2001.
33. Sorg, O. and Magistretti, P. J., Characterization of the glycogenolysis elicited by vasoactive intestinal peptide, noradrenaline and adenosine in primary cultures of mouse cerebral cortical astrocytes, *Brain Res.*, 563, 227, 1991.
34. Stella, N. et al., Glutamate-evoked release of arachidonic acid from mouse brain astrocytes, *J. Neurosci.*, 14, 568, 1994.
35. Cooper, J. R., Bloom, F. E., and Roth, R. H., *The Biochemical Basis of Neuropharmacology*, 7th ed., Oxford University Press, New York, 1996.
36. Lindvall, O., Ingvar, M., and Stenevi, U., Effects of methamphetamine on blood flow in the caudate-putamen after lesions of the nigrostriatal dopaminergic bundle in the rat, *Brain Res.*, 211, 211, 1981.
37. Lyons, D. and Porrino, L. J., Dopamine depletion in the rostral nucleus accumbens alters the cerebral metabolic response to cocaine in the rat, *Brain Res.*, 753, 69, 1997.
38. Faraci, F. M. and Brian, J. E. Jr., Nitric oxide and the cerebral circulation, *Stroke*, 25, 692, 1994.
39. Fillenz, M. et al., The role of astrocytes and noradrenaline in neuronal glucose metabolism, *Acta Physiol. Scand.*, 167, 275, 1999.
40. Iadecola, C., Regulation of the cerebral microcirculation during neural activity: is nitric oxide the missing link?, *Trends Neurosci.*, 16, 206, 1993.
41. Cohen, Z. et al., Serotonin in the regulation of brain microcirculation, *Prog. Neurobiol.*, 50, 335, 1996.
42. Sato, A. and Sato, Y., Cholinergic neural regulation of regional cerebral blood flow, *Alzheimer Dis. Assoc. Disord.*, 9, 28, 1995.
43. Vaucher, E., Linville, D., and Hamel, E., Cholinergic basal forebrain projections to nitric oxide synthase-containing neurons in the rat cerebral cortex, *Neuroscience*, 79, 827, 1997.
44. Elhusseiny, A. and Hamel, E., Muscarinic — but not nicotinic — acetylcholine receptors mediate a nitric oxide-dependent dilation in brain cortical arterioles: a possible role for the M5 receptor subtype, *J. Cereb. Blood Flow Metab.*, 20, 298, 2000.
45. Barbelivien, A. et al., Neurochemical stimulation of the rat substantia innominata increases cerebral blood flow (but not glucose use) through the parallel activation of cholinergic and non-cholinergic pathways, *Brain Res.*, 840, 115, 1999.
46. Head, R. J. et al., Isolated brain microvessels: preparation, morphology, histamine and catecholamine contents, *Blood Vessels*, 17, 173, 1980.
47. Jones, B. E., Relationship between catecholamine neurons and cerebral blood vessels studied by their simultaneous fluorescent revelation in the rat brainstem, *Brain Res. Bull.*, 9, 33, 1982.
48. Krimer, L. S. et al., Dopaminergic regulation of cerebral cortical microcirculation, *Nat. Neurosci.*, 1, 286, 1998.
49. Nehlig, A., Daval, J. L., and Debry, G., Caffeine and the central nervous system: mechanisms of action, biochemical, metabolic and psychostimulant effects, *Brain Res. Brain Res. Rev.*, 17, 139, 1992.
50. Gulbenkian, S., Uddman, R., and Edvinsson, L., Neuronal messengers in the human cerebral circulation, *Peptides*, 22, 995, 2001.
51. Orzi, F. et al., Comparative effects of acute and chronic administration of amphetamine on local cerebral glucose utilization in the conscious rat, *J. Cereb. Blood Flow Metab.*, 3, 154, 1983.
52. Trugman, J. M. and James, C. L., D1 dopamine agonist and antagonist effects on regional cerebral glucose utilization in rats with intact dopaminergic innervation, *Brain Res.*, 607, 270, 1993.
53. Wechsler, L. R., Savaki, H. E., and Sokoloff, L., Effects of *d*- and *l*-amphetamine on local cerebral glucose utilization in the conscious rat, *J. Neurochem.*, 32, 15, 1979.
54. Jones, S. R. et al., Mechanisms of amphetamine action revealed in mice lacking the dopamine transporter, *J. Neurosci.*, 18, 1979, 1998.

55. Sulzer, D., Maidment, N. T., and Rayport, S., Amphetamine and other weak bases act to promote reverse transport of dopamine in ventral midbrain neurons, *J. Neurochem.*, 60, 527, 1993.
56. Chen, Y. C. et al., Mapping dopamine D2/D3 receptor function using pharmacological magnetic resonance imaging, *Psychopharmacology (Berl)*, 2004, print ahead of time.
57. Ferre, S. et al., Antagonistic interaction between adenosine A2A receptors and dopamine D2 receptors in the ventral striopallidal system. Implications for the treatment of schizophrenia, *Neuroscience*, 63, 765, 1994.
58. Latini, S. et al., A2 adenosine receptors: their presence and neuromodulatory role in the central nervous system, *Gen. Pharmacol.*, 27, 925, 1996.
59. Sebastiao, A. M. and Ribeiro, J. A., Adenosine A2 receptor-mediated excitatory actions on the nervous system, *Prog. Neurobiol.*, 48, 167, 1996.
60. Quarta, D. et al., Opposite modulatory roles for adenosine A1 and A2A receptors on glutamate and dopamine release in the shell of the nucleus accumbens. Effects of chronic caffeine exposure, *J. Neurochem.*, 88, 1151, 2004.
61. Chen, Y. I., Choi, J. K., and Jenkins, B. G., Mapping interactions between dopamine and adenosine A2a receptors using pharmacologic MRI, *Synapse*, 55, 80, 2004.
62. Ferre, S. et al., The striopallidal neuron: a main locus for adenosine–dopamine interactions in the brain, *J. Neurosci.*, 13, 5402, 1993.
63. Villringer, A. et al., Dynamic imaging with lanthanidechelates in normal brain: contrast due to magnetic susceptibility effects, *Magn. Reson. Med.*, 6, 164, 1988.
64. Frank, J. A. et al., Measurement of relative cerebral blood volume changes with visual stimulation by 'double-dose' gadopentetate-dimeglumine-enhanced dynamic magnetic resonance imaging, *Invest. Radiol.*, 29 (Suppl. 2), S157, 1994.
65. Henriksen, L., Paulson, O. B., and Lassen, N. A., Visual cortex activation recorded by dynamic emission computed tomography of inhaled xenon 133, *Eur. J. Nucl. Med.*, 6, 487, 1981.
66. Greenberg, J. H. et al., Metabolic mapping of functional activity in human subjects with the [18F]fluorodeoxyglucose technique, *Science*, 212, 678, 1981.
67. Mazziotta, J. C. et al., Tomographic mapping of human cerebral metabolism: auditory stimulation, *Neurology*, 32, 921, 1982.
68. Phelps, M. E., Positron computed tomography studies of cerebral glucose metabolism in man: theory and application in nuclear medicine, *Semin. Nucl. Med.*, 11, 32, 1981.
69. Baron, J. C. et al., Noninvasive measurement of blood flow, oxygen consumption, and glucose utilization in the same brain regions in man by positron emission tomography: concise communication, *J. Nucl. Med.*, 23, 391, 1982.
70. Fox, P. T. et al., Nonoxidative glucose consumption during focal physiologic neural activity, *Science*, 241, 462, 1988.
71. Grafton, S. T., PET: activation of cerebral blood flow and glucose metabolism, *Adv. Neurol.*, 83, 87, 2000.
72. Lassen, N. A. and Ingvar, D. H., Brain regions involved in voluntary movements as revealed by radioisotopic mapping of CBF or CMR-glucose changes, *Rev. Neurol. (Paris)*, 146, 620, 1990.
73. Singer, J. R., *Science*, 130, 1652, 1959.
74. Dixon, W. T. et al., Projection angiograms of blood labeled by adiabatic fast passage, *Magn. Reson. Med.*, 3, 454, 1986.
75. Detre, J. A. et al., Perfusion imaging, *Magn. Reson. Med.*, 23, 37, 1992.
76. Ogawa, S. et al., Brain magnetic resonance imaging with contrast dependent on blood oxygenation, *Proc. Natl. Acad. Sci. U.S.A*, 87, 9868, 1990.
77. Turner, R. et al., Echo-planar time course MRI of cat brain oxygenation changes, *Magn. Reson. Med.*, 22, 159, 1991.
78. Bandettini, P. A. et al., Time course EPI of human brain function during task activation, *Magn. Reson. Med.*, 25, 390, 1992.
79. Davis, T. L. et al., Calibrated functional MRI: mapping the dynamics of oxidative metabolism, *Proc. Natl. Acad. Sci. U.S.A*, 95, 1834, 1998.
80. Hoge, R. D. et al., Investigation of BOLD signal dependence on cerebral blood flow and oxygen consumption: the deoxyhemoglobin dilution model, *Magn. Reson. Med.*, 42, 849, 1999.

81. Mandeville, J. B. et al., MRI measurement of the temporal evolution of relative CMRO(2) during rat forepaw stimulation, *Magn. Reson. Med.*, 42, 944, 1999.
82. Ogawa, S., Lee, R. M., and Barrere, B., The sensitivity of magnetic resonance image signals of a rat brain to changes in the cerebral venous blood oxygenation, *Magn. Reson. Med.*, 29, 205, 1993.
83. Fox, P. T. and Raichle, M. E., Focal physiological uncoupling of cerebral blood flow and oxidative metabolism during somatosensory stimulation in human subjects, *Proc. Natl. Acad. Sci. U.S.A*, 83, 1140, 1986.
84. Hyder, F. et al., Increased tricarboxylic acid cycle flux in rat brain during forepaw stimulation detected with 1H[13C]NMR, *Proc. Natl. Acad. Sci. U.S.A*, 93, 7612, 1996.
85. Hyder, F. et al., Oxidative glucose metabolism in rat brain during single forepaw stimulation: a spatially localized 1H[13C] nuclear magnetic resonance study, *J. Cereb. Blood Flow Metab.*, 17, 1040, 1997.
86. Chen, W. et al., Study of tricarboxylic acid cycle flux changes in human visual cortex during hemifield visual stimulation using (1)H-[(13)C] MRS and fMRI, *Magn. Reson. Med.*, 45, 349, 2001.
87. Chen, Y. C. et al., Improved mapping of pharmacologically induced neuronal activation using the IRON technique with superparamagnetic blood pool agents, *J. Magn. Reson. Imaging*, 14, 517, 2001.
88. Kennan, R. P. et al., Physiological basis for BOLD MR signal changes due to neuronal stimulation: separation of blood volume and magnetic susceptibility effects, *Magn. Reson. Med.*, 40, 840, 1998.
89. Mandeville, J. B. et al., Dynamic functional imaging of relative cerebral blood volume during rat forepaw stimulation, *Magn. Reson. Med.*, 39, 615, 1998.
90. van Bruggen, N. et al., High-resolution functional magnetic resonance imaging of the rat brain: mapping changes in cerebral blood volume using iron oxide contrast media, *J. Cereb. Blood Flow Metab.*, 18, 1178, 1998.
91. Mandeville, J. B. et al., Regional sensitivity and coupling of BOLD and CBV changes during stimulation of rat brain, *Magn. Reson. Med.*, 45, 443, 2001.
92. Taylor, A. M. et al., Use of the intravascular contrast agent NC100150 injection in spin-echo and gradient-echo imaging of the heart, *J. Cardiovasc. Magn. Reson.*, 1, 23, 1999.
93. Saini, S. et al., Multicentre dose-ranging study on the efficacy of USPIO ferumoxtran-10 for liver MR imaging, *Clin. Radiol.*, 55, 690, 2000.
94. Mandeville, J. B. et al., Exogenous contrast agent improves sensitivity of gradient-echo functional magnetic resonance imaging at 9.4 T, *Magn. Reson. Med.*, 52, 1272, 2004.
95. Prichard, J. et al., Lactate rise detected by 1H NMR in human visual cortex during physiologic stimulation, *Proc. Natl. Acad. Sci. U.S.A*, 88, 5829, 1991.
96. Chhina, N. et al., Measurement of human tricarboxylic acid cycle rates during visual activation by (13)C magnetic resonance spectroscopy, *J. Neurosci. Res.*, 66, 737, 2001.
97. Merboldt, K. D. et al., Decrease of glucose in the human visual cortex during photic stimulation, *Magn. Reson. Med.*, 25, 187, 1992.
98. Gruetter, R. et al., Observation of resolved glucose signals in 1H NMR spectra of the human brain at 4 Tesla, *Magn. Reson. Med.*, 36, 1, 1996.
99. Gruetter, R., Seaquist, E. R., and Ugurbil, K., A mathematical model of compartmentalized neurotransmitter metabolism in the human brain, *Am. J. Physiol. Endocrinol. Metab.*, 281, E100, 2001.
100. Mason, G. F. et al., Simultaneous determination of the rates of the TCA cycle, glucose utilization, alpha-ketoglutarate/glutamate exchange, and glutamine synthesis in human brain by NMR, *J. Cereb. Blood Flow Metab.*, 15, 12, 1995.
101. Guimaraes, A. R. et al., Echoplanar chemical shift imaging, *Magn. Reson. Med.*, 41, 877, 1999.
102. Hyder, F., Renken, R., and Rothman, D. L., In vivo carbon-edited detection with proton echo-planar spectroscopic imaging (ICED PEPSI): [3,4-(13)CH(2)]glutamate/glutamine tomography in rat brain, *Magn. Reson. Med.*, 42, 997, 1999.
103. Posse, S. et al., In vivo measurement of regional brain metabolic response to hyperventilation using magnetic resonance: proton echo planar spectroscopic imaging (PEPSI), *Magn. Reson. Med.*, 37, 858, 1997.
104. Loubinoux, I. et al., Cerebral metabolic changes induced by MK-801: a 1D (phosphorus and proton) and 2D (proton) in vivo NMR spectroscopy study, *Brain Res.*, 643, 115, 1994.

105. Petroff, O. A. and Rothman, D. L., Measuring human brain GABA in vivo: effects of GABA-transaminase inhibition with vigabatrin, *Mol. Neurobiol.*, 16, 97, 1998.
106. Kustermann, E. H. G. et al., Assessment of amphetamine induced stimulus using in vivo 13C MRS in rat brain, *International Society for Magnetic Resonance in Medicine*, Sydney, Australia, p. 1362, 1998.
107. Lin, Y. J. and Koretsky, A. P., Manganese ion enhances T_1-weighted MRI during brain activation: an approach to direct imaging of brain function, *Magn. Reson. Med.*, 38, 378, 1997.
108. Duong, T. Q. et al., Functional MRI of calcium-dependent synaptic activity: cross correlation with CBF and BOLD measurements, *Magn. Reson. Med.*, 43, 383, 2000.
109. Verity, M. A., Manganese neurotoxicity: a mechanistic hypothesis, *Neurotoxicology*, 20, 489, 1999.
110. Watanabe, T., Frahm, J., and Michaelis, T., Functional mapping of neural pathways in rodent brain in vivo using manganese-enhanced three-dimensional magnetic resonance imaging, *NMR Biomed.*, 17, 554, 2004.
111. Weckesser, M. et al., Functional imaging of the visual cortex with bold-contrast MRI: hyperventilation decreases signal response, *Magn. Reson. Med.*, 41, 213, 1999.
112. Gollub, R. L. et al., Cocaine decreases cortical cerebral blood flow but does not obscure regional activation in functional magnetic resonance imaging in human subjects, *J. Cereb. Blood Flow Metab.*, 18, 724, 1998.
113. Zaharchuk, G. et al., Cerebrovascular dynamics of autoregulation and hypoperfusion. An MRI study of CBF and changes in total and microvascular cerebral blood volume during hemorrhagic hypotension, *Stroke*, 30, 2197, 1999.
114. Kalisch, R. et al., Blood pressure changes induced by arterial blood withdrawal influence bold signal in anesthesized rats at 7 Tesla: implications for pharmacologic MRI, *Neuroimage*, 14, 891, 2001.
115. Longnecker, D. E. and Harris, P. D., Microcirculatory actions of general anesthetics, *Fed. Proc.*, 39, 1580, 1980.
116. Stullken, E. H. Jr. et al., The nonlinear responses of cerebral metabolism to low concentrations of halothane, enflurane, isoflurane, and thiopental, *Anesthesiology*, 46, 28, 1977.
117. Lindauer, U., Villringer, A., and Dirnagl, U., Characterization of CBF response to somatosensory stimulation: model and influence of anesthetics, *Am. J. Physiol.*, 264, H1223, 1993.
118. Hara, K. and Harris, R. A., The anesthetic mechanism of urethane: the effects on neurotransmitter-gated ion channels, *Anesth. Analg.*, 94, 313, 2002.
119. Anis, N. A. et al., The dissociative anaesthetics, ketamine and phencyclidine, selectively reduce excitation of central mammalian neurones by *N*-methyl-aspartate, *Br. J. Pharmacol.*, 79, 565, 1983.
120. Thomson, A. M., West, D. C., and Lodge, D., An *N*-methylaspartate receptor-mediated synapse in rat cerebral cortex: a site of action of ketamine?, *Nature*, 313, 479, 1985.
121. Hancock, P. J. and Stamford, J. A., Stereospecific effects of ketamine on dopamine efflux and uptake in the rat nucleus accumbens, *Br. J. Anaesth.*, 82, 603, 1999.
122. Ueki, M., Mies, G., and Hossmann, K. A., Effect of alpha-chloralose, halothane, pentobarbital and nitrous oxide anesthesia on metabolic coupling in somatosensory cortex of rat, *Acta Anaesthesiol. Scand.*, 36, 318, 1992.
123. Nieoullon, A. and Dusticier, N., Effects of alpha-chloralose on the activity of the nigrostriatal dopaminergic system in the cat, *Eur. J. Pharmacol.*, 65, 403, 1980.
124. Chen, Y. I., et al., Anesthetic filters for eliciting specific neurotransmitter effects in pharmacologic MRI, *Proceedings of the eighth annual meeting International Society of Magnetic Resonance in Medicine*, Denver, CO, p. 967, 2000.
125. Maekawa, T. et al., Local cerebral blood flow and glucose utilization during isoflurane anesthesia in the rat, *Anesthesiology*, 65, 144, 1986.
126. Lahti, K. M. et al., Comparison of evoked cortical activity in conscious and propofol-anesthetized rats using functional MRI, *Magn. Reson. Med.*, 41, 412, 1999.
127. Peeters, R. R. et al., Comparing BOLD fMRI signal changes in the awake and anesthetized rat during electrical forepaw stimulation, *Magn. Reson. Imaging*, 19, 821, 2001.
128. Dubowitz, D. J. et al., Functional magnetic resonance imaging in macaque cortex, *Neuroreport*, 9, 2213, 1998.
129. Leite, F. P. et al., Repeated fMRI using iron oxide contrast agent in awake, behaving macaques at 3 Tesla, *Neuroimage*, 16, 283, 2002.

130. Stefanacci, L. et al., fMRI of monkey visual cortex, *Neuron*, 20, 1051, 1998.
131. Vanduffel, W. et al., Visual motion processing investigated using contrast agent-enhanced fMRI in awake behaving monkeys, *Neuron*, 32, 565, 2001.
132. Schwarz, A. et al., Selective dopamine D(3) receptor antagonist SB-277011-A potentiates phMRI response to acute amphetamine challenge in the rat brain, *Synapse*, 54, 1, 2004.
133. Kleven, M. S. et al., Effects of repeated injections of cocaine on D1 and D2 dopamine receptors in rat brain, *Brain Res.*, 532, 265, 1990.
134. Letchworth, S. R. et al., Effects of chronic cocaine administration on dopamine transporter mRNA and protein in the rat, *Brain Res.*, 750, 214, 1997.
135. Bloom, A. S. et al., Determination of drug-induced changes in functional MRI signal using a pharmacokinetic model, *Hum. Brain Mapp.*, 8, 235, 1999.
136. Wise, R. G. et al., Combining fMRI with a pharmacokinetic model to determine which brain areas activated by painful stimulation are specifically modulated by remifentanil, *Neuroimage*, 16, 999, 2002.
137. Wise, R. G., Williams, P., and Tracey, I., Using fMRI to quantify the time dependence of remifentanil analgesia in the human brain, *Neuropsychopharmacology*, 29, 626, 2004.
138. Mulder, A. H. et al., Kappa- and delta-opioid receptor agonists differentially inhibit striatal dopamine and acetylcholine release, *Nature*, 308, 278, 1984.
139. Madras, B. K. et al., Cocaine receptors labeled by [3H]2 beta-carbomethoxy-3 beta-(4-fluorophenyl)tropane, *Mol. Pharmacol.*, 36, 518, 1989.
140. Endres, C. J. et al., Kinetic modeling of [11C]raclopride: combined PET-microdialysis studies, *J. Cereb. Blood Flow Metab.*, 17, 932, 1997.
141. Berntman, L. et al., Circulatory and metabolic effects in the brain induced by amphetamine sulphate, *Acta Physiol. Scand.*, 102, 310, 1978.
142. Perese, D. A. et al., A 6-hydroxydopamine-induced selective parkinsonian rat model, *Brain Res.*, 494, 285, 1989.
143. Bjorklund, L. M. et al., Embryonic stem cells develop into functional dopaminergic neurons after transplantation in a Parkinson rat model, *Proc. Natl. Acad. Sci. U.S.A*, 99, 2344, 2002.
144. Beauregard, M., Levesque, J., and Bourgouin, P., Neural correlates of conscious self-regulation of emotion, *J. Neurosci.*, 21, RC165, 2001.
145. Koepp, M. J. et al., Evidence for striatal dopamine release during a video game, *Nature*, 393, 266, 1998.
146. Blood, A. J. and Zatorre, R. J., Intensely pleasurable responses to music correlate with activity in brain regions implicated in reward and emotion, *Proc. Natl. Acad. Sci. U.S.A*, 98, 11818, 2001.
147. Loubinoux, I. et al., Cerebral functional magnetic resonance imaging activation modulated by a single dose of the monoamine neurotransmission enhancers fluoxetine and fenozolone during hand sensorimotor tasks, *J. Cereb. Blood Flow Metab.*, 19, 1365, 1999.
148. Sell, L. A. et al., Functional magnetic resonance imaging of the acute effect of intravenous heroin administration on visual activation in long-term heroin addicts: results from a feasibility study, *Drug Alcohol Depend.*, 49, 55, 1997.
149. Uftring, S. J. et al., An fMRI study of the effect of amphetamine on brain activity, *Neuropsychopharmacology*, 25, 925, 2001.
150. Breiter, H. C. et al., Functional imaging of neural responses to expectancy and experience of monetary gains and losses, *Neuron*, 30, 619, 2001.
151. Breiter, H. C. and Rosen, B. R., Functional magnetic resonance imaging of brain reward circuitry in the human, *Ann. NY Acad. Sci.*, 877, 523, 1999.
152. Chen, Y. I. et al., Improved mapping of pharmacologically induced neuronal activation using superparamagnetic iron blood pool agents, *International Society of Magnetic Resonance Medicine Seventh Annual Meeting*, Philadelphia, PA, p. 348, 1999.
153. Kaufman, M. J. et al., Cocaine-induced cerebral vasoconstriction differs as a function of sex and menstrual cycle phase, *Biol. Psychiatry*, 49, 774, 2001.
154. Breiter, H. C. et al., Acute effects of cocaine on human brain activity and emotion, *Neuron*, 19, 591, 1997.
155. Risinger, R. C. et al., Neural correlates of high and craving during cocaine self-administration using BOLD fMRI, *Neuroimage*, 26, 1097, 2005.

156. Garavan, H. et al., Cue-induced cocaine craving: neuroanatomical specificity for drug users and drug stimuli, *Am. J. Psychiatry*, 157, 1789, 2000.
157. Maas, L. C. et al., Functional magnetic resonance imaging of human brain activation during cue-induced cocaine craving, *Am. J. Psychiatry*, 155, 124, 1998.
158. Morgan, D. et al., Social dominance in monkeys: dopamine D2 receptors and cocaine self-administration, *Nat. Neurosci.*, 5, 169, 2002.
159. Volkow, N. D. and Fowler, J. S., Addiction, a disease of compulsion and drive: involvement of the orbitofrontal cortex, *Cereb. Cortex*, 10, 318, 2000.
160. Nestler, E. J., Molecular neurobiology of addiction, *Am. J. Addict.*, 10, 201, 2001.
161. Elman, I. et al., Clinical outcomes following cocaine infusion in nontreatment-seeking individuals with cocaine dependence, *Biol. Psychiatry*, 49, 553, 2001.
162. Bradberry, C. W. et al., Impact of self-administered cocaine and cocaine cues on extracellular dopamine in mesolimbic and sensorimotor striatum in rhesus monkeys, *J. Neurosci.*, 20, 3874, 2000.
163. Nyback, H. et al., Attempts to visualize nicotinic receptors in the brain of monkey and man by positron emission tomography, *Prog. Brain Res.*, 79, 313, 1989.
164. Domino, E. F. et al., Nicotine effects on regional cerebral blood flow in awake, resting tobacco smokers, *Synapse*, 38, 313, 2000.
165. Zubieta, J. et al., Regional cerebral blood flow effects of nicotine in overnight abstinent smokers, *Biol. Psychiatry*, 49, 906, 2001.
166. Sell, L. A. et al., Neural responses associated with cue evoked emotional states and heroin in opiate addicts, *Drug Alcohol Depend.*, 60, 207, 2000.
167. Fuller, S. A. and Stein, E. A., Effects of heroin and naloxone on cerebral blood flow in the conscious rat, *Pharmacol. Biochem. Behav.*, 40, 339, 1991.
168. Trusk, T. C. and Stein, E. A., Effect of intravenous heroin and naloxone on regional cerebral blood flow in the conscious rat, *Brain Res.*, 406, 238, 1987.
169. Xi, Z. X. et al., Opiate tolerance by heroin self-administration: an fMRI study in rat, *Magn. Reson. Med.*, 52, 108, 2004.
170. Robinson, T. E., Castaneda, E., and Whishaw, I. Q., Compensatory changes in striatal dopamine neurons following recovery from injury induced by 6-OHDA or methampehtamine: a review of evidence from microdialysis studies, *Can. J. Psychol.*, 44, 253, 1990.
171. Singer, T. P. and Ramsay, R. R., Mechanism of the neurotoxicity of MPTP. An update, *FEBS Lett.*, 274, 1, 1990.
172. Jenkins, B. G. et al., Mapping dopamine function in primates using pharmacologic magnetic resonance imaging, *J. Neurosci.*, 24, 9553, 2004.
173. Brownell, A.-L. et al., Cocaine congeners as PET imaging probes for dopamine terminals in normal and MPTP induced parkinsonism in nonhuman primate brain, *J. Nucl. Med.*, 37, 1186, 1996.
174. Albrecht, R. F. et al., Cerebral blood flow and metabolic changes from induction to onset of anesthesia with halothane or pentobarbital, *Anesthesiology*, 47, 252, 1977.
175. Cavazzuti, M. et al., Ketamine effects on local cerebral blood flow and metabolism in the rat, *J. Cereb. Blood Flow Metab.*, 7, 806, 1987.
176. Hougaard, K., Hansen, A., and Brodersen, P., The effect of ketamine on regional cerebral blood flow in man, *Anesthesiology*, 41, 562, 1974.
177. Takeshita, H., Okuda, Y., and Sari, A., The effects of ketamine on cerebral circulation and metabolism in man, *Anesthesiology*, 36, 69, 1972.
178. Stephan, H. et al., Effect of Disoprivan (propofol) on the circulation and oxygen consumption of the brain and CO_2 reactivity of brain vessels in the human, *Anaesthesist*, 36, 60, 1987.
179. Vandesteene, A. et al., Effect of propofol on cerebral blood flow and metabolism in man, *Anaesthesia*, (Suppl. 43), 42, 1988.
180. Algotsson, L. et al., Cerebral blood flow and oxygen consumption during isoflurane and halothane anesthesia in man, *Acta Anaesthesiol. Scand.*, 32, 15, 1988.
181. Drummond, J. C. et al., A comparison of the direct cerebral vasodilating potencies of halothane and isoflurane in the New Zealand white rabbit, *Anesthesiology*, 65, 462, 1986.
182. Todd, M. M. and Drummond, J. C., A comparison of the cerebrovascular and metabolic effects of halothane and isoflurane in the cat, *Anesthesiology*, 60, 276, 1984.

183. Cucchiara, R. F., Theye, R. A., and Michenfelder, J. D., The effects of isoflurane on canine cerebral metabolism and blood flow, *Anesthesiology*, 40, 571, 1974.
184. Hansen, T. D. et al., The role of cerebral metabolism in determining the local cerebral blood flow effects of volatile anesthetics: evidence for persistent flow–metabolism coupling, *J. Cereb. Blood Flow Metab.*, 9, 323, 1989.
185. Schmahl, F. W., Effects of anesthetics on regional cerebral blood flow and the regional content of some metabolites of the brain cortex of the cat, *Acta Neurol. Scand.*, (Suppl. 14), 156, 1965.

11 Brain fMRI in Clinical Pharmacological Studies

Irene Tracey, Petra Schweinhardt, and Chas Bountra

CONTENTS

11.1 INTRODUCTION

There is no doubt that the academic, industrial, and government communities are recognizing the enormous potential of human brain functional MRI (fMRI) in clinical pharmacological research and drug development. Most of the major pharmaceutical industries have embraced this new technology either via academic collaborations and/or by establishing the methodology in-house. The hope is that fMRI may allow us to demonstrate a functional effect with a potential drug (enhanced or reduced activation) in specific brain regions, in relatively small numbers of patients ($n = 10-12$). If this did prove to be feasible it offers the potential to evaluate many more molecules in clinical settings quickly. This is potentially very exciting, because one of the challenges faced by the pharmaceutical industry today is the great diversity of potential targets and even greater number of new chemical entities to evaluate in patients.

In this chapter, we will provide the reader with an introduction to the physiological basis of fMRI, its strengths and weaknesses with regard to clinical pharmacological studies, and take into account particular paradigm designs and data analysis issues that might affect the utility or efficacy of the read-out obtained. In addition, we will review the literature and discuss applications of the methodology, focusing most heavily on the field of pain but also discussing stroke, Alzheimer's disease, depression, and schizophrenia.

11.2 METABOLIC FUNCTIONAL IMAGING METHODS: PET AND FMRI

Functional brain imaging methods have revolutionized our understanding of how the human brain works, exploding onto the fields of neuroscience and medicine, giving us unprecedented

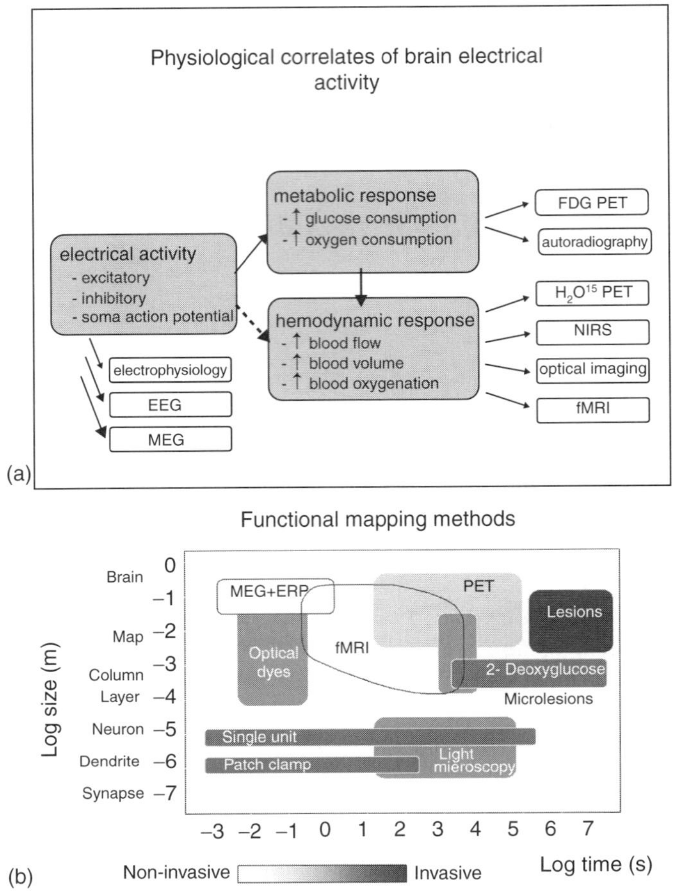

FIGURE 11.1 (a) Schematic drawing showing the physiological basis of what the major imaging methodologies measure during brain activation studies. Electroencephalography (EEG), magnetoencephalography (MEG), and invasive electrophysiology measure directly the electrical neuronal activity. In response to the neuronal electrical activity there is an increased metabolic response required to support the prior electrical activity, and several methods allow measurement of this aspect of neuronal activation; namely fluorodeoxyglucose positron emission tomography (FDG–PET) and autoradiography. Finally, to provide the oxygen and glucose needed for this increased metabolism, cerebral blood flow (CBF), blood volume (CBV), and blood oxygenation must increase, and H_2O^{15} PET, near-infrared spectroscopy, optical imaging and functional magnetic resonance imaging (fMRI) measure these changes. (b) Schematic drawing displaying key factors to be taken into consideration when performing a brain imaging experiment: spatial and temporal resolution as they relate to degree of invasiveness.

opportunities to see the human brain in action [1–3]. There is a growing range of methodologies available, each with pros and cons (see also Chapter 10, Section 10.1). Figure 11.1a displays the physiological correlates of brain electrical activity, and the corresponding available methods to measure them. Other methods not shown here but equally important for assessing function within the human brain include magnetic resonance spectroscopy (MRS) [4,5], diffusion weighted imaging, and tractography [6–8] (see also Chapter 10, Section 10.2.5). Their potential application to clinical pharmacological studies is similarly being realized at present but a discussion of this is outside the remit of this chapter.

There is considerable evidence that local cerebral blood flow (CBF) changes reflect variations in local synaptic activity, as measured using positron emission tomography (PET) [9].

Functional MRI is a method for determining which parts of the brain are activated by different types of physical sensation or activity, such as sight, sound, or movement of a subject, as well as areas responding to cognitive tasks and activation by other means (such as drug administration). The MR signal or brightness of functional MRI images depends on the local cerebral hemodynamics. The MR signal is strongly influenced by the oxygenation state of the blood, known as blood oxygen level dependency (BOLD). It is this endogenous image contrast which allows us to distinguish between active and less active brain regions both in space and time. Several physiological changes occur alongside an increase in brain activity. Glucose consumption, oxygen consumption, CBF, and cerebral blood volume (CBV) increase locally. The fraction of oxygen extracted from the blood increases, which leads to an over-compensatory increase in CBF. Consequently, the local ratio between oxyhemoglobin and deoxyhemoglobin actually rises. Oxy- and deoxyhemoglobin differ in their magnetic properties. Deoxyhemoglobin produces a greater loss of MR signal than oxyhemoglobin. The net effect of the increase in brain activity is thus a small rise in the MR signal. The peak of this signal typically occurs around 6 to 9 sec after a brief stimulus. These changes are commonly referred to as the BOLD response. The effects of local increases in blood flow and microvascular oxygenation in the region of activation are mapped as a change in raw image intensity. Therefore, the BOLD signal reflects simultaneously changes in local CBF and variations in the deoxyhemoglobin/oxyhemoglobin ratio [10]. Reviews by Howseman and Bowtell [11] and by Jezzard et al. [1] describe in detail these techniques, explaining the contrast mechanisms that enable signal detection (see also Section 10.2 of Chapter 10).

More recently, the neurophysiological basis of the BOLD response has been further investigated and the findings confirm that the BOLD contrast mechanism reflects the input and intracortical processing of a given brain area [12]. However, it should be recognized here that precise changes in neuronal activation or metabolism are not directly observed with fMRI. Indeed, the exact coupling mechanism between neuronal activity and the hemodynamic changes is not entirely understood. This is important when interpreting clinical pharmacological studies and the actual site of drug action. A change in local or global CBF might occur as a consequence of the drug that is unrelated to its direct effect on neuronal function. This would produce a change in the fMRI response (either in a baseline study or during an active paradigm to assess brain function to a task and its effect during drug administration) that is not specific to a drug-neuron interaction. Controlling for such confounds is critical if we are to interpret the data correctly and this will be discussed further in the next section (see also Chapter 10, Section 10.1).

Figure 11.1b displays how invasiveness, spatial, and temporal resolutions interact across various brain imaging methods, showing a clear trade-off between invasiveness and spatial/temporal resolution. It is clear from Figure 11.1b that fMRI scores reasonably well both spatially and temporally, and in addition is completely noninvasive. This is key to its application in clinical pharmacological studies where often the kinetics of drug action, experimental design issues, or access to patients means that multiple sessions are needed across a relatively long time period for the same subject. As fMRI is noninvasive this is of no consequence, short of patient or subject discomfort. Patients can therefore be followed and imaged several times during the course of their disease progression or therapeutic intervention.

The broad range of sophisticated cognitive and neurophysiological experiments that fMRI has allowed to be performed has expanded our knowledge of brain function and extended enormously the early PET literature. A review of the results of these experiments, along with the pros and cons of PET vs. fMRI, is not relevant here; however, there are several excellent reviews and books that cover the basic principles, methods, and scientific contributions that fMRI and PET have made to neuroscience [1–3,13–16].

11.3 PHARMACOLOGICAL FMRI, PARADIGM DESIGN, AND DATA ANALYSIS

Pharmacological fMRI (phFMRI) is the combination of administering drugs with the collection of fMRI data. Although this nomenclature is becoming widely used it is not yet fully accepted as the only term for combining drugs with MRI studies. Pharmacological fMRI may be used to study a range of effects that a particular drug may have on the brain, for example, the measurement of drug-induced CBF changes or metabolic changes as determined using MRS. In this chapter, we restrict our examination to fMRI techniques using endogenous image contrast, which are applied to study pharmacological effects. Such investigations aim to determine either a direct modulation of regional brain activation through centrally acting drugs or an indirect modulation of regional brain activation by altered afferent input after treatment with peripherally acting drugs. The techniques described may be used in future to investigate sites and mechanisms of drug action directly in humans and animals and to establish novel pharmacokinetic and pharmacodynamic parameters. We have been developing, with success, some of these novel methods using standard compounds during various proof-of-concept studies [17–21].

Centrally active drugs may produce one or more of the following effects that influence the fMRI BOLD image contrast within the brain (see also Chapter 10, Section 10.4):

1. Global changes in parameters such as CBF, CBV, and blood oxygenation, arising from physiological changes such as heart rate, blood pressure, or respiration rate
2. Local changes of the BOLD signal resulting from drug-induced alterations of the neurovascular coupling
3. Local changes in CBF or CBV resulting directly from local drug binding
4. Local changes in CBF or CBV resulting from modifications of neuronal activity

It is the last of these effects which is of most interest in human pharmacological studies. Experimentally, we may choose to control for or eliminate the effects of global changes so that they do not disrupt our observation of local changes reflecting the drug action on the functional neuroanatomy [22]. The need to isolate local changes resulting from drug administration, particularly in neuronal activity, has led to two basic approaches to phFMRI studies.

The simplest phFMRI approach employs a long resting or baseline fMRI image sequence taken during placebo followed by drug infusion. The placebo and drug infusion periods are then compared. There are several problems associated with this resting baseline, such as the reality of a resting baseline, ordering effects due to the kinetics of drug action, and subject motion to name a few [18]. Nevertheless, several studies have been conducted using this approach, and as long as care is taken when interpreting the data, useful information can be obtained. For example, Breiter et al. [23] looked at the acute effects of cocaine on human brain activity and emotion using a double-blind cocaine and saline infusion protocol in cocaine-dependent subjects while imaging the entire brain for 5 min before and for 13 min after infusion. This simple approach revealed focal signal increases and decreases in many brain areas suspected of being involved with feelings of rush, craving, and addiction (for example, ventral tegmentum, pons, nucleus accumbens, right parahippocampal gyrus, and amygdala). This study clearly demonstrated at an early point the ability of phFMRI to map dynamic patterns of brain activation following cocaine infusion and provided evidence of dynamically changing brain networks associated with cocaine-induced euphoria and cocaine-induced craving. Although the underlying cause of the fMRI signal change cannot be unequivocally assigned during these baseline studies, they nevertheless provide valuable human *in vivo* information for the pharmaceutical industry. First, they show that the drug has central effects that are large and measurable, although it should be remembered that this does not prove that the drug has bound centrally. This is important, as currently there are no noninvasive methods to determine whether a novel compound has measurable central effects in the human brain. Second, the spatial localization of fMRI allows these effects to be localized to regions approximately $3 \times 3 \times 3$ mm^3

large, which means that the specificity of the effect for novel compounds can also be determined. Finally, the temporal nature of fMRI means that the time course of action for the drug can be determined based on the brain signal change we measure rather than on direct binding data for the drug. To obtain this latter information the analysis of the data is more complex, and does not rely on simple subtraction of baseline data during placebo from data collected during drug infusion.

A more appropriate procedure for the analysis of phFMRI data from the resting baseline approach is the waveform analysis protocol (WAP) developed by Bloom et al. [24]. Their motivation for this novel procedure stems from the fact that a drug's pharmacokinetic or time-related changes in drug concentration in the blood stream or in other body compartments are measurable, predictable, and known for most commonly used drugs. Therefore, they devised an alternative means of signal detection using an input function relying on the single-dose pharmacokinetics of a drug of interest. They describe a waveform detection procedure based upon a pharmacokinetic algorithm and its application to detect changes in regional brain activation following acute nicotine administration. WAP is applied to every voxel within the brain to produce activation maps that can be displayed using any of the calculated waveform parameters.

A non-stimulation baseline phFMRI study to determine which brain areas respond to increasing, cumulative-dosing of nicotine has been performed by Stein et al. [25] using the WAP methodology. A dose-dependent increase in activation was found in the following areas: nucleus accumbens, amygdala, cingulate, and frontal lobes. They claim that activation in these structures is consistent with nicotine's behavior-arousing and behavior-reinforcing properties in humans, and again highlights the power of phFMRI and novel analysis methods to determine highly localized effects of drugs within the human brain noninvasively. In summary, resting phFMRI methods can produce useful results, but have yet to be exploited in drug discovery studies. Growing interest in this field means, however, that we can expect to see many such studies in the future.

The second phFMRI approach employs an activation paradigm specifically to highlight brain areas of activation to a specific cognitive, sensory, or motor task. The tasks are performed under the influence of both the drug and a suitable placebo and the task-related activity is compared during these two periods in controls and patients. This approach provides more specific results than the baseline resting method since it reveals the effects of the drug in question on the particular task-related functional neuroanatomy. Simplistically, there would be an influence of the drug on subject performance of the task, and the underlying brain changes accounting for this change in performance would then be identified.

"Functional MRI is limited by its ability to measure hemodynamic changes through the BOLD signal". However as mentioned earlier, if the drug has a global effect on the hemodynamic\ response, this confound must be removed prior to interpreting specific drug effects on areas of activation in response to the activation paradigm. Three strategies used to deal with this problem are:

1. To determine the BOLD changes without ANY activation paradigm (i.e., only off condition) with and without drug
2. Incorporate a control task, such as a visual checkerboard to determine nonspecific effects on activation due to the drug
3. Include other imaging sequences to determine general blood flow and blood volume changes due to the drug prior to performing more complex activation paradigms

For drugs of abuse, such as cocaine and heroin, as well as for anesthetics, where large physiological changes in, e.g., heart rate and blood pressure occur, these control conditions are especially important, as highlighted in a recent study [17]. In future studies it might therefore be necessary to include other imaging sequences to determine general blood flow, blood volume changes due to the drug prior to performing more complex activation paradigms.

There are two final methodological considerations which relate specifically to data analysis. The first is whether the drug is to be administered acutely or chronically. When given acutely within one imaging session, it is relatively easy to analyze the data off and on drug without confounds of changing task performance, scanner drift, shifting baseline, and signal-to-noise ratio that do certainly occur across time in a multiple-session design. However, for many compounds, particularly orally given drugs, the time courses preclude such simple designs and the data collected might be off or on drug (perhaps with the drug at different concentrations depending upon the kinetics) at different time points. As fMRI is not a quantitative procedure it has until recently been difficult to perform data analysis across sessions in a meaningful way so that these confounds and noise variances are removed and activation changes to a task on and off drug can be robustly compared across time [26]. To obtain meaningful data of drug action in an experimental group of controls or patients, the results of which can be extrapolated to a wider population statistically requires at least 12 subjects in each arm and an analysis of random group effects to be performed [26]. The second consideration is what to measure in the fMRI signal that might best reflect a drug effect. There are several obvious candidate markers:

- Volume of activation as defined either within a functional or anatomical mask
- Change in amplitude of signal change for all or a certain percentage of pixels with a functionally or anatomically defined region of interest
- Shift in position of peak of activation to a different area

Combinations of these markers have also been proposed, not necessarily with regard to phFMRI, but just in terms of defining differential task-induced brain activation changes in a quantitative fashion [1]. The problem of what to measure becomes acute when measuring a potentially small drug effect. Complexities of local or global confounds in the signal unrelated to the effect on function one wants to measure, noise due to multiple sessions, and differential effects in functional brain regions that may be large or small in spatial extent thereby producing different degrees of dilution or partial volume effects, has meant that no consensus within the fMRI community on how to proceed has been established. However, developments in analysis procedures are progressing [1].

Having given a background to the methodology we shall now discuss a spectrum of clinical pharmacological studies that have been performed to date.

11.4 APPLICATIONS OF PHARMACOLOGICAL FMRI IN CLINICAL RESEARCH AND DRUG DEVELOPMENT

Medical treatment, irrespective of the underlying disease, is predominantly directed towards restoration of function and alleviation of unpleasant symptoms (e.g., pain). FMRI and phFMRI of the human brain are potentially useful in all clinical studies aimed at one of these objectives. The following strategy is the most obvious and promising approach to investigate restoration of function through treatment: First, a sign that is both indicative of the disease and can be exploited in an imaging environment has to be determined. Good examples are declined working memory in Alzheimer's disease or ipsilateral motor cortex involvement during voluntary movement in subcortical stroke. The brain activation pattern characteristic for this task needs to be established in healthy volunteers, either prior to the investigation of patients or simultaneously. Also, unspecific drug effects should be characterized in healthy controls. Patients can be investigated either before and after treatment or at several time points during the course of therapy. Full or partial normalization of brain activity indicates successful treatment which can be simultaneously confirmed with improved task performance, in conjunction with clinical measures.

With regard to pain, the case is slightly different as clinical pain can only be mimicked inadequately in healthy subjects and therefore patients have to serve as their own controls.

11.4.1 Alzheimer's Disease and Mild Cognitive Impairment

Alzheimer's disease (AD) is clinically characterized by loss of mental functions and behavioral changes, dominated by progressive, chronic memory loss (see also Chapter 7, Section 7.3). Hippocampal atrophy and degeneration of cholinergic axons are the pathohistological hallmarks of the disease. Dying brain cells cause an increase in glutamate concentration which in turn can lead to death of formerly unaffected cells. Currently approved treatment strategies address these biochemical disturbances and either enhance cholinergic activity by inhibition of the enzyme acetylcholinesterase (AChE) (rivastigmine, donezepil, galantamine) or exhibit NMDA-receptor antagonism (memantine). Rivastigmine has been shown to provoke an increase of activation in prefrontal cortex and the face recognition area (fusiform gyrus) during a working memory task and a face encoding task, respectively [27]. This is of particular interest as subjects in this study received only a single dose of 3 mg, which is half of the minimum daily dosage that has been shown to be clinically effective in large multicenter trials [28,29]. Unfortunately, the MRI study suffered from patient drop out and was therefore not fully counterbalanced, but if results can be replicated in further studies, phFMRI has proved itself to be a more sensitive tool than some clinical outcome measures used in phase III drug development trials.

Mild cognitive impairment (MCI) is characterized in its typical amnestic form by isolated memory impairment and memory complaints in the context of otherwise normal cognition and normal daily functioning [30]. Structural changes are similar to those seen in AD, although less pronounced [31,32]. Approximately half of the patients diagnosed with MCI develop AD or another type of dementia within 5 years [30]. Saykin et al. [33] showed that working memory performance in patients with MCI improved on short-term treatment (6 weeks) with donezepil. The improvement in task performance was correlated with the increase in frontal fMRI activity, further supporting the hypothesis of affected frontal-temporal circuitry in impaired cognitive function [33].

11.4.2 Depression

Clinical depression is the most common psychiatric disorder. Pharmaceutical treatment strategies include tricyclic antidepressants, serotonin noradrenaline reuptake inhibitors (SNRIs), and selective serotonin reuptake inhibitors (SSRIs), all of them thought to restore neurotransmitter imbalances in the brain. Several studies to date have shown normalization of brain activation in patients treated with antidepressant agents [34–37]. Hyperactivity in limbic structures such as the amygdala in response to viewing pictures with negative valences has been shown to be reduced within 2 weeks of treatment with the SSRIs fluoxetine and sertraline, with evidence for further changes at 8 weeks [35,37]. This indicates that phFMRI is an adequate tool to study treatment effects in this patient population in a longitudinal study design. Furthermore, fMRI might be useful to predict effectiveness of a drug on a single-subject basis. In a well-conducted study, Davidson et al. [34] found that responsiveness of individual patients to venlafaxine was related to their baseline anterior cingulate gyrus activation. The possibility of tailoring therapy to an individual, based on an initial fMRI scan, would be of great clinical and economical benefit.

11.4.3 Schizophrenia

Schizophrenia is a mental illness that is among the world's top ten causes of long-term disability. The cause of the disease remains unknown and differentiating primary events from epiphenomena has been difficult [38,39]. Antipsychotic medications, in concert with psychosocial treatment, are the mainstay for managing schizophrenia. Efficacy of typical antipsychotic drugs, such as chlorpromazine and haloperidol, is highly correlated with their affinity for postsynaptic dopamine (D_2)-receptors [40], but the widespread dopaminergic antagonism frequently causes serious side effects, including parkinsonian symptoms and neuroleptic-induced tardive dyskinesia. The introduction of atypical antipsychotics has led to improved treatment efficacy and reduced side effects, but the neurobiological differences between the two classes of neuroleptics remain unknown.

PhFMRI offers the possibility of studying the different mechanisms of drug action and thereby deepening our understanding of the disease. Honey et al. [41] tested the hypothesis that substitution of typical with atypical antipsychotics reverses a hypodopaminergic state in the frontal cortex, held responsible for impaired cognitive performance which is a core symptom of schizophrenia (which was formerly termed dementia praecox). Using a verbal working memory task, they could show that frontal function in patients was significantly enhanced after drug substitution with the atypical antipsychotic risperidone, although no change in task performance could be detected [41]. However, cognitive improvement with risperidone had been shown previously in larger patient samples [42]. Taken together, this suggests a higher sensitivity of fMRI for detection of subtle treatment effects that are missed when using standard behavioral measures to assess disease load or treatment efficacy. A supplementary strategy of enhancing cognitive function in schizophrenic patients is the use of anticholinergic drugs, commonly used in AD (see Section 11.4.1). Donezepil, an AChE-inhbitor, did indeed enhance prefrontal activity in a verbal fluency task when added to atypical antipsychiotic treatment. This effect was still present when compared with placebo, which itself led to activity increases in various brain regions [43].

The next example emphasizes the importance of randomized and controlled conditions for the study of drug effects, although this is often difficult to achieve in clinical settings. When studying effects of neuroleptic medication, it is particularly important to control for unspecific drug effects as neuroleptics are known to alter cerebral metabolism and blood flow severely [44,45]. Including a control group in a study of drug-naive schizophrenic patients and treated patients using a simple motor task allowed the authors to differentiate between increased activation due to untreated schizophrenia and a deficit in activity due to neuroleptic agents [46].

It has been hypothesized that cortical cytoarchitectural abnormalities found in schizophrenia lead to abnormal neuronal connectivity [39]. FMRI findings in schizophrenia do indeed suggest a disruption in functional circuits [47], which is further supported by a phFMRI study showing partial restoration of cerebellar circuits by treatment with the atypical neuroleptic olanzapine [48].

11.4.4 Ischemic Stroke

It has been demonstrated that intracerebral reorganization occurs after stroke in humans [49,50], and many efforts have been made to modulate this reorganization in injured brains. The pharmacological agents amphetamine, methylphenidate, and the SSRI fluoxetine have all been shown to be beneficial for motor recovery in conjunction with physical therapy [51–53]. A prospective, double-blind, placebo-controlled crossover study combining fluoxetine and fMRI in response to a finger tapping task found that a single dose was enough to modulate cerebral sensory-motor activation in patients. This redistribution of activation toward the motor cortex output was associated with an enhancement of motor performance [54].

11.4.5 Pain

Over the past several decades, the pharmaceutical industry, government-funded research councils, charitable organizations, and a variety of patient bodies have funded novel analgesic drug discovery to the tune of several billion pounds. To date, the drugs available to patients consist of mu opioid agonists, nonsteroidal antiinflammatory drugs (NSAIDs) (e.g., aspirin, ibuprofen, and diclofenac, all inhibitors of both cyclooxygenase 1 and 2), selective inhibitors of cyclooxygenase 2 (e.g., celecoxib), paracetamol (which is not an inhibitor of either cyclooxygenase isoform), gabapentin, a variety of anticonvulsants (e.g., lamotrigine), and tricyclic antidepressants (e.g., amitryptilline). Other agents include local anesthetics, such as lidocaine (nonselective sodium channel blockers), which cannot be taken orally or in a chronic manner. For many of the above-mentioned clinically used medicines there is still much discussion about the mode (molecular target) or site of action (peripheral nerve terminal, dorsal root ganglion, second order dorsal horn neurones, supraspinal sites, or descending/ascending projections linking spinal cord and brain, or indeed peripheral immune cells) [55–57].

From a patient perspective, neither of these parameters is particularly important. All the patient is concerned with is efficacy (onset, ceiling, duration of action), safety, and tolerability. Of course, recognizing that most chronic pain sufferers are the elderly proportion of society (rheumatoid arthritis, osteoarthritis, chronic back pain, various neuropathies, e.g., postherpetic neuralgia, diabetic neuropathy), makes the safety and tolerability hurdle particularly challenging. Invariably these patients have other age-related conditions which may have a negative impact on the optimal functioning of major systems in the body.

The physician would like a drug that requires minimum dose titration and has an acceptable risk-benefit profile in a large proportion of patients. Researchers are interested in trying to identify novel molecular targets or combinations of targets that have an efficacy and/or safety advantage over existing treatments. Historically, this has proved to be not very easy. Academic and industrial partnerships have progressed several chemical entities, often with a novel mode of action (e.g., neurokinin NK1 receptor antagonists), into a variety of patient groups (migraine, neuropathic pain, pain associated with osteoarthritis or rheumatoid arthritis). These large clinical studies have been spectacularly unsuccessful and therefore, questions have been asked regarding the following potential problems associated with such studies.

(i) The Predictive Utility of Preclinical Models — In Terms of Both Efficacy and Safety

Often, preclinical efficacy studies are relatively acute (a few days, a maximum of a few weeks), whereas the patients we are trying to treat have often had progressively deteriorating conditions over several years, or indeed decades, and the behavioral readouts are prone to subjective error [58–60]. Another caveat of preclinical assay systems, i.e. animal models, is that changes in pain threshold to an exogenous stimulus (e.g., mechanical pressure or increased temperature) are assessed following a local inflammation or nerve injury. We cannot easily or reliably, in such systems, measure spontaneous or ongoing pain. It is this which is often most debilitating for patients.

(ii) Was the Dose Evaluated Clinically, Appropriate to Produce the Desired Pharmacological Effect at the Target Tissue?

This question is intellectually and technically very challenging. Often in such clinical studies the dose evaluated tends to be the maximum well-tolerated dose in young healthy volunteers (not patients). This dose in humans may not be sufficient to achieve the right concentration, at the right site (e.g., specific thalamic nuclei), for the right length of time to produce the desired pharmacodynamic effect. Indeed, in preclinical species it is sometimes feasible to escalate the dose in an acute setting, to produce an analgesic or antihyperalgesic effect. This may be possible because our ability to assess safety/tolerability in lower species is very limited (e.g., we cannot measure nausea or migraine) and the blood-brain barrier in animals may be less restrictive.

(iii) Was the New Molecule Evaluated in the Right Patient Group or Subgroup?

We all recognize that pain, as a symptom, is immensely heterogeneous. Patients can report hyperalgesia (exaggerated pain response to a normally painful stimulus), allodynia (painful response to a normally innocuous stimulus), spontaneous or ongoing pain, pain on contact (incident pain), pain at a noninjured site (referred pain), pain at the injured site (primary), or in its immediate vicinity (secondary). Many of these responses can be evoked or altered by environmental temperature changes, can alter during the course of the day or with changes in mood (depression, anxiety). This means that selection of a completely homogeneous group of patients is very difficult. This is in complete contrast to *in vivo* preclinical studies, where, for example rodents are of the same age and sex, have very similar weight, and have the same injury applied at approximately the same time, and so on. The understanding of this patient heterogeneity in terms of symptomatology, etiology, or indeed, pathophysiology is of great interest to all researchers. However, it also has major implications for the first clinical study to be conducted with a novel chemical entity.

FMRI being a functional readout can be applied to understand supraspinal mechanisms in volunteers, patients, and animals in a noninvasive manner [61,62]. This technique therefore gives us an opportunity to correlate objectively disease mechanisms in animals with those in human volunteers or patients [63]. Such understanding will undoubtedly help address the first and last points above. If we can use this technology, for example, to select a group or subgroup of patients exhibiting similar or supraspinal activation maps in response to a defined mechanical or thermal stimulus [56,64–73], then this will be a major advance for drug development. FMRI may also allow us to demonstrate a functional effect with a potential drug (enhanced or reduced activation) in specific brain regions, in relatively small numbers of patients ($n = 10–12$). Early studies suggest this might be true (see below), and if this does prove feasible it offers the potential to evaluate many more molecules in clinical settings quickly. This is relevant as there is a great diversity of potential targets and an even greater number of new chemical entities to evaluate in patients, therefore the challenge faced by the pharmaceutical industry is to get a fast and reliable, objective readout promptly so that reliable go or no-go decisions can be made.

To date, a few studies have been performed to evaluate the utility of phFMRI for assessing efficacy of analgesic compounds. Wise et al. [20] investigated the effect of the μ-opioid receptor agonist remifentanil on the fMRI response and pain perception of acute experimental pain in healthy volunteers. Increasing doses of the drug produced a cumulative reduction of activation in response to short noxious stimuli in pain-processing brain regions such as the insular cortex and cingulate gyrus. Interestingly, pertinent pain ratings decreased less than the amount of activation suggesting that the fMRI signal is a more sensitive measure of the drug effect than conscious pain perception [18,19]. This is a key observation that has important implications for proof-of-concept studies in the early phases of drug discovery (phase II), where the behavioral clinical measure could lack validity due to the wrong parameter being assessed or the measure could lack the sensitivity to detect subtle drug effects. Harnessing phFMRI at early stages could provide key data to support drug efficacy and guide dosing. Further studies of the same group enabled the development of a paradigm and analysis procedure to determine noninvasively and spatially a novel pharmacodynamic parameter based upon the time course of remifentanil effect on pain processing within the human brain [21]. Figure 11.2a and Figure 11.2b and Figure 11.3a and Figure 11.3b highlight some of the key findings from these studies.

Generally, the subjective perception of acute experimental pain is very well reflected by the hemodynamic response measured both with PET [74,75] and fMRI [76,77]. We recently confirmed a close relationship between the fMRI response and the subjective pain perception also for allodynic pain in neuropathic pain patients [78]. To date, only preliminary data of one study investigating the effect of analgesic agents on brain activation in a clinical population have been published [79]. Four fibromyalgia patients were studied before and after treatment with the

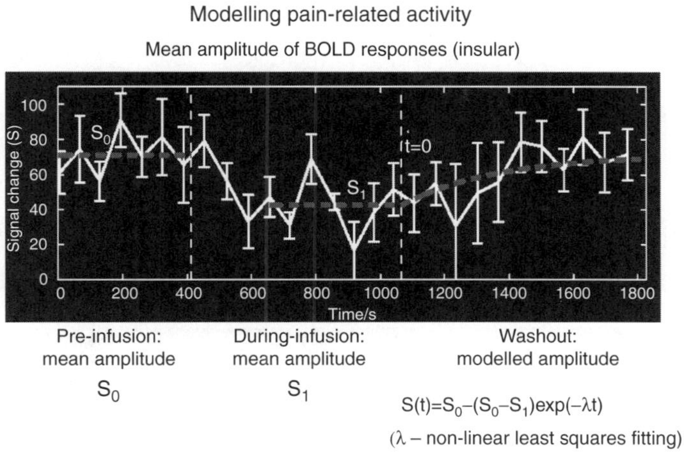

(a)

	fMRI BOLD response	Perceived pain intensity
Equilibration half-life($t_{1/2}I$) (min)	1.83 (–2.17, 5.83)	2.80 (–0.12, 5.73)
"Washout" half-life($t_{1/2}W$) (min)	3.07 (1.09, 5.05)	2.80 (1.12, 4.48)

$t_{1/2}$keo from: EEG 1.6 ± 0.9 min, analgesia 1.3 ± 1.5 min

(b) $t_{1/2}$ from: EEG 3-5 min, plasma conc 3.2 ± 0.9 min

FIGURE 11.2 (a) Time course of the mean amplitude of the BOLD response to pain during the course of remifentanil sessions. Each point represents the response to one stimulus. Error bars indicate the standard error (SE) of the mean across subjects. Vertical broken lines indicate the onset and cessation of remifentanil infusion, respectively. Heavy broken red lines indicate the fitted exponential models from which the onset equilibrium half-life and washout half-life of drug effect on pain activity were estimated. (b) Pharmacokinetic-pharmacodynamic parameters of remifentanil derived from fMRI BOLD response amplitude and reported pain intensity. (Reproduced from Wise, R. G., Williams, P., and Tracey, I., *Neuropsychopharmacology*, 29, 626, 2004. Courtesy of Wise, R. G. et al. With permission of Nature Publishing Group.)

5-HT_3-receptor antagonist tropisetron. Treatment reduced activation in response to a mechanical pain stimulus in pain-relevant areas, but yielded reduced pain ratings in only two patients. Although this is a potentially very interesting result, pointing at the high sensitivity of imaging, the order of the pre- and posttreatment scans was not randomized, a crucial prerequisite for the interpretation of such data. In a study from our own laboratory [78], pain intensity of neuropathic pain patients was modulated by alteration of the patients (co-) analgesic medication following a randomized protocol. The results not only show that the fMRI signal in pain-processing areas changes accordingly to changes in pain perception but also indicate a relatively larger change of the objective imaging measure than subjective perception. Further analysis is in progress but these findings again illustrate the utility of phFMRI for potentially providing an early readout of drug effect.

Finally, phFMRI has also been used with promising results in other disease entities, such as attention deficit hyperactivity disorder [80] and temporal lobe epilepsy [81], as summarized in a recent review by Honey and Bullmore [82]. Studies of Parkinsons's disease showed restoration of activation in motor cortex [83] and amygdala [84], and investigated presynaptic dopamine and cortical efficiency [85,86]. These applications and those more fully discussed above, highlight the fact that an improved understanding of clinical disease mechanisms will have a major impact on our

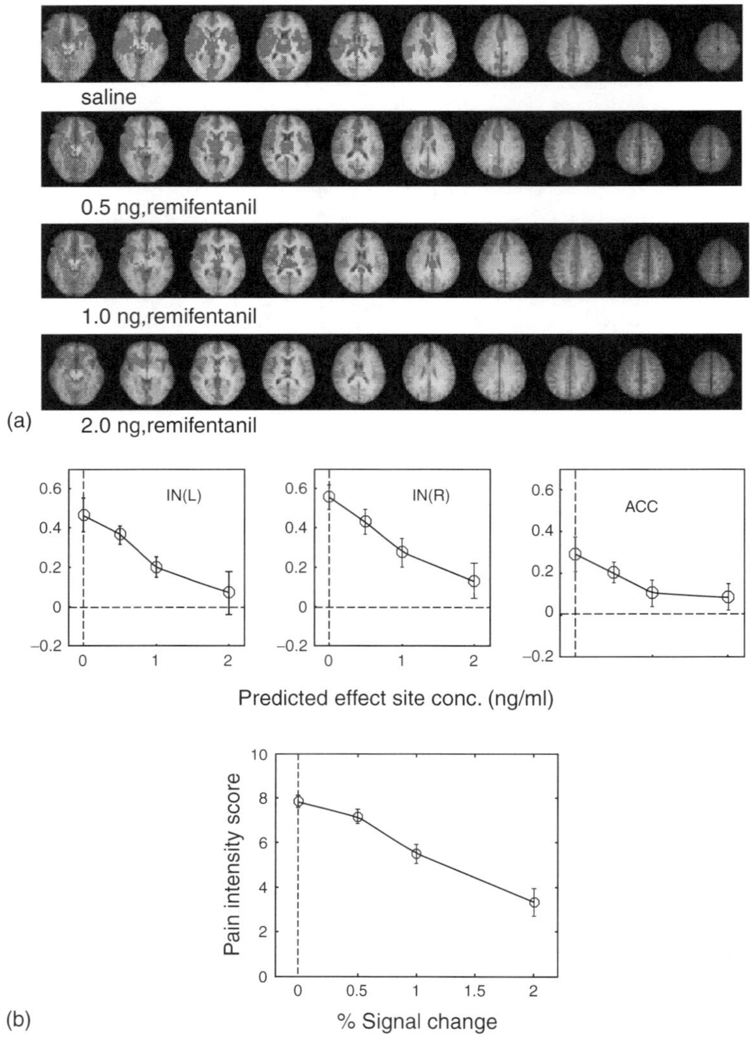

FIGURE 11.3 (a) Representative thermal pain related activity within a group of right-handed healthy subjects at increasing doses of remifenantil effector site concentration. (b) Representative group mean BOLD signal change against predicted effector site concentration. Only a few regions are shown (IN = insula cortex (left and right hemisphere); ACC = anterior cingulate cortex) to illustrate the sensitivity gains of fMRI vs. subjective rating. (Reproduced from Tracey, I. et al., Imaging analgesia: an FMRI study to investigate the relationship of increasing doses of remifentanil on pain-induced brain activation and perception, in review 2005. With permission.)

ability to identify new molecular targets and pathways for therapeutic intervention, or in pharmaceutical industry language, target identification or validation. There is no doubt that phFMRI will be an important tool in this process.

11.5 CONCLUSIONS

This chapter focused on pharmacological fMRI as a tool for the investigation of drug effects, but other methodologies, including MRS, Diffusion Tensor Imaging and EEG, are available and might have important roles to play in the development of pharmacological functional imaging. Combination of these techniques with phFMRI will increase our confidence in the conclusions we draw from phFMRI. For instance, it is of great importance to use direct measures of brain activity, such as EEG, to better understand the coupling between neuronal activity and the hemodynamic response to which fMRI is sensitive, i.e., the BOLD response, because it is the neuronal effects of centrally acting pharmacological agents that ultimately interest us. This coupling relationship has not yet been well characterized in humans under differing physiological conditions and we know little about how drug-induced changes in the fMRI response relate to non-neuronal drug effects rather than specific drug-induced changes in neuronal activity (see also Chapter 10, Section 10.1). Neurovascular coupling incorporates neurovascular signaling and vascular reactivity. The simultaneous collection of fMRI and EEG data will allow testing the hypothesis that complex neuronal responses do not show a fixed neurovascular coupling under the influence of physiological and pharmacological challenges. This will refine a future strategy for interpreting pharmacological fMRI studies, which are still in their infancy [87]. If we are to understand central drug effects then we have also to image functional activation within the human spinal cord. Such studies are feasible [88], however, to date there are no published studies combining fMRI of the spinal cord with a pharmacological challenge. There is an exciting future, however, for this field once technical and data analysis hurdles have been more fully overcome.

Brain phMRI has been performed in several major neurological and psychiatric diseases and has been proven to be an appropriate tool to monitor restoration of function due to pharmacological treatment. First results from studies investigating drug-induced pain alleviation are promising and show that phMRI will probably be equally useful in the study of analgesic agents. There are now several studies from a wide range of diseases indicating that phMRI and fMRI are more sensitive outcome measures than the behavioral measurements commonly used in drug trials. Moreover, the predictive potential of phMRI and fMRI for treatment efficacy would offer the possibility to tailor therapy individually and also allow a screening of compounds in early phases of drug development. It is thought that this technique offers the possibility of establishing a functional central nervous system effect with a new pharmacological entry. Of course, this may be mediated via a peripheral site of action (peripheral nerve terminals), but such early readouts of a pharmacodynamic effect could save the industry several tens of millions of pounds, and avoid the unnecessary exposure of patients/volunteers to molecules with limited or no therapeutic value. We are therefore optimistic regarding the utility of pharmacological fMRI in clinical studies, which is considered by the pharmaceutical industry as a key methodology for assessing drug action early in development.

REFERENCES

1. Jezzard, P., Matthews, P., and Smith, S. M., Eds., *Functional MRI: An Introduction to the Methods*, Oxford University Press, Oxford, 2001.
2. Mazziotta, J. C., Imaging: window on the brain, *Arch. Neurol.*, 57, 1413, 2000.
3. Ward, N. S. and Frackowiak, R. S., Towards a new mapping of brain cortex function, *Cerebrovasc. Dis.*, 17 (Suppl. 3), 35, 2004.
4. Di Costanzo, A. et al., High-field proton MRS of human brain, *Eur. J. Radiol.*, 48, 146, 2003.
5. Ross, A. J. and Sachdev, P. S., Magnetic resonance spectroscopy in cognitive research, *Brain Res. Brain Res. Rev.*, 44, 83, 2004.
6. Basser, P. J., Mattiello, J., and LeBihan, D., MR diffusion tensor spectroscopy and imaging, *Biophys. J.*, 66, 259, 1994.
7. Behrens, T. E. et al., Non-invasive mapping of connections between human thalamus and cortex using diffusion imaging, *Nat. Neurosci.*, 6, 750, 2003.
8. Conturo, T. E. et al., Tracking neuronal fiber pathways in the living human brain, *Proc. Natl. Acad. Sci. USA*, 96, 10422, 1999.

9. Sokoloff, L. et al., The [14C]deoxyglucose method for the measurement of local cerebral glucose utilization: theory, procedure, and normal values in the conscious and anesthetized albino rat, *J. Neurochem.*, 28, 897, 1977.
10. Rosen, B. R., Buckner, R. L., and Dale, A. M., Event-related functional MRI: past, present, and future, *Proc. Natl. Acad. Sci. USA*, 95, 773, 1998.
11. Howseman, A. M. and Bowtell, R. W., Functional magnetic resonance imaging: imaging techniques and contrast mechanisms, *Philos. Trans. R. Soc. Lond. B Biol. Sci.*, 354, 1179, 1999.
12. Logothetis, N. K. et al., Neurophysiological investigation of the basis of the fMRI signal, *Nature*, 412, 150, 2001.
13. Frackowiak, R., Friston, K. J., Frith, C. D., Dolan, R. J., and Mazziotta, J. C., Eds., *Human Brain Function*, Academic Press, San Diego, CA, 1997.
14. Mazziotta, J., Toga, A. W., Frackowiak, R. S. J., Eds., *Brain Mapping: The Disorders*, Academic Press, San Diego, CA, 2000.
15. Mazziotta, J. C., A century of imaging, *Arch. Neurol.*, 57, 58, 2000.
16. Peyron, R., Laurent, B., and Garcia-Larrea, L., Functional imaging of brain responses to pain. A review and meta-analysis (2000), *Neurophysiol. Clin.*, 30, 263, 2000.
17. Rogers, R. et al., An investigation to dissociate the analgesic and anesthetic properties of ketamine using functional magnetic resonance imaging, *Anesthesiology*, 100, 292, 2004.
18. Tracey, I., Prospects for human pharmacological functional magnetic resonance imaging (phMRI), *J. Clin. Pharmacol. Suppl.*, 41, 21S, 2001.
19. Tracey, I., Nociceptive processing in the human brain, *Curr. Opin. Neurobiol.*, 15, 478, 2005.
20. Wise, R. G. et al., Combining fMRI with a pharmacokinetic model to determine which brain areas activated by painful stimulation are specifically modulated by remifentanil, *Neuroimage*, 16, 999, 2002.
21. Wise, R. G., Williams, P., and Tracey, I., Using fMRI to quantify the time dependence of remifentanil analgesia in the human brain, *Neuropsychopharmacology*, 29, 626, 2004.
22. Stein, E. A., fMRI: a new tool for the in vivo localization of drug actions in the brain, *J. Anal. Toxicol.*, 25, 419, 2001.
23. Breiter, H. C. et al., Acute effects of cocaine on human brain activity and emotion, *Neuron*, 19, 591, 1997.
24. Bloom, A. S. et al., Determination of drug-induced changes in functional MRI signal using a pharmacokinetic model, *Hum. Brain Mapp.*, 8, 235, 1999.
25. Stein, E. A. et al., Nicotine-induced limbic cortical activation in the human brain: a functional MRI study, *Am. J. Psychiatry*, 155, 1009, 1998.
26. Smith, S. M., Overview of fMRI analysis, In *Functional MRI: An Introduction to Methods*, Jezzard, P. and Smith, S. M., Eds., Oxford University Press, Oxford, 2001.
27. Rombouts, S. A. et al., Alterations in brain activation during cholinergic enhancement with rivastigmine in Alzheimer's disease, *J. Neurol. Neurosurg. Psychiatry*, 73, 665, 2002.
28. Jann, M. W., Rivastigmine, a new-generation cholinesterase inhibitor for the treatment of Alzheimer's disease, *Pharmacotherapy*, 20, 1, 2000.
29. Spencer, C. M. and Noble, S., Rivastigmine. A review of its use in Alzheimer's disease, *Drugs Aging*, 13, 391, 1998.
30. Petersen, R. C. et al., Mild cognitive impairment: clinical characterization and outcome, *Arch. Neurol.*, 56, 303, 1999.
31. Du, A. T. et al., Magnetic resonance imaging of the entorhinal cortex and hippocampus in mild cognitive impairment and Alzheimer's disease, *J. Neurol. Neurosurg. Psychiatry*, 71, 441, 2001.
32. Jack, C. R. Jr. et al., Rates of hippocampal atrophy correlate with change in clinical status in aging and AD, *Neurology*, 55, 484, 2000.
33. Saykin, A. J. et al., Cholinergic enhancement of frontal lobe activity in mild cognitive impairment, *Brain*, 127, 1574, 2004.
34. Davidson, R. J. et al., The neural substrates of affective processing in depressed patients treated with venlafaxine, *Am. J. Psychiatry*, 160, 64, 2003.
35. Fu, C. H. et al., Attenuation of the neural response to sad faces in major depression by antidepressant treatment: a prospective, event-related functional magnetic resonance imaging study, *Arch. Gen. Psychiatry*, 61, 877, 2004.

36. Kalin, N. H. et al., Functional magnetic resonance imaging studies of emotional processing in normal and depressed patients: effects of venlafaxine, *J. Clin. Psychiatry*, 58 (Suppl. 16), 32, 1997.
37. Sheline, Y. I. et al., Increased amygdala response to masked emotional faces in depressed subjects resolves with antidepressant treatment: an fMRI study, *Biol. Psychiatry*, 50, 651, 2001.
38. Harrison, P. J. and Weinberger, D. R., Schizophrenia genes, gene expression, and neuropathology: on the matter of their convergence, *Mol. Psychiatry*, 10, 40, 2005.
39. Mueser, K. T. and McGurk, S. R., Schizophrenia, *Lancet*, 363, 2063, 2004.
40. Seeman, P. et al., Dopamine receptors in human and calf brains, using [3H]apomorphine and an antipsychotic drug, *Proc. Natl. Acad. Sci. USA*, 73, 4354, 1976.
41. Honey, G. D. et al., Differences in frontal cortical activation by a working memory task after substitution of risperidone for typical antipsychotic drugs in patients with schizophrenia, *Proc. Natl. Acad. Sci. USA*, 96, 13432, 1999.
42. Green, M. F. et al., Does risperidone improve verbal working memory in treatment-resistant schizophrenia?, *Am. J. Psychiatry*, 154, 799, 1997.
43. Nahas, Z. et al., Augmenting atypical antipsychotics with a cognitive enhancer (donepezil) improves regional brain activity in schizophrenia patients: a pilot double-blind placebo controlled BOLD fMRI study, *Neurocase*, 9, 274, 2003.
44. Bartlett, E. J. et al., Importance of pharmacologic control in PET studies: effects of thiothixene and haloperidol on cerebral glucose utilization in chronic schizophrenia, *Psychiatry Res.*, 40, 115, 1991.
45. Braus, D. F. et al., Antipsychotic drug effects on motor activation measured by functional magnetic resonance imaging in schizophrenic patients, *Schizophr. Res.*, 39, 19, 1999.
46. Muller, J. L. et al., Motor-induced brain activation in cortical, subcortical and cerebellar regions in schizophrenic inpatients. A whole brain fMRI fingertapping study, *Prog. Neuropsychopharmacol. Biol. Psychiatry*, 26, 421, 2002.
47. Yurgelun-Todd, D. A. et al., Functional magnetic resonance imaging of schizophrenic patients and comparison subjects during word production, *Am. J. Psychiatry*, 153, 200, 1996.
48. Stephan, K. E. et al., Effects of olanzapine on cerebellar functional connectivity in schizophrenia measured by fMRI during a simple motor task, *Psychol. Med.*, 31, 1065, 2001.
49. Chollet, F. et al., The functional anatomy of motor recovery after stroke in humans: a study with positron emission tomography, *Ann. Neurol.*, 29, 63, 1991.
50. Weiller, C. et al., Functional reorganization of the brain in recovery from striatocapsular infarction in man, *Ann. Neurol.*, 31, 463, 1992.
51. Dam, M. et al., Effects of fluoxetine and maprotiline on functional recovery in poststroke hemiplegic patients undergoing rehabilitation therapy, *Stroke*, 27, 1211, 1996.
52. Grade, C. et al., Methylphenidate in early poststroke recovery: a double-blind, placebo-controlled study, *Arch. Phys. Med. Rehabil.*, 79, 1047, 1998.
53. Walker-Batson, D. et al., Amphetamine paired with physical therapy accelerates motor recovery after stroke. Further evidence, *Stroke*, 26, 2254, 1995.
54. Pariente, J. et al., Fluoxetine modulates motor performance and cerebral activation of patients recovering from stroke, *Ann. Neurol.*, 50, 718, 2001.
55. Jones, A. K. and Derbyshire, S. W., Cerebral mechanisms operating in the presence and absence of inflammatory pain, *Ann. Rheum. Dis.*, 55, 411, 1996.
56. Millan, M. J., The induction of pain: an integrative review, *Prog. Neurobiol.*, 57, 1, 1999.
57. Porro, C. A. and Cavazzuti, M., Functional imaging studies of the pain system in man and animals, *Prog. Brain Res.*, 110, 47, 1996.
58. Czech, K. A. and Sagen, J., Update on cellular transplantation into the CNS as a novel therapy for chronic pain, *Prog. Neurobiol.*, 46, 507, 1995.
59. Dubuisson, D. and Dennis, S. G., The formalin test: a quantitative study of the analgesic effects of morphine, meperidine, and brain stem stimulation in rats and cats, *Pain*, 4, 161, 1977.
60. Tjolsen, A. et al., The formalin test: an evaluation of the method, *Pain*, 51, 5, 1992.
61. Chen, Y. C. et al., Detection of dopaminergic neurotransmitter activity using pharmacologic MRI: correlation with PET, microdialysis, and behavioral data, *Magn. Reson. Med.*, 38, 389, 1997.
62. Marota, J. J. et al., Cocaine activation discriminates dopaminergic projections by temporal response: an fMRI study in rat, *Neuroimage*, 11, 13, 2000.

63. Shah, Y. B. et al., Detection of cannabinoid agonist evoked increase in BOLD contrast in rats using functional magnetic resonance imaging, *Neuropharmacology*, 46, 379, 2004.
64. Binkofski, F. et al., Somatic and limbic cortex activation in esophageal distention: a functional magnetic resonance imaging study, *Ann. Neurol.*, 44, 811, 1998.
65. Davis, K. D. et al., fMRI of human somatosensory and cingulate cortex during painful electrical nerve stimulation, *Neuroreport*, 7, 321, 1995.
66. Davis, K. D., Functional MRI et al., of pain- and attention-related activations in the human cingulate cortex, *J. Neurophysiol.*, 77, 3370, 1997.
67. Davis, K. D. et al., Functional MRI study of thalamic and cortical activations evoked by cutaneous heat, cold, and tactile stimuli, *J. Neurophysiol.*, 80, 1533, 1998.
68. Hsieh, J. C. et al., Traumatic nociceptive pain activates the hypothalamus and the periaqueductal gray: a positron emission tomography study, *Pain*, 64, 303, 1996.
69. Jones, A. P. et al., Experiences with functional magnetic resonance imaging at 1 Tesla, *Br. J. Radiol.*, 71, 160, 1998.
70. Morrow, T. J. et al., Regional changes in forebrain activation during the early and late phase of formalin nociception: analysis using cerebral blood flow in the rat, *Pain*, 75, 355, 1998.
71. Porro, C. A. et al., Temporal and intensity coding of pain in human cortex, *J. Neurophysiol.*, 80, 3312, 1998.
72. Sweet, W. H., Pain — old and new methods of study and treatment, *Acta Neurochir. Suppl.*, 64, 83, 1995.
73. Xu, X. et al., Functional localization of pain perception in the human brain studied by PET, *Neuroreport*, 8, 555, 1997.
74. Coghill, R. C. et al., Pain intensity processing within the human brain: a bilateral, distributed mechanism, *J. Neurophysiol.*, 82, 1934, 1999.
75. Derbyshire, S. W. et al., Pain processing during three levels of noxious stimulation produces differential patterns of central activity, *Pain*, 73, 431, 1997.
76. Bornhovd, K. et al., Painful stimuli evoke different stimulus-response functions in the amygdala, prefrontal, insula and somatosensory cortex: a single-trial fMRI study, *Brain*, 125, 1326, 2002.
77. Craig, A. D. et al., Thermosensory activation of insular cortex, *Nat. Neurosci.*, 3, 184, 2000.
78. Peyron, R. et al., An fMRI study of cortical representation of mechanical allodynia in patients with neuropathic pain, *Neurology*, 63, 1838, 2004.
79. Koeppe, C. et al., The influence of the 5-HT3 receptor antagonist tropisetron on pain in fibromyalgia: a functional magnetic resonance imaging pilot study, *Scand. J. Rheumatol. Suppl.*, 119, 24, 2004.
80. Vaidya, C. J. et al., Selective effects of methylphenidate in attention deficit hyperactivity disorder: a functional magnetic resonance study, *Proc. Natl. Acad. Sci. USA*, 95, 14494, 1998.
81. Jokeit, H., Okujava, M., and Woermann, F. G., Carbamazepine reduces memory induced activation of mesial temporal lobe structures: a pharmacological fMRI-study, *BMC Neurol.*, 1, 6, 2001.
82. Honey, G. and Bullmore, E., Human pharmacological MRI, *Trends Pharmacol. Sci.*, 25, 366, 2004.
83. Buhmann, C. et al., Pharmacologically modulated fMRI — Cortical responsiveness to levodopa in drug-naive hemiparkinsonian patients, *Brain*, 126, 451, 2003.
84. Tessitore, A. et al., Dopamine modulates the response of the human amygdala: a study in Parkinson's disease, *J. Neurosci.*, 22, 9099, 2002.
85. Mattay, V. S. et al., Dopaminergic modulation of cortical function in patients with Parkinson's disease, *Ann. Neurol.*, 51, 156, 2002.
86. Peters, S. et al., Apomorphine reduces BOLD signal in fMRI during voluntary movement in Parkinsonian patients, *Neuroreport*, 14, 809, 2003.
87. Iannetti, G. D. et al., Simultaneous recording of laser-evoked brain potentials and continuous, high-field functional magnetic resonance imaging in humans, *Neuroimage*, 28, 708, 2005.
88. Stroman, P. W. et al., Mapping of neuronal function in the healthy and injured human spinal cord with spinal fMRI, *Neuroimage*, 17, 1854, 2002.

12 Imaging Inflammatory Processes of the Brain: Multiple Sclerosis as an Example

Martin Rausch, Iris-Katharina Penner, Cedric Berger, and Markus Rudin

CONTENTS

12.1 PHYSIOLOGICAL ASPECTS OF NEUROINFLAMMATORY PROCESSES

Several diseases of the central nervous system (CNS) are caused or at least accompanied by inflammatory processes. These processes comprise acute inflammatory events, which are supported by infiltration of brain tissue by different types of leukocytes but also by the transformation of brain residing microglia to an activated form and later also to phagocytotic cells. Immune defense in the CNS generally follows a typical layout in which the different cells of the immune system play their specific role. Immune responses are generally induced by the presence of a foreign antigen. Antigen-presenting cells (e.g., pericytes) present characteristic peptide-motifs of the antigen together with other surface signals to cells of the immune system, which consequently initiate their immunological/inflammatory response. Different types of T cells, such as cytotoxic T cells, T helper and plasma cells, are involved in this process. Moreover, cells of the monocyte phagocytic system comprising blood-borne monocytes and brain-residing microglial cells contribute to the proinflammatory processes as professional macrophages.

The recruitment of immune cells is mediated by a variety of chemotactic factors (chemokines) secreted into the circulation and of adhesion proteins (selectins, integrins) presented at the luminar surface of activated endothelial cells. The recognition of integrins by leukocytes is an important hallmark for the infiltration of inflammatory cells into the brain parenchyma (Figure 12.1a). For example, selectins such as E-selectin are responsible for tethering (slowing-down and capturing) of leukocytes in postcapillary venules, and intercellular adhesion molecules (ICAM) facilitate the arrest of leukocytes on the endothelial surface and mediate the transcytosis of leukocytes across the endothelial wall.

Inflammatory processes, and in particular neuroinflammation, are not only observed as a response to the presence of foreign antigens but also to endogenous antigens, e.g., due to mechanical damage and pathological alterations in the tissue state (see also Chapter 8, Section 8.2 and Section 8.5.5). Typically, inflammatory cells are observed in and around tumor tissue, hemorrhagic transformations, cell debris, and scar formation.

In the following we will focus on a specific neuroinflammatory disorder, multiple sclerosis (MS), which is associated with autoimmunity against myelin in the brain and spinal cord, and on the role of imaging for the characterization of the disease process and the evaluation of novel therapeutic interventions. MS comprises both neuroinflammatory and neurodegenerative aspects. While the initial phases are characterized by inflammatory events, i.e., activation of endothelium and infiltration of inflammatory cells, the chronic consequences of the disease are demyelination leading to impaired neuronal function due to compromised axonal signal processing, and finally irreversible loss of axons (Figure 12.1b).

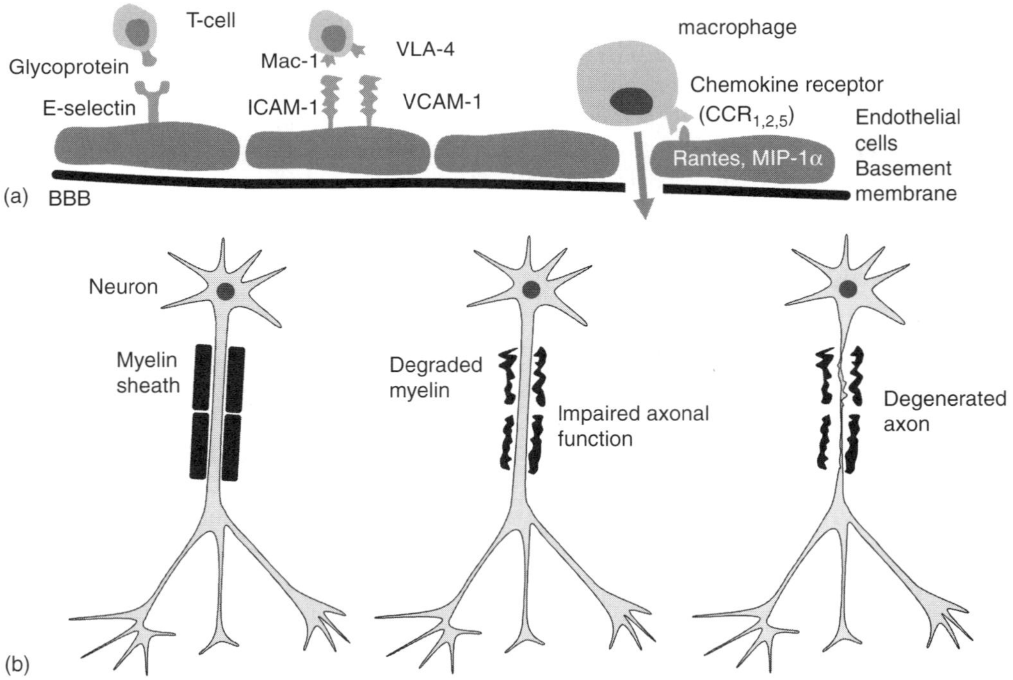

FIGURE 12.1 (a) Factors contributing to the recruitment of immune cells into the CNS. Selectins, integrins, and chemokines interact with specific receptors on leukocytes during the different stages of their recruitment. *In vivo* imaging aims at visualizing the cells themselves or the chemotactic factors. (b) Multiple sclerosis leads to the destruction of the myelin sheath of axons in the CNS and later to degeneration of axons and neurons. In a first stage, the myelin is degraded, which affects the efficient conductance of electrical signals along the axon. Later the axon itself is affected, which finally leads to necrosis of the neuron.

12.2 MULTIPLE SCLEROSIS: PATHOPHYSIOLOGY AND CLINICAL PRESENTATION

MS is an inflammatory and demyelinating disease of the CNS that predominately affects young adults and which has a genetic and environmental background. Typically, the disease is characterized by relapses where patients often present episodes of neurological and/or cognitive dysfunction. In the case of a relapsing remitting disease course these deficits can be transient and be followed by complete recovery. In the case of a progressive disease course, some deficits might persist and even aggravate with time. In fact, MS is a complex and heterogeneous disease with a phenotype that is not unitary. Not only do disease courses vary among relapsing remitting, primary progressive, and secondary progressive, but also clinical symptoms as well as domains of cognitive dysfunction. As the interpatient variability on the clinical side is high, identical therapeutic strategies cannot be applied to each individual. Pathologically, the variability is less pronounced. Characteristic features are perivascular inflammation, demyelination, and axonal loss. However, as described by Trapp and colleagues [1], different types of axonal damage can be observed in MS: inflammatory processes can lead to transient demyelination, followed by remyelination and restoration of function. But chronically demyelinated axons might also undergo degeneration and irreversible dissection. In the case of demyelination followed by regeneration, conduction slowing or failure may be a consequence that can be related to a slowing of the physical or mental abilities of patients. In the case of axonal loss, deficits may persist. The clinical or neurological deficits are quantified according to the expanded disability status scale (EDSS) [2]. However, the main tissue changes that take place within the disease process are located in the white matter. In the past, MRI has been employed as a valuable tool to detect and characterize those changes. Unfortunately, conventional MRI provides only low pathological specificity and correlations between lesion volume, atrophy, and lesion localization and clinical symptoms or cognitive measures are only moderate [3–5]. Other measures, such as functional magnetic resonance imaging (fMRI) or diffusion tensor imaging, (DTI) that focus on the brain function and fiber integrity provide more plausible data about brain damage and specific brain functions [6–8].

12.3 ANIMAL MODELS FOR MULTIPLE SCLEROSIS

In order to elucidate the underlying mechanisms of neuroinflammation a number of animal models for MS has been developed. The most prominent models are acute and chronic-relapsing experimental autoimmune encephalomyelitis (EAE) in mice, rats, and monkeys [9].

EAE can be induced by sensitization of animals with a myelin antigen, injected e.g., into the hind paw together with an adjuvant (actively induced EAE). The time course and pathology of the disease depend on the species and the type of antigen. For immunization one can either use homogenized spinal cord or myelin fragments such as myelin basic protein (MBP), proteolipid protein (PLP), or myelin-oligodendrocyte glycoprotein (MOG).

Another option is to induce EAE by administering $CD4^{+}$T cells that have been activated *in vitro* (adoptive transfer EAE). Here, the time course of the disease runs in a more synchronous mode. Moreover, this protocol highlights the importance of T cells for disease induction.

Although not being identical to all pathophysiological aspects of the human disease, EAE models nevertheless reproduce many aspects of MS [9]. While active EAE in Lewis rats induces a strong inflammatory response, it does not lead to chronic axonal damage as found in human MS. Active immunization of inbreed rats (Lewis, DA, BN) or mice (SJL, C57/Bl6 strains) leads to a relapsing-remitting time course and persistent damage of axons and is therefore more similar to the human pathology. Therefore, EAE models can be used to streamline the development and validation of novel imaging approaches suited for patient/therapy management and for testing novel therapeutic strategies.

12.4 *IN VIVO* MRI IN MULTIPLE SCLEROSIS

12.4.1 Concepts

Imaging of inflammatory events in the brain can be based on targeting various processes along the pathophysiological cascade:

1. *Targeting antigens or immune cells*: The immune cells themselves or chemokine receptors could serve as primary imaging targets, since their presence or activation in the brain is directly linked to the disease process and to the damage of brain tissue. However, due to limitations in sensitivity, cell-preparation and other technical drawbacks, *in vivo* cell tracking or receptor mapping is still a complex field, which, however, with modern target-specific imaging approaches will become feasible (see Chapter 25, Section 25.5.1).
2. *Targeting secondary markers of inflammation*: Imaging of neuroinflammation has emerged from the visualization of processes downstream of the initial inflammatory events, i.e., structural/microstructural changes in brain tissue. Markers of vascular edema, demyelination, and blood-brain barrier (BBB) damage have been extensively applied both in preclinical and clinical studies. Despite the fact that their specificity for the pathophysiology of MS remains questionable, these readouts have played, and still do, a tremendous role for the *in vivo* assessment of inflammatory diseases of the CNS due to their robustness and broad availability.

12.4.2 Imaging of Structural Changes

12.4.2.1 Assessment of BBB Leakage: Gd-Enhancing Lesions

The BBB delineates the vascular lumen from brain parenchyma and, in contrast to vessel walls in the periphery, only a few molecules can cross the intact BBB freely by diffusion. The barrier layers consist of endothelial cells with adjacent cells forming the tight junctions (*zonulae occludentes*). In addition, the BBB is composed of the basement membrane and astrocytic end-feets contacting the tight junctions from the abluminal side. While water and lipophilic substrates, such as O_2 and CO_2, can diffuse freely along their concentration gradient, uptake of nutrients such as glucose and amino acids depends on transporter systems, while other larger molecules might be taken up by specific receptor-mediated transcytosis [10,11].

Transcytosis of leukocytes from the circulation into the brain parenchyma and their associated inflammatory processes can interfere with the integrity of the BBB. This damage is specific for leukocyte infiltration under inflammatory conditions since the trans-endothelial migration of immune cells during immune surveillance does not lead to BBB damage [12]. Moreover, BBB breakdown can occur as a consequence of direct mechanic (hemorrhage) or ischemic damage of endothelial cells. BBB damage can be visualized by contrast-enhanced MRI using paramagnetic contrast agents (CAs). In most cases, low molecular weight CAs such as Gd-DOTA or Gd-DTPA are used, which have been approved for clinical use for almost two decades. These CAs are administered intravenously at a typical dose of 0.1 mmol/kg (clinical single dose). The intact BBB is impermeable for these molecules but in areas of acute inflammation CA can leak out of the blood vessels into the interstitial space, where it leads to an enhancement of longitudinal and transversal relaxation rates and therefore to a change in MR signal intensity.

Contrast-enhanced MRI plays a major role for the staging of active disease in MS patients, since it is superior in sensitivity compared with any other MRI technique, i.e., contrast-enhanced MRI detects more lesions [13]. However, the relevance of these lesions with regard to staging of MS patients and prognosis remains an open issue [14].

The ambiguous implications of Gd-enhanced MRI arise mainly from the unclear relation between lesion pathology and the mechanism of Gd-uptake [15]. In particular for neuroinflammatory diseases, the route by which CA enters the brain tissue is still not completely understood. In a study on BBB damage in an animal of chronic relapsing EAE in guinea pigs an increased number of endothelial vesicles containing Gd have been found. However, there was no evidence for opening of tight junctions in these areas [16]. Nevertheless, disruption of the tight junction complex might also contribute to the increased BBB permeability. Breakdown of occludin, zona coccludin protein ZO1, and fibrinolysis are possible factors leading to increased diffusion of molecules across the BBB [17,18]. Histological analysis of sections from EAE animals and biopsies taken from MS patients allowed comparison of regions of BBB damage with those displaying cell infiltrates. In a model of adoptive transfer EAE in the rat, during the late stage of the disease, areas of Gd-DTPA accumulation were found to match accurately regions characterized by high concentration of activated macrophages [19]. Similar results have been reported for MS patients, for whom macrophages loaded with MBP and MOG-positive degradation products were observed in tissue specimens collected from Gd-enhancing lesions. However, this study also demonstrated BBB damage for chronic MS lesions, i.e., scar tissue largely devoid of immune-competent cells [20]. This illustrates that visualization of increased BBB permeability provides a sensitive but not very specific marker for acute inflammatory processes. It should also be remembered that correlative studies of Gd-enhancement and cellular infiltration cannot provide the ultimate proof for a one-to-one correlation, because tissue samples are always taken from areas which show clear signal abnormalities in the MR images; hence, the available data are biased. The occurrence of inflammatory events of neurological relevance, i.e., infiltration of immune-competent cells into brain parenchyma, might not be associated with structural damage. At least for the rat EAE model it was shown that areas of macrophage infiltration were not affected by BBB damage as measured by administration of Gd-DOTA [21]. Such tissue areas have been defined normal-appearing white matter.

12.4.2.2 T_2 Hyperintense Lesions and Multicomponent T_2 Mapping

Enhanced transverse relaxation times (T_2) are one of the most characteristic hallmarks of MS lesions. T_2 is a sensitive but rather unspecific imaging readout [22]. Combined MRI and histopathological analysis has shown that T_2 hyperintensity can be observed during the acute, subacute, and chronic demyelinated or even remyelinated state of lesions [20]. Physiologically, T_2 prolongation can be observed as a consequence of vascular edema, which results from a redistribution of water from the vasculature into the tissue. Occurrence of a vascular edema is an important indicator of acute inflammatory processes accompanied by acute or persistent BBB damage (Figure 12.2). However, it does not necessarily imply permanent damage of white matter tracts. Staging of tissue or calculation of the lesion load on the basis of T_2-relaxation times might therefore lead to misleading results. Transition from T_2-weighted imaging to actual measurements of T_2-relaxation times might improve the tissue characterization; compartments with different pathology-specific T_2 components could be identified, which are derived from the analysis of multiexponential T_2 decay by acquiring a series of spin echoes with different echo delays [23]. The T_2-relaxation time of water protons depends on their microenvironment and decreases with decreasing overall water mobility, i.e., with increasing binding affinity to tissue. At least two components contribute to the overall T_2 values measured in affected tissue: a long T_2 component (70 to 95 msec) of (bulk) water in cytoplasmic and extracellular spaces and a short T_2 component (10 to 55 msec) associated with water molecules bound within myelin membranes. Protons of cerebrospinal fluid (CSF) have T_2 times of the order of 1 sec [24]. Although not prominent in the T_2 maps, the short T_2 component might play the relevant role for the distinction between acute inflammation and persistent degeneration. As shown for MS lesions in patients [24] and in animal

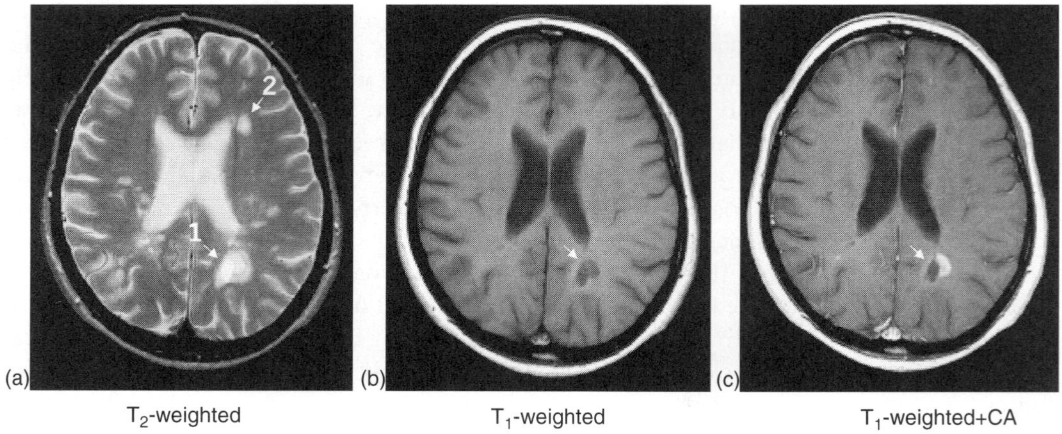

FIGURE 12.2 MR-images showing MS-lesions of different characteristics. (a) T_2-weighted image (TR = 2800 msec, TE = 45 msec). Two lesions are marked by arrows. (b) Same slice acquired with a T_1-weighted sequence (TR = 500 msec, TE = 15 msec) prior to administration and (c) after administration of a low molecular weight CA (Gd-DOTA). Only lesion 1 from the T_2-weighted scan appears hypointense on the T_1-weighted scan and takes up CA. Lesion 2 does not enhance CA. This set of images demonstrates the variable relationship of lesion type and MR parameters.

models of EAE [25], a decrease of the fast T_2 component has been observed for chronic lesions; this is interpreted as loss of myelin and reflects a chronic impairment of tissue function.

12.4.2.3 Magnetization Transfer Contrast

Magnetization transfer imaging can be used to assess the degradation of myelin in the brain of MS patients or in animal models [26,27]. The technique probes the transfer of longitudinal magnetization between two molecular partners that are coupled via chemical exchange, magnetic cross-correlation, or spin diffusion. For water exchange in biological tissue the process studied is the transfer of longitudinal magnetization between free protons and protons that are bound to immobile (macromolecular) surfaces such as the myelin sheath of axons. While free protons contribute to the MR signal, bound protons are invisible due to their very short T_2 value. In order to measure the magnetization transfer, nonequilibrium longitudinal magnetization has to be generated typically by applying an off-resonance (with respect to the free water resonance frequency) saturation pulse, which saturates the magnetization of macromolecule-bound water protons, but ideally does not affect the magnetization of the protons of bulk water. In the mixing interval, during which the saturation pulse is applied, longitudinal magnetization is exchanged between the free bound water proton pools, leading to a signal loss of the effective MR signal (due to bulk water). The degree of signal attenuation depends on the experimental conditions chosen, the rate constant k for the magnetization exchange, the length of the mixing period, and the longitudinal relaxation time of the bulk water protons. It is, however, independent of the size of the amount of bound water. The various exchange-relevant tissue parameters can be derived quantitatively when applying multiple mixing times. However, quantification is time-consuming and, therefore, a comparison of two images (one acquired with and the other without the saturating pulse) is used to detect changes from normal tissue composition. A drawback of this approach is that the extent of signal attenuation depends on other factors than just the exchange rate. Assuming a two-site exchange rate, the magnetization transfer ratio (MTR) also depends on the longitudinal relaxation rate $1/T_1$ of the free water protons. In a continuous wave experiment the magnetization transfer effect is

$$\frac{M_z(\infty)}{M_z(0)} = \frac{1}{1 + kT_1} \qquad (12.1)$$

and therefore a change of the T_1 values in the lesion will also translate into a change of apparent MTRs [28]. Hence, for obtaining a true measure of the exchange rates, acquisition of a T_1 map is required (see Chapter 22, Appendix 1). The difficult task is to relate the pseudo-first order rate constant k derived from magnetization transfer maps, or correspondingly the degree of signal attenuation of the bulk water signal (the magnetization transfer ratio), to a measure of the macromolecular content in the respective brain region. This requires profound knowledge of the exchange mechanism underlying the simple two-site exchange model commonly used to derive rate constants.

MTRs have been extensively used in clinical MS trials. Compared with BBB damage and edema, reduction of MTR has been associated with permanent loss of white matter integrity or at least with transient demyelination. Similar assumptions have been made for tissue damage due to ischemia [29]. However, as already discussed, even quantitative measurements of MTRs or of exchange rate constants cannot provide direct information on the reduction of myelin or other membrane elements. Degradation of these structures should be associated with a reduced amount of bound water, which, however, is invisible in MRI. The indirect visualization by imaging the interaction of bound and free water protons by the magnetization transfer effect underlies one severe limitation: changes in the empirical rate constant k (or in MTRs) can be due to changes in the density of the bound protons or the alteration of the effective exchange rate. Hence, a strict biophysical link between the empirical MRI-derived parameters to tissue degradation is not possible. Nevertheless, the assumption that reductions in MTR qualitatively reflect tissue damage is plausible, and the readout is considered of diagnostic value.

12.4.2.4 T_1-Hypointense Lesions

Chronic lesions can appear hypointense on postcontrast T_1-weighted images [22,30], and were therefore termed black holes. It has been proposed that this signal change is associated with hypocellularity, demyelination, axonal loss, and/or the presence of reactive astrocytes [31]. Hence, T_1 hypointensity should indicate severe, irreversible damage of brain tissue, actually neurodegeneration, which should be more closely related to the disability status as compared with the inflammation marker vascular edema or BBB damage. From a diagnostic point-of-view, however, T_1 hypointensity is considered just a qualitative measure for the presence or absence of a lesion. Since several different pathological processes can lead to this form of signal loss (or a decrease of the T_1-relaxation time corresponding to an increase in R_1 relaxivity), it is almost impossible to measure the status of a lesion or to predict its future development.

12.4.2.5 Neurodegeneration and Atrophy

Brain atrophy reflects the loss of brain volume as a consequence of irreversible loss of neuronal structures in gray and white matter. Brain atrophy has been studied intensively for Alzheimer's disease (see Chapter 7, Section 7.5) or MS, for which progression of neurological and cognitive disability has been shown to correlate with loss of brain volume. Cerebral atrophy should, therefore, be a more relevant indicator of neurological and cognitive decline than readouts of neuroinflammation. Atrophy can be assessed either by measuring the brain parenchymal fraction (BPF), which is the ratio of the parenchymal divided by the total brain volume, or alternatively by measuring cortical thickness. The decrease in BPF in MS patients depends on the state of the disease; it is typically less than 1% per year. BPF values are obtained by automatic or semiautomatic segmentation of MR images into volumes of gray and white matter, CSF, and the remaining brain structures. Analysis procedures of both types yielded a scan-rescan variability of 0.3 to 0.4% [32]. However, automatic procedures are prone to errors in the absolute quantification of BPF due to incidental false classification of brain tissue. Although correlations of BPF and EDSS are only moderate, longitudinal assessment of BPF values in individual patients can be used to evaluate the effects of treatment. For example, it was shown that the decrease of brain volume was smaller in MS patients treated over a two-year period with interferon beta-1a as compared with the control cohort [33].

There are no comparative preclinical studies assessing brain atrophy in EAE models. First of all, most EAE models are models of acute inflammation; they do not comprise a chronic neurodegenerative component, or the chronic component has never been studied. Second, immunohistochemistry techniques allow direct evaluation of the neuronal impairment (demyelination and axonal damage), not requiring the assessment of any secondary morphological readouts. Invasive preclinical techniques, therefore, provide superior information for the analysis of the disease process and therapeutic intervention. Nevertheless, chronic preclinical models might be of value to relate the various readouts of neurodegeneration such as degeneration of neurons/axons, gross-morphological brain atrophy, and functional deficits.

Another question concerning the role of brain atrophy is whether it is the global loss of cerebral tissue that is most relevant for neurological/cognitive decline or whether there are specific brain areas, which when affected, cause major functional impairment. It is known from fMRI studies that activation of brain areas in the frontal and parietal cortex during an alertness-demanding task correlate with attention deficits in MS patients. Local cortical thickness measurements revealed that in addition to a diffuse loss of gray matter volumes throughout the brain, areas in the frontal and temporal cortex were specifically affected by tissue degeneration [34]. These observations suggest that tissue loss in critical brain areas should have a larger effect on functional/cognitive impairment; global measurements of cortical atrophy would underestimate this effect.

12.4.2.6 Functional MRI

FMRI is a method that allows visualization of functional processes within the brain by utilizing the blood oxygenation dependent (BOLD) effect [35,36]. This effect refers to a coupling between regional cerebral blood flow and regional brain metabolism as it was first described by Roy and Sherrington in 1890. Meanwhile, fMRI is a well-accepted method to study brain function in the normal and also in the damaged brain (see also Chapter 10 and Chapter 11). FMRI can help understand the functional mechanisms underlying cognitive and sensory-motor disorders of the CNS. First fMRI studies in MS focused mainly on the motor system [37,38]. Here, increased functional activation in regions directly related to the motor system was accompanied by additional activation in nonmotor regions. It has been suggested that these changes in brain activation might represent adaptive cortical reorganization that supports compensation of existing deficits. If so, this hypothesis would favor the idea that spontaneous plasticity processes even take place in a disease with diffuse tissue damage. The results obtained from studies on the motor system were confirmed by studies on cognitive processes in MS [6,39]. However, these functional changes derived entirely from studies on mildly impaired MS patients. Recent studies investigated patients at the earliest stage of MS. These so-called clinically isolated syndrome patients also show cortical reorganization when studied on motor or cognitive functions, indicating that compensatory mechanisms occur even before brain pathology is expressed clinically [37,40]. Interestingly, patients with severe impairment are characterized by a lack of additional recruitment of brain areas [6] leading to the assumption that compensatory brain mechanisms in MS decrease within the disease process and are behaviorally expressed by deficits.

12.4.3 Receptor-Specific Contrast Agents

Imaging of receptor expression or the presentation of vascular adhesion molecules is possible by coupling a target-specific ligand to a reporter system, which can be either a MRI CA, a fluorochrome, or a radioactive tracer. This principle has already been used for many years in immunohistochemistry, which is considered the gold standard for visualizing the presence of a specific target. As the analysis is carried out on histological sections access of the specific probe to the target is not hampered by tissue barriers. Second, *ex vivo* preparation of tissue sections allows the use of amplification systems, which lead to a dramatic improvement in sensitivity. In this respect, target-specific *in vivo* imaging has to overcome the same hurdles that have to be addressed in drug development. This is true in particular for CNS probes: after systemic administration of the tracer, it would have to cross the BBB in order to interact with a potential extravascular receptor. CAs providing improved relaxivity are often based on macromolecules (e.g., paramagnetic dendrimers, gadolinium-encapsulating liposomes, perfluorocarbon particles, or superparamagnetic iron oxide nanoparticles), which under normal conditions do not penetrate the BBB. Another aspect to be considered is the signal to background ratio: this requires high target affinity, or to be more precise, a slow target-off rate, and a rapid clearance of the unbound fraction of the probe.

The most severe limitation of MRI-based receptor mapping is the inherently low sensitivity of the imaging technique, and for target-specific imaging in particular, the relatively low molar relaxivity of MRI CAs. In addition, MRI CAs are just modulating the MRI signal, i.e., there is an inherent strong background signal. Changes in contrast could be either caused by intrinsic alterations in tissue composition (e.g., edema formation, proton density) or by contrast generated by the target-specific interaction. In general, target-specific tracer accumulation is a slow process typically requiring several hours; thus, MRI pre- and postcontrast images have to be acquired in different imaging sessions. This is less an issue for the brain, for which proper coregistration procedures have been developed; however, for nonbrain regions contrast differences due to spatial misalignment might outweigh the effect of the specific CA. Owing to their prominent role in the pathophysiology of (neuro)inflammation, *in vivo* visualization of leukocyte recruitment would be of high relevance for monitoring disease progression and treatment efficacy.

As previously stated, adhesion molecules play an important role in the modulation of the immune response because they orchestrate leukocyte infiltration to the site of inflammation. First examples of successful application of MRI CA-labeled receptor ligands is the visualization of ICAM-1 expression in an animal model of chronic EAE [41]. Paramagnetic polymerized liposomes were conjugated with an anti-ICAM-1 antibody via an avidin-biotin coupling. This targeted CA was infused systemically into mice with EAE and control animals, and MR images of the excised brains were taken 1 day following tracer administration. At this time point, significantly increased signal intensity was observed in T_1-weighted MR images of the brains of EAE mice as compared with those of control animals, indicating an enhanced longitudinal relaxivity due to accumulation of the targeted contrast agent. Administration of a nontargeted antibody-CA construct did not yield any intensity differences between the EAE and the control group. Along similar lines, selectin expression was demonstrated using a sialyl Lewis X (sLex) coupled to Gd-DTPA [42,43]. sLex, a carbohydrate antigen, is found on activated leukocytes and is able to bind to selectins, which are expressed on the luminar surface of endothelial cells during inflammation.

Another elegant approach for direct visualization of inflammatory processes is to target the peripheral benzodiazepine receptor of activated microglia. This, however, requires the use of positron emission tomography (PET), as potential targeted ligands have to cross the BBB in order to reach the receptor, and the development of low molecular weight drug-like reporter compounds. A benzodiazepine receptor ligand that fulfills these criteria is PK11195, which when labeled with the PET radionuclide ^{11}C could be successfully applied to study activated microglia in MS and AD patients [44–46]. Comparing MRI and PET scans for MS patients, it could be demonstrated that lesions defined by T_2 hyperintensity are not necessarily linked to activated microglia. The relation of PK11195 uptake to disease progression has not been elucidated but interesting relations to other MRI-related parameters were reported: PK11195 uptake is enhanced in Gd-enhancing lesions and higher uptake was observed in T_2 lesions during an attack [44].

12.4.4 Cell Labeling

In the previous section we focused on visualizing aspects of immune cell recruitment, i.e., on the expression of antigens by endothelial cells in the affected region. *In vivo* tracking of immune cells *per se* would provide another relevant readout to evaluate inflammatory processes in the brain. As already discussed, there are two classes of immune cells: lymphocytes, which orchestrate the tissue response to inflammation and play a minor role in direct tissue destruction, and macrophages, which eliminate the antigen-expressing pathogen and are responsible for massive tissue damage. The majority of *in vivo* labeling studies has focused on macrophages, taking advantage of their phagocytotic activity. Macrophages recognize nanoparticles of a certain size, which have been opsonated by plasma proteins, as foreign antigens, and incorporate them into their lysosomes. This mechanism is rather established for labeling cells of the monocyte phagocytic system of the liver with superparamagnetic iron oxide-based nanoparticles (small particles of iron oxide, SPIOs). Efficient labeling of the different types of macrophages (e.g., lymphnode or blood-borne monocytes) requires sufficient exposure time for phagocytotic label uptake. Nanoparticles should not be rapidly cleared by Kupffer-cells of the liver, circulation time should be of the order of several hours. Ultrasmall particles of iron oxide (USPIOs) were originally designed for the demarcation of benign from malignant lymphnode lesions. However, due to their plasma half-life of 5 h, it could be demonstrated that these particles also allow visualization of blood-borne macrophages in animal models of stroke and EAE [47–52].

Visualization of infiltrating macrophages offers several advantages over imaging of downstream processes such as BBB damage. First, macrophages are the most relevant factor of tissue damage in (neuro)inflammation. Second, acute inflammatory activity is a transient process. In the rat EAE model it could be demonstrated that the infiltration of macrophages is closely linked to behavioral disability as reflected by a neurological score. BBB damage, on the other hand, appears to be a more persistent effect, which extends over several days [53]. This suggests that the BBB is leaky during several phases of the inflammatory cascade including the early interaction of leukocytes with endothelial cells, the opening of tight junctions due to transcytosis and potentially also tissue repair mechanisms. There is also experimental evidence that macrophage recruitment is not necessarily associated with BBB opening (Figure 12.3). A detailed analysis of Gd- and USPIO-enhancing lesions in a chronic relapsing rat EAE model has demonstrated a significant spatial mismatch between BBB permeability and monocyte infiltration [49]. Qualitatively, Gd enhancement also appeared more diffuse as compared with the distribution of USPIO-labeled cells, possibly because low molecular weight CAs passively diffuse within the interstitium. However, during the acute phase of EAE there was also a clear mismatch in some areas that showed either accumulation of USPIO or Gd-DOTA. During the chronic phase, only USPIO-induced enhancement has been observed. Although the EAE model cannot be translated in a one-to-one fashion to human MS, these findings raise the question whether BBB damage can, in fact, serve as a reliable readout for acute inflammation. This reservation is even more justified, since BBB damage as measured by Gd extravasation is often also poorly correlated with neurological function and disease outcome [14]. Whether the correlation between the lesion load as derived from USPIO-enhancing lesions, reflecting a high macrophage concentration and correspondingly high inflammatory activity, and the clinical status of MS patients will reveal a better prognostic value of the MRI readout remains to be shown.

Nonphagocytotic immune cells cannot be tracked *in vivo* using MRI as easily as macrophages because those do not take up nanoparticles from the circulation. Imaging of such cells requires harvesting cells from a donor animal followed by *ex vivo* labeling. The feasibility of T-cell labeling

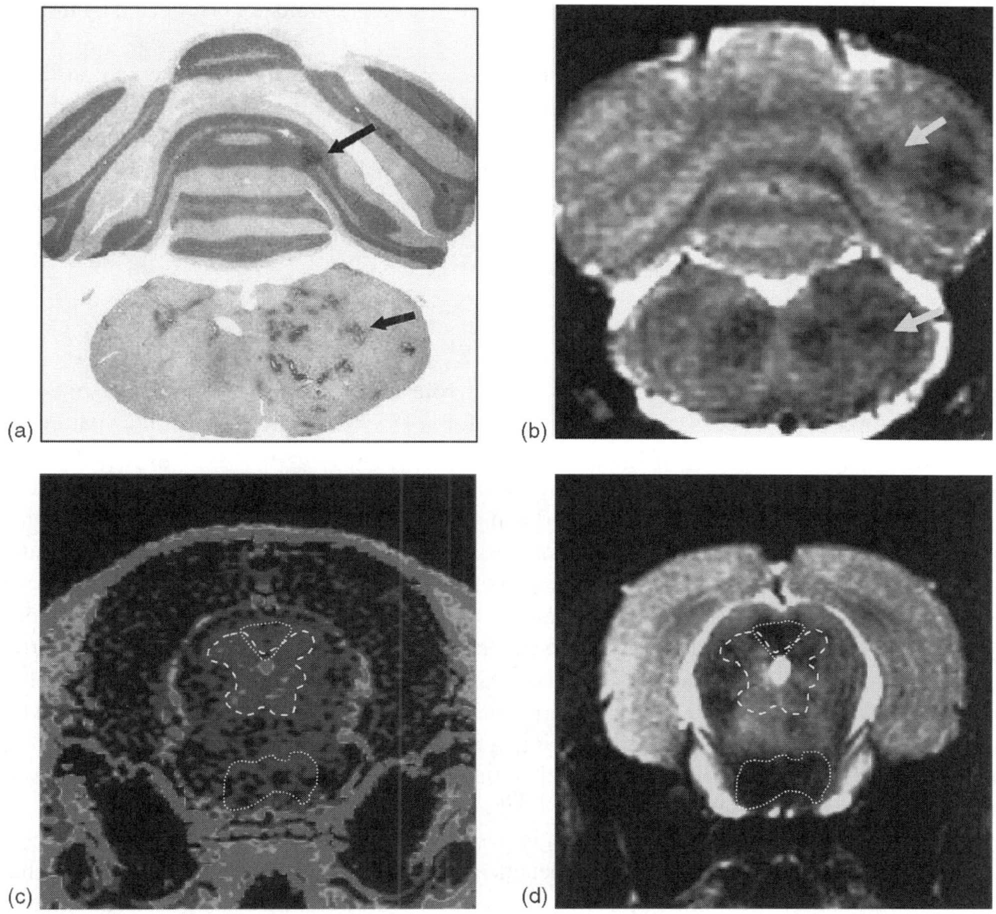

FIGURE 12.3 (See color insert following page 328.) Comparison of parametric images from one animal of the EAE group. (a) ED-1 stain demonstrating macrophages in the cerebellum and the medulla of an animal with acute EAE. (b) The T2 image displays hypo-intense areas, induced by accumulation of USPIO. (c) and (d) Corresponding slices from another animal with EAE demonstrating the mismatch of Gd and USPIO enhancements. Enhancement of Gd-DOTA is visible in structures of the midbrain. The discrepancy of spatial localization of USPIO and Gd-DOTA enhancement is demonstrated by the dotted and dashed lines. The area marked by the dotted line accumulated USPIO but no Gd-DOTA. The reverse situation can be observed in the area marked by the dashed line. (From Rausch, M. et al., *Magn. Reson. Med.*, 50, 309, 2003.)

by USPIOs was demonstrated: cells were incubated for several hours in medium containing the CA [54]. However, this approach proved to be not very efficient as the incorporation of CA by pinocytosis occurs at a rather low rate. Improved methods are based on conjugating nanoparticles with transfection agents, such as the trans-acting activator domain (TAT) of the human immune-deficiency virus [55], poly-L-lysine [56], or lipid-based transfection agents such as FuGENE [57], which serve as translocation signals and enhance the particle uptake (see also Chapter 25, Section 25.5). Alternatively, magnetodendrimers can be used, which tightly interact with the cell membrane [58]. Until now, *in vivo* tracking of labeled T cells has not been used extensively. The reason for that might be the relatively low sensitivity of MRI itself and the complex preparation of the cell cultures. Several factors have to be considered in this respect: first, T cells have to be myelin specific. For observation of bystander T cells, tremendous amounts of labeled cells must be administered because only a low fraction of these cells enter the brain. Second, clonal expansion will lead to label dilution, and finally, the specificity of T cells should not be affected by the labeling procedure.

Today, techniques to monitor migration of macrophages and lymphocytes are still in their infancy. Alternative imaging modalities are nuclear imaging using SPECT tracers such as ^{111}In oxime or ^{99m}Tc [59] or, at least for animal research, optical imaging in combination with stable expression of reporter genes. The advantage of the MR approach is high temporospatial resolution and the potential translatability to humans. It can be anticipated that imaging of monocyte infiltration, and eventually also lymphocyte recruitment, will have a profound influence on the diagnosis and management of MS patients.

12.4.5 Imaging of Drug Effects

In the previous section we focused on the role of MRI as a diagnostic method for neuroinflammatory processes, in particular for MS. In clinical practice, patients with neurodegenerative diseases, including MS, are typically diagnosed and staged on the basis of neurological or cognitive parameters, which are considered of high relevance and which can be easily assessed by a variety of standardized and validated neurological or neuropsychological test boxes. As mentioned previously, several comparisons between neurological parameters (indicative for disease progression) and imaging parameters have been evaluated for MS patients to assess the prognostic value of the MRI readouts. Generally, the correlation of the clinical status of patients and conventional imaging readouts was low to moderate. Provided that an imaging parameter can be assessed with sufficient accuracy, its poor correlation with disease outcome indicates that it is only in part relevant for the disease. Other parameters may also play a significant role, or the severity of the disease is determined by a complex interaction of different parameters. In order to use an imaging readout as a surrogate for the clinical outcome a high and robust correlation between the two measurements is mandatory.

One important objective for using imaging as a biomarker for therapy evaluation is that it is of predictive value, i.e., it should indicate a beneficial effect of a drug earlier than the established and well-accepted neurological or cognitive readouts. Moreover, it should be sensitive enough to detect positive effects of treatment from reasonable small cohorts, or in the best case, it should be able to predict the value of a certain medication for an individual patient. This last point is addressed by the concept of personalized medicine, which will gain greater importance as the number of possible medications increases. MRI readouts currently established in the clinics for the diagnosis of MS, such as lesion detection based on alterations of T_2 or T_1 contrast, BBB permeability, and MTR, do not fulfill these criteria. Even when analyzing data from large patient populations, the link of imaging readouts to clinical/neurological parameters is weak and the prognosis of disease progression for individual patients is almost impossible.

Second, imaging could be used to understand the effect of drugs on a mechanistic basis. This is particularly important for target validation, where *in vivo* imaging can help understand the importance of the target and evaluate the effect of the drug-target interaction on disease progression. However, advanced imaging approaches that are more intimately related to the pathophysiology of neuroinflammation, and which therefore might be more directly linked to the disease outcome, are still in the exploratory phase. They cannot be applied as diagnostic tools and for therapy evaluation as the majority of CAs allowing target- or cell-specific imaging are not yet approved for use in patients.

Labeling of cells with USPIO has proved to be a powerful tool to assess acute inflammation in preclinical research. In the case of treatment with the immunomodulator lovastatin, a significant reduction in USPIO accumulation was observed [53]. In another study, the compound FTY720 led to a complete abolishment of USPIO accumulation in treated animals [21]. However, disease staging on the basis of measuring BBB integrity in animals treated during the chronic phase of the disease resulted in a clear overestimation of the inflammatory process.

12.5 CONCLUSIONS

MRI has provided valuable information on neuroinflammatory processes in human CNS diseases. However, as MS is a very complex disease, the ultimate link between imaging parameters and patient outcome and prognosis is still weak. Hence, it is necessary to develop new imaging techniques or target-specific contrast agents for clinical staging and drug testing. Quantitative MRI with respect to MTR (demyelination) or T_1 mapping (scare formation) could be implemented without any need to approve new imaging agents. The use of new CAs, however, still requires intensive evaluation with respect to safety and efficacy before they can be used in clinical routine or drug studies. Moreover, fMRI can be used to study the functional consequences (cognitive or motor impairment) of tissue damage in specific brain areas. These data could be combined with structural analysis of white matter tracks by DTI or fiber tracking, which might help to understand the neurophysiologic link of axonal damage and cognitive impairment in individual patients.

To improve this situation for clinical research and drug development, animal models for neuroinflammation and degeneration such as the EAE model will continue to play an important role. First of all, it should be possible to use these models for further evaluation of conventional imaging readouts. They can be used to quantify the relation between the pathophysiology (e.g., demyelination, axonal loss, BBB damage) and the signal change in parametric images. Second, target-specific imaging methods based on novel CAs can be evaluated very well in experimental animal models. Therefore, the progress in clinical imaging and the development of new bio or surrogate markers relies critically on the effort and progress made in preclinical imaging research.

REFERENCES

1. Trapp, B. D., Ransohoff, R., and Rudick, R., Axonal pathology in multiple sclerosis: relationship to neurologic disability, *Curr. Opin. Neurol.*, 12, 295, 1999.
2. Kurtzke, J. F., Rating neurologic impairment in multiple sclerosis: an expanded disability status scale (EDSS), *Neurology*, 33, 1444, 1983.
3. Berg, D. et al., Lesion pattern in patients with multiple sclerosis and depression, *Mult. Scler.*, 6, 156, 2000.
4. Comi, G. et al., Brain magnetic resonance imaging correlates of cognitive impairment in multiple sclerosis, *J. Neurol. Sci.*, 115, S66, 1993.
5. Rovaris, M. et al., Relation between MR abnormalities and patterns of cognitive impairment in multiple sclerosis, *Neurology*, 50, 1601, 1998.
6. Penner, I. K. et al., Analysis of impairment related functional architecture in MS patients during performance of different attention tasks, *J. Neurol.*, 250, 461, 2003.
7. Filippi, M. et al., Correlations between structural CNS damage and functional MRI changes in primary progressive MS, *Neuroimage*, 15, 537, 2002.
8. Rocca, M. A. et al., Evidence for widespread movement-associated functional MRI changes in patients with PPMS, *Neurology*, 58, 866, 2002.
9. Gold, R., Hartung, H. P., and Toyka, K. V., Animal models for autoimmune demyelinating disorders of the nervous system, *Mol. Med. Today*, 6, 88, 2000.
10. Ballabh, P., Braun, A., and Nedergaard, M., The blood-brain barrier: an overview: structure, regulation, and clinical implications, *Neurobiol. Dis.*, 16, 1, 2004.
11. Abbott, N. J. et al., Delivery of imaging agents into brain, *Adv. Drug Deliv. Rev.*, 37, 253, 1999.
12. Gloor, S. M. et al., Molecular and cellular permeability control at the blood-brain barrier, *Brain Res. Brain Res. Rev.*, 36, 258, 2001.
13. Miller, D. H. et al., The role of magnetic resonance techniques in understanding and managing multiple sclerosis, *Brain*, 121, 3, 1998.
14. Kappos, L. et al., Predictive value of gadolinium-enhanced magnetic resonance imaging for relapse rate and changes in disability or impairment in multiple sclerosis: a meta-analysis. Gadolinium MRI meta-analysis group, *Lancet*, 353, 964, 1999.

15. Miller, D. H., Barkhof, F., and Nauta, J. J., Gadolinium enhancement increases the sensitivity of MRI in detecting disease activity in multiple sclerosis, *Brain*, 116, 1077, 1993.
16. Hawkins, C. P. et al., Duration and selectivity of blood-brain barrier breakdown in chronic relapsing experimental allergic encephalomyelitis studied by gadolinium- DTPA and protein markers, *Brain*, 113, 365, 1990.
17. Huber, J. D., Egleton, R. D., and Davis, T. P., Molecular physiology and pathophysiology of tight junctions in the blood-brain barrier, *Trends Neurosci.*, 24, 719, 2001.
18. de Vries, H. E. et al., The blood-brain barrier in neuroinflammatory diseases, *Pharmacol. Rev.*, 49, 143, 1997.
19. Morrissey, S. P. et al., In vivo MRI and its histological correlates in acute adoptive transfer experimental allergic encephalomyelitis, *Quantification of inflammation and oedema, Brain*, 119, 239, 1996.
20. Bruck, W. et al., Inflammatory central nervous system demyelination: correlation of magnetic resonance imaging findings with lesion pathology, *Ann. Neurol.*, 42, 783, 1997.
21. Rausch, M. et al., Predicability of FTY720 efficacy in experimental autoimmune encephalomyelitis bu in vivo macrophage tracking: clinical implications for ultrasmall superparamagnetic iron oxide-enhanced magnetic resonance imaging, *J. Magn. Reson. Imaging*, 20, 16, 2004.
22. Barkhof, F. and van Walderveen, M., Characterization of tissue damage in multiple sclerosis by nuclear magnetic resonance, *Philos. Trans. R. Soc. Lond. B Biol. Sci.*, 354, 1675, 1999.
23. Fischer, H. W. et al., Nuclear relaxation of human brain gray and white matter: analysis of field dependence and implications for MRI, *Magn. Reson. Med.*, 16, 317, 1990.
24. MacKay, A. et al., In vivo visualization of myelin water in brain by magnetic resonance, *Magn. Reson. Med.*, 31, 673, 1994.
25. Stewart, W. A. et al., Spin–spin relaxation in experimental allergic encephalomyelitis. Analysis of CPMG data using a non-linear least squares method and linear inverse theory, *Magn. Reson. Med.*, 29, 767, 1993.
26. Henkelman, R. M., Stanisz, G. J., and Graham, S. J., Magnetization transfer in MRI: a review, *NMR Biomed.*, 14, 57, 2001.
27. Graham, S. J. and Henkelman, R. M., Understanding pulsed magnetization transfer, *J. Magn. Reson. Imaging*, 7, 903, 1997.
28. Rudin, M. and Sauter, A., Measurement of reaction rates in vivo using magnetization transfer techniques, In *NMR: Basic Principles and Progress*, Vol. 27, Diehl, P., Ed., Springer, Heidelberg, p. 257, 1992.
29. Ordidge, R. J. et al., Investigation of cerebral ischemia using magnetization transfer contrast (MTC) MR imaging, *Magn. Reson. Imaging*, 9, 895, 1991.
30. Truyen, L. et al., Accumulation of hypointense lesions ("black holes") on T1 spin-echo MRI correlates with disease progression in multiple sclerosis, *Neurology*, 47, 1469, 1996.
31. van Walderveen, M. A. et al., Histopathologic correlate of hypointense lesions on T1-weighted spin-echo MRI in multiple sclerosis, *Neurology*, 50, 1282, 1998.
32. Zivadinov, R. et al., Reproducibility and accuracy of quantitative magnetic resonance imaging techniques of whole-brain atrophy measurement in multiple sclerosis, *J. Neuroimaging*, 15, 27, 2005.
33. Filippi, M. et al., Interferon beta-1a for brain tissue loss in patients at presentation with syndromes suggestive of multiple sclerosis: a randomised, double-blind, placebo-controlled trial, *Lancet*, 364, 1489, 2004.
34. Sailer, M. et al., Focal thinning of the cerebral cortex in multiple sclerosis, *Brain*, 126, 1734, 2003.
35. Kwong, K. K. et al., Dynamic magnetic resonance imaging of human brain activity during primary sensory stimulation, *Proc. Natl. Acad. Sci. USA*, 89, 5672, 1992.
36. Ogawa, S. et al., Intrinsic signal changes accompanying sensory stimulation: Functional brain mapping with magnetic resonance imaging, *Proc. Natl. Acad. Sci.* 89, 5951, 1992.
37. Filippi, M. et al., Simple and complex movement-associated functional MRI changes in patients at presentation with clinically isolated syndromes suggestive of multiple sclerosis, *Hum. Brain Mapp.*, 21, 108, 2004.
38. Reddy, H. et al., Evidence for adaptive functional changes in the cerebral cortex with axonal injury from multiple sclerosis, *Brain*, 123, 2314, 2000.

39. Staffen, W. et al., Cognitive function and fMRI in patients with multiple sclerosis: evidence for compensatory cortical activation during an attention task, *Brain*, 125, 1275, 2002.
40. Audoin, B. et al., Magnetic resonance study of the influence of tissue damage and cortical reorganization on PASAT performance at the earliest stage of multiple sclerosis, *Hum. Brain Mapp.*, 24, 216, 2004.
41. Sipkins, D. A. et al., ICAM-1 expression in autoimmune encephalitis visualized using magnetic resonance imaging, *J. Neuroimmunol.*, 104, 1, 2000.
42. Barber, P. A. et al., MR molecular imaging of early endothelial activation in focal ischemia, *Ann. Neurol.*, 56, 116, 2004.
43. Sibson, N. R. et al., MRI detection of early endothelial activation in brain inflammation, *Magn. Reson. Med.*, 51, 248, 2004.
44. Debruyne, J. C. et al., PET visualization of microglia in multiple sclerosis patients using [11C]PK11195, *Eur. J. Neurol.*, 10, 257, 2003.
45. Vowinckel, E. et al., PK11195 binding to the peripheral benzodiazepine receptor as a marker of microglia activation in multiple sclerosis and experimental autoimmune encephalomyelitis, *J. Neurosci. Res.*, 50, 345, 1997.
46. Cagnin, A. et al., In-vivo measurement of activated microglia in dementia, *Lancet*, 358, 461, 2001.
47. Rausch, M. et al., Dynamic patterns of USPIO enhancement can be observed in macrophages after ischemic brain damage, *Magn. Reson. Med.*, 46, 1018, 2001.
48. Rausch, M. et al., In-vivo visualization of phagocytotic cells in rat brains after transient ischemia by USPIO, *NMR Biomed.*, 15, 278, 2002.
49. Rausch, M. et al., MRI-based monitoring of inflammation and tissue damage in acute and chronic relapsing EAE, *Magn. Reson. Med.*, 50, 309, 2003.
50. Dousset, V. et al., Comparison of ultrasmall particles of iron oxide (USPIO)-enhanced T2-weighted, conventional T2-weighted, and Gadolinium-enhanced T1-weighted MR images in rats with experimental autoimmune Encephalomyelitis, *AJNR*, 20, 223, 1999.
51. Dousset, V. et al., *In vivo* macrophage activity imaging in the central nervous system detected by magnetic resonance, *Magn. Reson. Med.*, 41, 329, 1999.
52. Dousset, V. et al., Dose and scanning delay using USPIO for central nervous system macrophage imaging, *MAGMA*, 8, 185, 1999.
53. Floris, S. et al., Blood-brain barrier permeability and monocyte infiltration in experimental allergic encephalomyelitis: a quantitative MRI study, *Brain*, 127, 1, 2004.
54. Yeh, T. et al., *In vivo* dynamic MRI tracking of rat T-cells labeled with superparamagnetic iron-oxide particles, *Magn. Reson. Med.*, 33, 200, 1995.
55. Dodd, C. H. et al., Normal T-cell response and in vivo magnetic resonance imaging of T cells loaded with HIV transactivator-peptide-derived superparamagnetic nanoparticles, *J. Immunol. Methods*, 256, 89, 2001.
56. Frank, J. A. et al., Magnetic intracellular labeling of mammalian cells by combining (FDA-approved) superparamagnetic iron oxide MR contrast agents and commonly used transfection agents, *Acad. Radiol.*, 9, S484, 2002.
57. Arbab, A. S. et al., Comparison of transfection agents in forming complexes with ferumoxides, cell labeling efficiency, and cellular viability, *Mol. Imaging*, 3, 24, 2004.
58. Bulte, J. W. et al., Monitoring stem cell therapy in vivo using magnetodendrimers as a new class of cellular MR contrast agents, *Acad. Radiol.*, 9, S332, 2002.
59. Fulgenzi, A. et al., Technetium-99m scintigraphy to visualize T-cell homing in vivo: a preclinical study, *Nucl. Med. Biol.*, 30, 633, 2003.

Editorial Comments

Magnetic resonance (MR) techniques have the unique ability to measure *in vivo* the biochemical content of living tissue in the body in a dynamic, noninvasive and nondestructive manner. Fundamental for cancer research, serial investigations of steady-state tumor physiology and biochemistry are feasible, and in particular, the response of tumors to treatment can be studied noninvasively. Magnetic resonance imaging (MRI), magnetic resonance spectroscopy (MRS), and a combination of both approaches, spectroscopic imaging, allow some physiological parameters, for example pH, to be imaged. Important information on tissue bioenergetics and phospholipid membrane turnover, pH, hypoxia, oxygenation, as well as on various vascular aspects including blood flow, angiogenesis, permeability, and vascular volume may be derived using these methods. In addition, to some extent, MRS can be used to monitor anticancer drugs and their metabolites at the sites of action. The manifold uses of *in vivo* MR methodologies in the area of cancer are extensively discussed in Chapter 13 through Chapter 15 in view of providing noninvasive means for assessing new therapies.

13 Functional and Molecular Magnetic Resonance Imaging of Preclinical Cancer Models in Drug Discovery and Development

Zaver M. Bhujwalla, Kristine Glunde, Ellen Ackerstaff, Arvind P. Pathak, Barjor Gimi, Noriko Mori, Venu Raman, and Dmitri Artemov

CONTENTS

13.1 INTRODUCTION

Cancer cells exhibit typical characteristics (outlined in Table 13.1), which, although individually not dangerous, collectively make the disease life threatening and difficult to treat. Magnetic resonance (MR) methods can be applied to study several of these characteristics and their response to therapy, in the context of drug discovery and development. As a disease, cancer exhibits different levels of malignancy, starting with low grade tumors which tend to resemble normal cells and grow slowly, to high grade poorly differentiated or undifferentiated tumors, which do not resemble the tissue of origin [1], and are aggressive and grow rapidly. One of the challenges facing MR methods

TABLE 13.1
Characteristics of a Malignant Cell

Hallmarks of a Cancer Cell
Immortalization
Growth-factor-independent growth
Insensitivity to growth-inhibitory signals
Ability to invade and metastasize
Ability to secure nutrients by stimulating angiogenesis
Avoidance of apoptosis
Resistance to therapeutic measures

Source: From Kolch, W., et al., *Expert Rev. Mol. Med.*, 2002, 1, 2002 and Hanahan, D. and Weinberg, R. A., *Cell*, 100, 57, 2000. With permission of Cambridge University Press and Cell Press.

is to identify parameters, which closely reflect the grade or aggressiveness of tumors and the danger they pose. The paradigm shift of viewing cancer as a chronic disease, and the development of agents which control the tumor through therapies such as antiangiogenic drugs, differentiating agents, or specific molecular targeting, has resulted in a concurrent and urgent requirement to detect tumor response.

Within the past decade, a clearer picture has emerged of MR parameters that define the characteristics of a malignant lesion — the MR malignant phenotype. These identifying characteristics are critically important to understand the functional characteristics of tumor biogenesis, and to gain insight into the development of the malignant phenotype. Multiparametric molecular and functional magnetic resonance imaging (MRI) methods can thus reveal key targets for therapy, visualize delivery of the therapy, and assess the efficacy of treatment. Altered choline metabolism is a prime example of the identification of a common feature of neoplastic transformation revealed by magnetic resonance spectroscopy (MRS), which can be exploited for treatment, as discussed in this chapter.

MR methods traverse easily from bench to bedside, because it is possible to use these methods to study isolated cells, human tumor xenografts, and clinical tumors (see also Chapter 14). This ability to study isolated cells as well as tissues *in vivo* is important, since the tumor stromal components and microenvironment can significantly alter vascular and metabolic characteristics, as well as other phenotypic traits of cells in the tumor. As stated by Hanahan and Weinberg [2], "The field of cancer research has largely been guided by a reductionist focus on cancer cells and the genes within them — a focus that has produced an extraordinary body of knowledge. Looking forward in time, we believe that important new inroads will come from regarding tumors as complex tissues in which mutant cancer cells have conscripted and subverted normal cell types to serve as active collaborators in their neoplastic agenda. The interactions between the genetically altered malignant cells and these supporting coconspirators will prove critical to understanding cancer pathogenesis and to the development of novel, effective therapies."

The use of transgenic cells and tumor models provides an important bridge between preclinical and clinical studies to obtain insight into the effects of specific molecular alterations on the MR malignant phenotype detected in clinical studies. MR studies of transgenic cells and mouse models can be used to determine the consequences of overexpression, underexpression, or complete inactivation of molecular markers identified by genetic or histological analyses. Such studies enhance our understanding of the function of these markers, and how they act to influence the malignant phenotype. Information derived from transgenic models can lead to the development of therapies for cancer treatment.

In this chapter, we present data from the work carried out in our program to provide examples of how MR methods can play an important role, both in understanding cancer, as well as in drug discovery and development.

13.2 INTACT CELL PERFUSION STUDIES

13.2.1 STUDYING CANCER CELL INVASION

The ability of cancer cells to invade and metastasize is one of the most lethal aspects of cancer. Outlined in this section are examples to show how multiparametric MR methods can be applied to study cancer cell invasion, and to understand the effects of therapeutic interventions designed to reduce invasion. Cancer cells invade by secreting enzymes that degrade basement membrane. This invasive potential is commonly assayed by determining the penetration of cells into reconstituted basement membrane gel (Matrigel®). Invasion is quantified by counting the number of cells that invade Matrigel-coated filters over a period of 5–72 h [3,4]. These methods, however, do not permit evaluation of the metabolic state of tumor cells, nor do they allow invasion to be measured dynamically in the same sample, under controlled microenvironmental conditions or following therapeutic interventions.

We therefore developed an invasion assay system (Figure 13.1) to dynamically track invasion of cancer cells and simultaneously characterize oxygen tensions, and physiological and metabolic parameters [5,6]. We also incorporate perfluorotripropylamine (FTPA)-doped alginate beads in the MR tube and embed FTPA into the Matrigel layer to directly measure oxygen tensions in the sample from the T_1 relaxation time of FTPA (Figure 13.2). In this system, we can regulate oxygen tensions to less than 1.5%, which is necessary to evaluate the impact of the hypoxic tumor environment on cancer cell invasion. Typical invasion and metabolic data obtained with this assay for a noninvasive (DU-145) and an invasive (MatLyLu) prostate cancer cell line are shown in Figure 13.3.

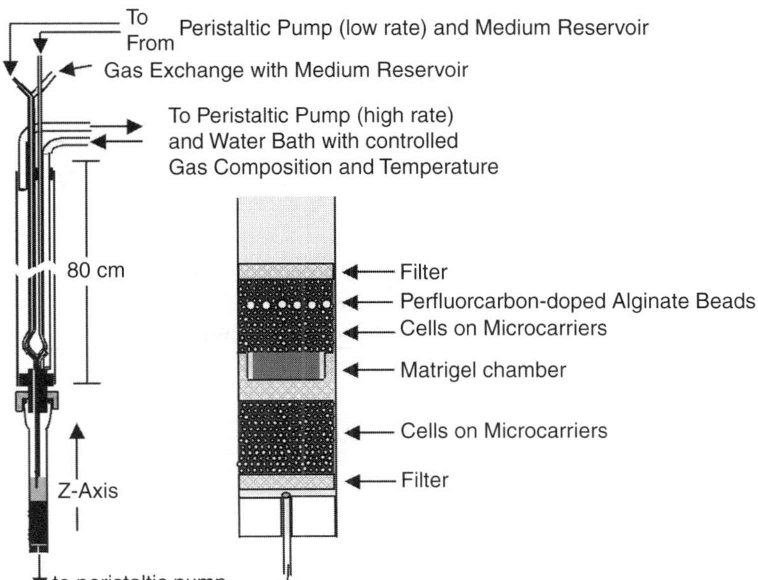

FIGURE 13.1 Schematic of metabolic Boyden chamber assay showing the reproducible layer of Matrigel® and (FTPA)-doped alginate beads. (Adapted from Pilatus, U., et al., *Neoplasia*, 2, 273, 2000. With permission of Neoplasia Press Inc. Copyright 2000.)

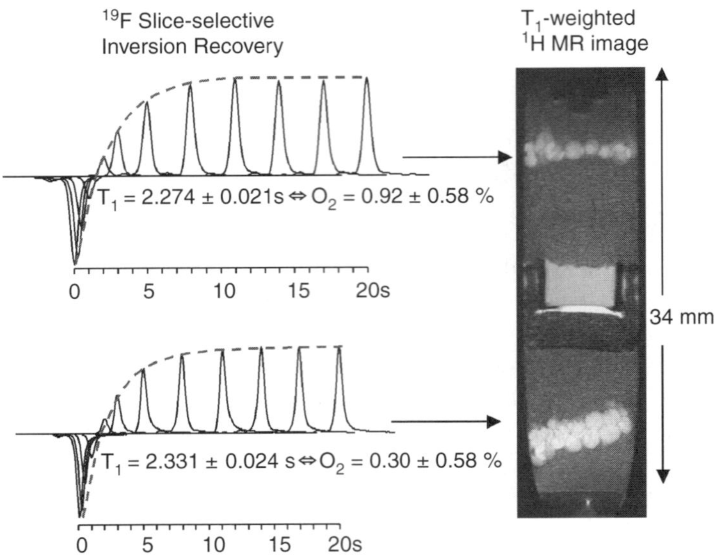

FIGURE 13.2 Characterization of oxygen tensions in the metabolic Boyden chamber perfusion system. (Adapted from Pathak, A.P., et al., *Methods Enzymol.*, 386, 3, 2004. With permission of Elsevier, Copyright 2004.)

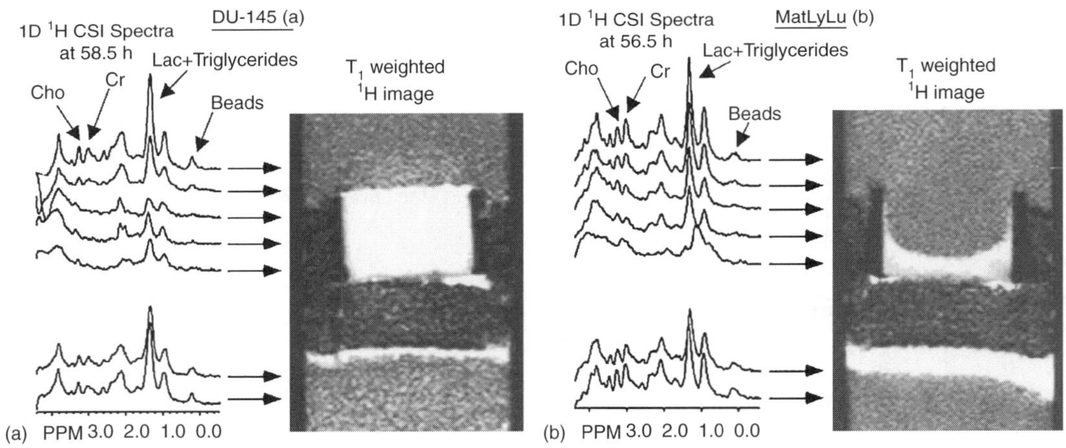

FIGURE 13.3 Expanded ^{1}H MR image of sample showing the Matrigel® layer for: (a) DU-145 and (b) MatLyLu cells at comparable time points. Images were obtained with TR = 1 sec, TE = 30 msec, FOV = 40 mm, slice thickness = 2 mm, resolution = 0.078 mm. ^{1}H MR spectra are from 0.31 mm thick localized slices from within the sample. (Adapted from Pilatus, U., et al., *Neoplasia*, 2, 273, 2000. With permission of Neoplasia Press Inc. Copyright 2000.)

Proton MR experiments with perfused cells in the metabolic Boyden chamber can be performed on a 400 MHz instrument (130 G/cm shielded gradient). A quantitative index of invasion is obtained from the intracellular water profiles, by using a single high-resolution profile to determine the number of cells in the Matrigel layer and in the entire sample. ^{31}P and ^{19}F MRS are performed during the course of a single experiment. ^{31}P MR spectra demonstrate the stability and viability of the cells in the perfusion system (Figure 13.4). The ability of this assay to detect differences in invasion is shown in Figure 13.5. We have added an extra level of complexity to this invasion assay

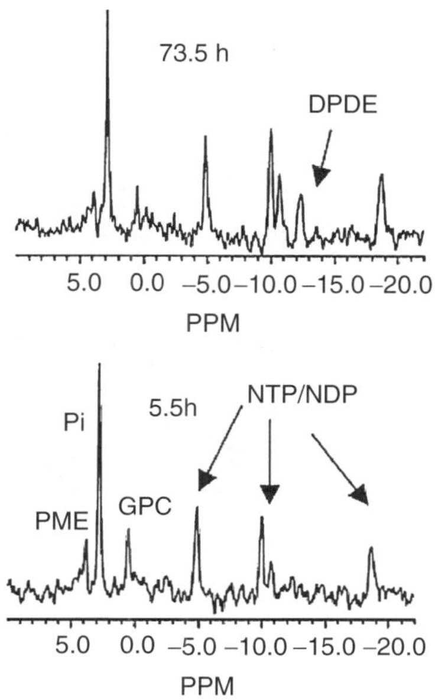

FIGURE 13.4 ^{31}P MR spectra obtained from a sample of DU-145 cells on Biosilon® beads 5 and 73 h after loading the cells. The ^{31}P MR spectra demonstrate the stability of the energy levels of the cells in this system over a period of 3 days. (From Pathak, A.P., et al., *Methods Enzymol.*, 386, 3, 2004. With permission of Elsevier, Copyright 2004.)

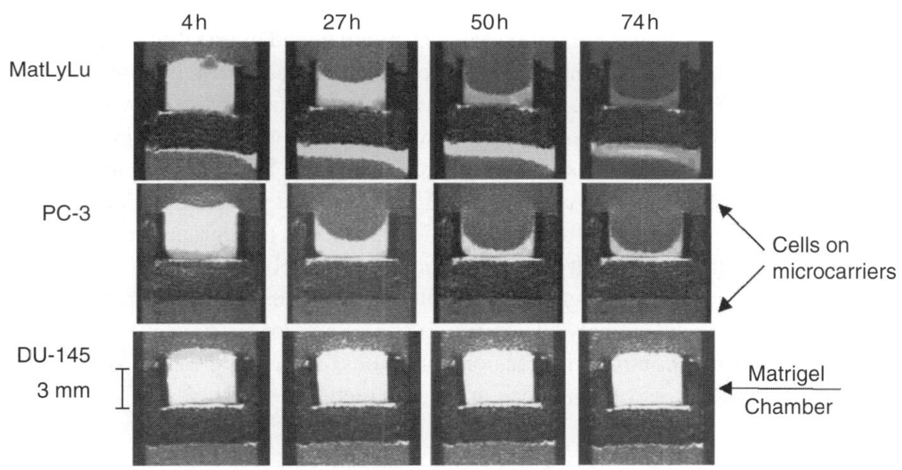

FIGURE 13.5 Metabolic Boyden chamber assay demonstrating differences in invasive characteristics of prostate cancer cell lines. The T_1 weighted ^1H MR images show the bright Matrigel layer that is significantly degraded by MatLyLu, and PC-3 cells, but not by DU-145 cells. (From Pathak, A.P., et al., *Methods Enzymol.*, 386, 3, 2004. With permission of Elsevier, Copyright 2004.)

by incorporating an endothelial cell layer between the Matrigel layer and the cancer cells [7]. This provides a closer simulation of the *in vivo* condition, since it is very likely that the interaction between endothelial cells and cancer cells contributes significantly to the invasive and metastatic process. We have also used this assay to determine the effect of hypoxia on cancer cell invasion. Preliminary results suggest that hypoxia reduces invasion, but the presence of endothelial cells, confers an advantage in invasion of cancer cells [7,8].

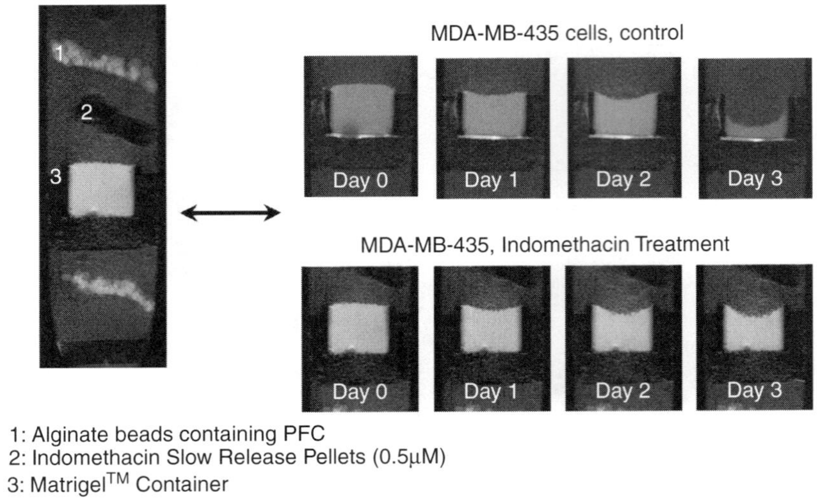

FIGURE 13.6 Representative T_1-weighted ^1H MR images demonstrating the effect of indomethacin treatment on degradation of Matrigel by MDA–MB-435 cells. Also shown in the panel on the left is the morphology of the sample during indomethacin treatment; from bottom to top: filter, cells, alginate beads, cells, Matrigel, cells, indomethacin pellets, cells, alginate beads, cells.

13.2.2 Studying Therapeutic Response

This assay can also be used to detect the effects of therapeutic agents designed to reduce invasion. Similar to wounded or injured tissue, the physiological microenvironment in most solid tumors is characterized by pro-inflammatory conditions such as hypoxia and extracellular acidosis [9,10]. In solid tumors, these environments can contribute to the upregulation of inflammatory pathways which may influence cell motility, invasion, vascularization, and metastatic dissemination [11–14]. We therefore evaluated the effects of the antiinflammatory agent indomethacin on invasion and metabolism of the malignant and invasive human breast cancer cell line MDA–MB-435 using our MR-compatible invasion assay [15]. As shown in Figure 13.6, the presence of indomethacin in the cell perfusion system reduced the ability of MDA–MB-435 cells to degrade the layer of Matrigel.

These data demonstrate the utility of multiparametric MRI of cells to understand factors influencing cancer invasion. Such an assay is valuable for testing the effects of metabolic inhibitors on cancer cell invasion or conversely, determining the effects of antiinvasive therapies on cell metabolism, under carefully controlled perfusion conditions. The cell perfusion system can also be used to directly study the effect of drugs on cancer cell metabolism.

13.3 *IN VIVO* HUMAN TUMOR XENOGRAFT STUDIES

13.3.1 Multiparametric MR Studies of Human Tumor Xenografts

Several MRI and MR spectroscopic imaging (MRSI) techniques have been developed and applied to study preclinical models of cancer. We, and others [6,16–18], have detected significant differences in vascular, physiological, and metabolic characteristics of metastatic and nonmetastatic cancer models with MRI and MRS. A unique aspect of MR is its ability to investigate the relationship between tumor vascularization, physiology, metabolism, and metastasis, and to understand how the abnormal vasculature impacts upon these (see also Chapter 14). While it is useful to study these as separate characteristics, the ability to relate metabolism and vascularization within the same region of interest adds a new dimension to our understanding of how one factor impacts on the other in tumor models with different vascular and metastatic characteristics.

Such combinations, if identified, may represent regions of high metastatic threat. For this purpose, we have developed combined vascular, metabolic, and extracellular pH (pH_e) imaging (Figure 13.7) [19], and we also perform combined vascular, metabolic, and optical imaging [20]. Such multiparametric imaging approaches can be used to identify patterns of vascularization and metabolism, characteristic of drug resistance, or radiation resistance.

13.3.2 Multiparametric/Multimodality Transgenic Tumor Model Studies

A tumor is a complex organization of cells with different genotypic as well as phenotypic characteristics. Although it is widely accepted that the malignant cell arises from genetic alterations, it is possible that several of the subsequent lethal phenotypic traits of cancer, such as invasion and metastasis, may arise from the unique physiological microenvironment of solid tumors frequently characterized by areas of poor blood flow, hypoxia, high lactate levels, and low pH_e [10,21–23]. The application of molecular biology techniques to multiparametric/multimodality imaging has provided unprecedented opportunities for understanding and characterizing the tumor microenvironment. We have combined optical, MRI, and MRSI techniques to understand the relationship between vascularization, metabolism, and hypoxia.

The hypoxia inducible factor (HIF-1) mediates the adaptive response of cells to hypoxia [24]. Under normoxic conditions, HIF-1α is subject to ubiquitination and proteosomal degradation [24]. Under hypoxic conditions, ubiquitination of HIF-1α is dramatically reduced and the activity of its transcriptional activation domain increases [25]. HIF-1 can act as a transcriptional activator for several key genes such as vascular endothelial growth factor (VEGF) and several glycolytic enzymes [26,27]. Each of these target genes contains hypoxia response elements (HREs), which include one or more HIF-1 binding sites. By placing enhanced green fluorescent protein (EGFP) expression under the control of an HRE (HRE–EGFP), it is possible to indirectly detect HIF-1 activity and hypoxia in tissues, as shown schematically in (Figure 13.8). PC-3 human prostate cancer cells stably transfected with HRE–EGFP, under oxygenation and 14 h after treatment with 10 μM cobalt chloride, which mimics hypoxia, are shown in Figure 13.9. A dramatic increase in fluorescence can be observed in Figure 13.9b, demonstrating the feasibility of using HRE–EGFP-transfected cells to detect hypoxia.

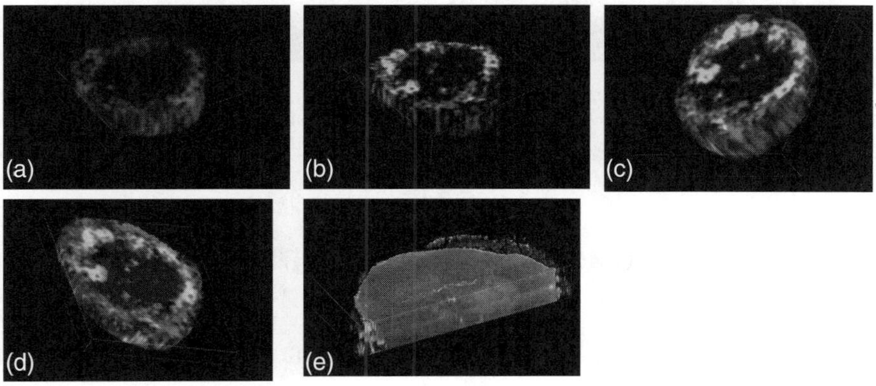

FIGURE 13.7 (See color insert following page 328.) Three-dimensional reconstructed maps obtained from a single MDA–MB-231 tumor (470 mm^3) of (a) MRI map of vascular volume (range 0 to 200 μl/g); (b) MRI map of vascular permeability (range 0 to 7 μl/g min); (c) fused map of vascular volume and permeability; (d) fused map of vascular volume, permeability and pH_e (range from 5.3 to 7.2); (e) hematoxylin and eosin stained histological sections. Spatial resolution of the vascular volume and permeability maps are 0.125 mm in plane with 1 mm slice thickness. The pH_e map was obtained with a spatial resolution of $1 \times 1 \times 4$ mm^3. (Adapted from Bhujwalla, Z. M., et al., *NMR Biomed.*, 15, 114, 2002. With permission of John Wiley & Sons. Copyright 2002.)

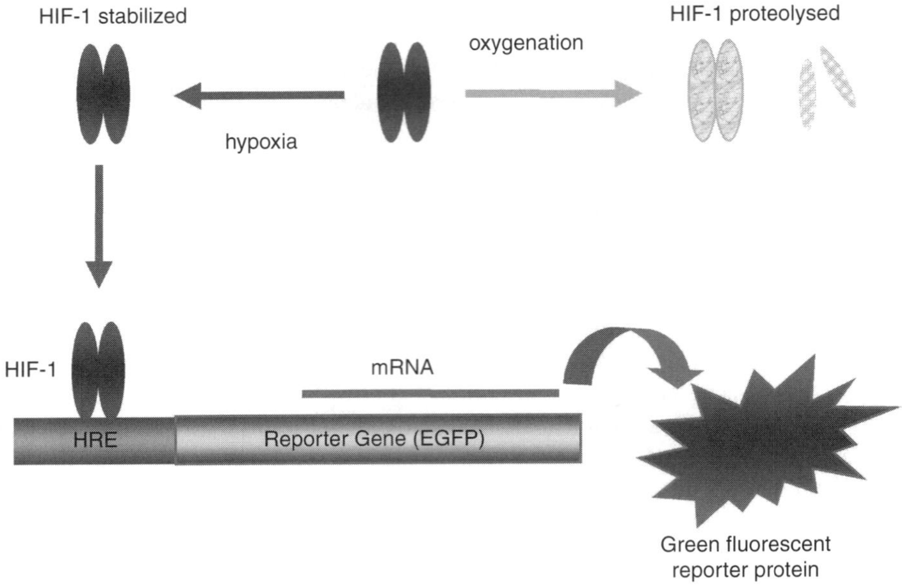

FIGURE 13.8 Schematic display of the formation of GFP under hypoxic conditions utilizing a construct with EGFP under the control of an HRE. (Reproduced from Winnard, P. Jr. and Raman, V. *J. Cell. Biochem.*, 90, 454, 2003. With permission of Wiley-Liss, Inc., a subsidiary of John Wiley & Sons. Copyright 2003.)

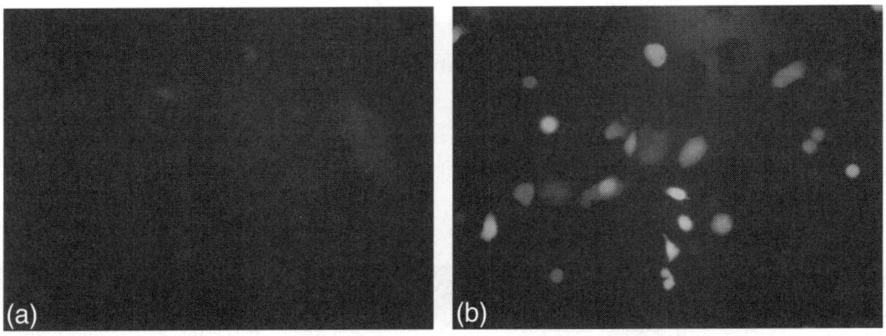

FIGURE 13.9 (See color insert following page 328.) (a) Stably transfected PC-3 cells expressing HRE–GFP under normoxic conditions (20× lens). (b) Stably transfected PC-3 cells expressing HRE–GFP following treatment with 14 h cobalt chloride (10 μM, 20 × lens).

We are currently using a multiparametric approach of combined vascular, spectroscopic, and optical imaging to obtain vascular, metabolic, and hypoxia maps, from co-localized regions within tumors derived from PC-3 clones stably expressing HRE–EGFP [20]. Data from these studies suggest that regions of low vascular volume are typically hypoxic and also exhibit high permeability, most likely due to increased expression of VEGF. These results demonstrate the use of such an approach to understand the dynamics of the relationship between vascularization and metabolism in tumors (see Figure 13.10). Such an approach is useful in the development and discovery of drugs targeting hypoxia and HIF-1.

In previous studies, we have routinely observed that areas of high vascular volume are typically found in viable tumor regions, whereas areas highly permeable to the macromolecular contrast agent albumin–GdDTPA were typically associated with poorly vascularized and dying regions of the tumor [6]. These data suggest that therapeutic anticancer agents of similar size (80 to 90 kD)

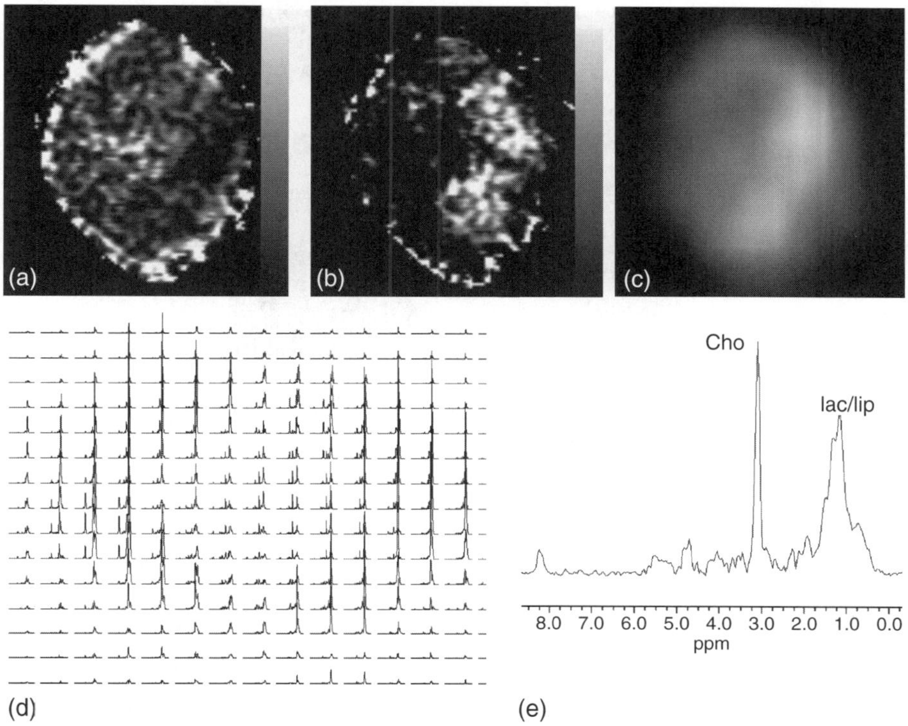

FIGURE 13.10 Co-registered maps of (a) vascular volume, (b) permeability surface area product (PSP) and (c) total choline obtained from the central slice of a transgenic PC-3 tumor (270 mm^3). Vascular volume ranged from 0 to 126 μl/g and PSP from 0 to 3.4 μl/g min. Proton chemical shift imaging spectra obtained from $1 \times 1 \times 4$ mm^3 voxels used to generate the total choline map are shown in (d), and an MR spectrum obtained from a single $1 \times 1 \times 4$ mm^3 voxel with elevated signals from total choline and lactate/lipid is shown in (e). (Adapted from Pathak, A. P., et al., *Methods Enzymol.*, 386, 3, 2004. With permission of Elsevier. Copyright 2004.)

would also most likely leak out in hypoxic dying regions, but not in well-vascularized viable regions of the tumor. By overexpressing VEGF in a cancer cell model, we observed that it was possible to significantly alter the vascular phenotype of tumors so that several regions of high vascular volume were also highly permeable.

VEGF (or VEGF-A) is a multifunctional cytokine that is expressed as several isoforms consisting of polypeptides of different sizes (121, 145, 165, 183, 189, and 206 amino acid residues), which are formed from the same gene by alternative splicing [28,29]. These isoforms have distinct but overlapping functions in angiogenesis. Dafni and colleagues [30] have used C6-pTET–$VEGF_{165}$ tumors, in which overexpression of $VEGF_{165}$ can be modulated *in vivo* by addition or withdrawal of tetracycline in the drinking water, to study the effect of sustained expression of VEGF on lymphatic drain. VEGF overexpressing tumors showed high blood volume fraction and high vessel permeability as detected by contrast enhanced MRI using biotin–BSA–GdDTPA. The rate of change in contrast enhancement was highest in the tumor at early time points, and progressively shifted from the tumor at later time points, in accordance with radial outward convection of the contrast agent [30].

We created stable clones of human breast and prostate cancer cells overexpressing $VEGF_{165}$. In solid tumors derived from these transgenic cells, we investigated the effect of VEGF overexpression on vascularization determined with contrast enhanced MRI using the macromolecular contrast agent albumin–GdDTPA. VEGF overexpression significantly increased vascular

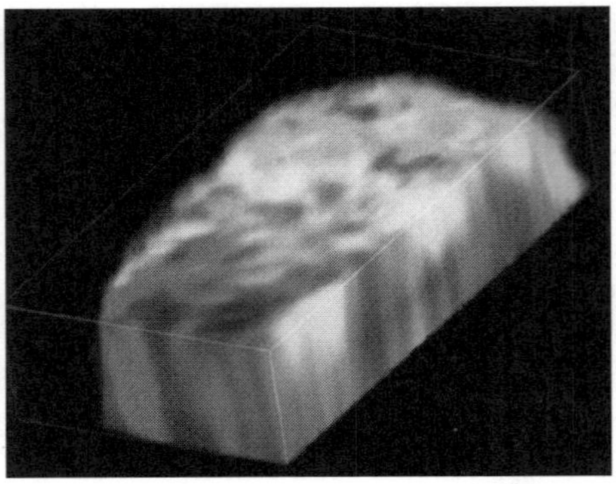

FIGURE 13.11 (See color insert following page 328.) Three-dimensional reconstructed fusion image of vascular volume (red) and permeability (green) from a human prostate cancer xenograft model overexpressing VEGF. Several regions exhibiting yellow are detected demonstrating that regions of high vascular volume are also highly permeable. In previous studies, we have routinely observed that regions of high vascular volume are not permeable [6]. Here, we have shown that VEGF overexpression significantly increases the permeability of well-vascularized regions. (Adapted from Bhujwalla, Z. M., et al., *Proceedings of International Society Magnetic Resonance Medicine*, 2003.)

volume and permeability. As shown in Figure 13.11, VEGF overexpression also significantly increased the permeability of regions with high vascular volume, which are not very permeable in wild type and control tumors [31], suggesting an important role for VEGF to mediate effective delivery of macromolecular therapeutic agents in solid tumors.

13.3.3 Imaging Interstitial Fluid Transport with MRI

The interstitial or extracellular matrix (ECM) of the tumor presents a barrier against the transport of macromolecules and against cancer cell dissemination. The ability to image and characterize the transport of macromolecular agents through the ECM or tumor interstitium can be used to understand factors affecting this transport, their role in macromolecular drug delivery, and in cancer cell dissemination [32,33]. Since the ease of transport of macromolecules through the matrix can be used as an index of its integrity, *in vivo* imaging can be used to design strategies for altering the porosity and integrity of the interstitial matrix, to improve delivery of therapeutic agents.

We have developed a technique to characterize delivery as well as interstitial transport of a macromolecular agent, albumin–GdDTPA, in human breast cancer models *in vivo*, using MRI [34]. The transport parameters derived include vascular volume, permeability-surface area product, macromolecular fluid exudate volume, and drainage and pooling rates [34]. The application of this analysis to identify pooling and draining voxels in multiple slices obtained through an MCF-7 tumor is shown in Figure 13.12.

13.3.4 Detecting Antiangiogenic Effects

Traditionally, a major promise of MR methods has been to detect response to cancer therapy. Several aspects of the use of MR in detecting therapeutic response have been addressed in Chapter 14. Since dynamic contrast enhanced MRI can measure vascular parameters such as vascular volume, permeability surface area product, and relative perfusion, this technique is especially useful for the discovery and development of antiangiogenic and antivascular therapy. Recent studies on dynamic contrast-enhanced-MRI evaluation of response to antiangiogenic and antivascular therapy using low and high molecular weight contrast agents are briefly summarized

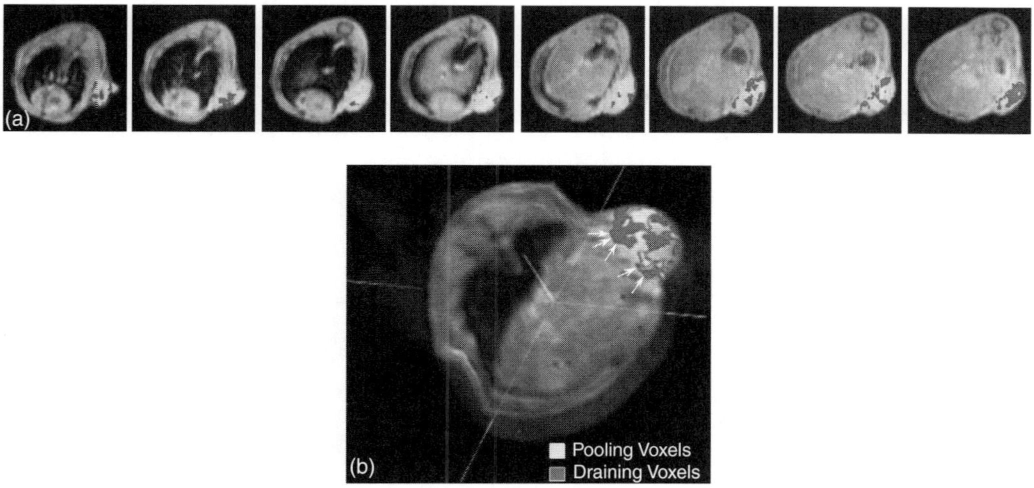

FIGURE 13.12 (See color insert following page 328.) (a) A montage of slices obtained from a severe combined immunodeficient mouse with an MCF-7 tumor in the mammary fat pad. M_0 maps for each slice were overlaid with a functional image, which displays the spatial distribution of draining (red) and pooling voxels (yellow). (b) 3-D reconstruction of the same montage using cubic interpolation, with a cutaway to illustrate drainage (arrows) at the tumor–host tissue interface. (Adapted from Pathak, A. P., et al., *Cancer Res.*, 65, 1425, 2005. With permission of the American Association for Cancer Research. Copyright 2005.)

in Table 13.2 and Table 13.3, respectively. A major advantage of MRI evaluation of antiangiogenic or antivascular therapy is that it provides spatial as well as temporal information following treatment with these agents.

We recently investigated the effect of the antiangiogenic agent TNP-470 on tumor vascular characteristics using MRI. TNP-470 is a fumagillin derivative and its antiangiogenic effects are thought to be due to inhibition of endothelial cell proliferation [35]. Representative vascular volume and permeability data obtained for a pair of volume-matched control and treated tumors are shown in Figure 13.13 and Figure 13.14, respectively. Treatment with TNP-470 resulted in a significant decrease in the permeable and vascular regions within the tumors [35]. However, a compensatory increase in levels of vascular volume and permeability was also apparent in some regions of the treated tumors, demonstrating the critical importance of imaging techniques, which provide spatial information in determining the effects of antiangiogenic therapy. These data demonstrate the ability of MRI to detect changes in tumor vasculature following treatment with antiangiogenic therapy.

13.3.5 MR Methods to Detect Drug Delivery

Poor drug delivery is a major problem in cancer chemotherapy. Restricted delivery of even low molecular weight drug molecules to tumor regions occurs in areas with reduced blood perfusion, low vascularization, and/or low permeability of the vasculature. MR methods can be used to directly determine the pharmacokinetics of a drug in the tumor. The development of specially designed surrogate markers of drug uptake labeled with MR contrast agents is an area of investigation which may yield major advantages in designing treatments optimizing drug delivery to tumors by selective modulation of the tumor vascular bed [36,37].

MR pharmacokinetic measurements of tumors *in vivo* have mainly been restricted to fluorinated drugs detected by ^{19}F MRS (see [38] for a review as well as Chapter 14, Section 14.3), although ^{13}C and ^{1}H MR have also been used to detect drug uptake and distribution [39]. ^{19}F MR has the advantage of relatively high sensitivity and no background signal, but the physicochemical and

TABLE 13.2
Representative MR Studies Using Low Molecular Weight (MW) Contrast Agents for Assessing the Efficacy of Antiangiogenic Therapy

Agent	Mechanism of Action	Low MW–MR Contrast Agent	MRI Parameter Assessed	Effect on MR Parameter	Study
ZD6126	Rapid and reversible tubulin binding leading to selective destabilization of tubulin cytoskeleton of neoendothelial cells	Gd–DTPA or Gd–DTPA–BMA	IAUC	ZD6126 eliminated contrast uptake in necrotic regions. Tumor IAUC decreased in a dose dependent manner. Rapid cell death and necrosis observed. Single dose treatment reduced tumor perfusion for more than 96 h	Evelhoch et al. [74], Robinson et al. [75], and McIntyre et al. [76]
Combrestatin A4 phosphate (CA4P)	Binds to colchicine binding site of tubulin, selectively causing depolymerization of microtubules in tumor vasculature	Gd–DTPA	K^{trans}	For both humans and rats, CA4P acutely reduced K^{trans} in tumors	Galbraith et al. [77]
EMD72000	Blocks epidermal growth factor (EGF) receptor	Gd–DTPA	K^{PS}, fPV	Lower K^{PS} and fPV seen posttreatment	Bangard et al. [78]
HuMV833	AntiVEGF antibody	Gd–DTPA–BMA	k_{fp}	k_{fp} decreased at 48 h posttreatment, with high interpatient variability and no dose response	Jayson et al. [79]
PTK787/ZK 222584	Inhibits VEGF-receptor tyrosine kinases VEGFR-1 (Flt-1) and VEGFR-2 (KDR)	Magnevist	K_i	Significant negative correlation between % of baseline K_i and increase in PTK/ZK dose. Nonprogressors had significantly greater reduction in K_i when compared with progressors	Morgan et al. [80]
Thalidomide	Directly inhibits angiogenesis induced by basic fibroblast growth factor, VEGF and endothelial cell activity	Gd–DTPA	First-pass peak enhancement, maximal enhancement, and the initial enhancement slope percentage	For tumor regions the decrease in slope percentage parameter after thalidomide treatment was of statistical significance, with the other parameters revealing no definite statistical difference	Wang et al. [81]

Monoclonal antibody against vascular endothelial growth factor	Anti-VEGF–antibody	Different contrast agents with MW ranging from 557 Da to 92 kDa	K^{PS}, fPV	Mean K^{PS} and fPV values decreased significantly in the mab-VEGF antibody-treated group compared to baseline values using intermediate or macromolecular contrast media, but did not change significantly using small molecular contrast media	Turetschek et al. [82]
DC101	VEGF receptor-2 antibody	Gd–DTPA	Signal amplitude, i.e., increase of signal intensity relative to precontrast value, k_{ep}	Amplitudes of treated tumors decreased posttreatment. The decrease in amplitude was most pronounced in tumor centers, consistent with change of microvessel density	Kiessling et al. [83]
Dexamethasone	Inhibition of VEGF and/or via vasoconstriction	Gd–DTPA	Gradient- (GE) and spin-echo (SE) relative cerebral blood volume (rCBV) maps	GE rCBV decreased and SE rCBV increased in animals treated with dexamethasone, suggesting a vessel-size selective effect	Badruddoja et al. [84]

fPV, fractional plasma volume; K_i, bi-directional transfer coefficient; K^{trans}, transfer constant; K^{PS}, k_{fp}, k_{ep}, transendothelial permeability; IAUC, initial area under the curve.

TABLE 13.3
Representative MR Studies Using High Molecular Weight Contrast Agents for Assessing the Efficacy of Antiangiogenic Therapy

Agent	Mechanism of Action	High MW–MR Contrast Agent	MRI Parameter Employed for Assessment	Effect on MR Parameter	Study
TNP-470	Inhibits endothelial cell proliferation	Albumin–GdDTPA	Vascular volume, PSP	Decrease in vascular volume; decrease in permeability in some regions, with a compensatory increase in others	Bhujwalla et al. [35]
Avastin	Humanized antiVEGF antibody	Novel protein-binding contrast agent B22956/1, ProHance, and albumin–GdDTPA also used for contrast	K^{PS}	Mean K^{PS} decreased significantly in treated group compared with baseline, and increased significantly in controls, when using B22956/1 contrast. No significant changes observed with ProHance and albumin–GdDTPA	Preda et al. [85]
SU6668	Inhibits VEGF-R2 receptor typrosine kinase (Flk-1/KDR), platelet-derived growth factor (PDGF) receptor, and fibroblast growth factor (FGF) receptor 1	Albumin–GdDTPA	kPS, fPV	Decrease in kPS and fPV observed 24 h post treatment, although a less pronounced effect was observed in the rim than in the core	Marzola et al. [86]

PSP, permeability surface area product; fPV, fractional plasma volume; K^{PS}, kPS, transendothelial permeability.

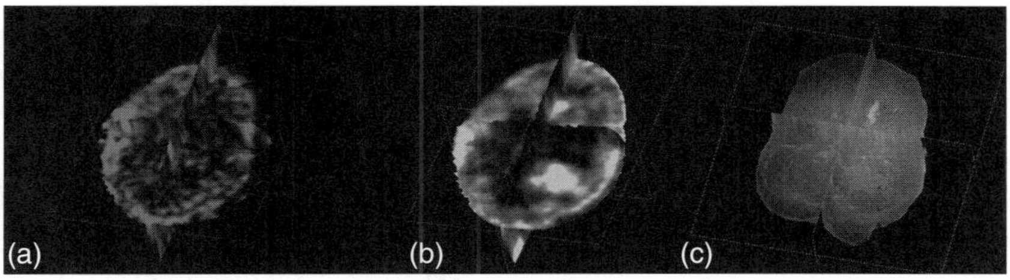

FIGURE 13.13 Triplanar views of 3-D reconstructed maps of (a) vascular volume, (b) permeability, and (c) hematoxylin and eosin stained histological sections for a control MatLyLu tumor (volume 405 mm^3). (Adapted from Bhujwalla, Z. M., et al., *Clin. Cancer Res.*, 9, 355, 2003. With permission of the American Association for Cancer Research. Copyright 2003.)

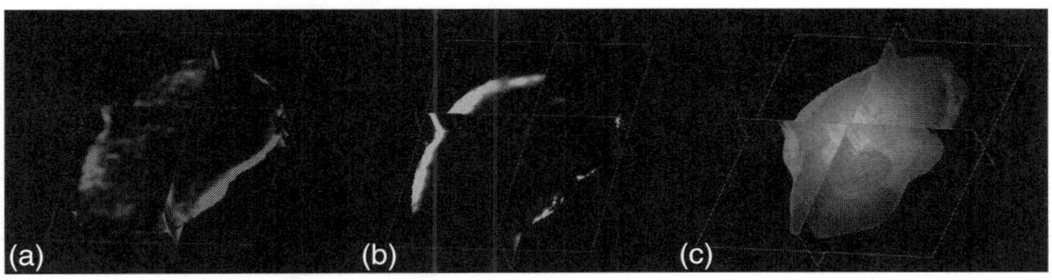

FIGURE 13.14 Triplanar views of 3-D reconstructed maps of (a) vascular volume, (b) permeability, and (c) hematoxylin and eosin stained histological sections for a MatLyLu tumor treated with TNP-470, 30 mg/kg every second day, total dose 90 mg/kg (volume 395 mm^3). (Adapted from Bhujwalla, Z. M., et al., *Clin. Cancer Res.*, 9, 355, 2003. With permission of the American Association for Cancer Research. Copyright 2003.)

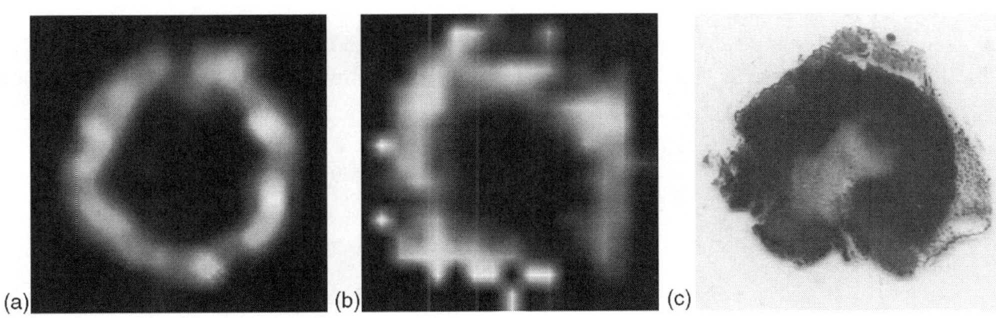

FIGURE 13.15 Maps of (a) contrast uptake, (b) drug uptake, and (c) hematoxylin and eosin stained histological section of the slice from an MDA–MB-435 tumor with a large central necrotic region. (Adapted from Artemov, D., et al., *Cancer Res.*, 61, 3039, 2001. With permission of the American Association for Cancer Research. Copyright 2001.)

pharmacological properties of the drug may be altered by fluorine labeling, for drugs lacking fluorine atoms. In such cases, ^{1}H MRS or ^{13}C MRS may be used, provided the drug has a well-resolved peak, and can be delivered at doses high enough to be detected within the sensitivity limitations of MRS (see [39] for a review). Unique MR-based technologies have been developed to detect ^{13}C labeled drug molecules *in vivo* [37]. As shown in Figure 13.15, these studies have demonstrated that low molecular weight MR contrast agents can be used as surrogate markers of drug delivery to solid tumors [37].

13.4 IDENTIFYING TARGETS WITH MR

The elevation of phosphocholine (PC) and total choline is one of the most widely established characteristics of cancer cells. Increased total choline (tCho: PC + glycerophosphocholine + free choline) and PC levels have been detected in the breast (Figure 13.16), prostate, and different types of brain tumors (see also Chapter 14, Section 14.3.3). Numerous *in vivo* and *in vitro* ^{1}H, ^{31}P, and ^{13}C MRS studies revealed high levels of PC or phosphoethanolamine (PE), or both, in several cancers, whereas low levels of these metabolites were found in corresponding normal tissues (reviewed in [40–42]). These studies demonstrate the significance of phospholipid precursors and catabolites as biochemical indicators of tumor progression and response to therapy.

Transgenic interventions, which increase the malignant characteristics of cancer cells, are found to increase PC or total choline, whereas the reverse is observed in transgenic interventions, which reduce the malignancy of cells. Mutations of the *ras* oncogene family are frequently detected in cancers. Ronen et al. [43] have studied NIH-3T3 fibroblasts transfected with mutant *ras*-oncogene using MRS, and detected significantly higher PC levels in the *ras*-transfected cells compared to the parental cell line. In our program, we have performed studies using transgenic models to further understand choline phospholipid metabolism. Human cancers that contain a *p53* mutation are more aggressive, and more often fatal. We characterized the choline phospholipids of HCT116 human colon cancer cells with ($p53^{+/+}$) and without *p53* ($p53^{-/-}$). As shown in Figure 13.17 and Figure 13.18, we observed that loss of p53 function resulted in increased levels of PC and total choline, which were consistent with increased malignancy [44].

We also studied transgenic breast cancer cell lines stably transfected with a metastasis suppressor gene (*nm23*). Transfection with *nm23* led to increased glycerophosphocholine (GPC) and decreased PC compared to vector transfected control cells, consistent with a reduction of the metastatic phenotype of the *nm23* transfected cells [45]. These changes in phospholipid metabolism detected following *nm23* transfection indicate that phospholipid metabolism mediated signaling may be involved in invasion and metastasis.

Overall, these data show that various molecular alterations, such as *nm23* expression, *p53* expression, and malignant transformation, arrive at a common endpoint in the choline phospholipid metabolism, and demonstrate the important role of choline phospholipids and their metabolites

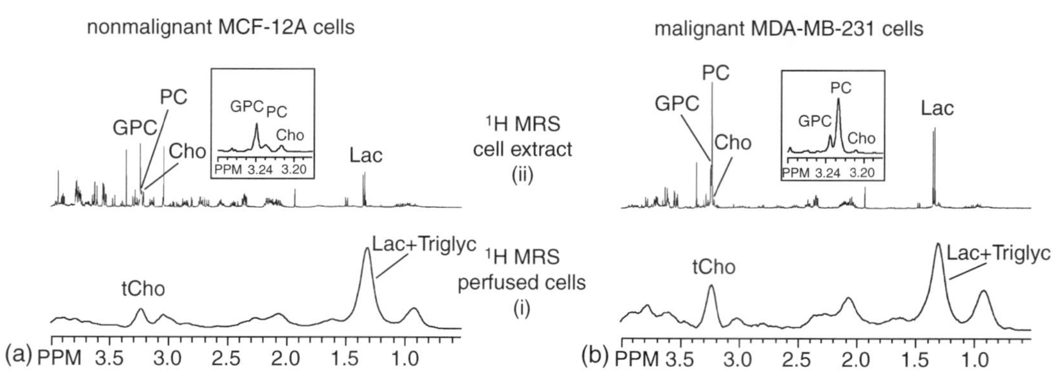

FIGURE 13.16 Representative ^{1}H MR spectra of (a) nonmalignant human mammary epithelial cells (HMECs, MCF-12A) and (b) malignant and invasive human breast cancer cells (MDA–MB-231). (i) ^{1}H MRS of perfused cells demonstrates the increased total choline (tCho: PC + glycerophosphocholine (GPC) + free Choline (Cho)) levels in breast cancer cells vs. nonmalignant HMECs. (ii) ^{1}H MRS of cell extracts demonstrates the increased PC levels in breast cancer cells compared to HMECs. (Adapted from Ackerstaff, E., et al., *J. Cell. Biochem.*, 90, 525, 2003. With permission of Wiley-Liss, Inc., a subsidiary of John Wiley & Sons. Copyright 2003.)

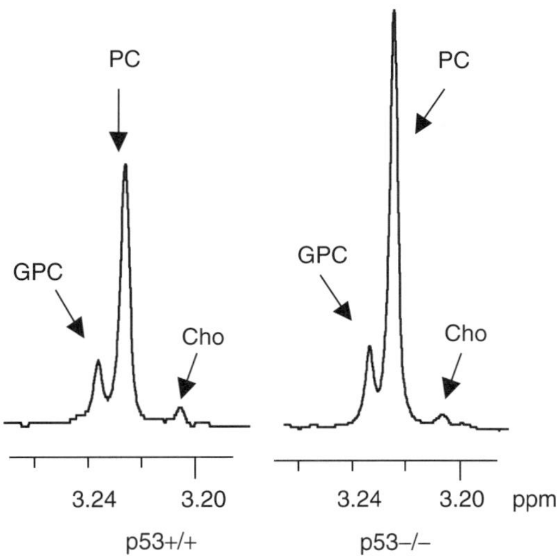

FIGURE 13.17 Representative ^{1}H MR spectra of the phospholipid region of HCT116 *p53* $^{+/+}$ (left) and *p53* $^{-/-}$ (right) cell extracts, obtained from identical cell numbers, demonstrating a significant increase of PC in the *p53* $^{-/-}$ cells. (Adapted from Mori, N., et al., *Mol. Imaging*, 3, 319, 2004. With permission of MIT Press. Copyright 2004 Massachusetts Institute of Technology.)

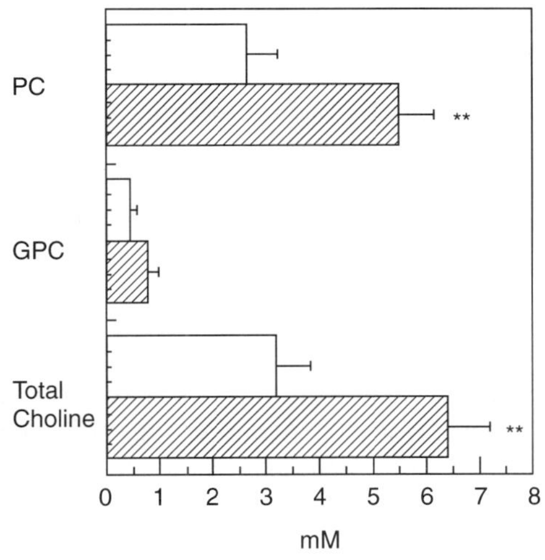

FIGURE 13.18 PC, GPC, and total choline (PC + GPC + Cho) levels measured in HCT116 *p53* $^{+/+}$ (white bars) and *p53* $^{-/-}$ cells (shaded bars) from ^{1}H spectra, showing significantly increased PC levels in *p53* $^{-/-}$ cells. The data represent the mean ± SE of seven cell extracts for each cell line; ** significantly different compared to *p53* $^{+/+}$ ($P < .01$). (Adapted from Mori, N., et al., *Mol. Imaging*, 3, 319, 2004. With permission of MIT Press. Copyright 2004 Massachusetts Institute of Technology.)

in cancer. Importantly, these observations raise the possibility that the alteration of choline phospholipid metabolism presents a unique target to exploit for therapy, and provide a strong rationale for targeting enzymes required for choline phospholipid metabolism in cancer cells. The enzymes involved in choline phospholipid metabolism are outlined in Figure 13.19.

Some of the potential mechanisms underlying the increased phosphocholine levels observed in cancer cells include increased expression and activity of choline kinase [46,47], a higher rate of

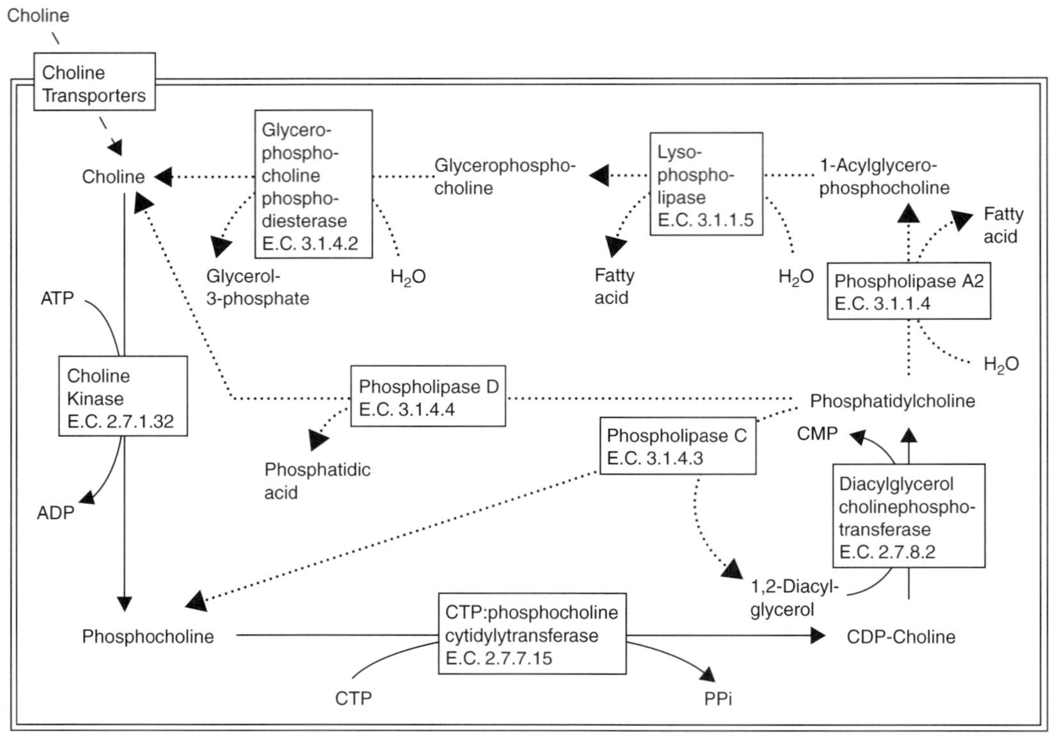

FIGURE 13.19 Schematic representation of enzymes involved in choline phospholipid metabolism. Solid arrows mark anabolic (biosynthetic) pathways, and catabolic (hydrolytic) pathways are marked by dotted arrows. CDP, cytosine diphosphate; CMP, cytosine monophosphate; CTP, cytosine triphosphate; PPi, pyrophosphate. (Adapted from Glunde, K., et al., *Cancer Res.*, 64, 4270, 2004. With permission of the American Association for Cancer Research. Copyright 2004.)

choline transport [48], and phospholipase activity [49,50]. To further understand the role of these enzymes and the mechanisms underlying the alterations in choline phospholipid metabolism, we performed microarray-based gene expression analysis to determine molecular differences in choline phospholipid metabolism between breast cancer cells and nonmalignant human mammary epithelial cells (HMECs) [51]. Microarray gene expression analysis was performed with the Human Genome U133 GeneChip Set from Affymetrix containing 39,000 transcripts. The data shown in (Table 13.4) demonstrate that breast cancer cells overexpressed choline kinase and phospholipase C, but underexpressed lysophospholipase 1, cytosolic calcium-dependent phospholipase A_2, and phospholipase D_1 [51]. The elevation of PC typically observed in tumor extracts is consistent with the overexpression of choline kinase detected in the microarray analyses [51].

Antisense RNAs [52] and ribozymes [53] have been widely used to inhibit gene expression. However, using antisense RNA or ribozyme to inhibit gene expression can be nonspecific and ineffective. It is possible to circumvent this by using small interfering RNAs (siRNAs) of 21 to 23 nucleotides, which mediate effective degradation of the endogenous homologous RNA [54]. The availability of siRNA technology to target specific gene expression has proved very successful [55], and provides new opportunities to target genes in choline phospholipid metabolism as well as other critical pathways identified by MR methods.

An example of human MDA–MB-231 breast cancer cells treated with siRNA designed to knock down choline kinase expression [56] is shown in Figure 13.20. A threefold or higher reduction in choline kinase mRNA was detected within 48 h of treatment with this choline kinase

TABLE 13.4
Gene Expression Differences in MDA–MB-231 Breast Cancer Cells vs. MCF-12A Human Mammary Epithelial Cells

Gene	MCF-12A	MDA–MB-231	Fold Change (90% CI)
Choline kinase (2 independent probe sets)	39 ± 13	166 ± 29	4.27 (2.44 to 9.91)
Lysophospholipase 1 (2 independent probe sets)	684 ± 29	174 ± 11	−3.94 (−3.47 to −4.50)
Phospholipase A2, group IVA (cytosolic, calcium-dependent)	98 ± 15	20 ± 3	−4.98 (−3.41 to −7.45)
Pancreas-enriched phospholipase C	19 ± 9	43 ± 8	2.28 (1.14 to 9.98)
Phospholipase C, beta 3, neighbor pseudogene	209 ± 45	577 ± 87	2.76 (1.82 to 4.51)
Phospholipase D1 (phosphatidylcholine-specific)	35 ± 4	12 ± 4	−2.85 (−1.78 to −5.89)

Significantly over- or under-expressed genes (more than twofold difference) involved in choline phospholipid metabolism are listed. Only well-characterized human genes are displayed. C.I. represents confidence interval. Expression index values are mean ± standard error.

Source: Adapted from Glunde, K., et al., *Cancer Res.*, 64, 4270, 2004. With permission of the American Association for Cancer Research. Copyright 2004.

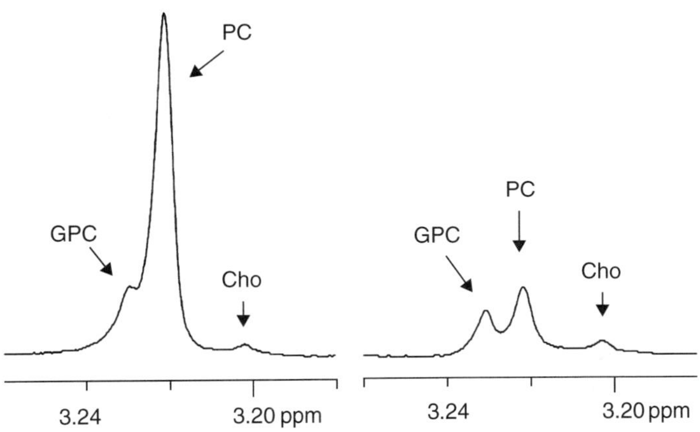

FIGURE 13.20 Proton spectra of cell extracts obtained from control MDA–MB-231 breast cancer cells (left spectrum, 5.8×10^7 cells) and MDA–MB-231 cells treated with siRNA designed to knock down choline kinase expression (right spectrum, 4.6×10^7 cells).

mRNA specific siRNA [57]. A significant reduction in PC is apparent in siRNA-treated MDA–MB-231 cells. We are currently investigating the effect of choline kinase knockdown on phenotypic changes in these cells. Chemically derived choline kinase inhibitors have been observed to exhibit an antimitogenic and antiproliferative effect in cells [58,59] and in tumors in mice [60]. These data demonstrate the feasibility of using MR methods to identify a key target, and to use MRS to determine the outcome of treatment.

13.5 MRI OF RECEPTOR AND GENE EXPRESSION

The development of smart contrast agents has revolutionized the application of MR methods to study cancer by detecting receptor expression and specific molecular targets. This new capability is particularly important in the discovery and development of highly specific drugs targeting molecules and pathways (see also Chapter 15, Section 15.3.1). The past few years have also seen the development of ingenious amplification strategies to increase the sensitivity to detect receptors and molecular targets.

Strategies for generating targeted contrast can be broadly categorized as: (i) where the contrast agent macromolecule is directed to a specific receptor using a high-affinity ligand such as a monoclonal antibody (mAb), (ii) where the number of MR reporter molecules increases with enzymatic activity, resulting in signal amplification, and (iii) where the presence of a targeted probe is detected through a decrease in the bulk water signal due to chemical exchange between protons of bulk water and those of the probe (see review by Pathak et al. [61]). The high detection sensitivity of the latter strategy is due to numerous water molecules interacting with a single molecule of the probe.

In one of the first examples of the use of MRI to detect gene expression, Weissleder and colleagues used 9L glioma cells genetically engineered to express the modified transferrin receptor, ETR, lacking a negative feedback regulation domain. Tumors derived from these cells exhibited significant shortening of T_2^* following administration of transferrin-monocrystalline iron oxide nanoparticles [62].

Detecting the expression of a specific reporter is another example of the application of MR imaging to transgenic cancer cells and tumor models. Artemov et al. [63] developed an MR-based approach to detect HER-2/neu receptor expression in a transgenic HER-2/neu overexpressing tumor model. A two-step labeling procedure permits separation of the targeted contrast agent complex into two components with relatively low molecular weight (160 kD for mAb, and 70 kD for avidin), which improves delivery. For *in vivo* studies, receptors were prelabeled with biotinylated anti-HER-2/neu mAb (biotinylated Herceptin), and probed with a GdDTPA–avidin conjugate 12 h later. A maximum labeling efficiency of 50 gadoliniums (Gd) per receptor was estimated, from an average of 12.5 Gd^{3+} per avidin and four biotins per mAb. Positive contrast in HER-2/*neu* overexpressing tumor xenografts was detected in T_1-weighted MR images using this approach [63]. Such an approach can be extended to image gene expression with MRI which, combined with the functional imaging capabilities of MR methods, can provide insight into the functional effects of a gene of interest.

Large Gd complexes, such as paramagnetic polymerized liposomes [64] and Gd–perfluorocarbon nanoparticles [65,66] targeted to $\alpha_v\beta_3$ integrin receptors, have also been used to image $\alpha_v\beta_3$ integrin receptors expressed on the angiogenic endothelium of tumors. Similarly, human folate receptors in ovarian xenografts were imaged using a folate-conjugated GdDTPA magnetic dendrimer CA [67].

The strategy of targeting iron-oxide nanoparticles to selected receptors using mAb has also been used to image HER-2/*neu* expression in malignant breast cancer cells with a two-step labeling process by conjugating biotinylated Herceptin® mAb and streptavidin–superparamagnetic iron oxide (SPIO) nanoparticles [68]. Strong T_2 contrast was detected in AU-565 cells with high levels of HER-2/*neu* receptor expression, as shown in Figure 13.21. Receptor targeting with iron-oxide nanoparticles has also been applied *in vivo*. Since the protein synaptotagmin binds to phosphatidylserine residues that relocate to the outer leaflet of the plasma membrane in apoptotic cells, SPIO particles conjugated to the C2 domain of synaptotagmin have been used to image apoptosis in solid tumors following chemotherapy [69].

Spectroscopic imaging can also be used to image gene and receptor expression. Stegman et al. [70] used bacterial or yeast cytosine deaminase (CD) to convert 5-fluorocytosine (5-FC) to 5-fluorouracil (5-FU) and detected the conversion *in vivo*. Solid tumors derived from yeast CD transfected cells were easily detected *in vivo*, with high specificity in a mammalian setting. In a study by Aboagye et al. [71], CD was covalently bound to a mAb specific to the L6 antigen expressed in tumors derived from human lung adenocarcinoma H2981 cells. Signal from 5-FU was detected in these tumors using ^{19}F MRSI, following administration of 5-FC.

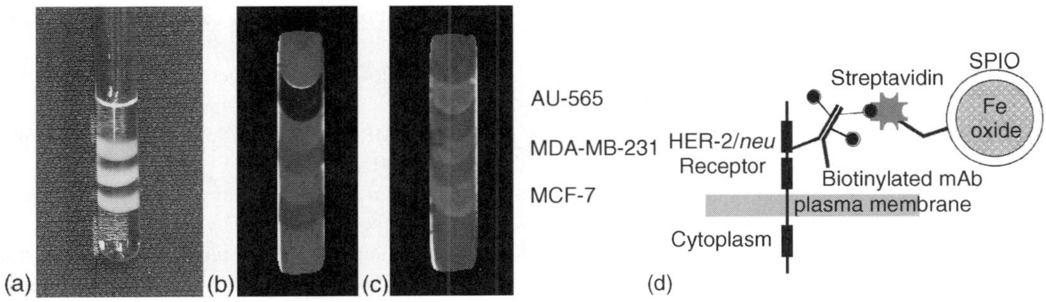

FIGURE 13.21 MR images of AU-565, MDA–MB-231, and MCF-7 breast cancer cells embedded in agarose gel in a 5-mm MR tube. (a) Layout of the cell sample. Cells were pretargeted with (b) biotinylated Herceptin, and (c) nonspecific biotinylated mAb (negative control), and probed with streptavidin SPIO microbeads as shown in (d). T_2 maps of the cell samples were reconstructed from eight T_2-weighted images acquired with a relaxation delay of 8 sec and TE in the range 20 to 250 msec. A T_2 map of a cell sample probed with Herceptin is shown in (b), and the control cell sample treated with a nonspecific biotinylated mAb is shown in (c). Expression level of the HER-2/*neu* receptor was 2.7×10^6 for AU-565, 8.9×10^4 for MCF-7, and 4×10^4 for MDA–MB-231 cells, respectively. (Adapted from Pathak, A. P., et al., *Methods Enzymol.*, 386, 3, 2004. With permission of Elsevier. Copyright 2004.)

These novel contrast agents and strategies used to detect genes and receptors have been applied in preclinical models. The translation of these techniques to the clinic, however, will require substantial improvements in CA chemistry and MR technology.

13.6 CONCLUSION

A wealth of spatial and temporal information on tumor vasculature, metabolism, and physiology can be obtained from noninvasive MRI and MRSI methods. Recent advances in the development of targeted CAs have increased the versatility of MR for molecular imaging, and make it an invaluable technique in drug discovery and development for a complex disease such as cancer. MR methods can provide multiple parameters from co-localized regions, allowing multivariate analyses of these parameters. The more information that can be gathered to characterize complex cancer lesions, the better informed the clinician or researcher will be in decisions on prognosis or response to therapy, or in determining how specific molecular alterations may alter function. Studies combining multiparametric/multimodality imaging and genomic as well as proteomic analyses [72] will play an important role in the ultimate characterization of the malignant phenotype with MR methods, and in successful drug discovery and development against cancer.

ACKNOWLEDGMENTS

Work from the authors' program was supported through funding by NIH grants 2R01 CA73850, 1R01 CA90471, 2R01 CA82337, P50 CA 103175, RO1 CA97310.

REFERENCES

1. DeMarzo, A. M. et al., Pathological and molecular aspects of prostate cancer, *Lancet*, 361, 955, 2003.
2. Hanahan, D. and Weinberg, R. A., The hallmarks of cancer, *Cell*, 100, 57, 2000.
3. Albini, A. et al., Comparison of the chemotactic response to conditioned medium of BALB/c3T3 fibroblasts and their SV 40 transformants, *Tumori*, 71, 97, 1985.

4. Gehlsen, K. R., Wagner, H. N. Jr., and Hendrix, M. J., Membrane invasion culture system (MICS), *Med. Instrum.*, 18, 268, 1984.
5. Pilatus, U. et al., Imaging prostate cancer invasion with multi-nuclear magnetic resonance methods: the metabolic Boyden chamber, *Neoplasia*, 2, 273, 2000.
6. Bhujwalla, Z. M. et al., Vascular differences detected by MRI for metastatic versus nonmetastatic breast and prostate cancer xenografts, *Neoplasia*, 3, 143, 2001.
7. Ackerstaff, E. et al., Endothelial cells promote cancer cell invasion under hypoxia, *Proceedings of International Society Magnetic Resonance Medicine, Glasgow*, 2001, p. 727.
8. Ackerstaff, E. et al., VEGF Overexpression increases invasion of a human prostate cancer cell line under hypoxia in the presence of endothelial cells, *Proceedings of International Society Magnetic Resonance Medicine*, 2004, p. 64.
9. Dvorak, H. F., Tumors: wounds that do not heal. Similarities between tumor stroma generation and wound healing, *N. Engl. J. Med.*, 315, 1650, 1986.
10. Vaupel, P., Kallinowski, F., and Okunieff, P., Blood flow, oxygen and nutrient supply, and metabolic microenvironment of human tumors: a review, *Cancer Res.*, 49, 6449, 1989.
11. Fulton, A. M., The role of eicosanoids in tumor metastasis, *Prostaglandins Leukot. Essent. Fatty Acids*, 34, 229, 1988.
12. Noguchi, M. et al., The role of fatty acids and eicosanoid synthesis inhibitors in breast carcinoma, *Oncology*, 52, 265, 1995.
13. Karmali, R. A. et al., Eicosanoids and metastasis: experimental aspects in Lewis lung carcinoma, *Cancer Biochem. Biophys.*, 9, 97, 1986.
14. Tsujii, M. et al., Cyclooxygenase regulates angiogenesis induced by colon cancer cells, *Cell*, 93, 705, 1998.
15. Ackerstaff, E. et al., Anti-inflammatory agent indomethacin reduces invasion and causes metabolic changes in a human breast cancer cell line, *Proceedings of International Society Magnetic Resonance Medicine*, 2004, p. 65.
16. Aboagye, E. O. and Bhujwalla, Z. M., Malignant transformation alters membrane choline phospholipid metabolism of human mammary epithelial cells, *Cancer Res.*, 59, 80, 1999.
17. Fan, X. et al., Differentiation of nonmetastatic and metastatic rodent prostate tumors with high spectral and spatial resolution MRI, *Magn. Reson. Med.*, 45, 1046, 2001.
18. Su, M. Y. et al., Characterization of N-ethyl-N-nitrosourea-induced malignant and benign breast tumors in rats by using three MR contrast agents, *J. Magn. Reson. Imaging*, 9, 177, 1999.
19. Bhujwalla, Z. M. et al., Combined vascular and extracellular pH imaging of solid tumors, *NMR Biomed.*, 15, 114, 2002.
20. Bhujwalla, Z. M. et al., Characterization of the tumor microenvironment using combined MRI, MRSI and optical imaging, *Proceedings of International Society Magnetic Resonance Medicine*, 2004, p. 219.
21. Brizel, D. M. et al., Tumor oxygenation predicts for the likelihood of distant metastases in human soft tissue sarcoma, *Cancer Res.*, 56, 941, 1996.
22. Hockel, M. et al., Tumor hypoxia in pelvic recurrences of cervical cancer, *Int. J. Cancer*, 79, 365, 1998.
23. Walenta, S. et al., High lactate levels predict likelihood of metastases, tumor recurrence, and restricted patient survival in human cervical cancers, *Cancer Res.*, 60, 916, 2000.
24. Semenza, G. L., HIF-1: mediator of physiological and pathophysiological responses to hypoxia, *J. Appl. Physiol.*, 88, 1474, 2000.
25. Semenza, G. L., Expression of hypoxia-inducible factor 1: mechanisms and consequences, *Biochem. Pharmacol.*, 59, 47, 2000.
26. Semenza, G. L. et al., Hypoxia response elements in the aldolase A, enolase 1, and lactate dehydrogenase A gene promoters contain essential binding sites for hypoxia-inducible factor 1, *J. Biol. Chem.*, 271, 32529, 1996.
27. Shibata, T., Giaccia, A. J., and Brown, J. M., Development of a hypoxia-responsive vector for tumor-specific gene therapy, *Gene Ther.*, 7, 493, 2000.
28. Neufeld, G. et al., Vascular endothelial growth factor (VEGF) and its receptors, *Faseb J.*, 13, 9, 1999.
29. Toi, M., Matsumoto, T., and Bando, H., Vascular endothelial growth factor: its prognostic, predictive, and therapeutic implications, *Lancet Oncol.*, 2, 667, 2001.

30. Dafni, H. et al., Overexpression of vascular endothelial growth factor 165 drives peritumor interstitial convection and induces lymphatic drain: magnetic resonance imaging, confocal microscopy, and histological tracking of triple-labeled albumin, *Cancer Res.*, 62, 6731, 2002.
31. Bhujwalla, Z. M. et al., MRI of prostate tumors overexpressing VEGF exhibit distinct alterations of vascular permeability, *Proceedings of International Society Magnetic Resonance Medicine*, 2003.
32. Jain, R. K., Vascular and interstitial barriers to delivery of therapeutic agents in tumors, *Cancer Metastasis Rev.*, 9, 253, 1990.
33. Jain, R. K., Physiological barriers to delivery of monoclonal antibodies and other macromolecules in tumors, *Cancer Res.*, 50, 814s, 1990.
34. Pathak, A. P. et al., Characterizing extravascular fluid transport of macromolecules in the tumor interstitium by magnetic resonance imaging, *Cancer Res.*, 65, 1425, 2005.
35. Bhujwalla, Z. M. et al., Reduction of vascular and permeable regions in solid tumors detected by macromolecular contrast magnetic resonance imaging after treatment with antiangiogenic agent TNP-470, *Clin. Cancer Res.*, 9, 355, 2003.
36. Taylor, J. S. and Reddick, W. E., Evolution from empirical dynamic contrast-enhanced magnetic resonance imaging to pharmacokinetic MRI, *Adv. Drug Deliv. Rev.*, 41, 91, 2000.
37. Artemov, D., Solaiyappan, M., and Bhujwalla, Z. M., Magnetic resonance pharmacoangiography to detect and predict chemotherapy delivery to solid tumors, *Cancer Res.*, 61, 3039, 2001.
38. Wolf, W., Presant, C. A., and Waluch, V., 19F-MRS studies of fluorinated drugs in humans, *Adv. Drug Deliv. Rev.*, 41, 55, 2000.
39. Griffiths, J. R. and Glickson, J. D., Monitoring pharmacokinetics of anticancer drugs: non-invasive investigation using magnetic resonance spectroscopy, *Adv. Drug Deliv. Rev.*, 41, 75, 2000.
40. de Certaines, J. D. et al., In vivo 31P MRS of experimental tumours, *NMR Biomed.*, 6, 345, 1993.
41. Negendank, W., Studies of human tumors by MRS: a review, *NMR Biomed.*, 5, 303, 1992.
42. Ackerstaff, E., Glunde, K., and Bhujwalla, Z. M., Choline phospholipid metabolism: a target in cancer cells?, *J. Cell. Biochem.*, 90, 525, 2003.
43. Ronen, S. M. et al., Magnetic resonance detects changes in phosphocholine associated with Ras activation and inhibition in NIH 3T3 cells, *Br. J. Cancer*, 84, 691, 2001.
44. Mori, N. et al., Loss of p53 function in colon cancer cells results in increased phosphocholine and total choline, *Mol. Imaging*, 3, 319, 2004.
45. Bhujwalla, Z. M. et al., Nm23-transfected MDA–MB-435 human breast carcinoma cells form tumors with altered phospholipid metabolism and pH: a 31P nuclear magnetic resonance study in vivo and in vitro, *Magn. Reson. Med.*, 41, 897, 1999.
46. Ramirez de Molina, A. et al., Overexpression of choline kinase is a frequent feature in human tumor-derived cell lines and in lung, prostate, and colorectal human cancers, *Biochem. Biophys. Res. Commun.*, 296, 580, 2002.
47. Ramirez de Molina, A. et al., Increased choline kinase activity in human breast carcinomas: clinical evidence for a potential novel antitumor strategy, *Oncogene*, 21, 4317, 2002.
48. Katz-Brull, R. and Degani, H., Kinetics of choline transport and phosphorylation in human breast cancer cells; NMR application of the zero trans method, *Anticancer Res.*, 16, 1375, 1996.
49. Noh, D. Y. et al., Overexpression of phospholipase D1 in human breast cancer tissues, *Cancer Lett.*, 161, 207, 2000.
50. Guthridge, C. J. et al., Phospholipases A2 in ras-transformed and immortalized human mammary epithelial cells, *Cancer Lett.*, 86, 11, 1994.
51. Glunde, K., Jie, C., and Bhujwalla, Z. M., Molecular causes of the aberrant choline phospholipid metabolism in breast cancer, *Cancer Res.*, 64, 4270, 2004.
52. Sokol, D. L. and Murray, J. D., Antisense and ribozyme constructs in transgenic animals, *Transgenic Res.*, 5, 363, 1996.
53. Marschall, P., Thomson, J. B., and Eckstein, F., Inhibition of gene expression with ribozymes, *Cell. Mol. Neurobiol.*, 14, 523, 1994.
54. Caplen, N. J. et al., Specific inhibition of gene expression by small double-stranded RNAs in invertebrate and vertebrate systems, *Proc. Natl. Acad. Sci. USA*, 98, 9742, 2001.
55. Xia, H. et al., siRNA-mediated gene silencing in vitro and in vivo, *Nat. Biotechnol.*, 20, 1006, 2002.

56. Glunde, K., Raman, V., and Bhujwalla, Z. M., Correlation between choline kinase mRNA and 1H MRS-detectable choline metabolite levels in stable choline kinase knock-down clones of a human breast cancer cell line, *Proc. Int. Soc. Magn. Reson. Med.*, 2004, p. 2029.
57. Glunde, K. et al., RNA interference-mediated choline kinase suppression in breast cancer cells induces differentiation and reduces proliferation, *Cancer Res.*, 65, 11034, 2005.
58. Hernandez-Alcoceba, R. et al., Choline kinase inhibitors as a novel approach for antiproliferative drug design, *Oncogene*, 15, 2289, 1997.
59. Campos, J. M. et al., Quantitative structure–activity relationships for a series of symmetrical bisquaternary anticancer compounds, *Bioorg. Med. Chem.*, 10, 2215, 2002.
60. Hernandez-Alcoceba, R., Fernandez, F., and Lacal, J. C., In vivo antitumor activity of choline kinase inhibitors: a novel target for anticancer drug discovery, *Cancer Res.*, 59, 3112, 1999.
61. Pathak, A. P. et al., Molecular and functional imaging of cancer: advances in MRI and MRS, *Methods Enzymol.*, 386, 3, 2004.
62. Weissleder, R. et al., In vivo magnetic resonance imaging of transgene expression, *Nat. Med.*, 6, 351, 2000.
63. Artemov, D. et al., Magnetic resonance molecular imaging of the HER-2/neu receptor, *Cancer Res.*, 63, 2723, 2003.
64. Sipkins, D. A. et al., Detection of tumor angiogenesis in vivo by alphaVbeta3-targeted magnetic resonance imaging, *Nat. Med.*, 4, 623, 1998.
65. Winter, P. M. et al., Improved molecular imaging contrast agent for detection of human thrombus, *Magn. Reson. Med.*, 50, 411, 2003.
66. Anderson, S. A. et al., Magnetic resonance contrast enhancement of neovasculature with alpha(v)beta(3)-targeted nanoparticles, *Magn. Reson. Med.*, 44, 433, 2000.
67. Konda, S. D. et al., Development of a tumor-targeting MR contrast agent using the high-affinity folate receptor: work in progress, *Invest. Radiol.*, 35, 50, 2000.
68. Artemov, D. et al., MR molecular imaging of the Her-2/neu receptor in breast cancer cells using targeted iron oxide nanoparticles, *Magn. Reson. Med.*, 49, 403, 2003.
69. Zhao, M. et al., Non-invasive detection of apoptosis using magnetic resonance imaging and a targeted contrast agent, *Nat. Med.*, 7, 1241, 2001.
70. Stegman, L. D. et al., Noninvasive quantitation of cytosine deaminase transgene expression in human tumor xenografts with in vivo magnetic resonance spectroscopy, *Proc. Natl. Acad. Sci. USA*, 96, 9821, 1999.
71. Aboagye, E. O. et al., Intratumoral conversion of 5-fluorocytosine to 5-fluorouracil by monoclonal antibody–cytosine deaminase conjugates: noninvasive detection of prodrug activation by magnetic resonance spectroscopy and spectroscopic imaging, *Cancer Res.*, 58, 4075, 1998.
72. Guccione, S. et al., Functional genomics guided with MR imaging: mouse tumor model study, *Radiology*, 228, 560, 2003.
73. Kolch, W. et al., The role of Raf kinases in malignant transformation, *Expert Rev. Mol. Med.*, 1, 2002, 2002.
74. Evelhoch, J. L. et al., Magnetic resonance imaging measurements of the response of murine and human tumors to the vascular-targeting agent ZD6126, *Clin. Cancer Res.*, 10, 3650, 2004.
75. Robinson, S. P. et al., Tumour dose response to the antivascular agent ZD6126 assessed by magnetic resonance imaging, *Br. J. Cancer*, 88, 1592, 2003.
76. McIntyre, D. J. et al., Single dose of the antivascular agent, ZD6126 (N-acetylcolchinol-O-phosphate), reduces perfusion for at least 96 hours in the GH3 prolactinoma rat tumor model, *Neoplasia*, 6, 150, 2004.
77. Galbraith, S. M. et al., Combretastatin A4 phosphate has tumor antivascular activity in rat and man as demonstrated by dynamic magnetic resonance imaging, *J. Clin. Oncol.*, 21, 2831, 2003.
78. Bangard, C. et al., Magnetic resonance imaging in an orthotopic rat model: blockade of epidermal growth factor receptor with EMD72000 inhibits human pancreatic carcinoma growth, *Int. J. Cancer*, 114, 131, 2005.
79. Jayson, G. C. et al., Molecular imaging and biological evaluation of HuMV833 anti-VEGF antibody: implications for trial design of antiangiogenic antibodies, *J. Natl. Cancer Inst.*, 94, 1484, 2002.

80. Morgan, B. et al., Dynamic contrast-enhanced magnetic resonance imaging as a biomarker for the pharmacological response of PTK787/ZK 222584, an inhibitor of the vascular endothelial growth factor receptor tyrosine kinases, in patients with advanced colorectal cancer and liver metastases: results from two phase I studies, *J. Clin. Oncol.*, 21, 3955, 2003.
81. Wang, J. et al., Dynamic contrast-enhanced MRI analysis of perfusion changes in advanced hepatocellular carcinoma treated with an antiangiogenic agent: a preliminary study, *Am. J. Roentgenol.*, 183, 713, 2004.
82. Turetschek, K. et al., Tumor microvascular changes in antiangiogenic treatment: assessment by magnetic resonance contrast media of different molecular weights, *J. Magn. Reson. Imaging*, 20, 138, 2004.
83. Kiessling, F. et al., Dynamic contrast-enhanced magnetic resonance imaging rapidly indicates vessel regression in human squamous cell carcinomas grown in nude mice caused by VEGF receptor 2 blockade with DC101, *Neoplasia*, 6, 213, 2004.
84. Badruddoja, M. A. et al., Antiangiogenic effects of dexamethasone in 9L gliosarcoma assessed by MRI cerebral blood volume maps, *Neuro-oncology*, 5, 235, 2003.
85. Preda, A. et al., MRI monitoring of Avastin antiangiogenesis therapy using B22956/1, a new blood pool contrast agent, in an experimental model of human cancer, *J. Magn. Reson. Imaging*, 20, 865, 2004.
86. Marzola, P. et al., In vivo assessment of antiangiogenic activity of SU6668 in an experimental colon carcinoma model, *Clin. Cancer Res.*, 10, 739, 2004.

14 MR for Clinical Pharmacological Studies in Cancer

Geoffrey S. Payne, David J. Collins, Elizabeth M. Charles-Edwards, Mounia Beloueche-Babari, and Martin O. Leach

CONTENTS

14.1 INTRODUCTION

Imaging, using CT or MRI, has provided a major endpoint of response assessment for clinical trials of conventional cytotoxic agents. Changes in bidirectional size (WHO criteria) or unidirectional size (of the maximum dimension) RECIST are used as measures of tumor response. While widely used, these measures are usually performed at the end of, typically, six courses of treatment, and do not provide an early assessment of response. Size is usually considered to encompass the whole observable volume, and does not provide an easy way of assessing the volume of viable tumor remaining, where there may also be areas of necrosis or cyst. While MRI, based on the water content of tissues, provides unrivaled morphological detail, it can also provide a number of functional measures of tissues. Contrast agents can change the MR properties of water, providing a means of probing the vascular function of tumors. While most contrast agents are passive, there is considerable research effort directed at active agents that will report on their local environment or cell surface receptors, or bioactive probes with signals that can be modulated by local biochemical activity. Diffusion of water can be measured, probing the extracellular space of tumors, providing information on cellularity and necrosis. These methods have been shown to inform on drug delivery, and response.

In addition to MRI, MRS provides a means of measuring both tissue and drug metabolism. ^{31}P and ^{1}H MRS provide information on metabolites involved in energy and lipid metabolism. ^{19}F and ^{31}P MRS can monitor the metabolism of drugs such as 5-fluoro-uracil (5FU) and cyclophosphamide. Where new drugs contain these nuclei, or are enriched with ^{13}C, there is the possibility to monitor their metabolism and their delivery to different tissues. MRS has been used to monitor response to conventional agents, showing early changes in phospholipid metabolism. Recent studies indicate a potential role for ^{31}P and ^{1}H MRS in the evaluation of novel pathway inhibitors. ^{19}F labeled compounds can be used to assess the delivery and activation of prodrugs by gene therapies, such as gene-directed enzyme prodrug therapy (GDEPT).

Cancer therapy is moving from conventional therapeutics, such as cytotoxic DNA-binding agents and anti-metabolites, to approaches based on our growing knowledge of the cancer genome, and the function of specific pathways (see also Chapter 13). Small molecule inhibitors are directed at pathways and processes upregulated or modified in cancer, such as Ras/Raf/MAPK and PI3K pathways, cell cycle control, cellular damage, repair and shutdown, angiogenesis, and vascular processes. Recent results have shown that MRS exhibits phospholipid metabolite changes that correlate with inhibition of target proteins in signaling cascades. The technology is available to translate this to clinical studies. MRI using dynamic contrast agents have been used in clinical trials to assess antiangiogenic and antivascular therapies.

In the following sections we consider functional MRI, using both intrinsic and extrinsic contrast mechanisms together with their applications, and then address developments in MRS and their application to the evaluation of cancer therapeutics.

14.2 FUNCTIONAL MAGNETIC RESONANCE IMAGING

14.2.1 Intrinsic Contrast Mechanisms

Intrinsic contrast MRI mechanisms, i.e., mechanisms exploiting endogenous tissue properties, can image therapeutic-induced changes in tumor function. In addition to the classic response end points associated with the size of a solid tumor, intrinsic contrast mechanisms can provide information regarding a tumor's microscopic cellular architecture, vascular supply, and oxygenation. The three mechanisms discussed in this section, diffusion-weighted MRI (DWMRI) and associated intravoxel incoherent motion (IVIM), arterial spin labeling (ASL) and blood oxygen-level dependent (BOLD) contrast are not an exhaustive list, rather they have been chosen for inclusion because they are widely available on clinical MRI scanners and their noninvasive nature makes them particularly attractive for repetitive clinical measurements. Significant possibilities lie in imaging nuclei critical to cellular processes other than hydrogen, such as sodium [1], and it is expected that all endogenous contrast mechanisms will benefit significantly from signal-to-noise increases associated with higher strength clinical MR scanners.

14.2.1.1 Diffusion-Weighted MRI

DWMRI uses water diffusion as a marker of tissue cellularity. DWMRI pulse sequences employ at least one diffusion-gradient comprising two equal but opposing polarity magnetic field gradients. The intensity of the MR signal is inversely dependent on the net distance traveled by protons in the direction of the gradient within the observation period (i.e., between application of the two diffusion gradients). A sequence's sensitivity to diffusion (its b-value) can be varied by the operator. Diffusion measures can be made directionally dependent or independent via careful combination of data from several diffusion gradient directions. Acquisition of images at multiple b-values enables calculation of a quantitative apparent diffusion coefficient (ADC) map. The ADC of a pixel in such a map is represented as the pixel's intensity, i.e., the mean ADC of a region of interest can be determined by obtaining the mean pixel intensity value.

If the observation period is sufficient to allow water molecules to migrate distances comparable with the spacing between cells, then it becomes feasible to observe the restrictive effects of cell membranes. Successful treatment of a tumor with a cytotoxic agent may result in a subsequent reduction in tumor cell density prior to bulk tumor size changes. The reduction in cell density effectively increases the fractional volume of the extracellular space, and hence extracellular water diffusion, reflected in an increase in ADC obtained using imaging sequences sensitized to the appropriate diffusion length scale. Areas of necrosis, which can impede drug delivery, exhibit high ADC values. As such, ADC measurements may be used for serial assessment of response to therapy designed to kill tumor cells [2] or to predict response to treatment [3].

14.2.1.2 IntraVoxel Incoherent Motion

A diffusion-based measurement can be used to investigate parameters associated with tumor vascularity. Blood flow through microscopic blood vessels results in a loss of signal and it is possible to model microvascular capillary flow as a fast diffusion process [4]. IVIM is sensitive to capillary level flow (of particular relevance to the delivery of drugs to tumor cells) and has been used to measure the effects of vasomodulators [5], but care must be taken to separate the slow flow effects from those caused by molecular diffusion [6].

The effect of subject motion can make diffusion-based measurements meaningless, a confounding factor when imaging patients. Very fast scanning techniques can minimize the effect of motion and the majority of diffusion-based measurements are made using fast echo-planar imaging (EPI). Whilst now widely available, EPI has a number of disadvantages including vulnerability to the effects of susceptibility mismatches in the subject (e.g., in areas of air-tissue interface) and eddy currents in the preceding diffusion-encoding gradients. The method of data acquisition can often lead to N/2 ghosting, a ghost image shifted by one half of the image field of view, image blurring and such an extensive fat, water shift that fat-suppressed imaging is required. These factors can reduce both the accuracy and the precision of the measurements being made. Thus, DWMRI-based acquisitions should be accompanied by an appropriate quality assurance programme [7]. EPI is an acoustically noisy technique with the potential to cause peripheral nerve stimulation, which, whilst not dangerous, can be a painful and disconcerting experience.

14.2.1.3 Arterial Spin Labeling

An alternative approach for quantifying microvascular flow involves magnetically tagging blood water proximal to, or in, the tissue of interest and using it as an endogenous tracer with the resulting regional concentration of labeled spins in tissue being a function of regional blood flow. ASL does not require the administration of an extrinsic tracer and so minimally disturbs the system being imaged. The perfusion-weighted image is available immediately after acquisition and can be repeated immediately if of unusable quality (e.g., due to the effect of patient motion). ASL may produce absolute perfusion related quantities allowing comparison of patients within a group or comparison of serial measurements. For quantitative imaging, small differences in T_1 have to be measured very precisely, and the low signal-to-noise ratio, an issue with all the endogenous contrast mechanisms, can adversely affect accuracy and precision. ASL can produce unrealistically high perfusion values arising from motion and negative perfusion in areas of very low or no perfusion. The model used in conjunction with ASL perfusion measurements generally assumes a fast diffusion exchange between capillary and extravascular space, which may not be the case in fast-flowing blood or in necrotic tumors. ASL has been used to quantify changes in perfusion resulting from radiotherapy in a group of patients with head-and-neck cancer [8] and its performance compared favorably with that of contrast-enhanced MRI in the estimation of blood flow within brain tumors [9].

14.2.1.4 Blood Oxygen-Level Dependent Contrast

The BOLD contrast mechanism originates from the dependency of hemoglobin's magnetic susceptibility upon its oxygenation state. Deoxyhemoglobin (deoxy-Hb) is more paramagnetic than oxyhemoglobin (HbO2). The paramagnetic deoxy-HB causes a magnetic field gradient between the blood vessel and the surrounding tissue, which causes a direct signal loss in T_2^* weighted MR images and in T_2 weighted images via a diffusion process. Whilst BOLD contrast MRI is used extensively in brain research, its use within the context of evaluating the oxygenation and vascular function of solid tumors is comparatively new and generally performed in conjunction with a controlled modulation of blood oxygenation (e.g., by inhalation of oxygen or carbogen, a mixture of approximately 95% oxygen and 5% carbon dioxide).

In animals, BOLD results derived from T_2^* weighted scans at 4.7 T were sensitive to a differential response to hypercapnia associated with mature vessels, whilst the BOLD response to hyperoxia was associated with total vascular function in tumor and wound-induced angiogenesis in animal models [10]. In another animal model, microvessel density was found to correlate inversely ($r = -0.89$, $p < .001$) with the increase in BOLD signal of head and neck carcinoma xenografts measured using a carbogen stimulus in conjunction with a T_2-weighted scan performed at 4.7 T [11]. T_2^* weighted BOLD can be dominated by the effects of large vessels distal to the tumor, but it has a significantly greater signal response to changes in oxygenation than does T_2 weighted BOLD imaging which may be of significance when imaging in the clinical environment at 1.5 T. In both clinical and preclinical scenarios, the requirement to alter levels of blood oxygenation leads to significant practical problems in fitting and using a mask system that can deliver gases whilst the subject is being scanned. T_2^* weighted BOLD imaging is often performed using an EPI sequence and consequently suffers from the effects discussed above.

14.2.2 Dynamic Contrast Enhanced MRI in Clinical Drug Trials

14.2.2.1 Low Molecular Weight Agents

Low molecular weight paramagnetic contrast agents, such as Gd-DTPA, are routinely used as diagnostic agents in radiology. Following intravenous bolus injection or infusion, they transit through the heart and lungs, causing some dispersion of the bolus, and enter the arterial supply. Where the vascular endothelium is permeable (for example, outside of the normal central nervous system) these contrast agents equilibrate with the extravascular extracellular space. Subsequently, the contrast agent is renally excreted. In cancer, the microvascular endothelium is often abnormal, containing large fenestrations in the vascular walls. At sites where the extracellular space is also increased, this can lead to significant extravasion of contrast agent. The effect of the paramagnetic contrast agent at typical tissue concentrations is to increase the rate of T_1 relaxation of water molecules, resulting in increased intensity in T_1 weighted images, and thus aiding identification and diagnosis of abnormality. The high concentration in the first pass bolus can also cause local T_2^* relaxation, resulting in a loss of signal on T_2^* weighted images. This latter phenomenon is seen only over tens of seconds, whereas the T_1 enhancement typically occurs over 30 sec and may persist for minutes, depending on the tissue characteristics.

By measuring the uptake and washout behavior of the contrast agent in tissue, it is possible to deduce a range of physiological descriptors of the tissue or tumor under evaluation, including aspects of vascular function. This is performed by repeating an identical measurement sequence many times during and following contrast bolus injection, providing a set of T_1 weighted dynamic contrast-enhanced images [12].

Dynamic contrast-enhanced MRI (DCE-MRI) using small molecular weight gadolinium chelates enables noninvasive imaging characterization of tissue vascularity. Depending on the measurement technique and pharmacokinetic model used, dynamic data parameters reflecting tissue perfusion (blood flow, blood volume, mean transit time), microvessel permeability surface area product and extracellular leakage space can be obtained. Typically, parameters reflecting tissue perfusion are obtained by so-called first pass bolus tracking T_2^* weighted measurements, which are sensitive to the high contrast agent concentration immediately following the bolus injection. Currently, bolus-tracking techniques are not in routine use outside of the brain or in clinical trials. This is due to the effects of magnetic field inhomogeneity in regions such as the pelvis and the extravasation of contrast agent outside of the brain. Potential clinical applications include screening for malignant disease, lesion characterization, monitoring lesion response to treatment, and assessment of residual disease. Newer applications include pharmacodynamic assessments of antivascular anticancer drugs and predicting efficacy of treatment.

DCE-MRI methods vary depending on the objectives of the study. High spatial resolution combined with volume coverage requires high signal-to-noise and a relatively long measurement sequence (>30 sec per volume), which has been a limitation, but advances in instrumentation and processing methods are now reducing this. DCE-MRI for pharmacokinetic analysis requires high temporal resolution (<5 sec per volume) of data volumes acquired before, during, and after the administration of a bolus of contrast agent, reducing the spatial resolution obtained. The performance of modern MRI scanners provides a widely available, robust, and reliable tool for DCE-MRI studies. As DCE-MRI is noninvasive, sequential studies can be performed on the same patient several times during treatment with novel therapeutic agents. The use of DCE-MRI in clinical trials of antiangiogenic and other therapeutic agents is increasing as DCE-MRI measurement and post-processing methods are developed.

14.2.2.2 Measurement Methodology

There are a number of requirements that need to be met when using T_1 based quantitative DCE-MRI methods to estimate vascular changes in clinical drug trials. A primary requirement for quantitative pharmacokinetic modeling of DCE-MRI data is to obtain a precontrast estimate of the native tissue T_1, as contrast agent induced signal intensity changes alone cannot be used due to complex relationships between measurement sequence parameters and initial tissue relaxation times [13]. It is then necessary to have an imaging sequence that estimates changes in T_1 relaxation for the subsequent dynamic time points. These are required for the subsequent quantification of the contrast agent concentration in tissues during the DCE-MRI study, which is assumed to have a linear relationship between tissue T_1 and contrast agent concentration [14].

There are a large number of MRI methods for obtaining precontrast enhanced T_1 ranging from inversion-recovery based methods using either echo planar imaging [15,16] or rapid fast gradient-echo measurements, or saturation recovery methods using gradient-echo measurements [17,18]. It is a requirement of these techniques that image intensities in serial images can be directly related to one another, by fixing image gain parameters, or by having knowledge of these where they vary. 2D and 3D gradient-echo T_1 weighted measurements are most common due to their standard availability on all MR scanners. The signal obtained from a gradient-echo sequence is given by the following expression:

$$S_{\rm fl} = \frac{K\rho\left[\sin(\alpha)\left(1 - e^{\frac{-TR}{T_1}}\right)\right]}{\left(1 - \cos(\alpha)e^{\frac{-TR}{T_1}}\right)} e^{\frac{-TE}{T_{2s}}} \tag{14.1}$$

where $S_{\rm fl}$ is the signal, K is the system dependent scaling factor (including receiver gain and image scaling factors), ρ is the tissue proton density, TR is the measurement sequence repetition time, α is the measurement sequence flip angle, TE is the measurement sequence echo time, T_{2s} is the native transverse relaxation time, and T_1 is the longitudinal relaxation time. Varying α in a number of measurements, and maintaining all other measurement parameters constant, allows tissue T_1 to be estimated. The method can be used efficiently with a minimum of two values of α to obtain the precontrast tissue T_1. Here, an initial proton density weighted image with $\alpha < 5°$ followed by a dynamic series with a larger value of α is used [13,19]. As there are known imperfections in clinical imaging systems, which result in nonuniform distributions in flip angle across the image slice (B1 inhomogeneity) and less than ideal measurement slice profiles, calibration procedures are required to identify and correct for these effects [20]. Quality control uses phantoms of known T_1 values to measure the accuracy of the measurement method and obtain the calibration values. The use of 3D measurement sequences reduces slice profile effects. 3D imaging sequences result in longer measurement acquisition times, although with the advent of partially parallel acquisition methods [21] these sequences are now able to provide excellent volume coverage of target regions within the acquisition times (<6 sec) required for pharmacokinetic analysis.

14.2.2.3 Pharmacokinetic Analysis

All currently approved Gd-based contrast agents are extracellular agents, which diffuse into the extracellular space following distribution in the vascular compartment. Therefore, the tracer pharmacokinetic models generally used consist of two compartments: the blood plasma compartment and the tissue extracellular, extravascular compartment. Approved Gd-based contrast agents are eliminated renally following intravenous administration. The contrast agent concentration in plasma ($C_{\rm p}$) following i.v. injection is described by a bi-exponential rate equation [22] and is often used in pharmacokinetic modeling as a generalized description of the plasma concentration. The rate equation describing the transport of Gd contrast between the plasma and extracellular compartments is [23]

$$\frac{dC_{\rm t}(t)}{dt} = K^{\rm trans}C_{\rm p}(t) - k_{\rm ep}C_{\rm t}(t) \tag{14.2}$$

where $C_{\rm t}$ is the tissue concentration, $C_{\rm p}$ is the plasma concentration, and $K^{\rm trans}$ and $k_{\rm ep}$ are, respectively, volume rate constants for exchange between central blood compartment and tissue compartments and vice versa, reflecting bulk tissue properties. Again, following Tofts, the extracellular extravascular space ($v_{\rm e}$) is defined as

$$v_{\rm e} = \frac{K^{\rm trans}}{K_{\rm ep}} \tag{14.3}$$

where $K^{\rm trans}$ is a composite parameter that is dependent on the extraction, flow, and other physiological properties of the tissue. $K^{\rm trans}$ is considered within a general mixed perfusion and permeability model to be equal to

$$E \times F \times \sigma(1 - \text{Hct}) \tag{14.4}$$

where E is the extraction fraction of the contrast agent, F is blood flow, σ is tissue density, and Hct is the hematocrit. When blood flow is adequate, the rate of extraction E is small compared to supply, K^{trans} is then largely equal to the product of the capillary permeability and surface area. If the delivery of the contrast agent to tissue is very low, then blood perfusion is the dominant factor. The extraction of low molecular weight agents (<2000 Da) is similar in both normal and cancerous tissue [24], indicating that changes in K^{trans} are largely flow related. A major difficulty for quantitative DCE-MRI is the determination of the blood plasma concentration C_p, required for model-based analysis. Measuring C_p (often called the arterial input function) using MRI requires measurement sequences, which are able to measure over a large range of contrast agent concentrations. Tissue concentrations typically range over 0 to 2 mM/ml and the concentration in plasma can exceed 10 mM/ml during the first pass of the contrast agent following a bolus injection. In an artery, C_p has to be sampled at sufficient temporal resolution to accurately characterize the change in concentration following a bolus injection, ideally less than 2 sec, which challenges spatial image resolution and coverage, although continued developments in MRI scanner technology will make this a possibility in the future. Further confounding factors in the measurement of C_p are flow artifacts and motion. Several approaches have been utilized for obtaining C_p based on DCE-MRI measurements, which accept the limitations described above but have the advantage of providing individual and patient specific arterial input functions. The most common method of applying the model is to use the general plasma concentration C_p, derived from published physiological data [22]. An alternative method is to derive an estimate of C_p from a reference tissue concentration C_t and known physiological parameters of the reference tissue [25,26]. The advantage of the reference tissue approach is that the temporal sampling can be relaxed, since the rate of change in tracer concentration in the reference tissue is not as rapid as in plasma following a bolus. The disadvantages of using a reference tissue are that clinical treatments, or other extraneous factors, may affect the reference tissue blood flow, and the reference tissue derived C_p may not accurately reflect delivery to the tissues of interest.

There are a number of nonmodel based parameters which have been used for the evaluation of DCE-MRI measurement data. These include maximum contrast agent concentration, initial slope of the concentration time curve, washout slope, and the initial area under the Gd curve (IAUGC). Of these, the most useful is the IAUGC as this is the simplest to calculate [27]. The exact physiological relevance of the IAUGC is unclear. It does, however, provide a basic and fundamental measurement of how much Gd is detected in a region within a fixed time interval and has been shown to be useful in clinical DCE-MRI trials [28–30].

14.2.2.4 Software Requirements for DCE-MRI

Suitable software tools are required for the analysis of DCE-MRI measurements [31,32]. The software must satisfy the following requirements: easy data import including calibration data, conversion of measured DCE-MRI time series data to contrast agent concentrations, user defined regions of interest tools, calculation or automated detection of an arterial input function, and pharmacokinetic modeling of individual pixels or regions of interest within the DCE-MRI data. For detailed data analysis, the generation of parametric images derived from the model fitting, statistical evaluation of the individual pixel derived parametric data, including mean, median values, ranges, histograms and errors, are required [33]. Nonmodel-based parameters, such as IAUGC and initial slope and peak amplitudes of the DCE-MRI time series data, provide additional useful parametric images. Examples of such parametric images are shown in Figure 14.1. As motion can significantly affect the quality of DCE-MRI data, it is essential that the data can be assessed for motion. Ideally, DCE-MRI data should be coregistered before analysis. This is particularly important when evaluating data from organs such as the liver [34].

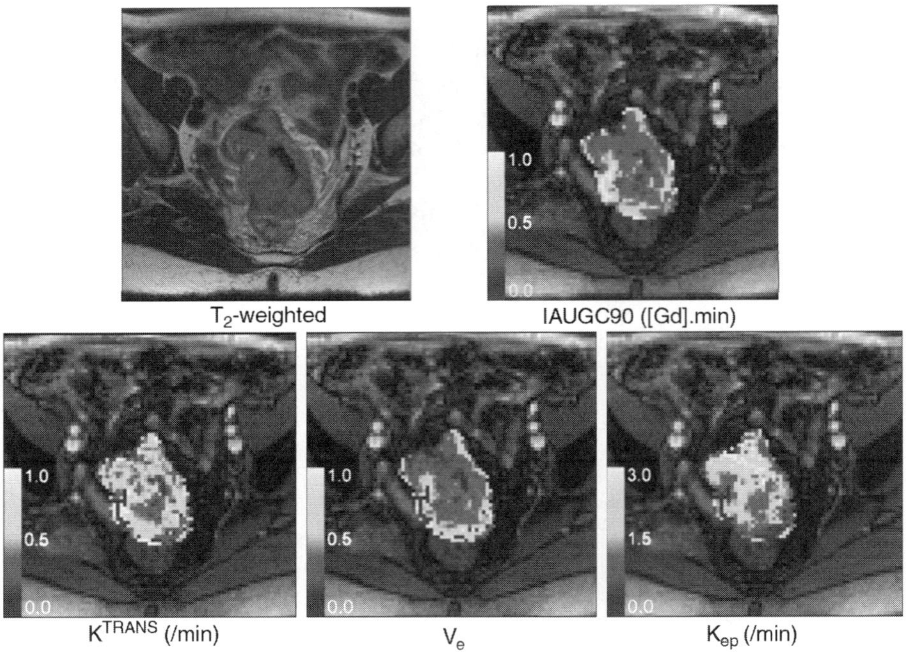

FIGURE 14.1 (See color insert following page 328.) (a) 3 mm axial T_2-weighted MR image showing a polypoidal tumor arising from the distal sigmoid. There is evidence of extramural invasion on the right. (b) Calculated map of initial area under the Gadolinium concentration curve (IAUGC) over 0–90 sec. (c), (d), and (e) Calculated maps of K^{trans}, v_e and K_{ep}, respectively.

14.2.2.5 Higher Molecular Weight Contrast Agents

As low molecular weight contrast molecules <1 kDa are readily transported across the vascular wall, in a range of normal and cancerous tissues [24], they have limited specificity to characterize the physiological properties of abnormal vasculature associated with cancer outside of the CNS. One of the principle motivations behind the development of larger molecular weight contrast agents is to develop a molecule with the size and properties to remain within the vascular space in normal tissues, but to enter the extracellular space of cancerous tissues. A significant number of agents have been developed and evaluated and a number of preclinical results indicate increased sensitivity for a range of contrast agents with increasing molecular weights. A macromolecular contrast molecule (MMCM) has a molecular weight of greater than 50 kDa and is too large to cross the normal microvascular endothelium, and generally too large for glomerular filtration. An MMCM is termed a slow clearance blood pool agent.

Intermediate molecular weight molecules (IMWM) of 1 to 50 kDa are eliminated by glomerular filtration. As IMWM are largely retained in the blood pool, but are sufficiently small to enable renal excretion, they are rapidly eliminated. The rate of elimination of IMWCM is faster than that of low molecular weight agents, which exchange with the extracellular space. Intermediate weight contrast media are known as rapid-clearance blood pool agents [35]. Low molecular weight molecules (LMWM) have high sensitivity but poor specificity as they readily enter the extravascular extracellular space. MMCM have poorer sensitivity as fewer molecules enter the extracellular space, although this is partially compensated by the relaxivity of MMCM, which is higher than LMWM. They have high specificity as they only enter the extravascular extracellular space where microvascular endothelia barriers are disrupted in malignant tumors.

Currently, no multicenter *in vivo* therapeutic drugs trials are in progress with MMCM as most of these agents are under investigation and development themselves. In preclinical studies of antiangiogenic treatments using MMCM, the published results indicate improved response assessments using MMCM over both LMWM and IMWM [36,37]. Potential disadvantages of using MMCM in clinical studies is that the rate of uptake in the malignant tissue is slow and several tens of minutes are required to obtain data required for the evaluation of transport kinetics. During this time, substantial patient motion can occur and scanning costs are increased as a result of lengthy examinations. The advantages are increased specificity, improved spatial resolution, and potentially simplified pharmacokinetic analysis.

14.2.2.6 Clinical Therapeutic Trials

DCE-MRI is particularly well suited for trials of new antiangiogenic or antivascular agents, where the method reports on one of the end points of therapeutic action. Several such trials have been published recently [38–42]. As the methodology develops, it is expected that such measurements will provide a wider range of physiological information that will benefit evaluation of a growing range of agents. A recent report has reviewed the requirements for MR methods used in early stage clinical trials of antiangiogenic or antivascular agents [43].

14.3 APPLICATIONS USING MAGNETIC RESONANCE SPECTROSCOPY

MRS can be applied in several distinct ways to aid pharmaceutical development in oncology. Firstly, it can be used to study uptake and metabolism of drugs directly (pharmacokinetics). Secondly, it can be used to look at the effect of the drug on tumor and normal tissue metabolism (pharmacodynamics) — both for conventional chemotherapeutic agents, and also for new treatments that target specific signaling pathways. Thirdly, some compounds are now being developed that report on specific characteristics of the tumor microenvironment, which in turn may help optimize pharmaceutical development. These applications are discussed and illustrated in the following sections, preceded by some general comments about the methodology required, and competing/complementary technologies. The methods described could be used both in developing new therapeutic agents, to assess general mechanisms and effects, but might also be used to tailor treatment for individual patients.

14.3.1 General Issues

The key property of MRS is the chemical shift that is produced between species of the same nuclear type, but experiencing different chemical environments. This enables different metabolites of endogenous and exogenous compounds to be distinguished, a feature that cannot be achieved with any radionuclide technique.

The main limitation of MRS is the high threshold of sensitivity — several orders of magnitude higher than for radiolabeled compounds. For studies of body fluids and tissue samples, this is not so critical as it is possible to perform measurements at high magnetic field with good spectral resolution. However, for clinical studies *in vivo*, where the noninvasive nature of MRS is so important, sensitivity can be a major problem. Apart from studies in the brain, most MRS studies therefore use surface coil receivers, to take advantage of their superior sensitivity for superficial tissues compared with volume coils. However, this then limits many studies to the evaluation of superficial lesions. Such studies also benefit from the use of adiabatic rf pulses to compensate for the nonuniform transmit fields of the coils. MRS data are acquired from either single voxels or grids of voxels (spectroscopic imaging), where the minimum size of the voxel is again determined by sensitivity considerations — concentration of the compounds being studied, distance from the receiver coil, magnetic field strength, and nuclear species being studied are the main factors.

TABLE 14.1
Relative Sensitivity of the NMR Nuclei Used in Pharmacological Research

Nucleus	Relative Sensitivity at a Given Magnetic Field Strength	Natural Abundance (%)	Absolute Sensitivity for Natural Abundance
^{1}H	1.00	99.98	1.00
^{19}F	0.83	100	0.83
^{31}P	0.0663	100	0.0663
^{13}C	0.0159	1.1	0.000176

Typical voxel sizes might be 1 to 2 cm for ^{1}H MRS and 3 to 4 cm for ^{31}P MRS. Table 14.1 lists the nuclei most often used for MRS *in vivo*. ^{1}H and ^{19}F are often the nuclei of choice, and, although carbon plays a major role in biological systems, it is very difficult to be detected unless enriched or highly concentrated compounds are available.

Clinical MRS examinations have been relatively complex compared with imaging, but with appropriate quality assurance, good results can be obtained from multicenter studies [44]. Standardization is an important issue which can contribute to transportable measurements [45]. Recent developments in hardware and in the magnetic fields available to clinical centers are leading to significant improvements in the ease and sensitivity of MRS measurements.

Some magnetic nuclei are coupled through bonds to other magnetic nuclei, known as J-coupling. In an AX system where one nucleus of interest (A) is coupled to a single additional nucleus (X), the spectral peak of A is split into two peaks of equal amplitude, for an AX_2 system there are three peaks (of ratio 1:2:1), and so on. This both broadens the peak and reduces the total amplitude. Most high-field MR systems (used for the study of fluid and tissue samples) but only a few clinical MR systems, have a technique available called decoupling to overcome this [46,47].

While in principle MR spectra may be quantified in absolute terms, this requires correcting for relaxation time constants of the nuclear species, and reference to some other compound within the same region of tissue of known concentration. It is often neither desirable nor necessary to obtain this information. For longitudinal studies it is often sufficient to look at changes in ratios of peak areas, while pattern recognition techniques can be used to evaluate spectra [48].

Radiolabeling has already been mentioned as a competing or complementary technique for measuring compounds in tissue noninvasively. The key differences are listed in Table 14.2.

TABLE 14.2
Key Characteristics of MRS and Radiolabeling for Measuring Compounds Noninvasively

	MRS	Radiolabeling
Sensitivity	Poor — require concentration ~ mM, and obtain resolution ~1–4 cm	Good — concentration threshold ~ pM and spatial resolution ~5 mm
Preparation	Generally use endogenous or exogenous compounds without any manipulation	Cannot see endogenous compounds. Exogenous compounds require radiochemistry
Quantitative	Yes	Yes
Metabolite discrimination	Yes	No

14.3.2 Drug Uptake and Metabolism

Where compounds are administered in sufficient quantities, MRS can be used to monitor the delivery and metabolism of the drug itself. All drugs contain ^{1}H nuclei and so may be detected with MRS. Since the ^{1}H MR-spectrum from tissue is quite crowded, it is often advantageous to use other nmr-nuclei that may be present (^{19}F, ^{31}P, or ^{13}C), even though these may be less sensitive, if they produce isolated signals that are easier to identify and quantify (see also Chapter 13, Section 13.3.5).

As mentioned above, while the concentration threshold for detection of MRS signals is several orders of magnitude lower than for radiolabeling studies, MRS has two unique advantages:

1. The drug can be used without any modification, as normally administered, and without the requirement for special preparation.
2. MRS is sensitive to the chemical environment of the observed nucleus. In many cases, drug metabolism leads to a sufficient change in chemical shift so that parent drug and metabolites may be distinguished. This property is not shared with any other noninvasive method, and is the driving motivation for most MRS studies of drug pharmacokinetics.

One drug which has been extensively studied in this way is 5FU and related compounds [49,50]. Although 5FU is one of the earlier chemotherapeutic drugs, it is still used as a primary treatment in several cancers including colorectal and breast. Since the drug contains ^{19}F, it can be detected using ^{19}F MRS. ^{19}F is a favorable nucleus to study, owing to the lack of background ^{19}F MRS signals from tissue, and relatively high sensitivity (Table 14.1). The metabolism of 5FU is quite complex, with at least two different anabolic pathways, as well as a catabolic pathway [50]. Several metabolites are characterized by well-resolved ^{19}F MRS signals and can be used to distinguish whether the required anabolic pathways are being followed [51]. Of particular interest in studies of 5FU is the co-administration of treatment modifiers, and the influence these have on metabolism [51]. MRS has followed uptake and metabolism following both bolus administration and following low-dose continuous infusion of 5FU. Long half-lives of 5FU following bolus administration suggested trapping within the tumor, and showed a strong correlation with treatment response [52]. In addition, it was localized ^{19}F MRS that first observed the biliary recirculation of fluoro-β-alanine, a catabolite of 5FU, into the gall bladder [53].

^{31}P MRS measurements of the alkylating agents ifosfamide and cyclophosphamide illustrate the breadth of studies that can be performed. Measurements of urine samples at high magnetic field strengths are simple to perform, give good signal-to-noise ratios and spectral resolution, and yield useful information on metabolism and elimination [54]. Plasma samples may also be studied in this way. ^{31}P-MRS has been used to detect and quantify ifosfamide in GH3 prolactinomas and N-methyl-N-nitrosourea induced mammary tumors, demonstrating the technical feasibility of detecting signals from the compound *in vivo*, and in particular the effect of blood flow modifiers on uptake [55]. Finally, it has been demonstrated that signals can be detected *in vivo* from patients undergoing standard treatments [56], although with current equipment the threshold is approximately 1000 mg/m^2. To date, no studies have been performed to investigate whether there is a correlation of uptake and metabolism with response.

^{13}C is less sensitive than ^{1}H, ^{19}F, or ^{31}P. However, by making use of polarization transfer techniques, signals can be increased by a factor of four or more. This has been applied in model systems to look at the pharmacokinetics of ^{13}C-enriched temozolomide in RIF-1 tumors [57].

MRS may also be useful in aiding evaluation of new treatments. One particular example is GDEPT, a new two-step treatment strategy. Firstly, a gene is targeted to the tumor where it expresses an enzyme. This enzyme then activates a nontoxic prodrug administered subsequently. Several prodrugs for carboxypeptidase G2 (one of the enzyme systems studied) contain ^{19}F detectable using MRS, and also demonstrate a sufficient chemical shift change on activation where prodrug and active compound may be distinguished [58]. Thus, both drug delivery and activation can be monitored. In addition, nontoxic analogues of the therapeutic compounds can be formed that may be used to verify that the gene has been delivered and expressed successfully before administration of the therapeutic agent. This application of MRS would not be possible using radio-isotopes.

14.3.3 Assessment of Treatment Response

Since MR spectra of tissue yield information on the biochemical composition, many studies have been performed to investigate the biochemical profiles of diseased tissues, and the changes induced in spectra by treatment. Since biochemical changes must necessarily precede cell death (whether by apoptosis or necrosis) and macroscopic tumor shrinkage, information from *in vivo* MR spectra should give an earlier indication to the oncologist regarding the effectiveness of a given treatment in a patient. Most early studies used ^{31}P MRS (see [59] for an excellent review) but technical advances, together with the greater sensitivity and increased availability of ^{1}H MRS, have recently made this a more popular probe of tumor behavior.

^{31}P MR spectra probe three complementary aspects of cell biochemistry:

1. Levels of ATP, phosphocreatine (PCr) and inorganic phosphate reflect cell energetics.
2. Levels of phosphomonoesters (PMEs, consisting of phosphocholine [PC] and phosphoethanolamine [PE]) and phosphodiesters (PDEs, consisting of glycerophosphocholine [GPC] and glycerophosphoethanolamine [GPE) reflect aspects of cell membrane metabolism and cell signaling.
3. The frequency (chemical shift) of the inorganic phosphate is a direct measure of intracellular pH.

It was originally anticipated that effective treatment would compromise the energy status of cells, resulting in low levels of cellular ATP. While to some extent this may be true, it can only be detected with careful quantitative measurements that must also take account of cell density. However, what is striking is that ^{31}P spectra of tumors tend to be characterized by elevated PMEs and PDEs compared with normal tissues [59], presumably a consequence of increased cell growth and therefore of demand for cell membranes. In addition, rather than exhibiting an acidic intracellular pH (expected for hypoxic cells undergoing anaerobic metabolism), the intracellular pH is often more alkaline than the corresponding tissue [59]. In patients who respond to treatment, there is a reduction in PME [60] or the ratio of PME to nucleotide triphosphate (NTP) [61–63].

The main characteristic peak in ^{1}H MR spectra associated with cancer is that of total choline (tCho), seen both in brain and in extracranial lesions such as breast (see also Chapter 13, Section 13.4). In normal breast, tCho is partly obscured by signals arising from lipids, but in cancer the peak is larger and easier to measure. One study has shown that in 89% of patients receiving neo-adjuvant chemotherapy for advanced breast cancer, the tCho peak is reduced or eliminated [64]. Another study of patients receiving doxorubicin as primary systemic therapy showed changes in tCho within 24 h that correlated strongly with change in lesion size ($p = .001$) [65]. Choline has also been shown to be reduced in brain lesions in response to chemotherapy [66,67] and radiation therapy [68], although the precise mechanism for this effect is yet to be elucidated. Similar effects have been observed in malignant lymphoma and germ cell tumors [69].

14.4 NOVEL THERAPEUTICS TARGETING MOLECULAR PROCESSES

Cancer drug development is witnessing a new era in which rational mechanism-targeted anticancer agents are playing an increasingly important role [70]. Indeed, much attention is currently focused on targeting signal transduction pathways that are frequently mutated in human cancers and are key to their development and progression [70,71]. Figure 14.2 illustrates some of the molecular targets

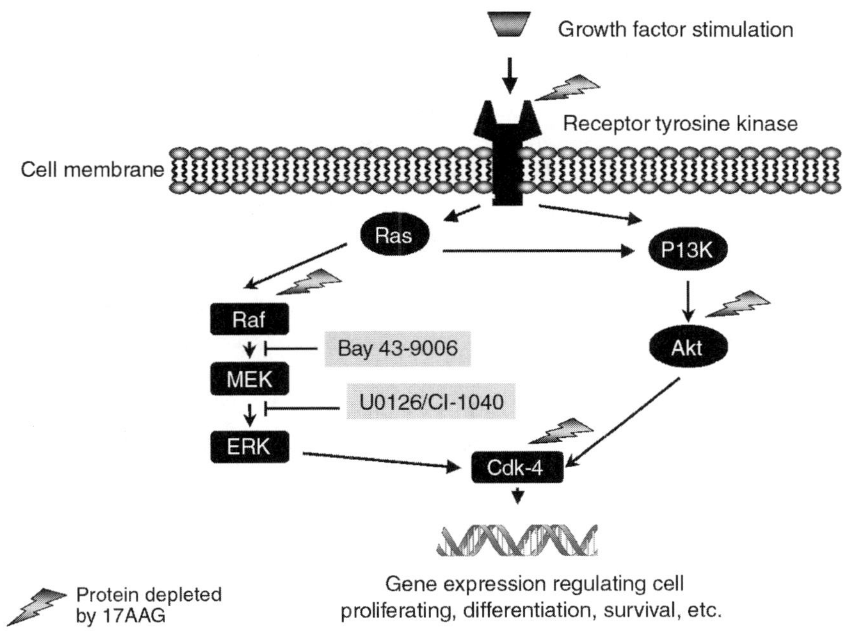

FIGURE 14.2 Examples of molecular targets for mechanism-based anticancer treatment.

of rational anticancer treatment. Two key pathways that are activated downstream of growth factor receptors are depicted, namely the Ras–Raf–MEK–ERK and the PI3K–Akt pathways. Because of their involvement in malignant transformation, these two signaling pathways constitute key targets for contemporary cancer drug development.

Detecting biomarkers of response to signaling inhibition will facilitate the clinical evaluation of this novel type of therapy, as blockade of the intended biochemical target can be monitored, and treatment efficacy assessed [71]. In this context, and as a noninvasive technique for studying tumor metabolism, MRS could, potentially, have a prominent role.

To date, however, most MR studies on mechanism-targeted cancer therapeutics have focused on preclinical models due, primarily, to the novelty of the field. Here, two specific examples are used to illustrate the use of MRS in monitoring the action of novel anticancer agents in preclinical models and how this can be translated to patient investigations.

14.4.1 MRS Monitoring of Ras–Raf–MEK–ERK Signaling Inhibition

The Ras–Raf–MEK–ERK (or MAPK) signaling pathway is deregulated in many human cancers and inhibitors of this pathway, such as the MEK inhibitor CI-1040 and the Raf-1 inhibitor BAY 43-9006 (Figure 14.2), which are now under clinical evaluation. ^{31}P MRS studies have shown that modulation of the MAPK pathway leads to alterations in phospholipid metabolism. In NIH3T3 murine fibroblasts, Ras activation was associated with an increase in PC levels and the PC/NTP ratio which were reversed upon treatment with broad spectrum Ras signaling inhibitors [72]. In this cell system, exposure to the prototype MEK inhibitor U0126 was also associated with a decrease in PC content and in the PC/NTP ratio [73]. Furthermore, inhibition with U0126 in human breast, as well as colon carcinoma cells, was also associated with a time-dependent drop in PC levels that correlated well with the decrease in P-ERK levels [74]. This effect on PC is likely to result from modulation of metabolic enzymes (e.g., choline kinase) by oncogenic proteins such as Ras [75]. Thus, PC could have potential as a noninvasive MRS pharmacodynamic marker for inhibition of Ras–Raf–MEK–ERK signaling.

14.4.2 MRS Monitoring of Hsp90 Inhibition

Heat shock protein 90 (Hsp90) is a molecular chaperone that maintains the proper folding of many cellular clients including oncogenic proteins such as Raf-1, Akt, and cell cycle kinases (e.g., Cdk-4) [76]. Inhibition of Hsp90 with agents such as 17-allylamino,17-demethoxygeldanamycin (17AAG) causes the simultaneous blockade of several oncogenic pathways (e.g., the MAPK and the PI3K–Akt pathway) that are critical for driving the malignant phenotype. This helps to bypass the mechanisms of resistance that often hamper the success of the more conventional cytotoxic therapies [76]. Inhibition of Hsp90 also results in up-regulation of Hsp70. 17AAG has shown potent antitumor activity both in *in vitro* and *in vivo* preclinical models, has undergone phase I clinical trials, and will shortly be undergoing phase II clinical evaluation [76].

^{31}P and ^{1}H MRS studies have shown that inhibition with 17AAG was associated with modulation of choline-containing metabolites in human cancer cell models *in vitro* and *in vivo* [77–79]. At conditions leading to Raf-1 and Cdk-4 depletion, and Hsp70 induction, 17AAG treatment caused, interestingly, an increase in PC and GPC levels in human melanoma, breast, and colon carcinoma cells *in vitro* [77–79]. In an *in vivo* colon carcinoma xenograft model, treatment with 17AAG was associated with a significant increase in the PME peak comprising PC and PE [78].

As part of the phase I/II clinical trials of 17AAG, ^{1}H decoupled ^{31}P chemical shift imaging has been deployed to investigate the effect of 17AAG on tumor metabolism in treated patients.

Figure 14.3 illustrates an example of a localized ^{31}P MR spectrum acquired from a sternal mass of a patient with renal cell carcinoma participating in the phase I trial of 17AAG. Several key metabolites including PMEs and NTP are readily detectable with very good signal-to-noise ratio. The aim of this study was to correlate the effect of the drug on its molecular targets (as determined from tumor biopsy samples) with potential changes in tumor phospholipid metabolism. It remains

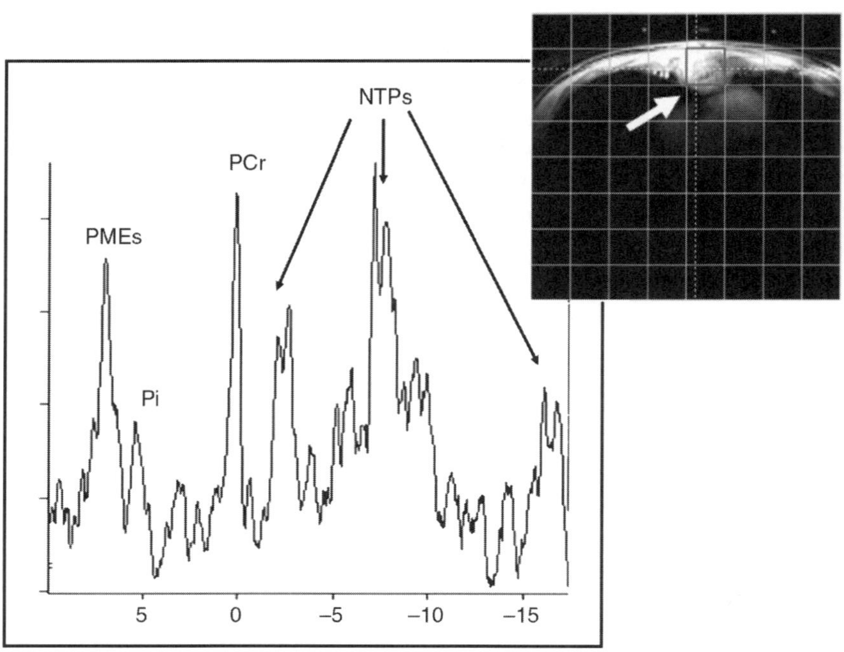

FIGURE 14.3 A localized spectrum from a sternal mass of a patient with renal cell carcinoma acquired using ^{1}H decoupled ^{31}P chemical shift imaging. PMEs: phosphomonoesters; NTPs: nucleotide triphosphates; PCr: phosphocreatine; Pi: inorganic phosphate.

to be seen whether MRS could be useful in detecting changes associated with response to treatment in patients from the phase II clinical trial of 17AAG.

The data available to date suggest that MRS could have a role in detecting noninvasive biomarkers of response to treatment with novel oncogenic pathway inhibitors in preclinical cancer models. If and when validated in patient studies, these noninvasive biomarkers could place MRS in a leading position over the currently implemented techniques for monitoring response to treatment during clinical trials with novel anticancer drugs.

14.4.3 Novel Diagnostic Agents for Evaluating the Tissue Microenvironment

Mention should be made of MRS compounds designed to report on a particular characteristic of the tissue microenvironment. A particular property of great importance in cancer growth and response is the hypoxic status, since regions of hypoxia are resistant to radiotherapy and many types of chemotherapy, as well as causing genetic instability, tumor progression, and angiogenesis [80]. The gold-standard for measurement of tumor oxygen tension is currently the Eppendorf microelectrode, but this is invasive, requires many tracks to obtain a useful estimate, is only useful for superficial lesions, and is prone to operator bias:

1. Use of perfluorocarbon emulsions to measure oxygen tension have been investigated for over 20 years. The ^{19}F T_1 is extremely sensitive to oxygen concentration. The main disadvantages relate to administration methods (intravenous delivery leads to low leakage into tumors of interest, while direct tumoral injection has many of the same problems as the Eppendorf electrode it seeks to replace) and to possible interference from other sources of relaxation (especially paramagnetic metals). Ref. [80] provides a good recent review.
2. Nitroimidazoles undergo irreversible bioreduction in the absence of oxygen, creating a highly reactive intermediate that binds to local macromolecules. Several fluorinated nitroimidazoles have been investigated as hypoxic markers, using the principle that they are only retained in hypoxic regions, with a ^{19}F nucleus included to be detectable by ^{19}F MRS. Examples include EF5 [81] and SR4554 [82]. A Phase 1 clinical trial of SR4554 shows it to be well-tolerated, with preliminary results suggesting increased retention in tumors compared with plasma levels [83]. Given the clinical importance of tumor hypoxia further developments in this area are to be expected.
3. Hyperpolarization of the ^{129}Xe nucleus has recently become possible, yielding signals 4 to 5 orders of magnitude larger than at thermal equilibrium. Among potential applications of this technology, it has been discovered that the Xe chemical shift in blood is extremely sensitive to the oxygen concentration [84], and may therefore give some indication of oxygen concentration of neighboring tissues.

14.5 CONCLUSIONS

In the above sections the potential and current applications of MR have been described. MR can evaluate conventional and novel therapeutics, with both imaging and spectroscopy methods applied in clinical studies. As detailed in Chapter 13, there is a much wider range of preclinical research in progress, identifying potential applications of this technology. One of the major strengths of MR is the growing ease of combining a range of functional and metabolic measurements, together with conventional morphology, into a single clinical measurement. MRI can evaluate morphology, aspects of vascular function such as perfusion and permeability affecting drug delivery as well as action, and descriptors of the tissue matrix such as water diffusion, which can provide information related to cellular density. An integrated examination can include ^{1}H or ^{31}P MRS to evaluate metabolic response, including action on specific targets. Continuing advances in instrumentation are aiding such multifunctional studies. Steps to standardize measurement approaches are in progress, and these will aid the use of these techniques in multicenter trials.

REFERENCES

1. Schepkin, V. D. et al., Sodium magnetic resonance imaging of chemotherapeutic response in a rat glioma, *Magn. Reson. Med.*, 53, 85, 2005.
2. Ross, B. D. et al., Evaluation of cancer therapy using diffusion magnetic resonance imaging, *Mol. Cancer Ther.*, 2, 581, 2003.
3. Dzik-Jurasz, A. et al., Diffusion MRI for prediction of response of rectal cancer to chemoradiation, *Lancet*, 360, 307, 2002.
4. Le Bihan, D. et al., Separation of diffusion and perfusion in intravoxel incoherent motion MR imaging, *Radiology*, 168, 497, 1988.
5. Wang, Z. et al., Effect of vasodilator hydralazine on tumor microvascular random flow and blood volume as measured by intravoxel incoherent motion (IVIM) weighted MRI in conjunction with Gd-DTPA-Albumin enhanced MRI, *Magn. Reson. Imaging*, 19, 1063, 2001.
6. Fujita, N. et al., Separation of diffusion and slow flow effects by use of flow rephasing and dephasing, *Magn. Reson. Med.*, 24, 109, 1992.
7. Delakis, I. et al., Developing a quality control protocol for diffusion imaging on a clinical MRI system, *Phys. Med. Biol.*, 49, 1409, 2004.
8. Schmitt, P. et al., Quantitative tissue perfusion measurements in head and neck carcinoma patients before and during radiation therapy with a non-invasive MR imaging spin-labeling technique, *Radiother. Oncol.*, 67, 27, 2003.
9. Warmuth, C., Gunther, M., and Zimmer, C., Quantification of blood flow in brain tumors: comparison of arterial spin labeling and dynamic susceptibility-weighted contrast-enhanced MR imaging, *Radiology*, 228, 523, 2003.
10. Neeman, M. et al., In vivo BOLD contrast MRI mapping of subcutaneous vascular function and maturation: validation by intravital microscopy, *Magn. Reson. Med.*, 45, 887, 2001.
11. Bhattacharya, A. et al., Lack of microvessels in well-differentiated regions of human head and neck squamous cell carcinoma A253 associated with functional magnetic resonance imaging detectable hypoxia, limited drug delivery, and resistance to irinotecan therapy, *Clin. Cancer Res.*, 10, 8005, 2004.
12. Collins, D. J. and Padhani, A. R., Dynamic magnetic resonance imaging of tumor perfusion, *IEEE Eng. Med. Biol. Mag.*, 23, 65, 2004.
13. Hittmair, K. et al., Method for the quantitative assessment of contrast agent uptake in dynamic contrast-enhanced MRI, *Magn. Reson. Med.*, 31, 567, 1994.
14. Donahue, K. M. et al., Studies of Gd-DTPA relaxivity and proton exchange rates in tissue, *Magn. Reson. Med.*, 32, 66, 1994.
15. Gowland, P. et al., Dynamic studies of gadolinium uptake in brain tumors using inversion-recovery echo-planar imaging, *Magn. Reson. Med.*, 26, 241, 1992.
16. Gowland, P. A. and Leach, M. O., Fast and accurate measurements of T_1 using a multi-readout single inversion-recovery sequence, *Magn. Reson. Med.*, 26, 79, 1992.
17. Haacke, M. E., *Magnetic Resonance Imaging: Physical Principles and Sequence Design*, John Wiley & Sons. Inc., New York, 1999.
18. Parker, G. J. et al., Improving image quality and T(1) measurements using saturation recovery turboFLASH with an approximate K-space normalisation filter, *Magn. Reson. Imaging*, 18, 157, 2000.
19. Wang, H. Z., Riederer, S. J., and Lee, J. N., Optimizing the precision in T_1 relaxation estimation using limited flip angles, *Magn. Reson. Med.*, 5, 399, 1987.
20. Parker, G. J., Barker, G. J., and Tofts, P. S., Accurate multislice gradient echo T(1) measurement in the presence of non-ideal RF pulse shape and RF field nonuniformity, *Magn. Reson. Med.*, 45, 838, 2001.
21. Pruessmann, K. P. et al., SENSE: sensitivity encoding for fast MRI, *Magn. Reson. Med.*, 42, 952, 1999.
22. Weinmann, H. J., Laniado, M., and Mutzel, W., Pharmacokinetics of GdDTPA/dimeglumine after intravenous injection into healthy volunteers, *Physiol. Chem. Phys. Med. NMR*, 16, 167, 1984.

23. Tofts, P. S. et al., Estimating kinetic parameters from dynamic contrast-enhanced T(1)-weighted MRI of a diffusable tracer: standardized quantities and symbols, *J. Magn. Reson. Imaging*, 10, 223, 1999.
24. Gerlowski, L. E. and Jain, R. K., Microvascular permeability of normal and neoplastic tissues, *Microvasc. Res.*, 31, 288, 1986.
25. Kovar, D. A., Lewis, M., and Karczmar, G. S., A new method for imaging perfusion and contrast extraction fraction: input functions derived from reference tissues, *J. Magn. Reson. Imaging*, 8, 1126, 1998.
26. Yang, C. et al., Estimating the arterial input function using two reference tissues in dynamic contrast-enhanced MRI studies: fundamental concepts and simulations, *Magn. Reson. Med.*, 52, 1110, 2004.
27. Evelhoch, J. L., Key factors in the acquisition of contrast kinetic data for oncology, *J. Magn. Reson. Imaging*, 10, 254, 1999.
28. Medved, M. et al., Semiquantitative analysis of dynamic contrast enhanced MRI in cancer patients: variability and changes in tumor tissue over time, *J. Magn. Reson. Imaging*, 20, 122, 2004.
29. Padhani, A. R. et al., Dynamic contrast enhanced MRI of prostate cancer: correlation with morphology and tumour stage, histological grade and PSA, *Clin. Radiol.*, 55, 99, 2000.
30. Engelbrecht, M. R. et al., Discrimination of prostate cancer from normal peripheral zone and central gland tissue by using dynamic contrast-enhanced MR imaging, *Radiology*, 229, 248, 2003.
31. Parker, G. J. et al., Probing tumor microvascularity by measurement, analysis and display of contrast agent uptake kinetics, *J. Magn. Reson. Imaging*, 7, 564, 1997.
32. Parker, G. J. et al., MRIW: parametric analysis software for contrast-enhanced dynamic MR imaging in cancer, *Radiographics*, 18, 497, 1998.
33. Leach, M. O. et al., Assessment of antiangiogenic and antivascular therapeutics using MRI: recommendations for appropriate methodology for clinical trials, *Br. J. Radiol.*, 76(Suppl. 1), S87, 2003.
34. White, M. J. et al., Diaphragm alignment of multiple breath-hold dynamic contrast-enhanced MRI of the liver for quantitative parameter estimation, *Proc. Intl. Soc. Magn. Reson. Med.*, 2665, 2004.
35. Bourasset, F. et al., Comparison of plasma and peritoneal concentrations of various categories of MRI blood pool agents in a murine experimental pharmacokinetic model, *MAGMA*, 12, 82, 2001.
36. Roberts, T. P. et al., Tumor microvascular changes to anti-angiogenic treatment assessed by MR contrast media of different molecular weights, *Acad. Radiol.*, 9 (Suppl. 2), S511, 2002.
37. Turetschek, K. et al., Tumor microvascular changes in antiangiogenic treatment: assessment by magnetic resonance contrast media of different molecular weights, *J. Magn. Reson. Imaging*, 20, 138, 2004.
38. Galbraith, S. M. et al., Effects of 5,6-dimethylxanthenone-4-acetic acid on human tumor microcirculation assessed by dynamic contrast-enhanced magnetic resonance imaging, *J. Clin. Oncol.*, 20, 3826, 2002.
39. Galbraith, S. M. et al., Combretastatin A4 phosphate has tumor antivascular activity in rat and man as demonstrated by dynamic magnetic resonance imaging, *J. Clin. Oncol.*, 21, 2831, 2003.
40. Jayson, G. C. et al., Molecular imaging and biological evaluation of HuMV833 anti-VEGF antibody: implications for trial design of antiangiogenic antibodies, *J. Natl Cancer Inst.*, 94, 1484, 2002.
41. Morgan, B. et al., Dynamic contrast-enhanced magnetic resonance imaging as a biomarker for the pharmacological response of PTK787/ZK 222584, an inhibitor of the vascular endothelial growth factor receptor tyrosine kinases, in patients with advanced colorectal cancer and liver metastases: results from two phase I studies, *J. Clin. Oncol.*, 21, 3955, 2003.
42. Yang, J. C. et al., A randomized trial of bevacizumab, an anti-vascular endothelial growth factor antibody, for metastatic renal cancer, *N. Engl. J. Med.*, 349, 427, 2003.
43. Leach, M. O. et al., The assessment of antiangiogenic and antivascular therapies in early-stage clinical trials using magnetic resonance imaging: issues and recommendations, *Br. J. Cancer*, 92, 1599, 2005.
44. Arias-Mendoza, F. et al., Methodological standardization for a multi-institutional in vivo trial of localized 31P MR spectroscopy in human cancer research. In vitro and normal volunteer studies, *NMR Biomed.*, 17, 382, 2004.
45. Leach, M. O. et al., International workshop on standardization in clinical magnetic resonance spectroscopy measurements: proceedings and recommendations, *Acad. Radiol.*, 1, 171, 1994.
46. Freeman, D. M. and Hurd, R., Decoupling: theory and practice. II. State of the art: in vivo applications of decoupling, *NMR Biomed.*, 10, 381, 1997.

47. Freeman, R. and Kupce, E., Decoupling: theory and practice. I. Current methods and recent concepts, *NMR Biomed.*, 10, 372, 1997.
48. Tate, A. R. et al., Automated classification of short echo time in in vivo 1H brain tumor spectra: a multicenter study, *Magn. Reson. Med.*, 49, 29, 2003.
49. Findlay, M. P. and Leach, M. O., In vivo monitoring of fluoropyrimidine metabolites: magnetic resonance spectroscopy in the evaluation of 5-fluorouracil, *Anticancer Drugs*, 5, 260, 1994.
50. McSheehy, P. M. and Griffiths, J. R., 19F MRS studies of fluoropyrimidine chemotherapy. A review, *NMR Biomed.*, 2, 133, 1989.
51. Findlay, M. P. et al., The non-invasive monitoring of low dose, infusional 5-fluorouracil and its modulation by interferon-alpha using in vivo 19F magnetic resonance spectroscopy in patients with colorectal cancer: a pilot study, *Ann. Oncol.*, 4, 597, 1993.
52. Presant, C. A. et al., Association of intratumoral pharmacokinetics of fluorouracil with clinical response, *Lancet*, 343, 1184, 1994.
53. Dzik-Jurasz, A. S. et al., Gallbladder localization of (19)F MRS catabolite signals in patients receiving bolus and protracted venous infusional 5-fluorouracil, *Magn. Reson. Med.*, 44, 516, 2000.
54. Martino, R. et al., A new approach to the study of ifosfamide metabolism by the analysis of human body fluids with 31P nuclear magnetic resonance spectroscopy, *J. Pharmacol. Exp. Ther.*, 260, 1133, 1992.
55. Rodrigues, L. M. et al., In vivo detection of ifosfamide by 31P-MRS in rat tumours: increased uptake and cytotoxicity induced by carbogen breathing in GH3 prolactinomas, *Br. J. Cancer*, 75, 62, 1997.
56. Payne, G. S. et al., Initial measurements of ifosfamide and cyclophosphamide in patients using (31)P MRS: pulse-and-acquire, decoupling, and polarization transfer, *Magn. Reson. Med.*, 44, 180, 2000.
57. Artemov, D. et al., Pharmacokinetics of the 13C labeled anticancer agent temozolomide detected in vivo by selective cross-polarization transfer, *Magn. Reson. Med.*, 34, 338, 1995.
58. Mancini, L. et al., GDEPT pharmacokinetics studied with 19F-MRS for validating gene and prodrug delivery and prodrug activation, *Proc. Intl. Soc. Magn. Reson. Med.*, 2610, 2005.
59. Negendank, W., Studies of human tumors by MRS: a review, *NMR Biomed.*, 5, 303, 1992.
60. Leach, M. O. et al., Measurements of human breast cancer using magnetic resonance spectroscopy: a review of clinical measurements and a report of localized 31P measurements of response to treatment, *NMR Biomed.*, 11, 314, 1998.
61. Karczmar, G. S. et al., P-31 spectroscopy study of response of superficial human tumors to therapy, *Radiology*, 179, 149, 1991.
62. Arias-Mendoza, F. et al., Preliminary results of a multi-institutional trial to demonstrate clinical predictive value of in vivo localized ^{31}P MR spectroscopy data in human non-Hodgkin's lymphoma, *Proc. Int. Soc. Magn. Reson. Med.*, 1, 98, 2000.
63. Maldonado, X. et al., 31Phosphorus magnetic resonance spectroscopy in the assessment of head and neck tumors, *Int. J. Radiat. Oncol. Biol. Phys.*, 40, 309, 1998.
64. Jagannathan, N. R. et al., Evaluation of total choline from in-vivo volume localized proton MR spectroscopy and its response to neoadjuvant chemotherapy in locally advanced breast cancer, *Br. J. Cancer*, 84, 1016, 2001.
65. Meisamy, S. et al., Neoadjuvant chemotherapy of locally advanced breast cancer: predicting response with in vivo (1)H MR spectroscopy–a pilot study at 4 T, *Radiology*, 233, 424, 2004.
66. Lichy, M. P. et al., Monitoring individual response to brain-tumour chemotherapy: proton MR spectroscopy in a patient with recurrent glioma after stereotactic radiotherapy, *Neuroradiology*, 46, 126, 2004.
67. Murphy, P. S. et al., Monitoring temozolomide treatment of low-grade glioma with proton magnetic resonance spectroscopy, *Br. J. Cancer*, 90, 781, 2004.
68. Nelson, S. J. et al., In vivo molecular imaging for planning radiation therapy of gliomas: an application of 1H MRSI, *J. Magn. Reson. Imaging*, 16, 464, 2002.
69. Schwarz, A. J. et al., Early in vivo detection of metabolic response: a pilot study of 1H MR spectroscopy in extracranial lymphoma and germ cell tumours, *Br. J. Radiol.*, 75, 959, 2002.
70. Gibbs, J. B., Mechanism-based target identification and drug discovery in cancer research, *Science*, 287, 1969, 2000.
71. Gelmon, K. A. et al., Anticancer agents targeting signaling molecules and cancer cell environment: challenges for drug development?, *J. Natl. Cancer Inst.*, 91, 1281, 1999.

72. Ronen, S. M. et al., Magnetic resonance detects changes in phosphocholine associated with Ras activation and inhibition in NIH 3T3 cells, *Br. J. Cancer*, 84, 691, 2001.
73. Beloueche, M. et al., Ras transformation and metabolism: an MRS investigation, *Proc. Int. Soc. Magn. Reson. Med.*, 9, 2216, 2001.
74. Beloueche-Babari, M. et al., Magnetic resonance spectroscopy monitoring of MAPK signalling inhibition, *Cancer Res.*, 65, 3356, 2005.
75. Ramirez de Molina A., Rodriguez-Gonzalez, A., and Lacal, J. C., From Ras signalling to ChoK inhibitors: a further advance in anticancer drug design, *Cancer Lett.*, 206, 137, 2004.
76. Maloney, A. and Workman, P., HSP90 as a new therapeutic target for cancer therapy: the story unfolds, *Expert Opin. Biol. Ther.*, 2, 3, 2002.
77. Beloueche, M. et al., Inhibition of Ras signalling pathways by the HSP90 inhibitor 17AAG in human breast cancer cells increases MRS observable phospholipid signals, *MAGMA*, 15, 86, 2002.
78. Chung, Y. L. et al., Magnetic resonance spectroscopic pharmacodynamic markers of the heat shock protein 90 inhibitor 17-allylamino,17-demethoxygeldanamycin (17AAG) in human colon cancer models, *J. Natl. Cancer Inst.*, 95, 1624, 2003.
79. Beloueche-Babari, M. et al., Identifying biomarkers reflecting the action of the Hsp90 inhibitor 17AAG in malignant human melanoma cells prior to clinical evaluation, *Proc. Int. Soc. Magn. Reson. Med.*, 13, 2042, 2005.
80. Robinson, S. P. and Griffiths, J. R., Current issues in the utility of 19F nuclear magnetic resonance methodologies for the assessment of tumour hypoxia, *Philos. Trans. R. Soc. Lond. B Biol. Sci.*, 359, 987, 2004.
81. Lord, E. M., Harwell, L., and Koch, C. J., Detection of hypoxic cells by monoclonal antibody recognizing 2-nitroimidazole adducts, *Cancer Res.*, 53, 5721, 1993.
82. Aboagye, E. O. et al., Preclinical evaluation of the fluorinated 2-nitroimidazole N-(2-hydroxy-3,3,3-trifluoropropyl)-2-(2-nitro-1-imidazolyl) acetamide (SR-4554) as a probe for the measurement of tumor hypoxia, *Cancer Res.*, 57, 3314, 1997.
83. Seddon, B. M. et al., A phase I study of SR-4554 via intravenous administration for noninvasive investigation of tumor hypoxia by magnetic resonance spectroscopy in patients with malignancy, *Clin. Cancer Res.*, 9, 5101, 2003.
84. Wolber, J. et al., Hyperpolarized 129Xe NMR as a probe for blood oxygenation, *Magn. Reson. Med.*, 43, 491, 2000.

15 Molecular Imaging in Cancer Therapies of the Future

Chrit Moonen

CONTENTS

15.1 INTRODUCTION

Molecular imaging is thought to play a major role in the characterization and measurement of biological processes at the cellular and molecular level [1–4]. Molecular imaging has attracted much attention recently, in particular since it is expected to become one of the major tools for individualized medicine in diagnosis, as well as for guidance of therapy. Nuclear medicine techniques have always been based on radiotracers incorporated in specific molecules [5], and are thus early examples of molecular imaging. However, the field is developing rapidly as a multimodality endeavor. Ultrasound imaging, MRI, optical imaging, and CT contribute to molecular imaging and complement PET and SPECT in this field. Apart from some of the nuclear medicine techniques, molecular imaging has started in the basic sciences. Many of the novel tools and contrast agents will continue to be developed firstly for small animals. However, the transition towards clinical research and clinical practice is happening at an increasingly rapid pace. The translational aspects will thus play an important role in molecular imaging. The objective of this chapter is to illustrate the different aspects of molecular imaging in the field of cancer.

It is instructive to analyze the recent attention to molecular imaging in the general context of genome-based medicine. It is well accepted that gene defects (acquired or hereditary) are at the basis of all major forms of cancer (and many other diseases). The complete deciphering of the human genome in healthy subjects [6] has become a major goal of health-related research for all diseases in which gene defects are suspected. Following the conclusion of this huge effort (at least for healthy subjects), it has become increasingly clear that this major achievement is only the beginning of the field of novel, genome-based, therapies. For example, despite small gene defects, gene expression patterns can be altered tremendously in cancer. The modified gene expression (and, as a result, also the modified protein and metabolite concentrations) alters the drug sensitivity and thus presents new opportunities in specific treatment. For example, the increased expression of the gene coding for the receptor Her-2/neu in approximately 25% of breast cancers [7] increases the prospects of treatment with the drug herceptin. Similarly, the drug Gleevec is acting specifically on a protein kinase overexpressed in some forms of leukemia [8].

New technologies have allowed very rapid determination of gene expression of hundreds of genes from a small biopsy [9]. The hope is that knowledge of expression patterns will lead to specific therapy optimized for each individual patient. Every week, papers are published with detailed analyses of expression at different stages of pathologies. Despite the expectations of these new technologies, some of their limitations should be addressed. Tumors are known to be very heterogeneous, and gene expression patterns follow this heterogeneity. In addition, gene expression patterns change upon therapy. Therefore, there is a clear need for a spatial and temporal understanding of gene expression. This objective cannot be realistically met by classical methods based on gene chips and biopsies. Therefore, molecular imaging approaches, based on contrast agents reporting on local gene expression or on its physiological consequences via indirect biomarker read-outs, hold tremendous promise.

15.2 DEFINITION OF MOLECULAR IMAGING

From the introduction above, the meaning of molecular imaging has probably become fairly evident. Nevertheless, it is worthwhile reflecting on the proper definition. Whereas it is evident that FDG–PET is a molecular imaging technique, it is less clear whether a PET study of perfusion by ^{18}O labeled water can also be classified as a molecular imaging study, since the purpose of the assay is not to give information on a molecular or cellular event. Also, whereas it is clear that MR spectroscopic imaging is a molecular imaging technique since the purpose is the mapping of specific metabolites, it is less clear whether contrast-enhanced MRI can be classified as such. If the purpose is the analysis of the blood-brain-barrier breakdown or the membrane permeability in tumors, it is doubtful whether it may be called a molecular imaging technique. Of course, the image contrast in such MR images is still based on the molecule water (or more precisely, of the water hydrogens). If the purpose is tracking of labeled stem cells or macrophages, most researchers in the field would probably call it a molecular imaging technique. Therefore, it is important to begin with a sound definition of molecular imaging, especially to distinguish it from functional and physiological imaging.

Several definitions have been offered in the literature [1–4]. The definition recently adopted at a meeting organized by the Radiological Society of North America and the Society of Nuclear Medicine [10] will be followed here:

> Molecular Imaging techniques directly or indirectly monitor and record the spatio-temporal distribution of molecular or cellular processes for biochemical, biological, diagnostic, or therapeutic applications.

In the context of genome-based therapy, particular attention will be paid here to gene expression.

15.3 IMPROVED DIAGNOSTICS BY MOLECULAR IMAGING FOR INDIVIDUALIZED THERAPY

15.3.1 SEEING GENES IN ACTION

15.3.1.1 Expression of Exogenous Genes

One of the most direct ways of analyzing gene expression is by using specific contrast agents that report, via a molecular imaging technique, directly on the concentration of gene products: the proteins. If a transfected cell line is used, and the objective is the analysis of the transgene expression, a gene coding for a marker gene may be added. If the expression of the transgene is coupled to that of another transgene (TG), the analysis of the expression of the marker gene can be extrapolated to the expression of TG. Several examples have been reported in the literature with the choice of the marker gene depending on the molecular imaging technique and the particular application (see also Chapter 13, Section 13.5).

The gene coding for the luciferase enzyme is a very powerful molecular imaging marker for optical imaging [11] (see also Chapter 2, Section 2.2.5). The concentration of the luciferase enzyme can be probed *in vivo* using the substrate luciferine. Together with the intracellular substrates ATP and oxygen, bioluminescence is generated that can be quantified using a highly sensitive CCD camera. Tumor cell lines can be transfected with the luciferase gene. Thus, tumor growth and metastasis formation can be probed noninvasively with bioluminescense imaging. However, diffraction of light generally limits its application to mice and small rats.

Nuclear medicine techniques employ different marker genes. The expression of the marker gene coding for thymidine kinase can be probed with substrate analogues, such as FIAU, that will not be further metabolized, but become trapped intracellularly [12]. This approach has been used recently in clinical research. Other marker techniques may be used, such as those coding for unique cross-membrane transporters.

MRI lacks the sensitivity of bioluminescence and nuclear medicine techniques. Hence, amplification techniques have to be developed to obtain the sensitivity and specificity of those molecular imaging techniques. The first approach is based on the specific design of a shielding cage for MRI contrast agents. The cage consists of galactose units. With the cage intact, the internal Gd contrast agent is shielded from tissue water. Hence, no relaxation of water hydrogens is observed. When the enzyme galactosidase is present, the galactose units are cleaved and the contrast agent is accessible for water. Relaxation effects are then observed. The gene coding for galactosidase can therefore be used as a MR marker gene, in conjunction with contrast agents shielded by cleavable galactose units [13].

Alternative approaches for MRI marker genes are based on genes coding for transport of iron (transferrin) from the extracellular spaces across the cell membrane [14]. The resulting intracellular accumulation of iron (either with or without administration of iron particles) results in local susceptibility differences, hence in the loss of local magnetic field homogeneity, and thus in MR signal decrease (Figure 15.1).

For quantification of expression of transgenes via the use of marker enzymes, it must be assured that conditions are met for a correlation of signal changes with gene expression. In general, the more indirect the detection method is, and the more amplification procedures are used, the more attention must be paid that quantification is indeed feasible.

15.3.1.2 Expression of Endogenous Genes

In the case of expression of endogenous genes, the convenience of marker genes is generally not available. The general approach is the design of specific contrast agents that report, via the molecular imaging technique, directly on the concentration of the proteins which are relevant to the particular type of tumor. Several genes are of direct importance for diagnosis and therapy.

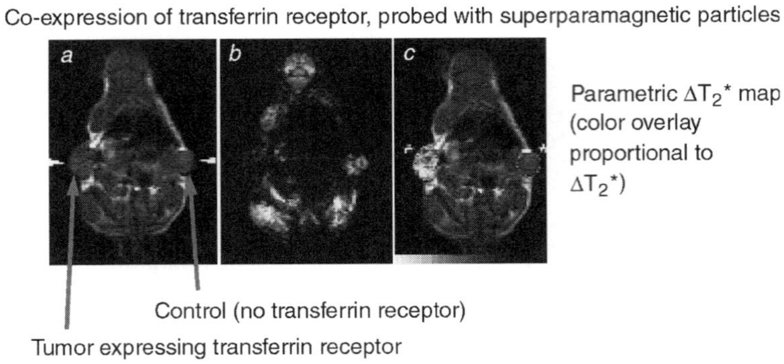

FIGURE 15.1 (See color insert following page 328.) Molecular imaging with MRI: Use of marker gene coding for transferrin, probed with super-paramagnetic articles. (From Weissleder, R. et al., *Nat. Med.*, 6, 351, 2000. Courtesy of R. Weissleder. With permission of Nature America Inc. Copyright 2000.)

Some genes are relevant for almost all tumors, for example the genes that are involved in common processes such as (i) angiogenesis in order to provide adequate perfusion to the growing tumor, (ii) breakdown of the extracellular matrix for infiltration of the tumor, and (iii) removal of dying tumor cells (triggered by apoptosis processes). Several growth factors, such as the vascular endothelial growth factor (VEGF), promote angiogenesis. Specific contrast agents are being developed to probe the presence of the VEGF receptor [15] (see also Chapter 13, Section 13.3.2). The invading tumor requires several proteases to allow penetration. The large class of matrix metalloproteases (MMP), and others such as cathepsin, are targets for molecular imaging contrast agents. An example is the use of an MMP optical contrast agent [16] whose fluorescence is quenched because of the two proximity of its two fluorophores. Upon cleavage of the molecule by MMP, the two fluorophores diffuse away from each other and a strong fluorescence is observed (Figure 15.2).

As mentioned previously, MRI requires amplification strategies for analysis of expression using specific contrast agents. Such contrast agents generally contain a specific part, such as a monoclonal

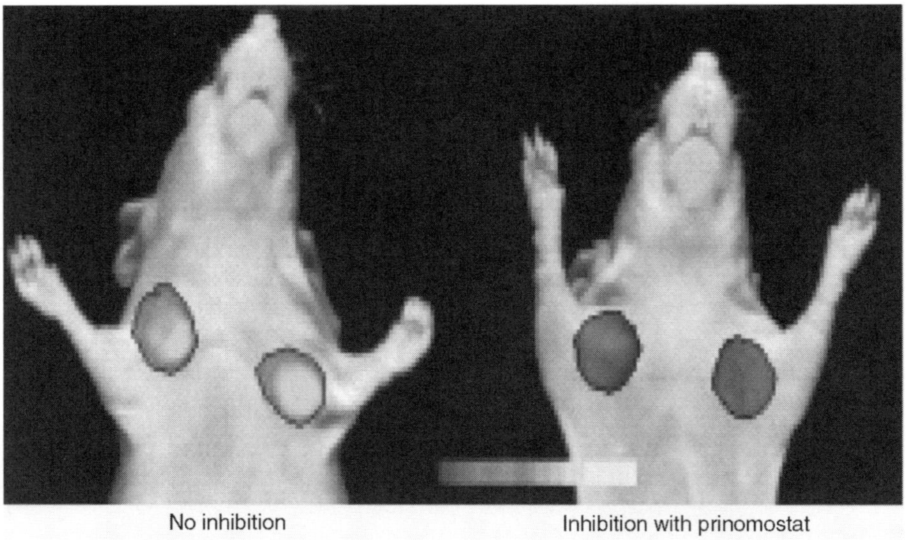

FIGURE 15.2 (See color insert following page 328.) Molecular imaging using specific optical contrast agent: Detection of MMP probed with fluorescent MMP substrates which become fluorescent upon chemical modification catalyzed by MMP. (From Bremer, C. et al., *Nat. Med.*, 7, 743, 2001. Courtesy of R. Weissleder. With permission of Nature America Inc. Copyright 2001.)

antibody, or a fragment thereof, or peptides with specific affinity. Recently, aptamers (small DNA or RNA strings) have shown potential in this field. The specific part is linked to a nanoparticle containing several contrast agent moieties. Either conventional molecules based on paramagnetic Gd^{3+} can be used, or (ultrasmall) superparamagnetic iron oxide (SPIO and USPIO) particles in order to fulfil the required amplification criteria. An example is shown in Figure 15.3 for the detection of $\alpha\nu\beta3$ integrin [17]. Such contrast agents can be rather large. When transport across

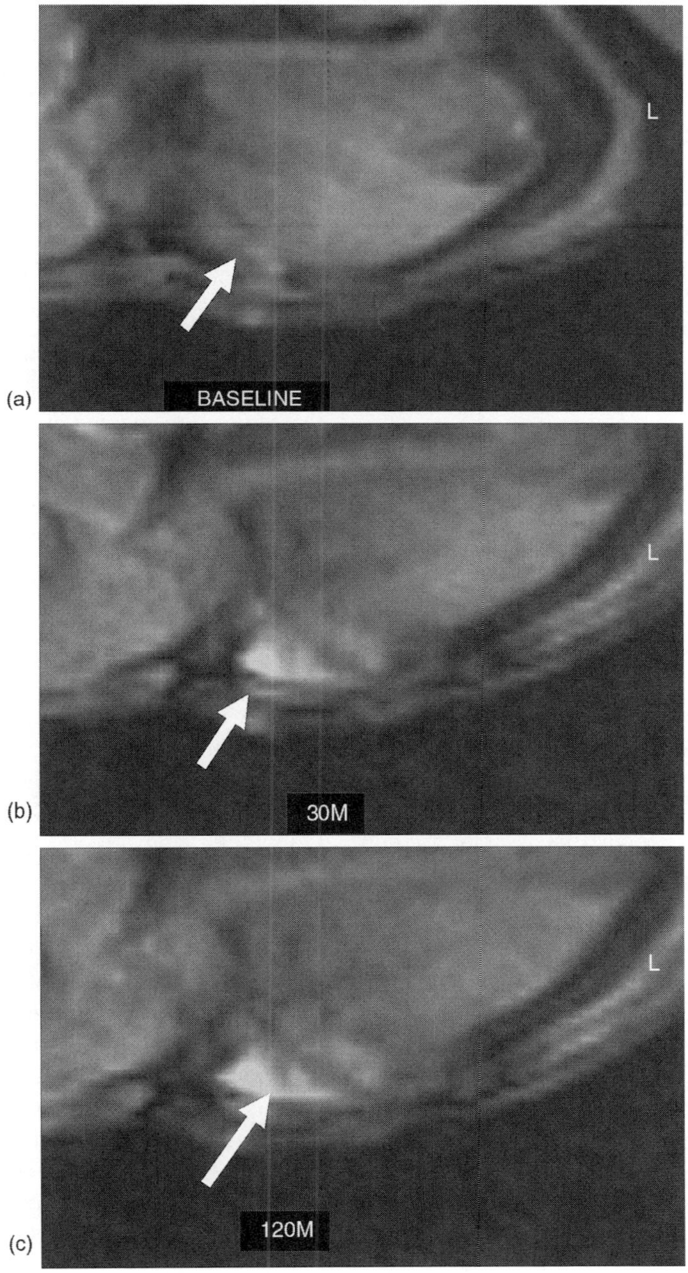

FIGURE 15.3 Molecular imaging with MRI using specific contrast agent: Detection of *avb3 Integrin* with targeted paramagnetic nanoparticles. (From Schmieder, A. H. et al., *Magn. Reson, Med.*, 53, 621, 2005. Courtesy of G. Lanza. With permission of Wiley-Liss Inc. Copyright 2005.)

membrane barriers is limited, the use of such agents may be restricted to membrane proteins directly accessible from the blood circulation. Such problems may not play a large role in tumors because of the leakiness of their vessel walls.

The development of specific ultrasound contrast agents follows a similar approach as those for MRI. Again, a specific part is linked to a particle visible by ultrasound imaging. Such particles may be (partially air-filled) microbubbles based on liposomes [18].

Analysis of expression of several specific genes may play a decisive role in stratification of patients. The example of the presence of the Her-2/neu receptor opens the possibility of treatment with herceptin. A recent study has demonstrated the feasibility of specific MRI contrast agents in the detection of the Her–Neu receptor in a melanoma cell line [19]. Receptor mapping has been a field of excellence for nuclear medicine approaches. Of particular interest in the cancer field (see below) is the mapping of somatostatin receptors in endocrine tumors [20].

15.3.2 Seeing Drugs in Action

Molecular imaging is becoming a very important tool for the pharmaceutical industry. Tumor growth and metastasis formation can be followed noninvasively in mice using optical imaging in combination with tumor cell lines containing the marker gene luciferase (see above). Animal models can thus be followed longitudinally, and potential drugs may be screened rapidly on a rather small number of animals [21].

The efficacy of cancer therapy has traditionally been assessed through morphological changes of the tumor in combination with clinical symptoms. Molecular imaging approaches show great potential in the very early assessment of drug efficacy. For instance, mapping of choline containing metabolites with MR spectroscopic imaging in prostate cancer is showing great promise [22] (see also Chapter 13, Section 13.4).

Molecular imaging and physiological imaging approaches are increasingly suggested as surrogate endpoints in the evaluation of drug efficacy. Perfusion studies allow early assessment of anti-angiogenesis therapies. Imaging of water diffusion has also shown great potential in the early evaluation of drug response. Strictly speaking, such studies belong to the class of physiological and functional imaging and not to the class of molecular imaging according to the definition given above.

15.4 THERAPY GUIDED BY MOLECULAR IMAGING

15.4.1 Combined Diagnostic and Therapeutic (Contrast) Agents

Once a molecular imaging contrast agent has been shown to accumulate at or near the tumor, a therapeutic agent may be added, or the molecular imaging marker may be replaced by the therapeutic agent assuming a similar biodistribution. An example is in the field of endocrine tumors in which the gene coding for the somatostatin receptor is overexpressed. Specific contrast agents containing a labeled somatostatin analogue were used in the clinic to demonstrate the high concentration of the receptor and the resulting concentration of the contrast agent. Then, replacement of the weak emitter for PET detection by a strong emitter was used for radiotherapeutic purposes. Excellent results have been obtained in this way [23].

Similarly, specific MRI and ultrasound contrast agents using nanoparticles visible by MRI and U.S. can be combined with the presence of therapeutic agents in the nanoparticles [24]. Internalization of the contents occurs, probably initiated by membrane fusion of the cell membrane and liposome wall. Also, in the case of U.S., the pressure wave may lead to a temporary increase of membrane permeability. This cavitation effect may be accentuated by the presence of air bubbles [25].

15.4.2 Local Drug Delivery Guided by Molecular Imaging

As said before, therapeutic agents can be combined with specific contrast agents for local drug delivery assisted by U.S. (see also Chapter 2, Section 2.2.4). Since a local pressure wave propagating from an ultrasound transducer may open up a drug nano-carrier, local drug delivery may be realized even without specific contrast agents with high affinity for a molecular target, so long as the ultrasound beam can be directed to a clearly defined region-of-interest (ROI). Such an approach is feasible with so-called focused ultrasound technology. Instead of a parallel or diverging ultrasound beam as is used in U.S. imaging, the beam is now converging into a focal area. The size of the focal area depends on the size of the transducer, on its aperture, and on the wavelength of the ultrasound. Molecular imaging can add a significant aspect to this development using contrast agents that are coreleased with the therapeutic agent [26,27]. This novel approach allows, in principle, an assessment of the bio-distribution and kinetics of the therapeutic agent so long as those parameters mimic closely those of the contrast agent.

Ultrasound assisted local drug delivery, guided by molecular imaging, may be based on two different classes of nano-carriers. The first approach consists of heat-sensitive carriers with the walls becoming leaky near the critical temperature [26]. In this case, focused ultrasound is used to heat up tissue in the ROI, and the nanocarriers release their contents where the temperature is above the critical temperature. The critical temperature of liposomes used for this purpose can be adjusted based on the composition of the lipid bilayer. A second approach is based on nano-carriers that become leaky because of the cavitation effect.

15.4.3 Image Guided Spatio-Temporal Control of Gene Expression

The ability of focused ultrasound to heat up tissue deep inside the body can be used to control transgene expression when the gene is placed under control of a heat-sensitive promoter (Figure 15.4). Such promoters are widely present in nature. For example, all mammals use them when they have a fever in order to produce protecting proteins, the so-called heat-shock proteins. The use of such promoters for control of expression of therapeutic genes requires tight temperature control in the ROI. MRI can be used for rapid temperature mapping, and has therefore been utilized for feedback control of the heating procedure. It has been demonstrated that local over-expression of a marker gene in a modified glioma cell line is feasible using this technology [28].

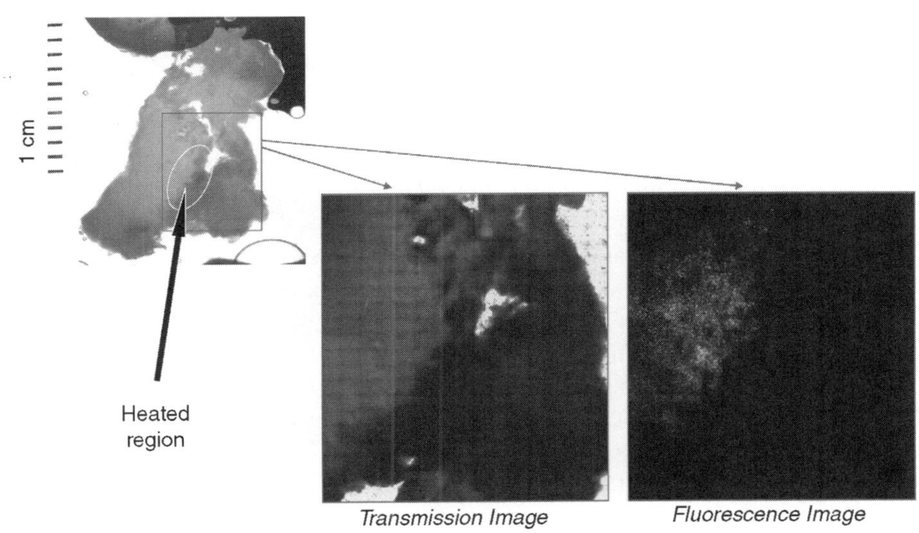

FIGURE 15.4 (See color insert following page 328.) Spatio-temporal control of transgene expression using MRI-guided focused ultrasound in combination with a heat-sensitive promoter. Analysis of GFP gene expression using confocal microscopy.

15.4.4 Tracking of Labeled (Stem) Cells

The ability of molecular imaging to track cells noninvasively is expected to have a large impact (see also Chapter 25). We will briefly address the issue of stem cell and macrophage tracking.

Stem cells and progenitor cells constitute nature's repair shop and have shown great therapeutic potential in animal models following transplantation [29]. Injection of stem cells has already been applied in clinical research in order to assess its potential following cardiac ischemia. Despite the ongoing human applications, many basic questions still remain. Molecular imaging will likely play an essential role in answering typical questions such as:

- When and how do stem cells migrate to their target tissue?
- When and how do stem cells differentiate *in vivo*?
- What is the timeframe of stem cell multiplication and functional recovery at the target site?
- Can we influence stem cell behavior/differentiation *in vivo* for gene therapy purposes?

Techniques have been developed to isolate stem cells, grow them in cell culture, label them with iron particles, and re-inject them into the tissue or into the bloodstream to allow tracking with MRI [30,31] (see also Chapter 25). It has been shown, in an animal ischemia model, that stem cells can home into the lesion site. Stem cells can also be labeled with the marker gene coding for luciferase [32] and tracked using bioluminescence imaging (Figure 15.5). Such molecular imaging techniques allow increased insight into the fate of stem cells, and may help the development of improved therapeutic strategies.

Macrophages can be labeled *in situ* by simple i.v. injection of USPIOs. It has been shown that macrophages accumulate in tissue as a result of inflammation [33], and in tumor tissues. Also, labeled macrophages can be used to visualize and analyze lymph nodes for the presence of metastases [34]. Since macrophages accumulate in tumor tissue, such an approach may also be used for local drug delivery.

15.5 CONCLUSION

Molecular imaging shows great promise in preclinical and clinical research. It is probably only at the beginning of its development. Specific contrast agents have been developed for a small number of proteins and processes. Despite these limited successes, molecular imaging has raised high expectations in many fields of interest, in particular in the cancer field. At present, molecular imaging has allowed promising developments towards:

- Noninvasive spatio-temporal evaluation of (trans)gene expression
- Noninvasive characterization of disease processes on the molecular level *in vivo*
- Translational research from animal models to clinical research and human application
- Early evaluation of drug efficacy in pre-clinical research and clinical applications
- Stratification of patient populations towards individualized therapies
- The rapid development of new treatment strategies such as gene and cell-based therapies

It is also increasingly evident that molecular imaging will influence the way health care and clinical research is organized. The following aspects have become clear:

- The field shows a need for specialists and teams understanding molecular biology, imaging and chemistry.
- There is an increased blurring between diagnostics and treatment.

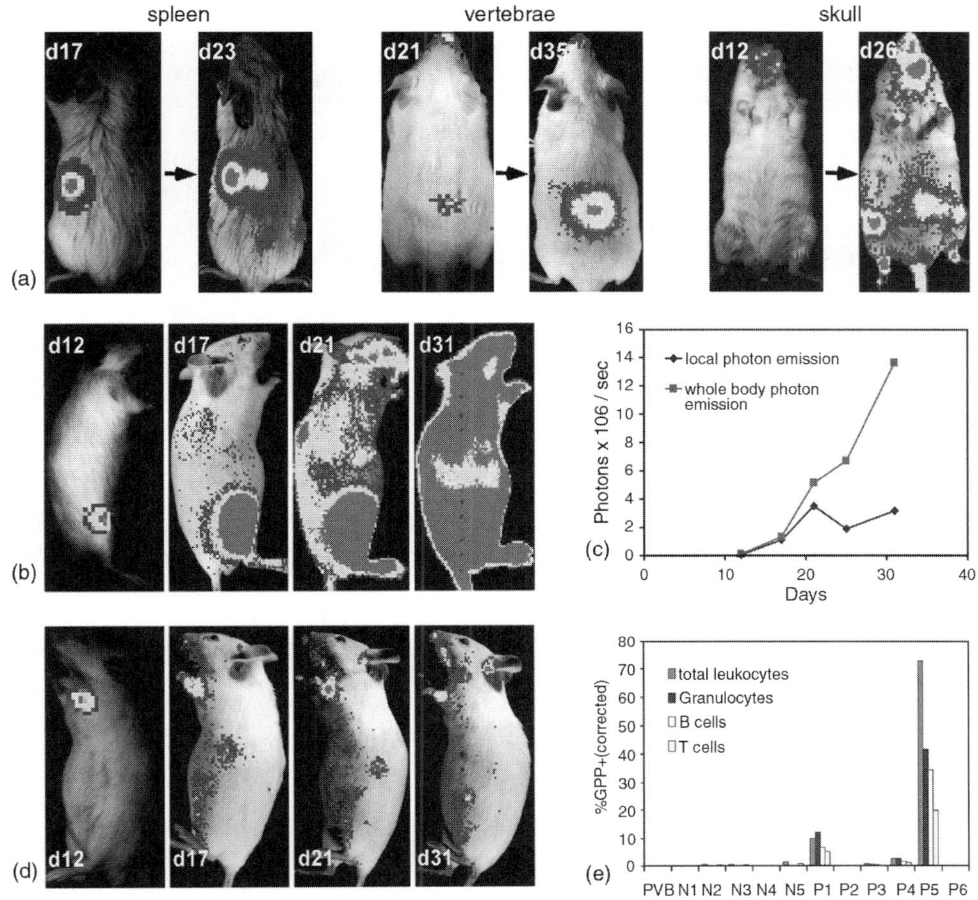

FIGURE 15.5 (See color insert following page 328.) Tracking of stem cells using bioluminescence imaging: Reconstitution of immune system following injection of hematopoietic stem cell transfected with the gene coding for luciferase. (From Cao, Y. A. et al., *Proc. Natl. Acad. Sci. USA*, 101, 221, 2004. Courtesy of C. Contag. With permission of The National Academy of Sciences. Copyright 2004.)

- Molecular imaging is accelerating the development of novel clinical and preclinical imaging instruments with combined technologies: MRI/(focused)ultrasound; PET/CT; MRI/PET.
- There is a large role for optical molecular imaging of mice in basic and in pharmaceutical research.
- Molecular imaging is part of a paradigm shift in health care towards early molecular diagnostics and image guided molecular therapy.

ACKNOWLEDGMENTS

European Union, NoE "Diagnostic Molecular Imaging;" Ligue National Contre le Cancer, Conseil Régional d'Aquitaine.

REFERENCES

1. Weissleder, R. and Mahmood, U., Molecular imaging, *Radiology*, 219, 316, 2001.
2. Rudin, M. and Weissleder, R., Molecular imaging in drug discovery and development, *Nat. Rev. Drug Discov.*, 2, 123, 2003.

3. Choy, G., Choyke, P., and Libutti, S. K., Current advances in molecular imaging: noninvasive in vivo bioluminescent and fluorescent optical imaging in cancer research, *Mol. Imaging*, 2, 303, 2003.
4. Hildebrandt, I. J. and Gambhir, S. S., Molecular imaging applications for immunology, *Clin. Immunol.*, 111, 210, 2004.
5. Phelps, M. E., Positron emission tomography provides molecular imaging of biological processes, *Proc. Natl. Acad. Sci. USA*, 97, 9226, 2000.
6. International Human Genome Sequencing Consortium, Initial sequencing and analysis of the human genome, *Nature*, 409, 860, 2001.
7. Blay, J. Y. et al., Targeted cancer therapies, *Bull. Cancer*, 92, E13, 2005.
8. Noble, M. E., Endicott, J. A., and Johnson, L. N., Protein kinase inhibitors: Insights into drug design from structure, *Science*, 303, 1800, 2004.
9. Jain, K. K., Role of pharmacoproteomics in the development of personalized medicine, *Pharmacogenomics*, 5, 331, 2004.
10. Adopted during molecular imaging summit, Radiological Society of North America and Society of Nuclear Medicine, Oak Brook, USA, April 21–22, 2005.
11. Edinger, M. et al., Advancing animal models of neoplasia through in vivo bioluminescence imaging, *Eur. J. Cancer*, 38, 2128, 2002.
12. Gambhir, S. S. et al., Imaging of adenoviral-directed herpes simplex virus type 1 thymidine kinase reporter gene expression in mice with radiolabeled ganciclovir, *J. Nucl. Med.*, 39, 1998, 2003.
13. Louie, A. Y. et al., In vivo visualization of gene expression using magnetic resonance imaging, *Nat. Biotechnol.*, 18, 321, 2000.
14. Hogemann-Savellano, D. et al., The transferrin receptor: a potential molecular imaging marker for human cancer, *Neoplasia*, 5, 495, 2003.
15. Li, S. et al., Characterization of (123)I-vascular endothelial growth factor-binding sites expressed on human tumour cells: possible implication for tumour scintigraphy, *Int. J. Cancer*, 91, 789, 2001.
16. Bremer, C., Tung, C. H., and Weissleder, R., In vivo molecular target assessment of matrix metalloproteinase inhibition, *Nat. Med.*, 7, 743, 2001.
17. Schmieder, A. H. et al., Molecular MR imaging of melanoma angiogenesis with alphanubeta3-targeted paramagnetic nanoparticles, *Magn. Reson. Med.*, 53, 621, 2005.
18. Morawski, A. M., Lanza, G. A., and Wickline, S. A., Targeted contrast agents for magnetic resonance imaging and ultrasound, *Curr. Opin. Biotechnol.*, 16, 89, 2005.
19. Artemov, D. et al., Magnetic resonance molecular imaging of the HER-2/neu receptor, *Cancer Res.*, 63, 2723, 2003.
20. Eriksson, B. et al., Role of PET in localization of neuroendocrine and adrenocortical tumors, *Ann. N.Y. Acad. Sci.*, 970, 159, 2002.
21. Roda, A. et al., Bioluminescence and chemiluminescence in drug screening, *Anal. Bioanal. Chem.*, 377, 826, 2003.
22. Kurhanewicz, J. et al., Combined magnetic resonance imaging and spectroscopic imaging approach to molecular imaging of prostate cancer, *J. Magn. Reson. Imaging*, 16, 451, 2002.
23. Waldherr, C. et al., Tumor response and clinical benefit in neuroendocrine tumors after 7.4 GBq (90)Y-DOTATOC, *J. Nucl. Med.*, 43, 610, 2002.
24. Lanza, G. M. et al., Novel paramagnetic contrast agents for molecular imaging and targeted drug delivery, *Curr. Pharm. Biotechnol.*, 5, 495, 2004.
25. Dijkmans, P. A. et al., Microbubbles and ultrasound: from diagnosis to therapy, *Eur. J. Echocardiogr.*, 5, 245, 2004.
26. De Zwart, J.A. et al., On the Feasibility of local drug delivery using thermo-sensitive liposomes and MR-guided focused ultrasound, *Proceedings of the International Society of Magnetic Resonance Medicine*, Denver, 2000.
27. Bos, C. et al., Simultaneous Monitoring of Temperature and T_1: Methods and Preliminary Results of Application to Drug Delivery using Thermosensitive Liposomes, *Magn. Reson. Med.*, 54, 1020, 2005.
28. Guilhon, E. et al., Image-guided control of transgene expression based on local hyperthermia, *Mol. Imaging*, 2, 11, 2003.
29. Daley, G. Q., Goodell, M. A., and Snyder, E. Y., Realistic prospects for stem cell therapeutics, *Hematology (Am. Soc. Hematol. Educ. Program)* 2003, 398, 2003.

30. Frank, J. A. et al., Clinically applicable labeling of mammalian and stem cells by combining superparamagnetic iron oxides and transfection agents, *Radiology*, 228, 480, 2003.
31. Hoehn, M. et al., Monitoring of implanted stem cell migration in vivo: a highly resolved in vivo magnetic resonance imaging investigation of experimental stroke in rat, *Proc. Natl. Acad. Sci. USA*, 99, 16267, 2002.
32. Cao, Y. A. et al., Shifting foci of hematopoiesis during reconstitution from single stem cells, *Proc. Natl. Acad. Sci. USA*, 101, 221, 2004.
33. Hauger, O. et al., Nephrotoxic nephritis and obstructive nephropathy: evaluation with MR imaging enhanced with ultrasmall superparamagnetic iron oxide-preliminary findings in a rat model, *Radiology*, 217, 819, 2000.
34. Harisinghani, M. G. et al., Noninvasive detection of clinically occult lymph-node metastases in prostate cancer, *N. Engl. J. Med.*, 348, 2491, 2003.

Editorial Comments

Based on data provided to the World Health Organization by 112 member states, the following table shows estimates for the ten leading causes of death in the year 2000:

Developed Countries % of Total Deaths	Developing Countries % of Total Deaths
Ischemic heart disease 23.3%	Ischemic heart disease 9.2%
Cerebrovascular disease 13.4%	Cerebrovascular disease 8.4%
Trachea, bronchus, lung cancers 4.4%	Lower respiratory infections 7.9%
Lower respiratory infections 3.6%	Perinatal conditions 6.0%
COPD 3.2%	HIV/AIDS 6.0%
Colon and rectum cancers 2.3%	COPD 5.2%
Self-inflicted injuries 1.8%	Diarrheal diseases 4.6%
Diabetes mellitus 1.7%	Tuberculosis 3.6%
Stomach cancer 1.7%	Malaria 2.7%
Hypertensive heart disease 1.7%	Road traffic accidents 2.4%

Despite great advances in its diagnosis, treatment, and prevention, heart disease is since long the leading cause of death in the world.

A first fundamental step in heart disease diagnosis was the introduction of cardiac catheterization in the 1950s, a procedure that involves threading a slender tube into the heart to take measurements and identify blocked arteries. This technique led to a new era in surgical treatment of coronary heart disease. Bypass operations, performed since 1967, involve the creation of new routes for blood supply to reach blood-starved heart muscles. In balloon angioplasty, developed a decade later, a deflated balloon is inserted into a narrowed artery. The balloon is then inflated at the site of the narrowing to widen it. Other surgical advances include replacement of diseased heart valves with artificial valves, implantation of pacemakers that maintain normal heart rhythm, use of temporary artificial hearts, and methods for correcting hereditary defects in the heart.

Drugs developed to treat angina pectoris, high blood pressure, dangerous abnormalities in heart rhythm, or high blood cholesterol levels, were shown to reduce the risk of heart attacks or stroke. In the 1980s, aspirin went into wide use to prevent blood clots that cause many heart attacks.

Identification of high blood pressure, high blood cholesterol, cigarette smoking, diabetes, obesity, and lack of exercise as risk factors led to the establishment of public health programs aiming to help reduce heart disease risks. Such preventive programs seem to be working — according to the American Heart Association, the death rate from coronary heart disease declined 26% between 1988 and 1998.

Cardiovascular MRI has rapidly evolved over the last two decades. As a noninvasive imaging modality, it is unrivaled in its ability to characterize soft-tissue structures and in its versatility, making it an ideal tool for studying patients with cardiovascular disease. As discussed in Chapter 17, left ventricular (LV) structure, function, perfusion, and viability can be evaluated within one examination with a high degree of precision while avoiding the harmful effects of ionizing radiation and nephrotoxic contrast agents.

Cardiac MRI on small animals is also feasible (Chapter 16). Approaches were developed to obtain a reliable cardiac trigger in both rats and mice despite the high heart beating rates. Assessments of ventricular function and mass have been well validated and are routinely performed by several research groups. Even advanced techniques such as perfusion imaging, delayed enhancement, or tagging are emerging.

The development of new therapies to treat heart disease is profiting from the progress in human and animal cardiac MRI. The accuracy and reproducibility provided by the technique in assessments of cardiac function are invaluable for the diagnosis and the evaluation of a patient's response to therapy. On the other hand, high-resolution cardiac MRI in small rodents opens the perspective to noninvasive drug profiling in animal models of disease. In particular, noninvasive analyses of transgenic models are enhancing our understanding of cardiovascular disease.

16 Cardiac MR Techniques Applied to Small Rodents

Matthias Nahrendorf and Wolfgang R. Bauer

CONTENTS

16.1 INTRODUCTION

Cardiac MRI is evolving as a powerful diagnostic tool in humans (see Chapter 17). It has the highest accuracy in measuring cardiac function, e.g., ejection fraction and myocardial mass [1], and it bears the potential to combine several modalities in one session, e.g., determination of myocardial viability, mechanical function, and perfusion status.

Besides human applications, the impact of cardiac MRI in small animals is also growing. There are several reasons why small animals are chosen: space in most laboratories is limited, which does not allow studies with larger animals. Meanwhile, the facilities and equipment necessary to perform the experiments (anesthesia, operation techniques, monitoring) have developed to such a state that handling of small animals is often easier compared to larger animals. Development of transgenic animal models is mainly carried out in mice, and to a lesser extent in rats, due to their fast reproduction cycle.

Small animal cardiac MRI mainly addresses the following topics:

1. Pathophysiology of the cardiovascular system
   a. Mechanistic insight
   b. Development of new therapies
2. Phenotypization of transgenic mice models
3. Development and validation of new cardiac MR techniques

16.2 CINE MRI FOR ASSESSMENT OF MORPHOLOGY AND FUNCTION OF THE LEFT VENTRICLE

Cine MRI has evolved to be the most exact tool to quantify cardiac morphology and function, characterized by small inter- and intraobserver variability [2,3] (see also Chapter 17, Section 17.4.1). Compared to invasive methods to assess cardiac function, it is more exact and can be performed repetitively, e.g., to follow the course of a disease or to monitor therapy [4,5]. Usually, segmented gradient-echo sequences are employed [6]. Comparable to most other applications for small animal imaging, it is desirable to perform these investigations in high field scanners, which are equipped with strong gradient systems and dedicated cardiac rat or mouse coils. This setup ensures sufficient signal-to-noise ratio (SNR) as well as spatial and temporal resolution. Nevertheless, modern clinical scanners have been shown to deliver sufficient image quality too [7].

The heart rates of rats (300 to 400/min) and mice (500 to 600/min) are high, therefore, sufficient temporal resolution is imperative to avoid motion artifacts and to allow for exact volumetry. The maximal acquisition window for one frame should be in the range of 6 to 8 msec, which would allow 12 to 16 image frames to be acquired to cover the cardiac cycle. Spatial in plane resolution for volumetry should be in the range of 100 to 150 μm in square for mice [2,3], which have a wall thickness of approximately 1 mm, and not more than 250 μm for rats, which have a wall thickness of up to 2 mm [5]. For certain experiments, such as assessment of cardiac anatomy in newborn mice [2], even better in-plane resolutions of less than 100 μm in plane are desirable. Usually, the slice thickness is around 1 mm for mice and 1 to 2 mm for rats. Since the left ventricle (LV) is covered by contiguous short axis slices from the base to the apex, this makes the acquisition of 10 to 20 slices mandatory.

Since real time imaging has not yet been established with spatial resolutions mandatory for mouse or rat heart imaging, ECG triggering is a prerequisite for good image quality. Even more so than in human cardiac MRI, this is hampered by the strong changing magnetic fields, especially caused by the powerful gradient systems used in high resolution MRI. These problems need to be addressed by a couple of solutions. First, good electrical contact has to be established between the ECG electrodes and the paws of the animal, for instance by using dedicated paste or gel. Connecting the right fore paw and the left hind leg may help to achieve the highest signal amplitude due to the main direction of the vector of the ECG. To avoid motion of the ECG leads, they should be immobilized, e.g., by taping them down on the animal holder. A position in the middle of the magnet bore, and avoiding forming loops of the leads, may further reduce artifacts induced by the gradient switching. ECG leads may be shielded to avoid picking up gradient noise. The use of commercially available carbon pediatric ECG leads has shown good results in rats. The trigger unit should be equipped with powerful, adjustable filter systems to facilitate the necessary clear ECG signal for optimal triggering. For some delicate applications, such as imaging of valves, additional respiratory gating can be helpful. This may be established by placing a pressure sensor on the chest wall of the mouse. The resulting pressure curve can then be used to gate the image acquisition to the end expiratory phase. To ensure physiologically valid measurements and stable conditions with respect to heart rate and cardiac output, the animal should be kept warm inside the cooled gradient system using a warming pad or a warm air blower, and the temperature should be monitored.

The use of surface coils has been widely propagated for cardiac MRI, since an improved SNR may be achieved. However, for applications involving semiautomatic or automatic post processing software, which uses the signal intensity to identify the blood-myocardium border, volume coils may be the better choice, since they do not suffer from signal intensity gradients (Figure 16.1).

Up to date postprocessing software should enable image segmentation to be performed in an automated fashion, relying on measurement of signal intensities and use of predefined likely shapes

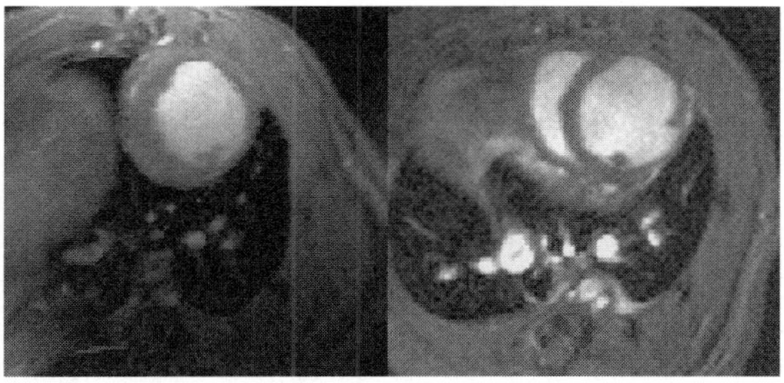

FIGURE 16.1 Diastolic short axis slices of rat hearts, acquired using a 7 T system. The left image of a rat heart 8 weeks after coronary ligation was acquired with a cardiac surface coil. Close to the coil, signal intensity is high, and diminishes towards the posterior wall of the left ventricle. The image on the right, acquired with a volume coil, displays no signal gradient.

and modeling, which help to detect the more difficult interfaces such as the LV anterior wall close to the body wall with similar signal intensity. In fact, clinical software is extremely suitable for performing the post processing, if available. Frequently, the raw data from experimental MR scanners has to be transformed into the DICOM format to use clinical segmentation software.

For the postprocessing, it is necessary to identify three different volumes in every short axis slice: the end-diastolic myocardial volume, the end-diastolic ventricular volume, and the end-systolic ventricular volume. To do so, the cine frames with the largest (diastolic) and smallest (systolic) chamber volume are selected (Figure 16.2). Once the area of these compartments has been determined, the area is multiplied by the slice thickness to yield the slice volume (Figure 16.3). This procedure has to be performed in every slice. Finally, slice volumes are summed up. For myocardial mass, the myocardial volume is multiplied by its gravity (1.05 g/cm^3).

16.3 MYOCARDIAL MOTION ANALYSIS BY TAGGING TECHNIQUES

Using a similar approach as in humans, the feasibility of myocardial motion analysis by tagging has been demonstrated in rats [8] and mice [9]. The principle of tagging consists of a localized saturation of the myocardium prior to read out with a cine gradient-echo sequence. It results in a grid of lines with low (saturated) signal, which move with the myocardium and can be followed by a cine sequence read out. In a study by Epstein et al. [9], a spatial modulation of magnetization (SPAMM) RF pulse with a duration of 4.8 msec was applied immediately after the ECG trigger. The intersections of the gridlines are then used to analyze the direction and magnitude of

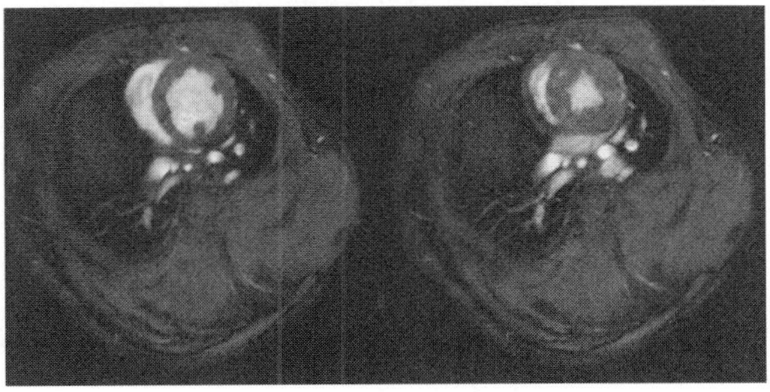

FIGURE 16.2 Diastolic and systolic frames of a mouse at midventricular level.

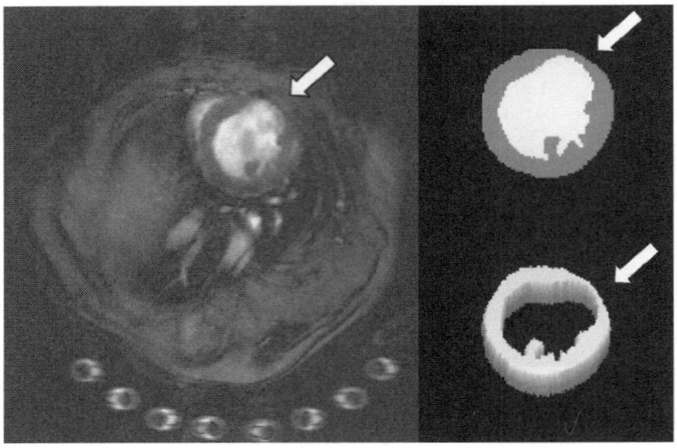

FIGURE 16.3 Left: diastolic short axis frame of a mouse 8 weeks after anterolateral myocardial infarction (arrow). Right upper panel: 2D result of segmentation process. Right lower panel: final myocardial compartment.

myocardial motion. Although this technique is robust and worked to detect lower and aberrant myocardial motion in mice after coronary ligation [9], it is limited by its rather low spatial resolution. Since the left ventricular wall of a mouse is only 1 mm thick, a maximum of two gridlines per direction can be achieved. The shortest reported distance between the gridlines has been 0.7 mm, close to the wall thickness of the mouse [9]. So far, these techniques have not been used to detect differences caused by pharmacotherapy or manipulation of the genome.

16.4 MYOCARDIAL MOTION ANALYSIS BY PHASE CONTRAST TECHNIQUES

The problem of the limited spatial resolution for motion analysis by tagging may be overcome by motion encoding with phase contrast MRI. Using this technique, the signal phase is influenced by bipolar gradient pulses, causing a linear dependence to the motion velocity of the corresponding voxel. Motion velocities and directions can be analyzed on a pixel-by-pixel basis, achieving an in plane resolution as high as $234 \times 234\ \mu m^2$ [10,11], enabling the detection of abnormal motions in mouse infarcted hearts (Figure 16.4).

16.5 CINE MRI FOR ASSESSMENT OF RIGHT VENTRICULAR FUNCTION AND MORPHOLOGY

Assessment of right ventricular function may be performed in a parallel fashion to the LV. A slightly adapted slice angulation has been proposed for the short axis slices for RV volumetry, e.g., perpendicular to the interventricular septum [3]. However, since MRI is a true 3D method, it is sufficient to use the standard LV short axis slices [12]. This approach considerably shortens scan time, because one set of short axis stacks may be used for segmentation of both ventricles. In addition, the assessment of both the left and right ventricular volume in the same image set enables the study of interventricular relations [12].

The right ventricular roof is slightly more cranial then the LV, therefore acquisition of two to three additional short axis slices in head direction is necessary. Parallel to the situation in humans, the assessment of right ventricular mass may be hampered by the small wall thickness of the RV. However, if a higher spatial resolution is used, this may be feasible [3].

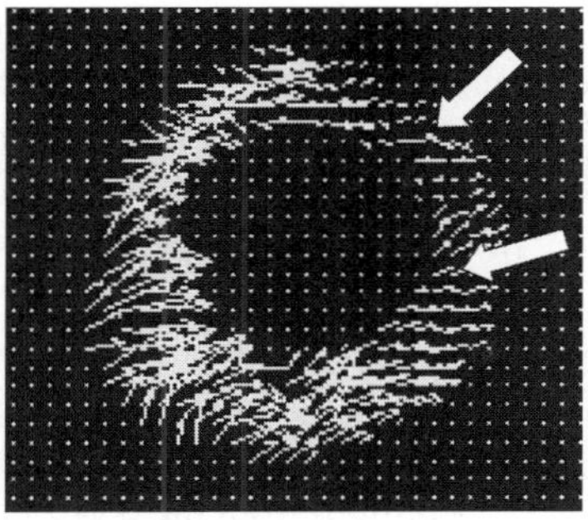

FIGURE 16.4 Vector map derived from phase contrast MRI, acquired during systole at midventricular level of a mouse 4 weeks after myocardial infarction (arrow). The length of the arrow encodes for the amplitude of the myocardial velocity, the shape for the direction of the motion. In the remote region, the arrows are pointed inwards, and are larger than in the hypokinetic infarct zone. Since the thickness of the infarct scar at 4 weeks is in the sub millimeter range, high spatial resolution is mandatory.

16.6 MEASUREMENT OF BLOOD SUPPLY TO THE MYOCARDIUM

Determination of blood supply to the myocardium is of paramount interest for the evaluation of ischemic heart disease and of other forms of heart disease, e.g., hypertrophy, in which an alteration of the microcirculation is considered to be responsible for the impairment of cardiac function. Measurement of blood supply may be performed at different levels of magnitude of the supplying vessel (see also Chapter 17, Section 17.4.2.2). As in humans, coronary arteries may be imaged in intact mice by the inflow effect [13], i.e., the vessels reveal high signal intensity whereas the stationary surrounding tissue exhibits low signal intensity. Isotropic spatial resolution up to 100 μm has been achieved by 3D flash techniques [13].

MR coronary angiography in intact mice and rats faces the same problems as in humans: superposition of cardiac movement and breathing, problems of quantification of vessel size and stenosis in low flow areas. Additionally, heart rate is in the range of 500 to 600 beats/min in mice and the diameter of proximal coronary vessels is lower than 200 μm, i.e., in the range of the achievable spatial resolution. Measurements on isolated hearts are less problematic. In 1991 Burstein [14] determined flow velocity in isolated rat hearts by bolus tracking techniques. Meanwhile, cine-FLASH phase contrast imaging provides time resolved flow measurements with a spatial resolution of $70 \times 70 \times 500\ \mu m^3$ [15] in nonstenotic and stenotic arteries.

A parameter quantifying the tissue supply by blood is perfusion. It is defined as the amount of blood flow within a tissue region normalized to the mass or volume of this tissue region. This parameter reflects the state of tissue supply better than the morphology or flow in larger coronary arteries, since the latter does not consider collateralization within the coronary system. Determination of myocardial perfusion is definitely the domain of MRI which combines noninvasiveness and functional information with a high spatial resolution. Especially in small animal models, these features make it superior to other imaging modalities, e.g., nuclear techniques, or the invasive determination of perfusion with microspheres.

In humans and larger animals, myocardial perfusion is mainly determined by first pass imaging techniques. A bolus of an MR contrast agent is applied, and the kinetics of signal intensity in the tissue and blood of the LV is related to perfusion. In small animals, less literature is available for this technique [16]. The first pass technique is hampered by the following constraints: the low fraction of blood volume in the myocardium implies an only moderate increase of signal intensity during the first pass, i.e., determination of perfusion is susceptible to measuring faults.

If one applies the conventional extracellular contrast agents, signal intensity depends, in a rather complex way, on perfusion and extracapillary penetration of contrast agent. Though quantification of perfusion may in principle be accomplished, one prefers semiquantitative methods, e.g., the slope to the maximum of signal intensity in the myocardium. Though these techniques are routinely used in humans (and larger animals), their application was not widely accepted for small animal imaging.

Intravascular contrast agents would, in principle, considerably facilitate the determination of perfusion from signal intensity time curves, as long as one considers it from the standpoint of tracer kinetics, i.e., concentration time curves in myocardium and blood. However, the determination of the concentration time curve in the myocardium from the corresponding signal intensity time curve is not trivial. The high amplitude of the concentration in the microcirculation during the first pass implies that different dynamic regimes of the transcapillary proton exchange have to be considered, i.e., quantification of the concentration is hampered.

An alternative to the first pass methods are spin labeling techniques which do not rely on a contrast agent. These techniques label inflowing arterial spins and observe this effect on signal intensity of tissue. In 1992, Williams et al. [17] demonstrated that the signal intensity in the brain depends on perfusion when the arterial spins, flowing into the brain, are continuously inversed. Though this technique also works in the isolated heart [18], it cannot be transferred to the intact heart, since the complex geometry/topology of blood supply by the coronary arteries in relation to the LV does not allow a simple inversion of arterial spins outside the imaging plane. An alternative is not to label the inflowing arterial spins, but those of the imaging slice by slice selective inversion. In this setup, inflow of native (noninversed) arterial spins into the imaging slice apparently accelerates longitudinal relaxation in the imaging slice (Figure 16.5).

The effect on T_1 mainly depends on perfusion and the transcapillary exchange of water protons. The magnitude of the latter is high enough that one obtains in myocardium a simple dependence of T_1 on perfusion, i.e.,

$$\Delta(1/T_1) = \Delta(\text{perfusion})/\lambda \qquad (16.1)$$

where $\Delta(1/T_1)$ is the change in longitudinal relaxation rate and λ is the partition coefficient of water between blood and tissue. This technique has been established and validated in the isolated rat heart [19,20], and in the intact rat [21–25], and mice heart [26,27].

Another parameter quantifying blood supply in myocardium is the intramyocardial relative blood volume (RBV), defined as the volume of blood in a sample of myocardium per volume (or mass) of this sample. It is worth noting that the RBV mainly resides in the capillaries, i.e., it mainly reflects the volume of the capillaries, and hence is a parameter of the myocardial microcirculation. Since it is discussed that alterations of the capillary supply is involved in many pathological processes, e.g., reduction of the capillary density during hypertrophy, the potential role of the parameter RBV is evident. The RBV may also be determined by first pass techniques, however, the constraints mentioned above for perfusion imaging are the same. An alternative are techniques working with intravascular contrast agent in the steady state. These contrast agents are confined to the intravascular space, e.g., conventional Gd-DTPA contrast agent linked to macromolecules (albumin), or larger superparamagnetic particles. They have the advantage that one can repeat measurements and that only a dynamic regime of transcapillary proton exchange has to be considered. The basic idea is that an intravascular contrast, though confined to the intravascular space, spreads its effect on relaxation by transcapillary spin exchange. Thus, even a small volume fraction of intracapillary blood volume filled with contrast agent considerably accelerates relaxation of extracapillary nuclear magnetization (Figure 16.6) and the apparent T_1 in myocardium becomes a function of the RBV [28,29].

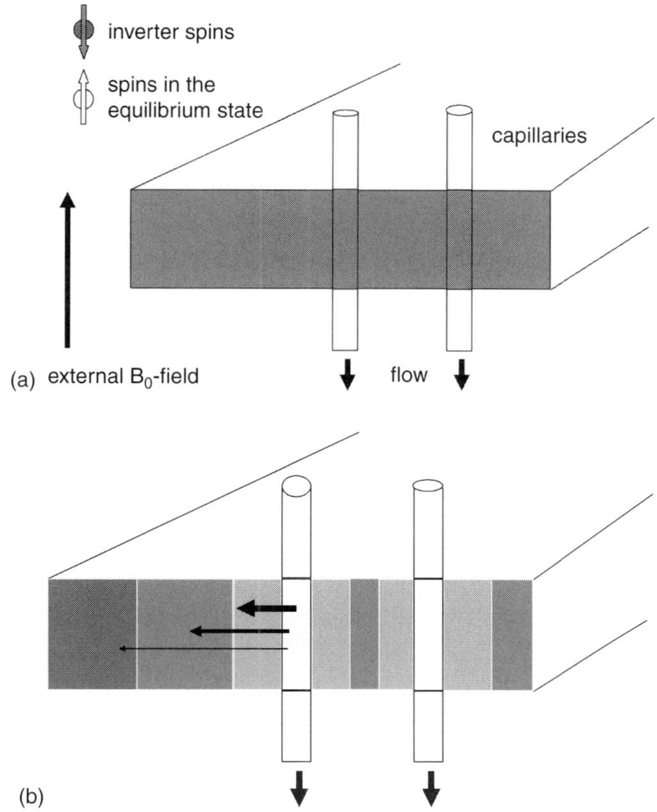

FIGURE 16.5 Principle of spin labeling perfusion measurement by slice selective spin inversion. Shown is a section of myocardium with its capillaries which is the dominating type of vessel here (~90Vol. %). (a) Spins are selectively inverted in the imaging plane, and thereafter start to relax towards equilibrium. (b) Additionally, spins in the thermo-magnetic equilibrium state enter the imaging slice by capillary inflow and transcapillary exchange. Therefore, longitudinal relaxation is apparently accelerated, i.e., T_1 is a function of perfusion and transcapillary exchange.

In many cases, the dynamics of spin exchange is in such a range that the simple relation

$$RBV/\lambda = \Delta(1/T_1\text{myocardium})/\Delta(1/T_1\text{blood}) \tag{16.2}$$

holds, where λ is the partition coefficient of water between blood and tissue and $\Delta(1/T_1)$ is the increase of the longitudinal relaxation rate after application of the contrast agent [22,29].

16.7 PATHOPHYSIOLOGY OF THE CARDIOVASCULAR SYSTEM, MYOCARDIAL INFARCTION, AND ISCHEMIA

The rat model of myocardial infarction, which is induced by coronary ligation after thoracotomy, has proven its value for decades. The landmark study of Pfeffer et al. [30] testing the use of ACE inhibitors after myocardial infarction in rats, may serve as one important example. By treating rats with coronary ligation with an ACE inhibitor, hitherto only used to treat hypertension, it was shown that the LV of rats did not dilate as fast as in the placebo group. Later on, the same effect was seen in patients [31] (see also Chapter 17, Section 17.4.3). Nowadays, every patient after MI receives ACE inhibitor treatment if no contraindication exists. Recently, the mouse model of MI has been

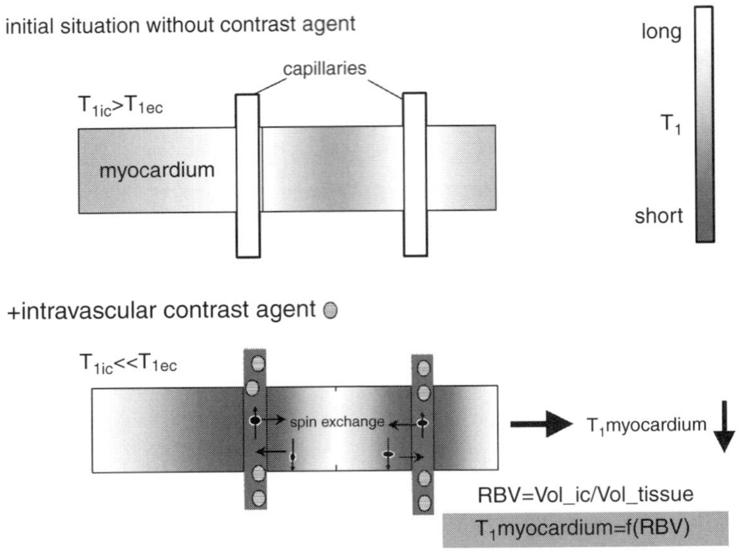

FIGURE 16.6 The intrinsic intracapillary longitudinal relaxation time T_1ic is moderately longer than that of the extracapillary space T_1ec (above). Adding of an intravascular contrast agent reverses this relation (below). Though confined to the intravascular space, the contrast agent exerts its effect on extracapillary relaxation by spin exchange. By this, even a small intracapillary volume fraction induces a considerable amount of decrease of T_1myocardium. The difference T_1moycardium pre, and post application of the contrast agent is a function of the relative intracapillary blood volume, i.e., RBV.

established to address pharmacological questions. Its major importance though is to test the role of single factors in the post MI remodeling process, e.g., enzymes [32] using genetically modified mouse models such as knock out mice.

Models of temporary ischemia, such as ischemia reperfusion, are also of interest and can be assessed by MR read outs. In addition, the rat model of coronary stenosis has been helpful in developing and validating novel MRI methods, such as spin labeling perfusion [24] or spectroscopic imaging [33]. On the other hand, application of these methods helped to better understand pathophysiology and metabolism in this frequent disease (Figure 16.7).

With the advantage of its noninvasive character, MRI allows for serial investigations in the same animal. Hence, changes due to interventions as coronary ligation can be monitored closely and more exactly. Small differences can be detected, and the number of animals to be sacrificed for research purposes is reduced [5]. In contrast to 2D echocardiography, MRI volumetry works without geometrical assumptions and therefore offers a high degree of accuracy in measurements of cardiac output and LV volumes; this is especially important in hearts deformed by asymmetric dilation after MI.

The most relevant parameters that determine left ventricular remodeling are the end-diastolic volume and the myocardial mass. Both these parameters may be determined in a serial fashion, with at least two measurement time points. It is advantageous to choose one very early time point, e.g., one day after MI, and a later time point, which may be 6 weeks in mice and 12 weeks in rats, to cover detectable changes in volumes within a reasonable time frame. In doing so, the opportunity arises to monitor the change of parameters such as LV end-diastolic volume. This approach makes a study powerful to detect small differences between treatment groups, even with a relatively small number of six to eight animals. Treatment groups have to be matched carefully with respect to infarct size, since this parameter determines the degree of LV dilatation and hypertrophy [5].

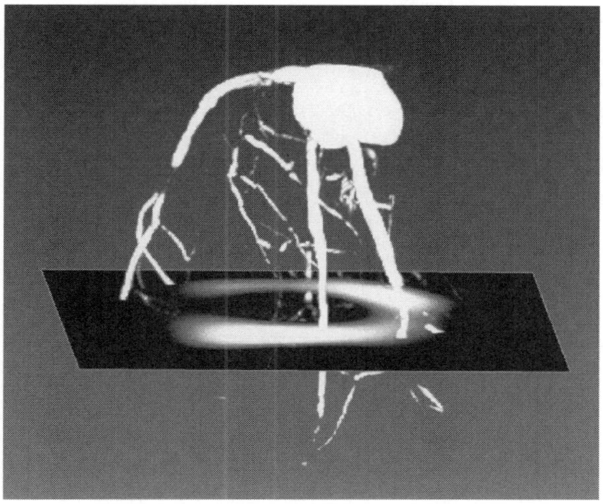

FIGURE 16.7 Fusion image of an isolated rat heart 2 weeks after induction of cronic coronary stenosis, acquired in a 12 T AMX. An ATP metabolite map, acquired with spatially resolved phosphorous spectroscopic imaging, was fused with a coronary MR angiogram. The possibility of visualizing the pathoanatomy (culprit lesion) and the metabolic impact of the disease envisions future imaging strategies to simplify clinical decision making.

MRI can be applied to assess the effects of therapeutical or other agents on infarct size, cardiac geometry, and function with high precision [34]. Thus, MRI bears a great potential to substantially contribute to the understanding of the underlying pathomechanisms in the development of chronic heart failure and can help to evaluate new therapy options.

16.8 REMODELING OF MICROCIRCULATION AFTER MYOCARDIAL INFARCTION

Whereas remodeling of the left ventricular geometry and function after myocardial infarction has been evaluated extensively, microcirculation and its potential implication on impairment of LV function has been less studied. There exist morphometric data, demonstrating a reduced capillary density in the hypertrophied residual myocardium after infarction, which suggest an impairment of the capillary blood supply in relation to the hypertrophied myocytes. Functional data on microcirculation are rare, however, especially, serial data do not exist. This is due to the fact that there exists no conventional measurement technique assessing noninvasively cardiac microcirculation. Above, we discussed how myocardial blood supply, and, hence, microcirculation, may be determined by MRI, with the key parameters perfusion and RBV. The latter is almost equivalent to the relative intracapillary blood volume, since the volume fraction of the latter in relation to total intramyocardial blood volume is $\sim$90% [35].

Serial measurements of perfusion in rats after myocardial infarction of intermediate size revealed a continuous decrease in the residual myocardium under baseline conditions and after maximum vasodilation (Figure 16.8) [23]. It is a well-known fact that residual myocardium develops a compensatory hypertrophy after infarction. A close correlation of baseline and maximum perfusion with the degree of hypertrophy could be demonstrated. It is noteworthy that other hemodynamic parameters, such as left ventricular pressure and heart rate, did not differ from control animals. This indicates that the decline of perfusion was due to an increase of the coronary resistance (Figure 16.9) [23]. The fact that this decline was also present after maximum vasodilation, i.e., when coronary resistance is clearly dominated by that of the capillaries,

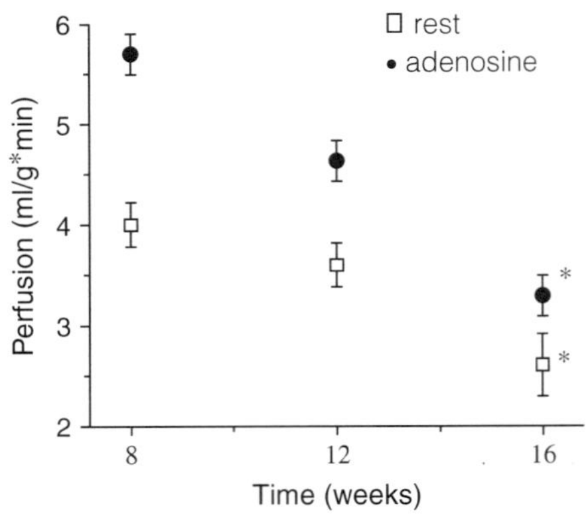

FIGURE 16.8 Myocardial perfusion (ml/g min) of infarcted animals from 8 to 16 weeks after MI. The level of significance *.05 $< p <$ .01 refers to comparisons of the values at 8 and 16 weeks.

demonstrates that the capillary resistance in the residual myocardium increases during hypertrophy after myocardial infarction. This could be due to an increase of the functional capillary length, but further investigations are necessary to clarify this observation.

16.9 PHENOTYPISATION OF TRANSGENIC ANIMALS

The noninvasive and exact character of MRI makes it the ideal tool for phenotyping transgenic mice models [36–38], only hampered by its relatively high costs and limited availability. Initial visions of using cardiac MRI to perform high throughput screenings of large quantities of living transgenic mice to identify a cardiac phenotype have so far not been realized (see also Chapter 5). A study by Schneider et al. [39] came closest to that vision, screening at high spatial resolution 32 mouse embryos after formalin fixation in one imaging session of 12 h duration (Figure 16.10).

Once a cardiac phenotype has been identified, MRI is the most exact tool to characterize it thoroughly. Its noninvasive character is of additional value, since serial investigations to follow the manifestation of a phenotype, due to switching of genes or to monitor changes after onset of therapeutic intervention, are possible. Using multiple MRI modalities (e.g., cine, perfusion, phase

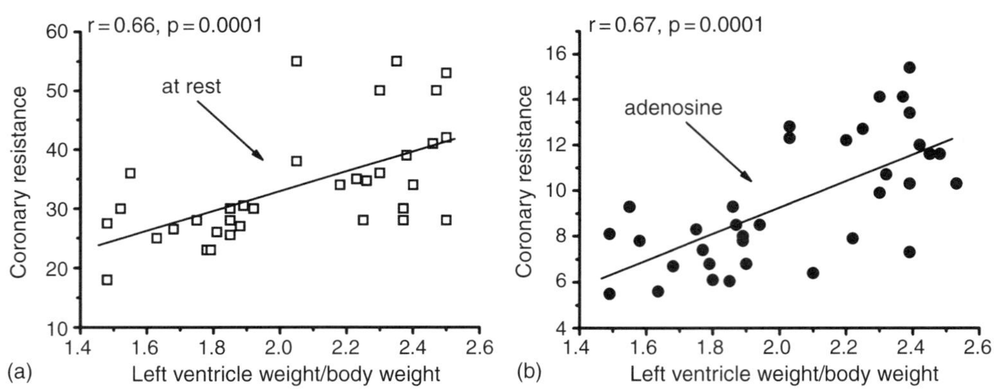

FIGURE 16.9 Linear regression analysis of LV weight/body weight (mg/g) and coronary resistance (mm Hg/g min ml) of infarcted animals under resting conditions and during vasodilation (adenosine).

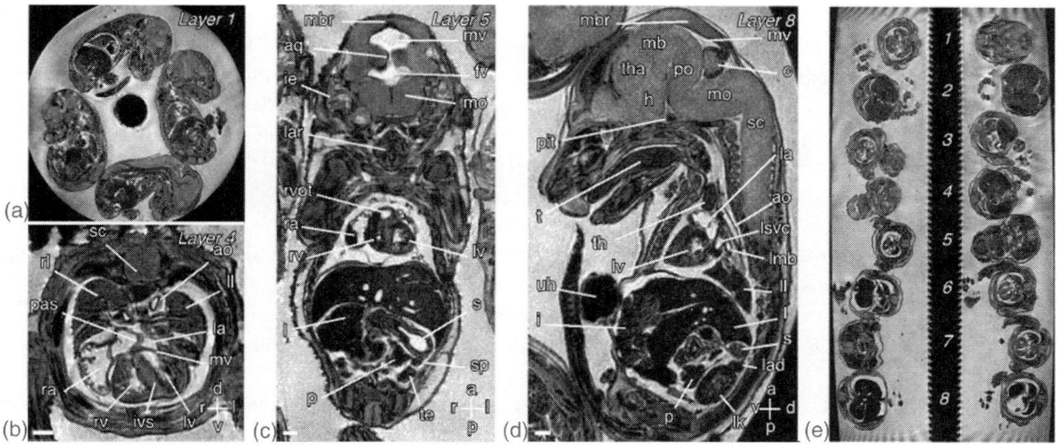

FIGURE 16.10 High-throughput high-resolution magnetic resonance microscopy on fixed mouse embryos: 32 embryos were stacked in eight layers (four embryos each) in a single MR tube. A major advantage of this approach is the ability to easily ship fixed embryos from referring laboratories to the laboratory that performs the MRI analysis. This minimizes the expense of animal relocation, rederivation, and breeding required to generate the embryos, and significantly reduces animal experimentation. (a) Transverse section through the top layer (layer 1) showing the four embryos in this layer. (b–d) Transverse, coronal, and sagittal sections through individual embryos in layers 4, 5, and 8, respectively. The voxel size is $25.4 \times 25.4 \times 24.4\ \mu m^3$. (e) Longitudinal view through the entire stack. Structures indicated in the axial views are the spinal cord (sc), the right and left lungs, atria and ventricles (rl, ll, ra, la, rv, lv), primary atrial and interventricular septa (pas, ivs), mitral valve (mv), midbrain roof (mbr), midbrain (mb), mesencephalic vesicle (mv), thalamus (tha), hypothalamus (h), pons (po), cerebellum (c), medulla oblongata (mo), pituitary (pit), tongue (t), thymus (th), left superior vena cava and main bronchus (lsvc, lmb), aorta (ao), liver (l), stomach (s), left adrenal and kidney (lad, lk), pancreas (p), intestines (i), umbilical hernia (uh), aqueduct of Sylvius (aq), fourth ventricle (fv), inner ear (ie), larynx (lar), right ventricular outflow tract (rvot), spleen (sp), and testes (te). Scale bars = 500 μm; axes: d — dorsal; v — ventral; r — right; l — left; a — anterior, p — posterior. (Reproduced from Schneider et al., *BMC Dev. Biol.*, 4, 16, 2004. Courtesy of J.E. Schneider, S. Neubauer, and S. Bhattacharya. With permission. Copyright 2004 licensee BioMed Central Ltd.)

contrast MRI) in one imaging session will allow a fast, precise, and comprehensive morphological and functional phenotyping. MRI spares the life of the often valuable transgenic mice, which then can be used for other assays, such as molecular biology read outs.

16.10 CONCLUSIONS

The existing armamentarium of imaging methods provide a comprehensive assessment of cardiac anatomy, function, perfusion, and motion in small animal models of heart failure. The noninvasive, exact character of cardiac MRI provides the research community with a diagnostic tool that promises to answer relevant questions exactly without sacrifice of the animal. This has been shown to be particularly valuable in the assessment of potential future therapies and the phenotyping of transgenic mice. Furthermore, the use of animal models has facilitated the evolvements of new imaging techniques and strategies, which can then be used for diagnostic cardiac MRI in patients.

REFERENCES

1. Grothues, F. et al., Comparison of interstudy reproducibility of cardiovascular magnetic resonance with two-dimensional echocardiography in normal subjects and in patients with heart failure or left ventricular hypertrophy, *Am. J. Cardiol.*, 90, 29, 2002.

2. Wiesmann, F. et al., Developmental changes of cardiac function and mass assessed with MRI in neonatal, juvenile, and adult mice, *Am. J. Physiol. Heart Circ. Physiol.*, 278, H652, 2000.
3. Wiesmann, F. et al., Analysis of right ventricular function in healthy mice and a murine model of heart failure by in vivo MRI, *Am. J. Physiol. Heart Circ. Physiol.*, 283, H1065, 2002.
4. Nahrendorf, M. et al., In vivo assessment of cardiac remodeling after myocardial infarction in rats by cine-magnetic resonance imaging, *J. Cardiovasc. Magn. Reson.*, 2, 171, 2000.
5. Nahrendorf, M. et al., Serial cine-magnetic resonance imaging of left ventricular remodeling after myocardial infarction in rats, *J. Magn. Reson. Imaging*, 14, 547, 2001.
6. Ruff, J. et al., Magnetic resonance microimaging for noninvasive quantification of myocardial function and mass in the mouse, *Magn. Reson. Med.*, 40, 43, 1998.
7. Franco, F. et al., Magnetic resonance imaging and invasive evaluation of development of heart failure in transgenic mice with myocardial expression of tumor necrosis factor-alpha, *Circulation*, 99, 448, 1999.
8. Rehwald, W. G. et al., Techniques for high-speed cardiac magnetic resonance imaging in rats and rabbits, *Magn. Reson. Med.*, 37, 124, 1997.
9. Epstein, F. H. et al., MR tagging early after myocardial infarction in mice demonstrates contractile dysfunction in adjacent and remote regions, *Magn. Reson. Med.*, 48, 399, 2002.
10. Streif, J. U. et al., In vivo time-resolved quantitative motion mapping of the murine myocardium with phase contrast MRI, *Magn. Reson. Med.*, 49, 315, 2003.
11. Gilson, W. D. et al., Complementary displacement-encoded MRI for contrast-enhanced infarct detection and quantification of myocardial function in mice, *Magn. Reson. Med.*, 51, 744, 2004.
12. Nahrendorf, M. et al., Time course of right ventricular remodeling in rats with experimental myocardial infarction, *Am. J. Physiol. Heart Circ. Physiol.*, 284, H241, 2003.
13. Ruff, J. et al., Magnetic resonance imaging of coronary arteries and heart valves in a living mouse: techniques and preliminary results, *J. Magn. Reson.*, 146, 290, 2000.
14. Burstein, D., MR imaging of coronary artery flow in isolated and in vivo hearts, *J. Magn. Reson. Imaging*, 1, 337, 1991.
15. Köhler, S. et al., Time resolved flow measurement in the isolated rat heart: characterization of left coronary artery stenosis, *Magn. Reson. Med.*, 50, 449, 2003.
16. Burstein, D., Taratuta, E., and Manning, W. J., Factors in myocardial perfusion imaging with ultrafast MRI and Gd-DTPA administration, *Magn. Reson. Med.*, 20, 299, 1991.
17. Williams, D. S. et al., Magnetic resonance imaging of perfusion using spin inversion of arterial water, *Proc. Natl Acad. Sci. USA*, 89, 213, 1992.
18. Williams, D. S. et al., Magnetic resonance imaging of perfusion in the isolated rat heart using spin inversion of arterial water, *Magn. Reson. Med.*, 30, 361, 1993.
19. Bauer, W. R. et al., The effect of perfusion on T_1 after slice selective spin inversion in the isolated cardioplegic rat heart: measurement of a lower bound of intracapillary–extravascular water proton exchange, *Magn. Reson. Med.*, 38, 917, 1997.
20. Bauer, W. R. et al., Fast high resolution imaging demonstrates fractality of myocardial perfusion in microscopic dimensions, *Circ. Res.*, 88, 340, 2001.
21. Belle, V. et al., In vivo quantitative mapping of cardiac perfusion in rats using a non invasive MR spin-labeling method, *J. Magn. Reson. Imaging*, 6, 1240, 1998.
22. Waller, C. et al., Myocardial perfusion and intracapillary blood volume in rats at rest and with coronary dilatation: MR imaging in vivo with use of a spin-labeling technique, *Radiology*, 215, 189, 2000.
23. Waller, C. et al., Serial MR imaging of microvascular adaptation in the infarcted rat heart, *Circulation*, 103, 1564, 2001.
24. Waller, C. et al., Impaired resting perfusion in viable myocardium distal to chronic coronary stenosis in rats, *Am. J. Physiol. Heart Circ. Physiol.*, 288, H2588, 2005.
25. Kober, F. et al., High-resolution myocardial perfusion mapping in small animals in vivo by spin-labeling gradient-echo imaging, *Magn. Reson. Med.*, 51, 62, 2004.
26. Kober, F. et al., Myocardial blood flow mapping in mice using high-resolution spin labeling magnetic resonance imaging: influence of ketamine/xylazine and isoaflurane anesthesia, *Magn. Reson. Med.*, 53, 601, 2005.

27. Streif, J. U. et al., Magnetic resonance perfusion imaging in microscopic dimensions: application to the murine myocardium, *Magn. Reson. Med.*, 53, 584, 2005.
28. Kahler, E. et al., Quantitative regional blood volume studies in rat myocardium in vivo, *Magn. Reson. Med.*, 40, 517, 1998.
29. Kahler, E. et al., Perfusion corrected mapping of regional blood volume in rat moycardium in vivo, *Magn. Reson. Med.*, 42, 500, 1999.
30. Pfeffer, J. M., Pfeffer, M. A., and Braunwald, E., Influence of chronic captopril therapy on the infarcted left ventricle of the rat, *Circ. Res.*, 57, 84, 1985.
31. Pfeffer, M. A. et al., Effect of captopril on mortality and morbidity in patients with left ventricular dysfunction after myocardial infarction. Results of the survival and ventricular enlargement trial. The SAVE investigators, *N. Engl. J. Med.*, 327, 669, 1992.
32. Heymans, S. et al., Inhibition of plasminogen activators or matrix metalloproteinases prevents cardiac rupture but impairs therapeutic angiogenesis and causes cardiac failure, *Nat. Med.*, 5, 1135, 1999.
33. Nahrendorf, M. et al., Chronic coronary artery stenosis induces impaired function of remote myocardium: MRI and spectroscopy study in rat, *Am. J. Physiol. Heart Circ. Physiol.*, 285, H2712, 2003.
34. Nahrendorf, M. et al., Impact of cerivastatin on left ventricular remodeling in rats with experimental myocardial infarction, *J. Am. Coll. Cardiol.*, 40, 1695, 2002.
35. Kassab, G. S., Lin, D. H., and Fung, Y. C., Morphometry of pig coronary venous system, *Am. J. Physiol. Heart Circ. Physiol.*, 267, H2100, 1994.
36. Wiesmann, F. et al., Dobutamine-stress magnetic resonance microimaging in mice: acute changes of cardiac geometry and function in normal and failing murine hearts, *Circ. Res.*, 88, 563, 2001.
37. Yang, Z. et al., Angiotensin II type 2 receptor overexpression preserves left ventricular function after myocardial infarction, *Circulation*, 106, 106, 2002.
38. Nahrendorf, M. et al., Creatine kinase knockout mice show left ventricular hypertrophy and dilatation, but unaltered remodeling post-myocardial infarction, *Cardiovasc. Res.*, 65, 419, 2005.
39. Schneider, J. E. et al., Identification of cardiac malformations in mice lacking Ptdsr using a novel high-throughput magnetic resonance imaging technique, *BMC Dev. Biol.*, 4, 16, 2004.

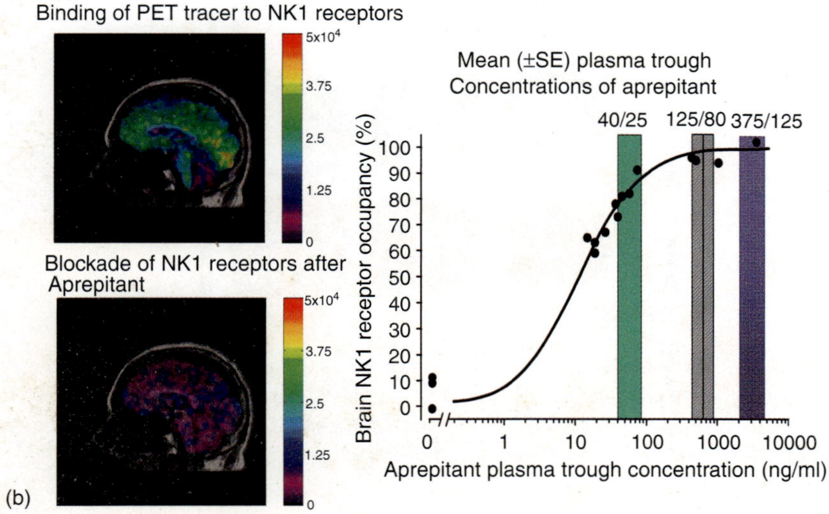

FIGURE 3.2 (b) PET plasma concentration CNS NK1 receptor occupancy for Aprepitant. It is clear that the dose response against emesis is likely to be related to CNS occupancy with the best dose being 125/80 mg as this achieves essentially the same therapeutic response as the higher dose of 375/2125 mg with lower drug exposure, thereby opening the therapeutic window. (Adapted from Bergstrom, M. et al., *Biol. Psychiat.*, 55, 1007, 2004. With permission of the Society of Biological Psychiatry Copyright 2004.)

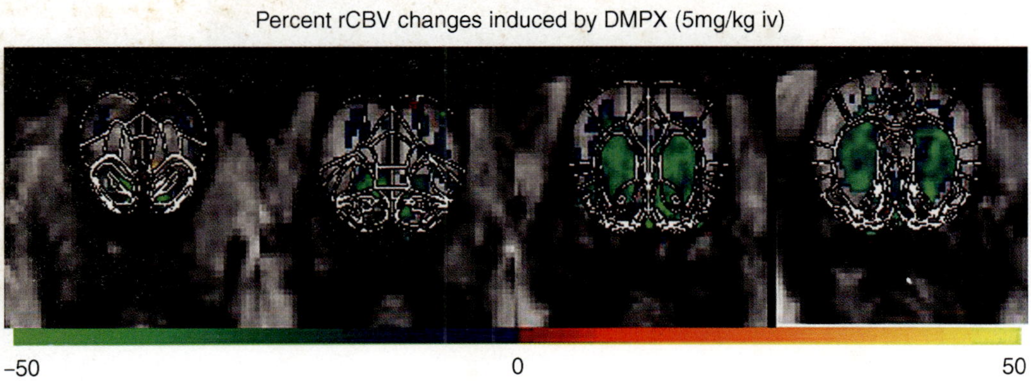

FIGURE 10.2 Illustrative map of rCBV changes induced in the rat brain by the A2a antagonist DMPX. The rCBV changes induced by this drug are negative. The rCBV map is shown overlaid on a gradient-echo image. Also overlaid on the image is a coregistered rat anatomic template demonstrating that the rCBV changes induced by DMPX are almost exclusively found in the caudate/putamen and nucleus accumbens consistent with the distribution of A2a receptors in the brain.

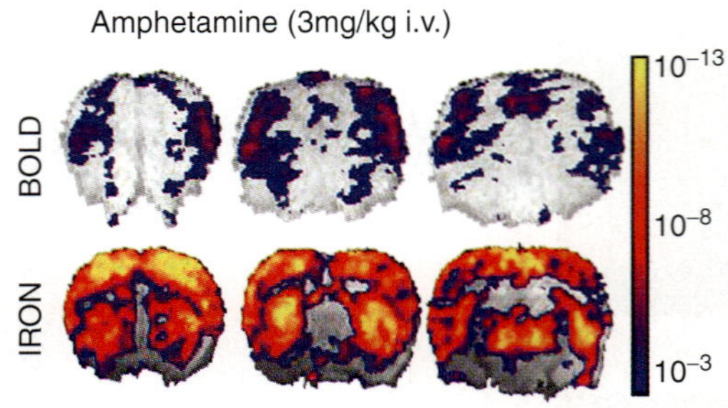

(a)

FIGURE 10.6 (a) Comparison of BOLD and IRON images at 4.7 T at the same statistical threshold derived from a student's *t*-test after administration of 3 mg/kg amphetamine in a rat. Note the nearly ten orders of magnitude decrease in the *p*-value for the IRON technique compared with the BOLD technique (both data sets were collected with the same number of images and identical imaging parameters).

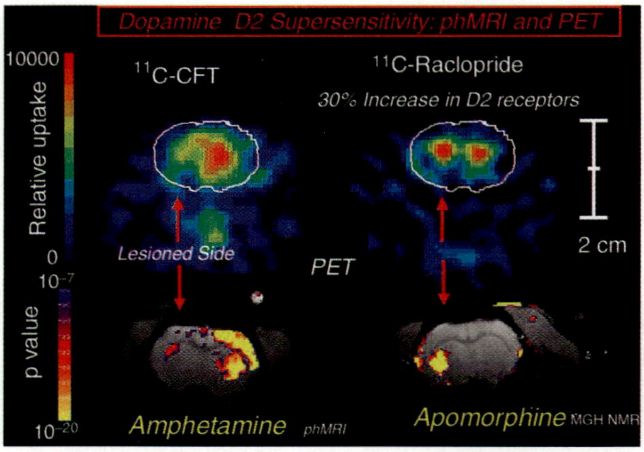

FIGURE 10.12 Comparisons of PET and phMRI data of the same rat unilaterally lesioned with 6-OHDA scanned with four different drugs showing binding of ^{11}C-CFT to presynaptic DAT terminals (top left) or ^{11}C-raclopride to postsynaptic D2 receptors (top right). On the bottom is the rCBV response to amphetamine (left) or apomorphine (right). The loss of ^{11}C-CFT binding indicates loss of presynaptic DA terminals. Conversely, the ^{11}C-raclopride data indicate upregulation of postsynaptic D2 receptors. These findings correlate well with the amphetamine data where the lesioned side shows loss of presynaptic dopamine release. Apomorphine stimulation leads to increased rCBV on the lesion side only (apomorphine is an indirect dopamine agonist with lower affinity than dopamine, thus in the presence of the high levels of dopamine on the intact side apomorphine has little effect). These data indicate the sensitivity of phMRI to dopaminergic supersensitivity. (From Nguyen, T. V. et al., *Synapse*, 36, 57, 2000. With permission.)

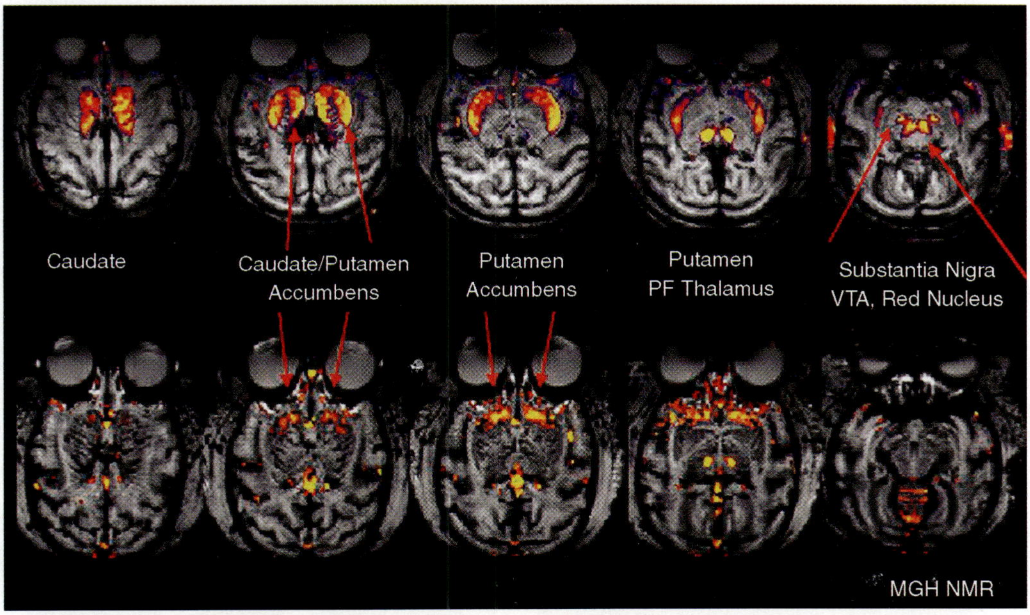

FIGURE 10.13 Maps of amphetamine stimulation in cynomolgus macaques. The response to 2.5 mg/kg amphetamine is shown on the top. Note the large increases in rCBV in the dopaminergic circuitry including the caudate, putamen, nucleus accumbens, parafascicular thalamus, substantia nigra, and ventral tegmental area. The bottom of the figure shows the response to amphetamine after long-term chronic treatment with low-dose MPTP. Note the response to amphetamine is lost in most regions except for the nucleus accumbens and the parafascicular thalamus. The data were acquired at 3 T using the IRON technique and spatial resolution of 0.7 mm in plane with 1.5 mm slices.

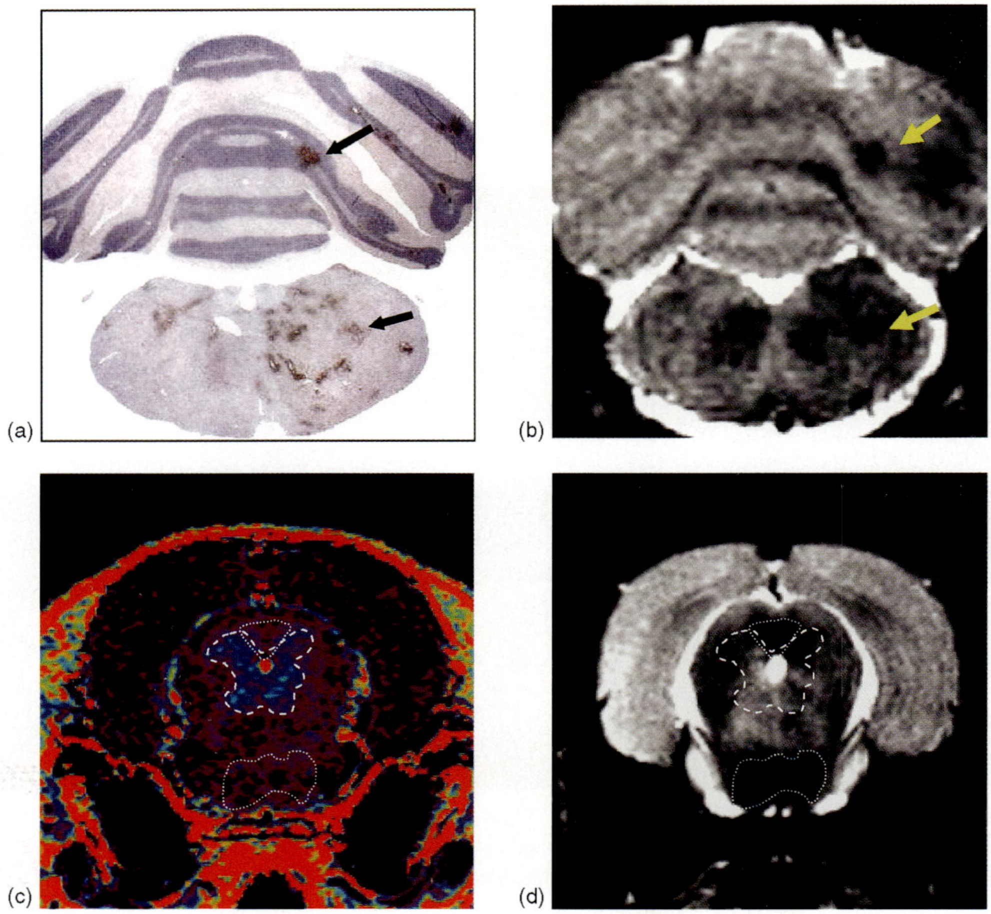

FIGURE 12.3 Comparison of parametric images from one animal of the EAE group. (a) ED-1 stain demonstrating macrophages in the cerebellum and the medulla of an animal with acute EAE. (b) The T2 image displays hypo-intense areas, induced by accumulation of USPIO. (c) and (d) Corresponding slices from another animal with EAE demonstrating the mismatch of Gd and USPIO enhancements. Enhancement of Gd-DOTA is visible in structures of the midbrain. The discrepancy of spatial localization of USPIO and Gd-DOTA enhancement is demonstrated by the dotted and dashed lines. The area marked by the dotted line accumulated USPIO but no Gd-DOTA. The reverse situation can be observed in the area marked by the dashed line. (From Rausch, M. et al., *Magn. Reson. Med.*, 50, 309, 2003.)

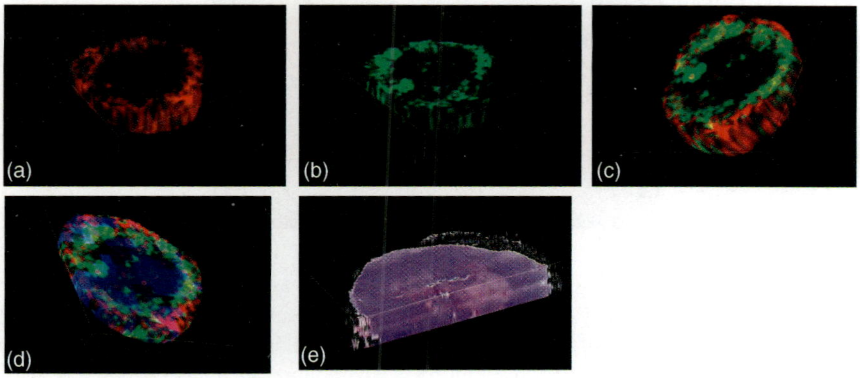

FIGURE 13.7 Three-dimensional reconstructed maps obtained from a single MDA–MB-231 tumor (470 mm^3) of (a) MRI map of vascular volume (range 0 to 200 μl/g); (b) MRI map of vascular permeability (range 0 to 7 μl/g min); (c) fused map of vascular volume and permeability; (d) fused map of vascular volume, permeability and pH_e (range from 5.3 to 7.2); (e) hematoxylin and eosin stained histological sections. Spatial resolution of the vascular volume and permeability maps are 0.125 mm in plane with 1 mm slice thickness. The pH_e map was obtained with a spatial resolution of $1 \times 1 \times 4$ mm^3. (Adapted from Bhujwalla, Z. M., et al., *NMR Biomed.*, 15, 114, 2002. With permission of John Wiley & Sons. Copyright 2002.)

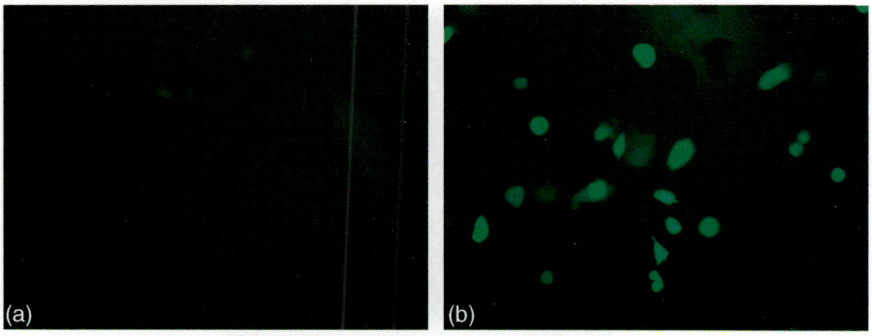

FIGURE 13.9 (a) Stably transfected PC-3 cells expressing HRE–GFP under normoxic conditions (20× lens). (b) Stably transfected PC-3 cells expressing HRE–GFP following treatment with 14 h cobalt chloride (10 μM, 20 × lens).

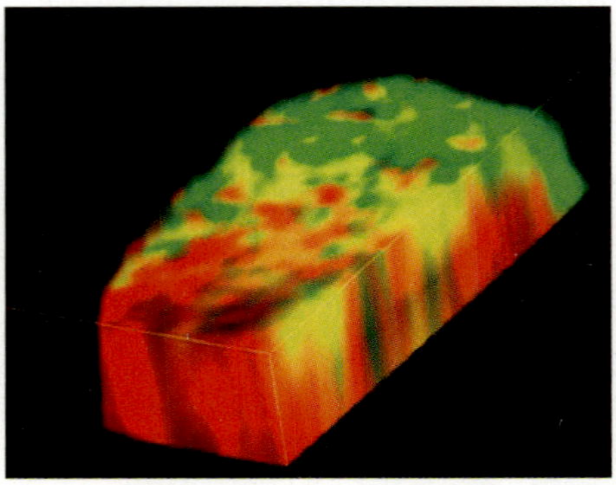

FIGURE 13.11 Three-dimensional reconstructed fusion image of vascular volume (red) and permeability (green) from a human prostate cancer xenograft model overexpressing VEGF. Several regions exhibiting yellow are detected demonstrating that regions of high vascular volume are also highly permeable. In previous studies, we have routinely observed that regions of high vascular volume are not permeable [6]. Here, we have shown that VEGF overexpression significantly increases the permeability of well-vascularized regions. (Adapted from Bhujwalla, Z. M., et al., *Proceedings of International Society Magnetic Resonance Medicine*, 2003.)

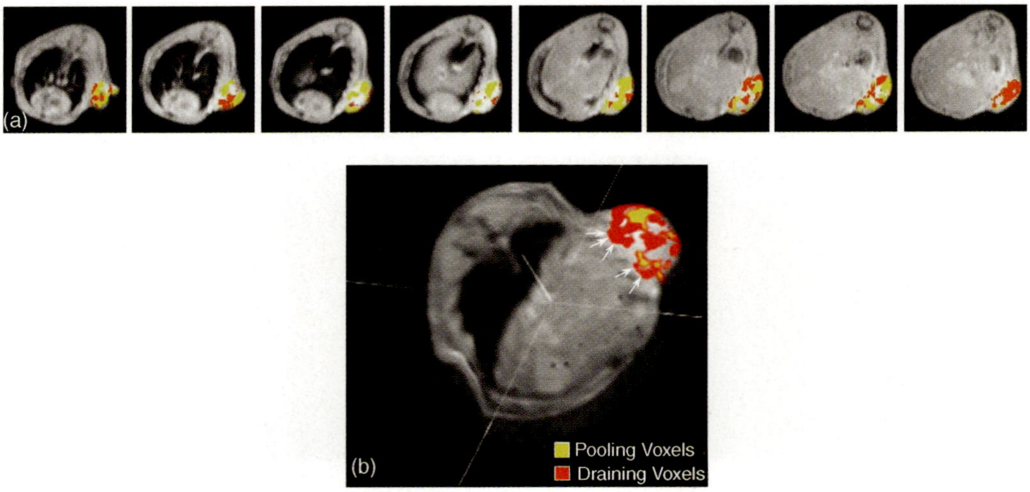

FIGURE 13.12 (a) A montage of slices obtained from a severe combined immunodeficient mouse with an MCF-7 tumor in the mammary fat pad. M_0 maps for each slice were overlaid with a functional image, which displays the spatial distribution of draining (red) and pooling voxels (yellow). (b) 3-D reconstruction of the same montage using cubic interpolation, with a cutaway to illustrate drainage (arrows) at the tumor–host tissue interface. (Adapted from Pathak, A. P., et al., *Cancer Res.*, 65, 1425, 2005. With permission of the American Association for Cancer Research. Copyright 2005.)

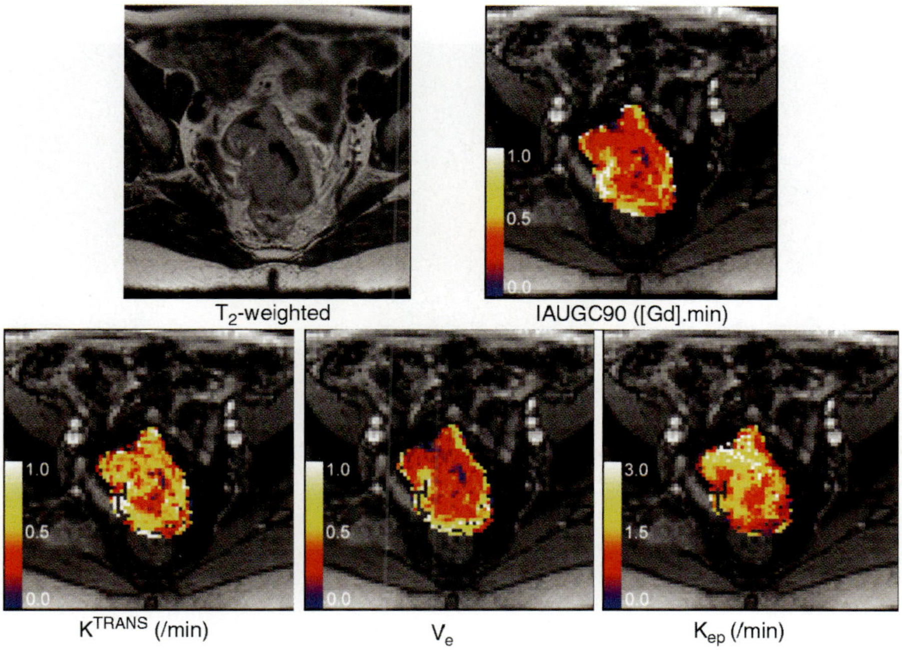

FIGURE 14.1 (a) 3 mm axial T_2-weighted MR image showing a polypoidal tumor arising from the distal sigmoid. There is evidence of extramural invasion on the right. (b) Calculated map of initial area under the Gadolinium concentration curve (IAUGC) over 0–90 sec. (c), (d), and (e) Calculated maps of K^{trans}, v_e and K_{ep}, respectively.

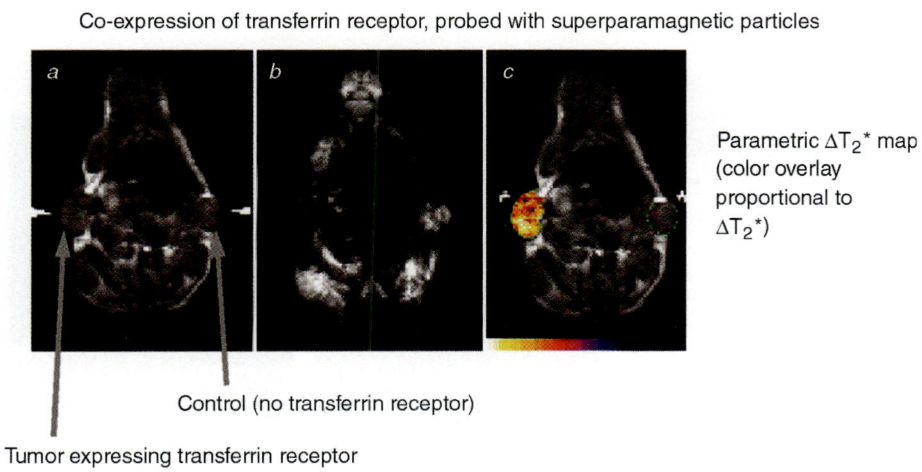

FIGURE 15.1 Molecular imaging with MRI: Use of marker gene coding for transferrin, probed with superparamagnetic articles. (From Weissleder, R. et al., *Nat. Med.*, 6, 351, 2000. Courtesy of R. Weissleder. With permission of Nature America Inc. Copyright 2000.)

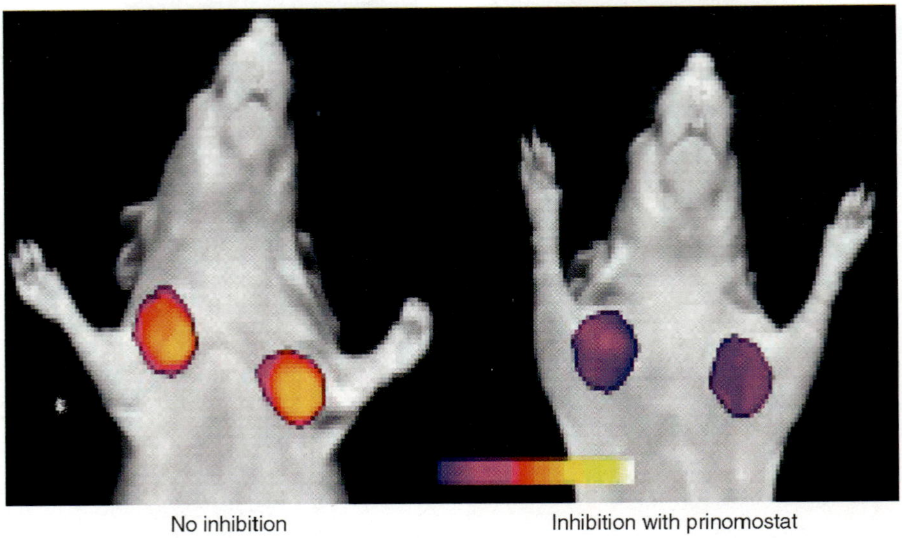

FIGURE 15.2 Molecular imaging using specific optical contrast agent: Detection of MMP probed with fluorescent MMP substrates which become fluorescent upon chemical modification catalyzed by MMP. (From Bremer, C. et al., *Nat. Med.*, 7, 743, 2001. Courtesy of R. Weissleder. With permission of Nature America Inc. Copyright 2001.)

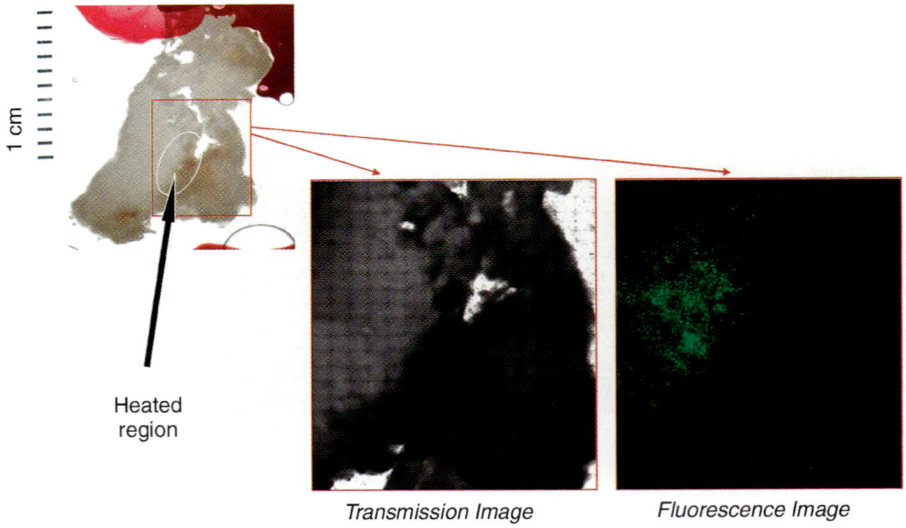

FIGURE 15.4 Spatio-temporal control of transgene expression using MRI-guided focused ultrasound in combination with a heat-sensitive promoter. Analysis of GFP gene expression using confocal microscopy.

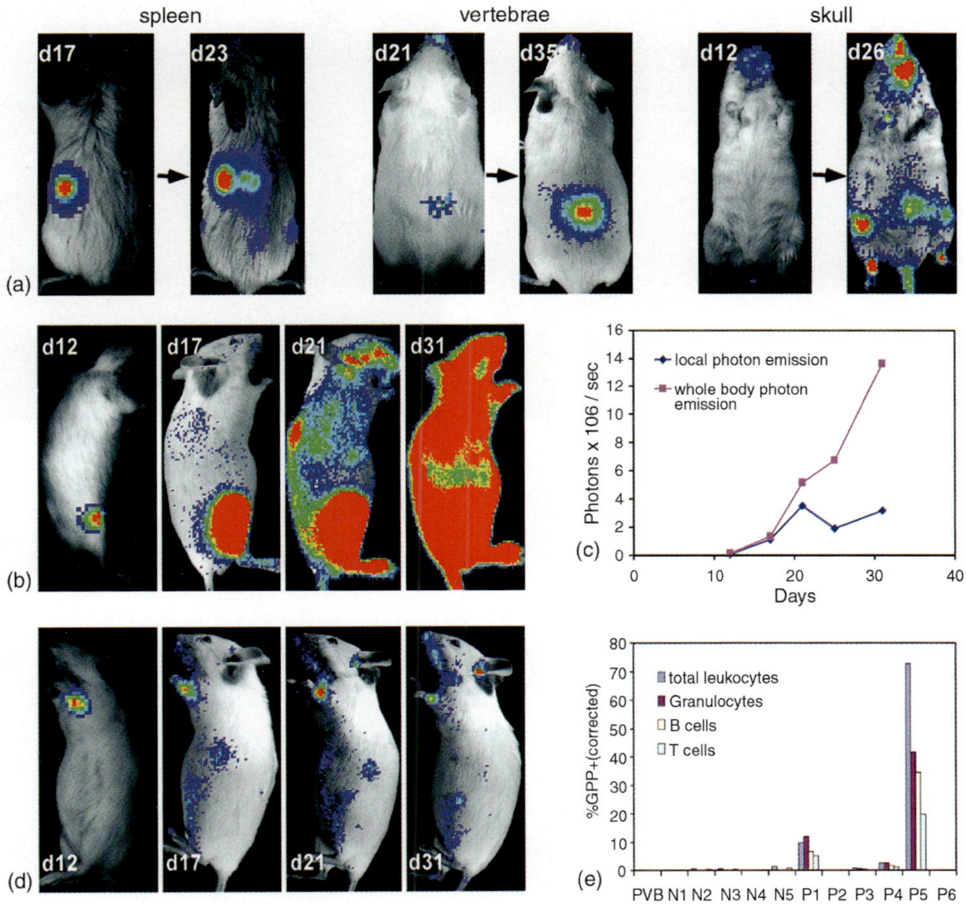

FIGURE 15.5 Tracking of stem cells using bioluminescence imaging: Reconstitution of immune system following injection of hematopoietic stem cell transfected with the gene coding for luciferase. (From Cao, Y. A. et al., *Proc. Natl. Acad. Sci. USA*, 101, 221, 2004. Courtesy of C. Contag. With permission of The National Academy of Sciences. Copyright 2004.)

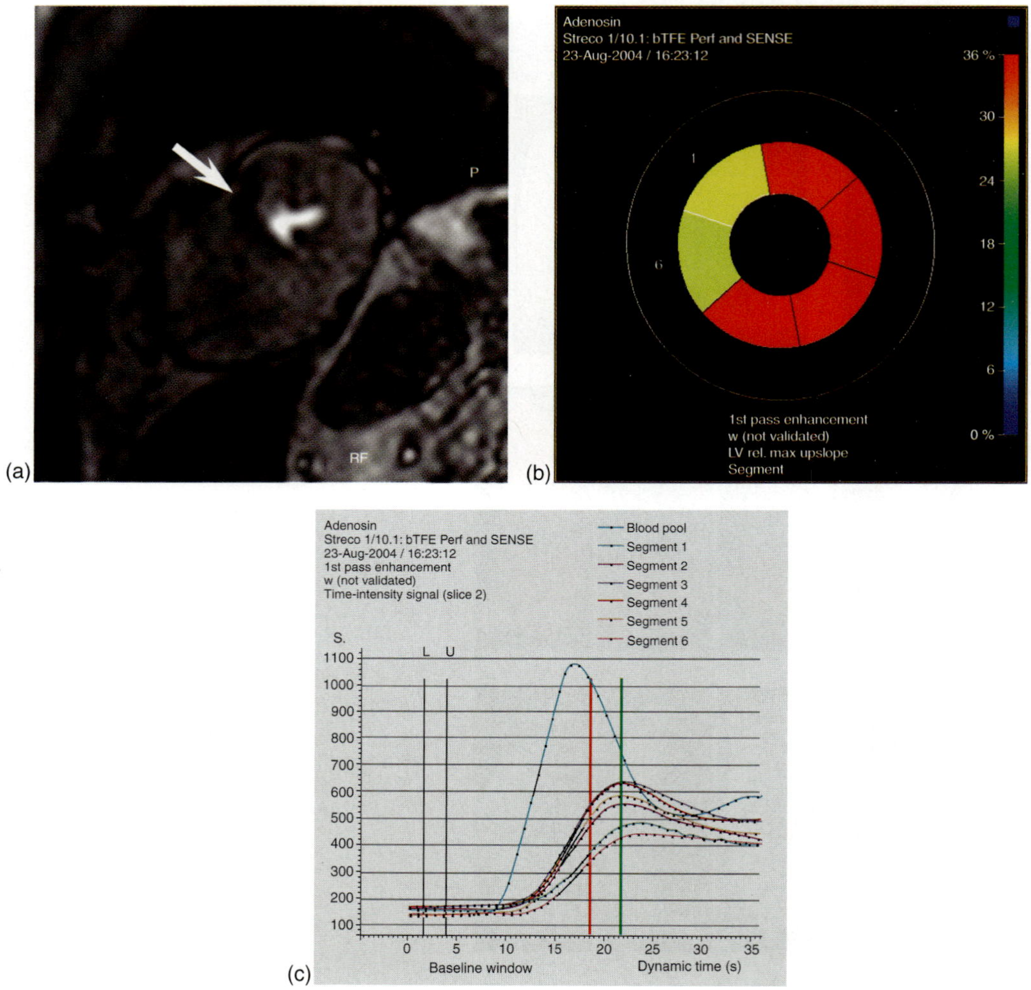

FIGURE 17.4 (a) A subendocardial adenosin induced perfusion defect of an extent of approximately 50% is clearly visualized in the anteroseptal and anterior segment (white arrow). A balanced TFE-technique used, TR/TE/alpha = 2.8 ms/1.4 ms/50 degrees, slice thickness of 10 mm. (b) Bull's eye shows changes of colour as signs of reduced myocardial perfusion at previously described segments. (c) Time–intensity curves show reduced signal intensity at the described segments, characterized as lower rise of the curves for segments 1 and 6.

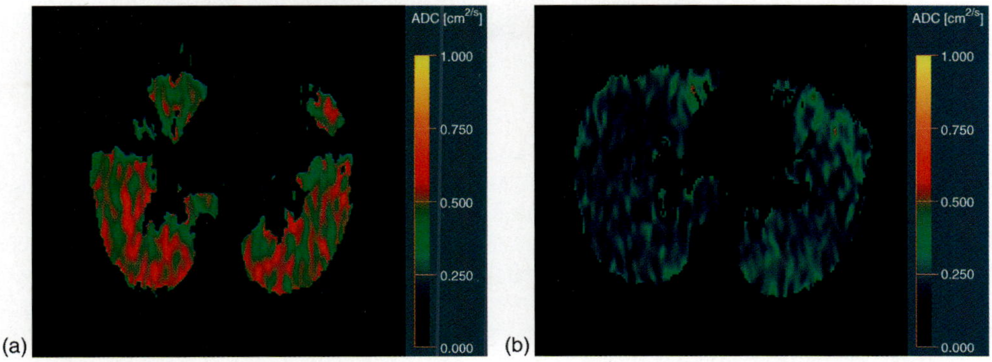

FIGURE 19.1 Color-coded parametric maps of the apparent diffusion coefficient (ADC) obtained from diffusion-weighted 3-He MRI in a patient with emphysema (a) and a healthy volunteer (b). In the patient with emphysema ventilated air spaces show higher ADC values (red) indicating structural lung changes with enlarged air spaces. In addition, nonventilated lung regions can be observed (arrows).

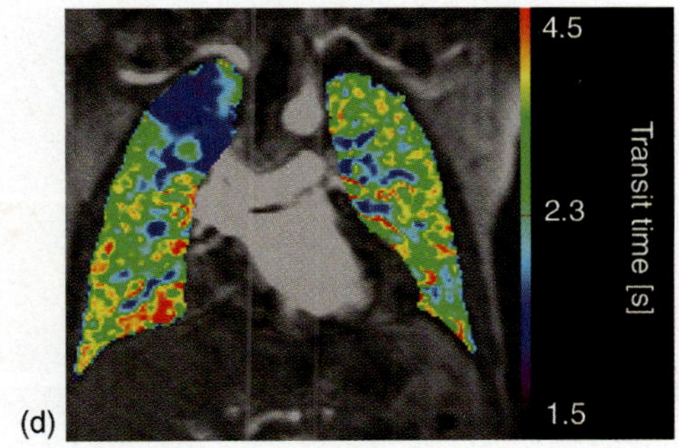

FIGURE 19.7 Color-coded map of pulmonary transit time (d) calculated from time-resolved MRA shows decreased transit time in that area compared to the rest of the lung.

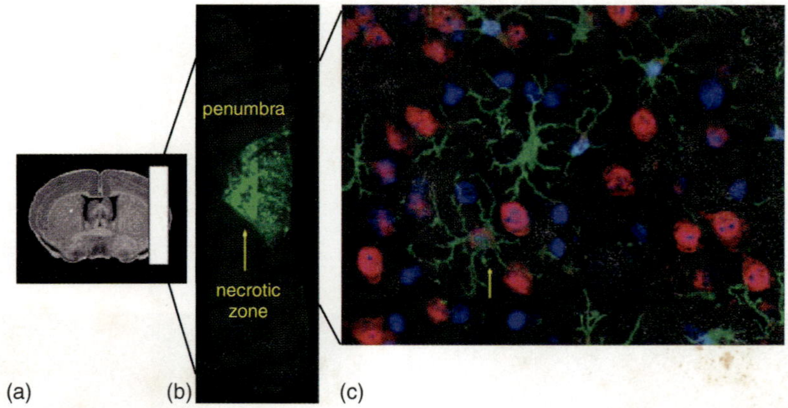

FIGURE 25.5 Transdifferentiation of bone marrow stem cells. Histological images of adult mouse brain following lethal irradiation and rescue with a bone marrow transplant from a transgenic green fluorescent (GFP) mouse. Four months later the animal underwent a middle cerebral artery occlusion to induce a stroke lesion. Three months after stroke induction, histological analysis revealed infiltration of GFP + (green) donor derived cells into the stroke lesion (b). Most of the cells differentiated into glial cells, but a low percentage also expressed neuronal nuclear antigens (C: red cells = anti-NeuN; blue = nuclei (DAPI)) suggesting that circulating stem cells originating from bone marrow can contribute to brain remodeling. (Reproduced from Szentirmai, O. and Carter, B. S., *Neurosurgery*, 55, 283, 2004. With permission. Copyright 2004. Lippincott Williams and Wilkins.)

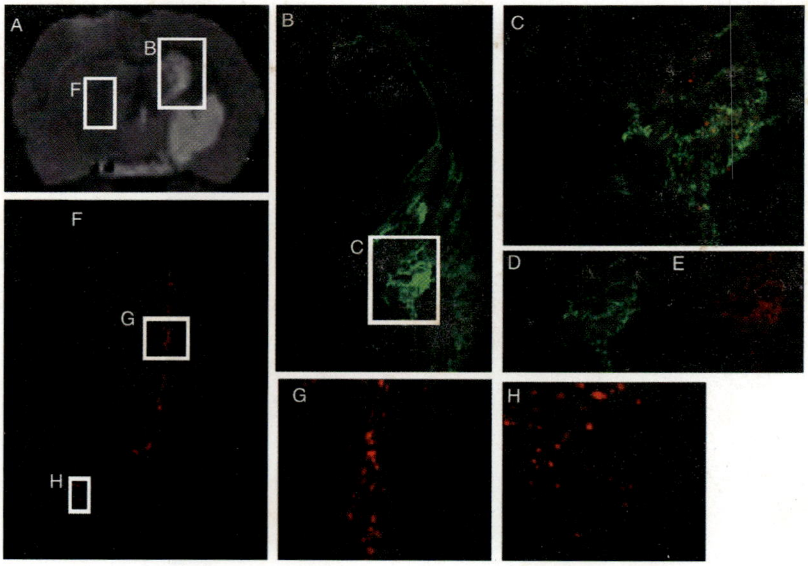

FIGURE 25.7 MRI of cellular migration in a rat stroke model. Neural stem cells labeled with gadolinium- and rhodamine-containing dextran polymers were transplanted into the brain hemisphere contralateral to the stroke lesion 3 months after induction. T_2-weighted MRI, obtained 14 days after injection, revealed hypointense regions in proximity to the stroke lesion, indicating infiltration by grafted cells (A). Fluorescent microscopy (C–H) confirmed the presence of rhodamin labeled cells (red) within or close to the lesion, which was filled with astrocytic scar tissue (green, anti-GFAP staining). This labeling strategy allows for convenient bimodal imaging of transplanted cells. (Reproduced from Modo, M. et al., *Neuroimage*, 21, 311, 2004. With permission. Copyright 2004. Elsevier.)

17 Cardiac MRI Techniques for Clinical Drug Trials

Sebastian Kelle and Eike Nagel

CONTENTS

17.1 INTRODUCTION

Cardiac magnetic resonance imaging (MRI) has gained widespread acceptance for the assessment of patients with a wide variety of diseases. This chapter cannot describe all these indications in detail, which has been done elsewhere [1,2]. In addition, it cannot replace extensive books on cardiac diseases; however, some basic principles of cardiac disease can be given here to facilitate the understanding of which parameters we measure and why we do this in cardiac patients.

17.2 PATHOPHYSIOLOGY OF CARDIAC DISEASE

The basic function of the heart is to supply the body with a sufficient amount of oxygenated blood and to supply the lung with a sufficient amount of deoxygenated blood for reoxygenation. Several mechanisms are available to keep up optimal function in different disease states.

17.2.1 VOLUME OVERLOAD

Volume overload occurs, if the heart needs to pump a larger amount of blood than it can physiologically handle. This may occur in patients with valvular insufficiency (leading to regurgitation of blood which needs to be pumped forward again), or in patients with shunts (i.e., a pathologic connection between the right and the left side of the heart, e.g., atrial septal defect, ventricular septal defect, fistulas, or congenital heart disease).

As a consequence of the increased blood volume, the heart increases its size before ejection (end-diastolic volume), which leads to an increase of the amount of blood pumped forward during each heart beat (stroke volume) due to the so-called Frank-Starling mechanism. However, this mechanism works best for short-term changes of blood volumes, it can only partially compensate for long-term alterations or large changes. In these cases not only the end-diastolic volume, but also the volume of the heart at the end of ejection (end-systolic volume) will increase, causing a reduction of cardiac performance, which shows clinically as a reduction of the patient's ability to exercise and, at a later stage, to exert him/herself at all. Whereas these changes can be reversed at an early stage, they become rapidly irreversible [3,4]. Thus, it is highly important to detect the underlying disease at an early stage, and to define the optimal time-point for a cure, e.g., a valve replacement or shunt-closure. The more exact a test is, the better this decision can be made in an individual patient.

17.2.2 PRESSURE OVERLOAD

Pressure overload occurs if the heart needs to overcome an increased pressure, normally in the arterial system of the body. The underlying disease comprises usually a reduction of size within the outflow of the left ventricle (e.g., aortic stenosis, hypertrophic obstructive cardiomyopathy) or an increase of pressure in the arterial system (arterial hypertension); however, both aortic valve stenosis and arterial hypertension are also quite common in the general and especially in the older population [4–7]. When the World Health Organization definition of hypertension is used, approximately 50% of middle-aged people (50–69 years of age) have hypertension [8]. The prevalence of aortic valve sclerosis and aortic valve stenosis increase with age, being present in 48 and 4%, respectively, of adults over 85 years of age [9,10]. In these cases the compensatory mechanism is to increase the pressure in the heart and — to overcome the increased force on the muscle — to increase left ventricular wall thickness resulting in proliferation of muscle mass. This mechanism is very effective and can compensate pressure overload for a long time [3]. Similarly to volume overload, it is usually reversible as long as no dilation of the ventricle has occurred. However, once ventricular dilation has started, the process becomes irreversible, and, thus, early detection of this time-point is essential in optimal handling of the patient.

17.2.3 CORONARY ARTERY DISEASE

Coronary artery disease (CAD) is a chronic progress, starting with thickening of the coronary artery wall and plaque development. These plaques usually grow outwards, not causing luminal area reduction in their early and intermediate states (the so-called positive remodeling). The disease can then progress in two opposite directions, either a plaque suddenly ruptures, causing myocardial infarction (see Section 17.2.4), or the lumen of the coronary arteries is more and more reduced, causing chronic myocardial ischemia. Since blood flow to the myocardium can be increased by a factor of approximately four in young and healthy persons (e.g., during physical exercise), blood flow at rest is only reduced if the lumen of the coronary artery is reduced by at least 80% [11]. Milder grades of coronary artery stenoses have no hemodynamic consequences at rest and can only be detected during stress.

17.2.4 Myocardial Infarction/Viability

In some patients myocardial infarction occurs due to chronic occlusion of a coronary artery; most patients, however, suffer from an acute cardiac event (i.e., plaque rupture resulting in coronary artery thrombosis). A critical reduction of blood flow and myocardial oxygenation will have two consequences. First, the myocardial cells stop contracting, but preserve their cellular integrity (stunning). If blood flow is restored, these areas return to normal function. If blood flow remains at a reduced level, these cells will remain viable, but without function, the so-called hibernating myocardium. Again, these areas return to normal after normalization of blood flow. On the contrary, however, if blood flow is further reduced, the cells will no longer be able to preserve their integrity, thus becoming irreversibly damaged. Such areas do not improve after revascularization. In most patients with myocardial infarction necrotic areas are surrounded by hibernating myocardium.

17.2.5 Systemic Disease/Cardiomyopathies

Many other noncardiac diseases lead to alterations of myocardial blood flow or of the myocardium itself [3,12–15]. The most important diseases and the resulting pathologies are listed in Table 17.1.

TABLE 17.1
Most Important Noncardiac Diseases and Their Characteristic Underlying Pathology as Well as Clinical Signs of Cardiac Involvement

Disease	Pathology; Signs of Cardiac Involvement
Sarcoidosis	Chronic granulomatous disease; cause cardiac failure, cor pulmonale, ventricular arrhythmias, heart block, sudden death
Hemochromatosis	Intracardial extensive iron deposits; gallop rhythm, ventricular arrhythmias, signs of heart failure
Fabry disease	Intracellular accumulation of a neutral glycolipid, widespread involvement of the myocardium, vascular endothelium, valves; multiple cardiovascular manifestations
Infective (viral)	Hearts in acute cases are flubby, focal hemorrhages; in chronic cases the heart is enlarged and hypertrophied; range of signs from asymptomatic patient, focal inflammation to fulminant fatal congestive heart failure due to diffuse myocarditis
Systemic lupus erythematosus	Deposition of immune complexes in the capillaries of visceral organs, possible inflammatory reaction of the pericardium, myocardium and the valves; multiple cardiovascular manifestations
Löffler's fibroplastic endocarditis	Mural endocardial thickening of the inflow portions and apex of the ventricles, endomyocardial fibrosis, myocarditis, endocardial thrombosis, eosinophilic endocarditis; cardiomegaly, congestive heart failure
Amyloidosis	Amyloid deposits in the walls of the small vessels of the heart; produce occlusive disease from the vasculitis as well as restrictive disease from the deposition, may produce restrictive cardiomyopathy

TABLE 17.2
Important Cardiomyopathies and Their Morphological and Functional Abnormalities, Listed are Dilated Cardiomyopathy (DCM), Hypertrophic Cardiomyopathy (HCM) with and without Obstruction and Restrictive Cardiomyopathy (RCM)

	DCM	H(O)CM	RCM
Morphology			
LV and RV size	+++	−	−
Hypertrophy	+	+++	−/+
Atrial dilation	++	+	++
Pleural effusion	+	−/+	+
Pericardial effusion	+	−	+
Ventricular thrombus	+	−	−
SVC/IVC dilation	+	−	+++
Myocardial function			
Global dysfunction	+++	+	+
Segmental dysfunction	+	+++	+
Diastolic dysfunction	+	++	+++
Valvular function			
Mitral regurgitation	+	++	+
Tricuspid regurgitation	+	−	+

Source: Modified from Nagel, E., Rossum, A. V., and Fleck, E., *Cardiovascular Magnetic Resonance*, Steinkopff, Darmstadt, Germany 2004. With permission.

Cardiomyopathies are diseases of the myocardium itself. The major exception is ischemic cardiomyopathy, which results from chronic myocardial ischemia and represents large areas of hibernating or necrotic myocardium. Important cardiomyopathies are characterized as shown in Table 17.2 [2].

17.3 DIAGNOSTIC OPTIONS

Several techniques are available to analyze patients with cardiac diseases. The first test, which is easy, can be rapidly performed and yields a high amount of information is the electrocardiogram (ECG). Certain criteria allow for the detection of left ventricular hypertrophy, myocardial infarction or increased stress in the myocardial wall. The test, however, does not allow detection of chronic ischemia or yield specific information on the disease. If performed during ergometric stress, the ECG allows for a detection of myocardial ischemia and is used as a screening test in large groups of patients. Its major limitation is the relatively low sensitivity (68%) and specificity (77%) [16] for the given low pretest probability in the large majority of patients used.

Echocardiography is used to gain more specific information on the presence, extent, and differential diagnosis of diseases. It allows for a rapid, bedside analysis of the left and right ventricle (dimensions, wall thickness, global and regional function), and, if performed during ergometric or pharmacological stress (e.g., with dobutamine), enables the detection of stress-induced ischemia, which can be seen as wall motion abnormalities during maximal exercise or high dose of dobutamine (e.g., 40 μg/kg body weight/min).

An additional limitation of echocardiography — both at rest and stress — is the difficulty in achieving an adequate image quality, especially in patients with adipositas or pulmonary disease. In addition, inferior segments and the epicardial wall are difficult to visualize in many patients despite considerable improvements with the introduction of second harmonic imaging.

Nuclear techniques are routinely applied to determine perfusion and viability. SPECT, however, has a spatial resolution of approximately $10 \times 10\ \text{mm}^2$, which is insufficient to detect subendocardial disease, and is limited by attenuation artefacts. PET has a spatial resolution of approximately $5 \times 5\ \text{mm}^2$ — still inadequate to detect subendocardial disease — and is only available at a limited number of centers.

Recently, several studies have shown a value of biochemical markers to detect and quantify cardiac disease [17–20]. *N*-terminal pro-brain natriuretic peptide (NT-pro-BNP) concentrations are high across the entire spectrum of CAD and parallel its clinical or angiographic severity [17]. NT-pro-BNP was shown to be a marker of long-term mortality in patients with stable coronary disease and can provide prognostic information [21]. C-reactive protein (CRP) levels predict future cardiovascular events independently of CAD severity and correlate with a number of angiographically complex coronary artery stenoses in patients with acute coronary syndrome. CRP has been shown to be a marker of atheromatous plaque vulnerability and CAD activity [18]. Both tests have the advantage of providing a rapid diagnosis by a simple blood sample analysis; however, they are limited by their inability to assess the definitive disease location and the underlying pathology.

17.4 CLINICAL APPLICATIONS

17.4.1 CARDIAC MR FOR THE ASSESSMENT OF LEFT VENTRICULAR MASS/VOLUMES/FUNCTION

Cardiac MRI is regarded as the reference standard for the determination of left ventricle (LV) and right ventricle (RV) mass, volumes, and function. This is due to its three-dimensionality, independency from imaging windows, high spatial and temporal resolution, as well as good contrast between blood vs. endocardium and epicardium vs. surrounding tissue [22].

Today's state of the art approach is based on 1.5 T imaging with dedicated cardiac coils using steady-state free precession (SSFP) techniques during breath holding. To image accurately LV anatomy and function in plane resolution should be more than 2 mm, slice thickness ≤ 10 mm and temporal resolution ≤ 40 msec. Basic coverage of the LV consists of three short axis and three long axis (two-, three-, and four-chamber) views (Figure 17.1). Three-dimensional models may then be applied to calculate the desired parameters [23]. The most accurate results, however, have been reported for complete LV coverage in a series of short axis views. Each slice is evaluated semiautomatically at end-diastole and at end-systole for LV area and myocardial area (papillary muscles are excluded from the LV-volume and added to the muscle mass). Functional parameters are determined as:

$$\text{LV volume}_{\text{(ED or ES)}} = \Sigma^{i}_{\text{all slices}}(\text{LV area}_{\text{slice I}}) \times \text{slice distance}$$

$$\text{LV}_{\text{(end-diastolic)}}\ \text{mass} = \text{LV}_{\text{(muscle tissue)}}\ \text{volume} \times 1.05\ \text{g/cm}^3$$

$$\text{stroke volume} = \text{LV}_{\text{end diastolic volume}} - \text{LV}_{\text{end systolic volume}}$$

$$\text{cardiac output} = \text{stroke volume} \times \text{heart rate}$$

$$\text{ejection fraction}(\%) = 100 \times (\text{stroke volume}/\text{LV}_{\text{end-diastolic volume}})$$

The specific weight of muscle tissue is defined as $1.05\ \text{g/cm}^3$ [2]. In direct comparison to echocardiography, a much higher reproducibility has been reported for cardiac MR (CMR), resulting in a significant reduction of sample size for a given statistical power [24,25] (Table 17.3). This high accuracy makes MR the method of choice to monitor the effects of drug therapy or other interventions.

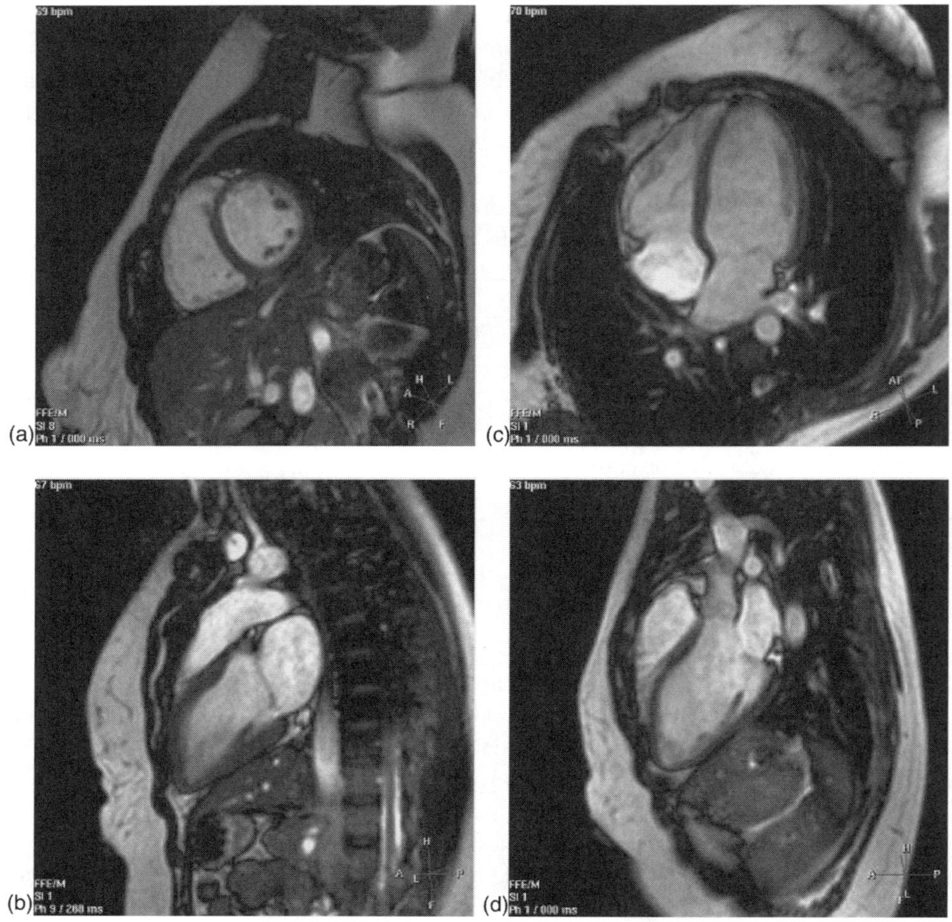

FIGURE 17.1 Standard views are used to visualize most parts of the left ventricle and to assessment all 17 segments. Images shows short-axis view (a), four-chamber view (b), two-chamber view (c), and three-chamber view (d). Images have been aquired using an SSFP technique with TR/TE/alpha = 3.2 ms/1.6 ms/60 degrees, and slice thickness of 5 mm.

Possible limitations are the need to systematically include or exclude trabeculae and the risk to include LV atrial volumes into the ESV due to through-plane motion of the valvular apparatus. Careful analysis, however, circumvents these problems [2]. Future directions are aiming at fully automated segmentation and single breath hold imaging for complete LV coverage [26]. With the advent of reliable and rapid flow sequences, these may be increasingly used for a basic determination of SV and cardiac output with a single scan of aortic flow.

17.4.2 Cardiac MR for the Detection of Coronary Artery Disease

Different approaches are available for the assessment of patients with known or suspected CAD. The major strategies are:

- The assessment of wall motion at rest and high dose dobutamine stress
- The assessment of myocardial blood flow (perfusion) at rest and adenosine vasodilation
- The direct visualization of the coronary artery lumen for the detection of luminal stenosis

TABLE 17.3
Sample Size Required to Detect the Same Change by Echo, CMR with a Power of 90% and $p < 0.05$

Clinical Change	Echo		CMR		% Reduction in Sample Size
	S.D.	*n*	S.D.	*n*	
EDV, 10 ml	23.8	121	7.4	12	90
ESV, 10 ml	15.8	53	6.5	10	81
EF, 3% (abs)	6.6	102	2.5	15	85
Mass, 10 g	36.4	273	6.4	9	97

In this study calculations showed that for the left ventricle, CMR requires a small number of patients to detect a 10-mL change in end-diastolic volume (EDV) and end-systolic volume (ESV); respectively, to detect a minimal change in ejection fraction (EF); and change of ventricular mass. The percentage reduction in sample size were compared with echocardiographic measurements from Ref. [24]. S.D., standard deviation; *n*, number of subjects.

Source: Reproduced from Bellenger, N., et al., *J. Cardiovasc. Magn. Reson.*, 2, 271, 2000. With permission of Taylor & Francis Copyright 2000.

Future directions include:

- Direct imaging of the vessel wall
- Direct imaging (and characterization) of coronary artery plaques
- Spectroscopic analysis of cardiac metabolites and energy state

None of these methods is perfect; they are, nevertheless, superior to most alternatives.

17.4.2.1 Dobutamine Stress MR

Technically dobutamine stress MR (DSMR) is relatively simple. Today's 1.5 T MR scanners are widely equipped to allow for rapid imaging of LV function (again using SSFP sequences; see Section 17.4.1). The major difference to standard LV imaging at rest is the use of high-dose dobutamine stress, which is a routine procedure in stress echo cardiography. Indeed, DSMR protocols are mirrored from dobutamine stress echocardiography (DSE). The monitoring requirements are listed in Table 17.4 [2], while contraindications and termination criteria can be found in Table 17.5 and Table 17.6 [2]. A standard set-up is shown in Figure 17.2.

TABLE 17.4
Monitoring Requirements for Stress MR Imaging

	Dobutamine + Atropine
Heart rate and rhythm (single lead ECG)	Continuously
Blood pressure	Every minute
Pulse oximetry[a]	Continuously
Symptoms	Continuously
Wall motion abnormalities	Every dose increment

[a] When the vector-ECG is used, pulse oximetry is not required.

Source: Modified from Nagel, E., Rossum, A.V., and Fleck, E., *Cardiovascular Magnetic Resonance*, Steinkopff, Darmstadt, 2004. With permission.

TABLE 17.5
Contraindications for MR Stress Tests

Severe arterial hypertension ($\geq$220/120 mmHg)
Unstable angina pectoris
Significant aortic stenosis (aortic valve gradient >50 mmHg or aortic valve area <1 cm^2)
Complex cardiac arrhythmias
Significant hypertrophic obstructive cardiomyopathy
Myocarditis, endocarditis, pericarditis
Other major disease

Source: Modified from Nagel, E., Rossum, A. V., and Fleck, E., *Cardiovascular Magnetic Resonance*, Steinkopff, Darmstadt, 2004. With permission.

TABLE 17.6
Dobutamine MR Stress Test Termination Criteria

Submaximal heart rate reached [(220 − age)0.85]
Blood pressure decrease >20 mmHg systolic below baseline systolic blood pressure or decrease >40 mmHg
from a previous level
Blood pressure increase >240/120 mmHg
Severe angina pectoris
Severe dyspnea
Global reduction reduction of LV function
New or worsening wall motion abnormalities in at least two adjacent left ventricular segments (out of 17)
Complex cardiac arrhythmias

Source: Modified from Nagel, E., Rossum, A. V., and Fleck, E., *Cardiovascular Magnetic Resonance*, Steinkopff, Darmstadt, 2004. With permission.

Several studies have shown the accuracy of DSMR for the detection of significant coronary artery disease in comparison to invasive angiography and the superiority in comparison to echocardiography [28,29]. This superiority is due to the better image quality of MR vs. echocardiography [30] (Figure 17.3). In patients with suboptimal echocardiographic image quality MR should be routinely used [27]. Similarly, in clinical trials DSMR allows for a much smaller sample size in comparison to DSE if proof of ischemia is a required parameter. Safety of DSMR is identical to that of DSE [31].

Limitations are the lack of large prospective trials to determine prognosis of patients with a negative DSMR study and the assessment of data. First reports, however, have shown that patients with a negative DSMR study or a LVEF >40% had fewer cardiac events in comparison to patients with a positive DSMR study or a LVEF <40% [32]. An unpublished study from our institution on the reproducibility of blinded multicenter DSMR reads has shown very good congruence of experienced readers.

Current work is focused on a user-independent quantitative evaluation of wall motion using tagging techniques in combination with HARP [33–35] (see also Chapter 16, Section 16.3). This may also allow facilitation of the evaluation of diastolic function [36].

17.4.2.2 Perfusion

The major advantage of perfusion imaging is the ability to measure one of the earliest steps within the ischemic cascade, the reduction of blood flow itself [37] (see also Chapter 16,

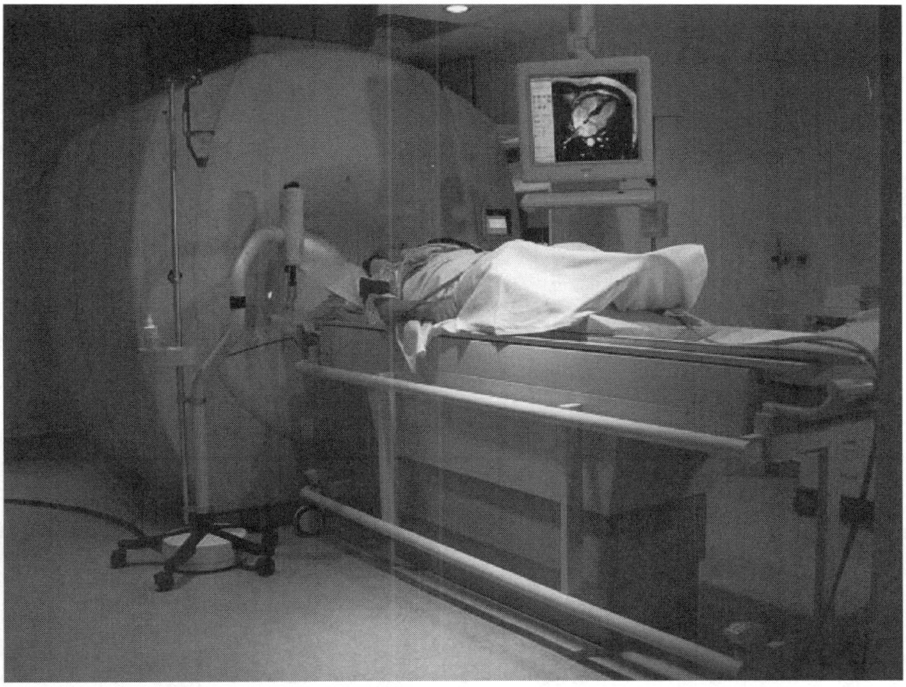

FIGURE 17.2 Set-up for a dobutamine stress MR examination. For fast patient evacuation, a trolley is placed under the table. In the scanner room, continuous respiratory monitoring and vector-ECG; outside the scanner room, blood pressure monitoring and infusion pump for dobutamine.

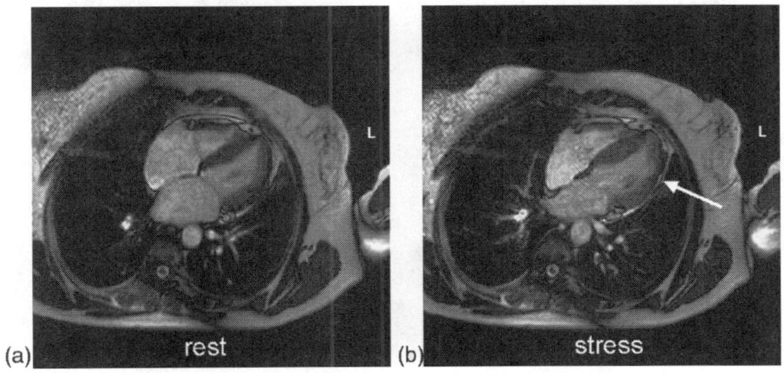

FIGURE 17.3 End-systolic acquired cine images at rest (a) and under 40 μg dobutamine (b). At rest normal wall motion, under high-dose dobutamine increase in wall thickening at septum, but occurrence of akinesia of the lateral wall (white arrow). All images were aquired with an SSFP technique at 1.5 T.

Section 16.6). Its major challenge is the difficulty to acquire artefact-free images within the limits of time available.

For perfusion imaging a dynamic dataset (complete multislice dataset every or every other heart beat) is acquired during the first passage of a peripherally injected contrast agent bolus. Usually this dataset consists of three to five slices, the higher diagnostic accuracy seems to be achieved with fewer slices and a higher in-plane resolution. To generate contrast between areas supplied by stenotic coronary arteries and areas supplied by normal coronary arteries a T_1-shortening contrast agent is injected during adenosine stimulation (140 μg/kg body weight/min for 4-max of 6 min). A strongly T_1 weighted imaging technique (usually SSFP or turbo-gradient-echo with a saturation prepulse) is used for imaging during the inflow of the contrast agent. Since current Gd-based contrast agents rapidly diffuse from the vessels into the interstitium, the first dynamics after contrast agent arrival are used to make a diagnosis. Areas with slower contrast agent wash-in (reduced upslope) or reduced amount (lower peak signal intensity) of contrast agent are regarded as pathologic (Figure 17.4). Data can be analyzed visually (comparison to normal segments), semiquantitatively (comparison to rest and normal values) or as absolute values (after extensive modeling). Due to

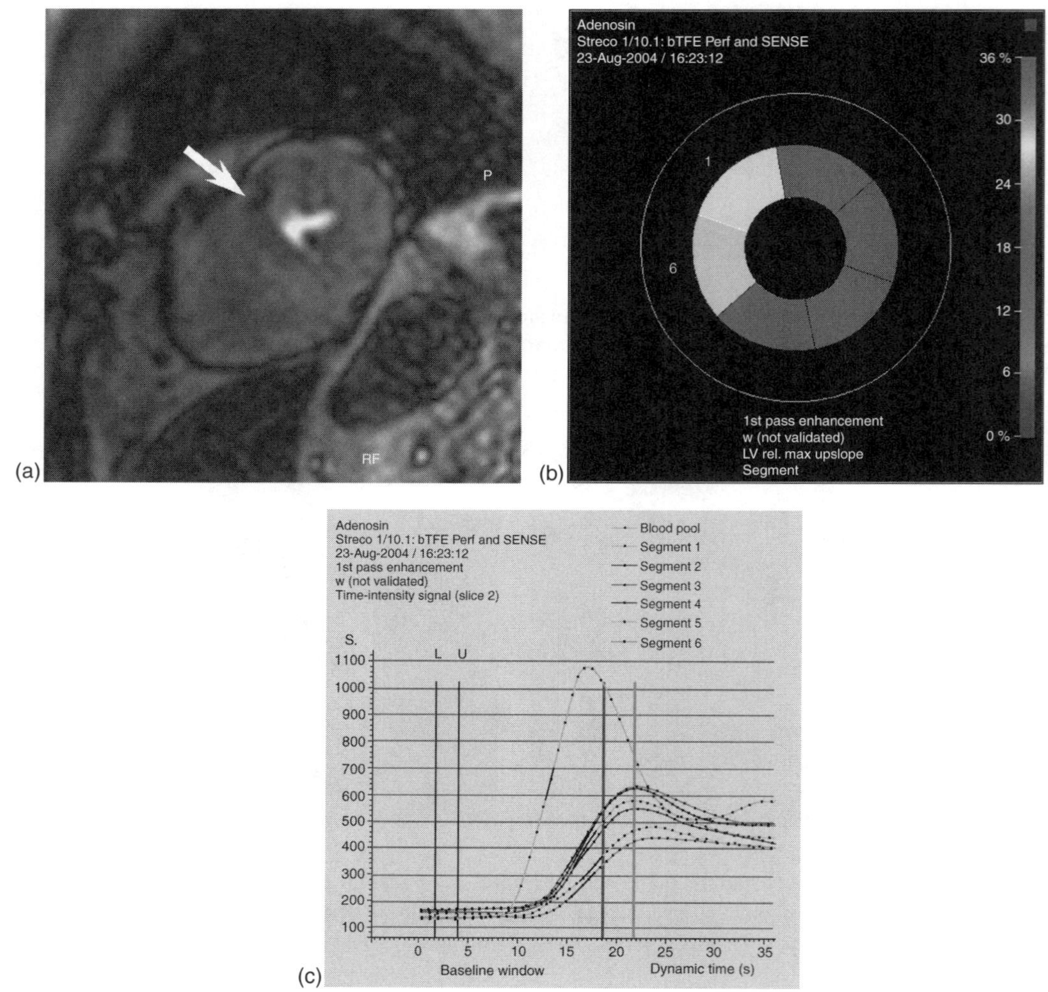

FIGURE 17.4 (See color insert following page 328.) (a) A subendocardial adenosin induced perfusion defect of an extent of approximately 50% is clearly visualized in the anteroseptal and anterior segment (white arrow). A balanced TFE-technique used, TR/TE/alpha = 2.8 ms/1.4 ms/50 degrees, slice thickness of 10 mm. (b) Bull's eye shows changes of colour as signs of reduced myocardial perfusion at previously described segments. (c) Time–intensity curves show reduced signal intensity at the described segments, characterized as lower rise of the curves for segments 1 and 6.

technical difficulties in image generation, no standardized data acquisition or evaluation scheme has been accepted up to now.

Published data show a high diagnostic accuracy of current MR perfusion approaches in comparison to cardiac catheterization [38] and PET [39]. This is due to the much higher spatial resolution of MR perfusion (in a range of 2–3 mm in plane) [2,40] in comparison to SPECT (4 to 8 mm in plane pixel size) [40,41], therefore allowing the detection of subendocardial defects, which are most sensitive to a reduction of blood flow [42].

First multicenter data of optimal dose finding are available and demonstrate using optimal dose a high sensitivity (93%) and specificity (75%) in comparison to cardiac catheterization [43,44].

Current research is focused on improving imaging sequences, on standardizing contrast-injection schemes (dose and administration speed), as well as on improving postprocessing.

17.4.2.3 Coronary Artery Imaging

MRI of coronary arteries — by some regarded as the holy grail, by others as superfluous since the proof of ischemia, rather than luminography should be required — remains an area of enormous interest, also triggered by recent advances of multislice capabilities.

In principle, two different strategies can be envisaged, the first being a replacement of invasive angiography and the second being an accurate visualization or exclusion of stenoses, which can be treated by a percutaneous coronary intervention.

Whereas the first is far away at the moment, since it requires grading of stenoses in tiny vessels and an image quality sufficient to base surgery upon, the second seems achievable with today's (prototype) techniques. Visualization of proximal and medial main vessels as well as major (>2 mm) side branches and proof or exclusion stenoses in these segments would allow detection of almost all patients with treatable CAD [45]. Such a dataset can be acquired using a large three-dimensional volume (whole heart) (Figure 17.5). The major technical challenge is to minimize artefacts from cardiac and respiratory motions. Artefacts from coronary motion are optimally suppressed by individual determination of the mid-diastolic coronary rest period for each patient and consecutive use of this information for image generation. Unfortunately, imaging time for high resolution scanning is of the order of minutes rather than seconds, prohibiting the use of

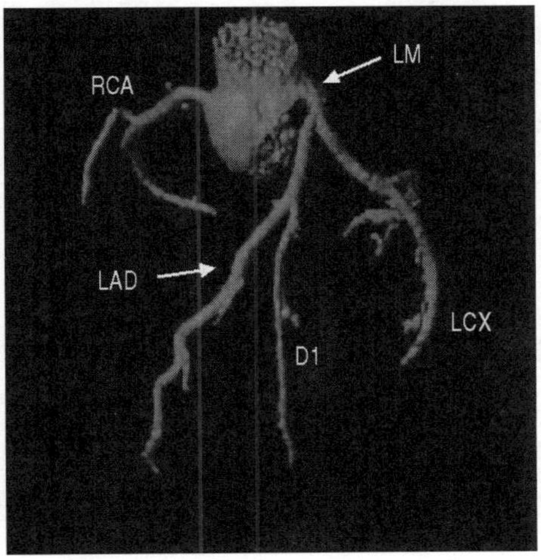

FIGURE 17.5 Three-dimensional visualization of the coronary artery tree by a native whole heart imaging in a healthy volunteer. All three major coronaries are clearly depicted. Right coronary artery (RCA); left anterior descending artery (LAD); left main stem (LM); left circumflex artery (LCX), and first diagonal branch (D1).

breath-holding in most patients with current state-of-the-art techniques. Alternatively navigator techniques can be applied, which allow detection — and correction — breathing motion during scanning [46]. These highly sophisticated methods which include affine transformation algorithms allow for an efficient visualization of a large volume within 10–15 min. This approach has been shown to be superior to breath-holding and — in combination with SSFP — allows for a high diagnostic accuracy. Unfortunately, the only multicenter trial on MRI of coronary arteries clearly shows that these techniques do not yet reach an adequate quality for routine clinical use [47].

17.4.2.4 Vessel Wall Imaging

The same technical challenges described for MRI of coronary arteries apply for the visualization of vessel wall and plaque. However, advances achieved with sophisticated motion suppression allow for an accurate and reproducible determination of vessel wall thickness. Since thickening of the wall precedes the formation of a hemodynamically significant luminal area reduction, the use of this strategy to detect patients at risk for a major coronary event and to measure the influence of therapy is intriguing [48–51] (Figure 17.6).

The next steps would be the visualization and characterization of plaque for the assessment of potential plaque instability. Since today's spatial resolution is far too low to accurately visualize different plaque components, the major hope is to develop contrast agents delineating the plaque and adhering to specific endothelial components of an unstable plaque. In the future such specific contrast agents may be combined with specific therapeutic components [52–54].

17.4.3 Cardiac MR for the Assessment of Myocardial Infarction and Viability

17.4.3.1 Contrast Enhancement

Contrast enhanced MR techniques for the detection of necrosis and viability are based on the behavior of T_1-shortening Gd-based contrast agents. These agents diffuse from the vascular space into the interstitium but not into viable cells. At any time-point after myocardial infarction the

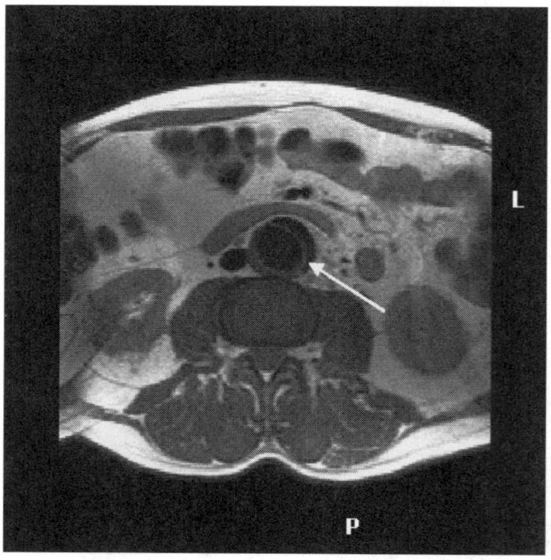

FIGURE 17.6 Transversal slice of the abdominal aorta in black-blood imaging technique shows dilatation of the aorta and a great plaque of the aortic wall at 6 and 9 o'clock with dissection and a small membrane (arrow). Image was performed with a proton-dense-weighted (PD), turbo-spin-echo (TSE), black-blood-sequence, TR/TE = 1500 ms/27 ms.

distribution volume for the contrast agent is increased in irreversible infarct areas either due to necrosis (contrast agent can pass into the damaged cells) or fibrosis (relative increase of interstitium vs. intracellular volume by replacement of large myocytes with small fibrocytes) [55]. Such relative accumulation of contrast agent can be visualized about 10–15 min after contrast agent injection (thus, the term late or delayed enhancement) with a heavily T_1-weighted technique using an inversion prepulse to null the signal of normal myocardium. Imaging is technically simple as is image interpretation due to the extreme contrast. In general, the slogan bright is dead seems to hold true for most instances and has been proven in a wide variety of animal models [55,56]. Due to the high spatial resolution the technique is clearly superior to PET and SPECT for the detection of irreversibly damaged myocardium and can be regarded as the reference standard [41,57] (Figure 17.7).

Using contrast-enhanced MRI, Kim et al. [58] have been able to show that the likelihood of functional improvement of areas with wall motion abnormalities at rest depends on the transmurality of necrosis — an information not available with any other technique. Again, the unprecedented accuracy of MR makes this method optimally suited to monitor the effects of treatment on the presence and size of myocardial necrosis and remodeling [59]. Delayed enhancement techniques are also increasingly used to assess patients with cardiomyopathies or inflammation (see Section 17.4.4).

17.4.3.2 Inotropic Stress

In areas with wall motion abnormalities at rest, two questions are to be asked: (1) how much necrotic (dead) tissue is in this area? and (2) will function improve after revascularization? Whereas the first question can be answered with delayed enhancement (see Section 17.4.3.1), the second question depends partially on the transmurality of necrosis and partially on the geometry

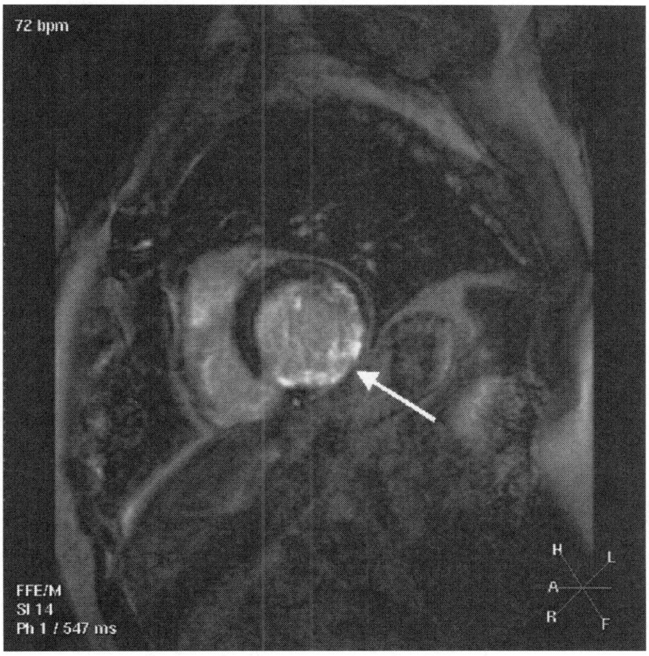

FIGURE 17.7 In the equatorial short-axis view, a transmural scar in the inferior wall is clearly delineated by delayed enhancement as high signal intensity (arrow). T_1-weighted imaging after application of a gadolinium-containing contrast agent.

(fiber arrangement) of the remaining viable myocardium. Although the amount of viable myocardium can be best determined with delayed enhancement, especially in nontransmural infarction a test which simulates function after restoration of blood flow may be better suited. Such a simulation can be performed with low-dose dobutamine stress. This test has been used in combination with echocardiography and non breath-hold MR imaging with a high predictive value [60]. Imaging is robust and simple, being performed at rest and during low dose dobutamine (5–10 μg dobutamine/kg body weight/min for 3–10 min) stress. Whereas the technique is well suited to give a binary answer on the question of whether or not functional improvement after revascularization is to be expected (superior to delayed enhancement), it does not give any information on the extent of necrosis. Its major limitation is the visual assessment of wall motion with the need to decide on sometimes small differences between rest and low-dose stress.

17.4.4 Cardiac MR in Systemic Disease/Cardiomyopathies

CMR is not only optimally suited to determine and follow patients with cardiac involvement due to systemic disease and cardiomyopathies (using LV volume and muscle mass assessment), but may yield an additional wealth of information when combined with the delayed enhancement technique [2]. Since this technique allows accurate determination and quantification of areas of fibrosis, different underlying pathologies can be differentiated according to typical patterns of fibrosis distribution [61]. In addition, the amount of fibrosis correlates with the outcome in patients with hypertrophic cardiomyopathy [62,63]. The accumulation of Gd-DTPA provides an estimate of the sum of increased blood flow, acute cell damage, and extravasation of fluid in areas of inflammation. Friedrich et al. concluded that MRI performed in patients with acute myocarditis with gadolinium-induced signal enhancement is an excellent candidate as a marker of inflammation. The option of longitudinal follow-up of the same patient with a changing clinical picture and suspicion of recurrence or persistence of disease makes MRI an attractive diagnostic tool [64].

17.4.5 Plaque Imaging

In the early stage of atherosclerosis, the vessel lumen is usually preserved by outward (positive) arterial remodeling, with relative preservation of lumen diameter [65]. It is of high clinical importance to recognize subclinical CAD, because acute coronary artery syndromes frequently result from rupture of an atherosclerotic plaque in an area of only mild-to-moderate luminal narrowing. MR can assess morphological alterations of the coronary vessels by measuring coronary arterial lumen and plaques. It was demonstrated, that in patients with atherosclerotic risk factors, the vessel wall area and therapy-induced changes can be registered with a high sensitivity by MRI [66,67]. The potential of MR plaque imaging has mainly been investigated in carotid and aortic atherosclerosis [49,51]. Coronary MRI can demonstrate vessel wall abnormalities and plaques since the high soft tissue contrast inherent to the MR method in combination with three-dimensional imaging is well suited for volume measurements to determine plaque burden [68]. Furthermore, MR vessel wall and plaque imaging with the advent of target specific contrast agents may lead to further extension [69].

17.5 DISCUSSION

Clinical applications of CMR enclose nearly every disease affecting the heart. The advantages of CMR are that it is noninvasive, free of ionizing radiation, has a high resolution, the ability to depict soft tissues and is independent of geometric assumptions and acoustic windows. Accurate and reproducible assessment of cardiac function is essential for the diagnosis, the assessment of

TABLE 17.7
Validation of MR Techniques

LV-mass/function/volume	Validated in multiple studies, reproducibility shown, high confidence, proven superiority to echocardiography
Dobutamine stress MR	Validated in single center trials in comparison to invasive angiography; superiority to echocardiography shown; good reproducibility of multicenter blinded reading shown in preliminary data
Myocardial perfusion	Validated in multiple studies, two multicenter trials show high accuracy available; comparison with SPECT on its way in MC trials; excellent validation in experimental animals
Coronary artery imaging	Validated in multiple studies, one MC trial shows high negative predictive value in comparison to invasive angiography
Scar imaging/viability	Validated in muliple studies, high accuracy for detection of fibrosis and remodeling; excellent validation in experimental animals
Vessel wall imaging	Validated in single center studies, low inter- and intraobserver variability

prognosis and evaluation of a patient's response to therapy and can serve as an endpoint for clinical drug trials. Validation of MR techniques is listed in Table 17.7. CMR has excellent interstudy reproducibility in normal, dilated, and hypertrophic hearts, and is superior to two-dimensional echocardiography [30,70,71]. The calculated sample sizes in patients to detect small changes in CMR of left ventricular volumes and function were found to be substantially smaller than recently published values for two-dimensional echocardiography (reduction of 81–97%) [66,72]. Compared to other imaging techniques, Mahrholdt et al. found that in assessment of the size of healed infarcts the reproducibility of ceMRI is superior to that of 99mTc sestamibi SPECT. The authors conclude that MRI reduces the number of patients needed for a clinical trial to 42% of that needed if infarct size is determined by SPECT [73]. The possibility of reproducible assessment of myocardial iron loading in thalassemia between two different manufacturers' scanners was demonstrated suggesting that it is possible to perform multicenter studies [74]. Due to the high reproducibility of CMR measurements [70], it appears ideally suited for use as a surrogate outcome. These observations show that CMR can reduce the necessary and sufficient sample sizes by as much as tenfold and decrease overall cost by as much as 80% [72]. Since MRI has no side-effects and the contrast agents used are extremely well tolerated with minimal influence on laboratory parameters, MRI can be used in combination with new drugs during phase I to III pharmacological trials. Even through stress MR (with dobutamine or adenosine) has side-effects in most patients during stress, these resolve rapidly after test and should, thus, not prohibit the combination of stress MR and pharmacological trials in most instances. Using simple cost calculations, approximately 5–11% of drug development costs may be saved thus providing substantial reductions in costs to society [1]. Economic value may be achieved by developing a single, noninvasive test that assesses all aspects of the heart, and CMR has the potential to provide this comprehensive examination in one sitting. With rapid imaging techniques, it should be possible to complete a comprehensive study in as little as 1 h. Operating costs derived from multiple sources and different countries estimated median cost of €435, which can, however, vary widely dependent on local conditions [1]. The effect of this initial test cost may be offset by a reduction in downstream utilization of other redundant imaging tests. Using a rudimentary cost analysis, adding the ability of CMR to perform multiple test functions may therefore provide cost savings to the healthcare system [1].

With the advent of faster scanners, automated analysis, increasing availability, and reducing costs, CMR is rapidly becoming a clinically tenable reference standard for the assessment of cardiovascular disease [75].

REFERENCES

1. Pennell, D. J. et al., Clinical indications for cardiovascular magnetic resonance (CMR): consensus panel report, *Eur. Heart J.*, 25, 1940, 2004.
2. Nagel, E., Rossum, A. v., and Fleck, E., *Cardiovascular Magnetic Resonance*, Steinkopff, Darmstadt, 2004.
3. Sokolow, M., McIlroy, M. B., and Cheitlin, M. D., *Clinical Cardiology*, 5th ed., Lange Medical Publications, 1990.
4. Kazzam, E. et al., Hypertension — still an important cause of heart failure?, *J. Hum. Hypertens.*, 19, 267, 2005.
5. Dahlström, U., Frequent non-cardiac comorbidities in patients with chronic heart failure, *Eur. J. Heart Fail.*, 7, 309, 2005.
6. Kaplan, N. M., Systemic hypertension: mechanisms and diagnosis, In *Braunwald — Heart Disease*, Braunwald, E., Ed., WB Saunders Co, Philadelphia, PA, pp. 817–851, 1992.
7. Braunwald, E., Valvular heart disease, In *Braunwald — Heart Disease*, Braunwald, E., Ed., WB Saunders Co, Philadelphia, PA, pp. 1007–1077, 1992.
8. Wilson, P. W., An epidemiologic perspective of systemic hypertension, ischemic heart disease, and heart failure, *Am. J. Cardiol.*, 80, 3J, 1997.
9. Otto, C. M. et al., Association of aortic-valve sclerosis with cardiovascular mortality and morbidity in the elderly, *N. Engl. J. Med.*, 341, 142, 1999.
10. Stewart, B. F. et al., Clinical factors associated with calcific aortic valve disease, *J. Am. Coll. Cardiol.*, 29, 630, 1997.
11. Gould, K., Kirkeeide, R., and Buchi, M., Coronary flow reserve as a physiologic measure of stenosis severity, *J. Am. Coll. Cardiol.*, 15, 459, 1990.
12. Mahrholdt, H., Wagner, A., and Sechtem, U., Congenital heart disease and cardiomyopathies, In *Cardiovascular Magnetic Resonance*, Nagel, E., van Rossum, A. C., and Fleck, E., Eds., Steinkopf, Darmstadt, pp. 105–132, 2004.
13. Wynne, J. and Braunwald, E., The cardiomyopathies and myocarditis: toxic, chemical, and physical damage to the heart, In *Braunwald — Heart Disease*, Braunwald, E., Ed., WB Saunders Co, Philadelphia, PA, pp. 1394–1450, 1992.
14. Maceira, A. M. et al., Cardiovascular magnetic resonance in cardiac amyloidosis, *Circulation*, 111, 186, 2005.
15. Vignaux, O., Cardiac sarcoidosis: spectrum of MRI features, *Am. J. Roentgenol.*, 184, 249, 2005.
16. Kuntz, K. M. et al., Cost-effectiveness of diagnostic strategies for patients with chest pain, *Ann. Intern. Med.*, 130, 709, 1999.
17. Ndrepepa, G. et al., Plasma levels of *N*-terminal pro-brain natriuretic peptide in patients with coronary artery disease and relation to clinical presentation, angiographic severity, and left ventricular ejection fraction, *Am. J. Cardiol.*, 95, 553, 2005.
18. Arroyo-Espliguero, R. et al., C-reactive protein elevation and disease activity in patients with coronary artery disease, *Eur. Heart J.*, 25, 401, 2004.
19. Johnson, B. D. et al., Serum Amyloid A as a predictor of coronary artery disease and cardiovascular outcome in women: the national heart, lung, and blood institute-sponsored women's ischemia syndrome evaluation (WISE), *Circulation*, 109, 726, 2004.
20. Clejan, S. et al., Blood histamine is associated with coronary artery disease, cardiac events and severity of inflammation and atherosclerosis, *J. Cell. Mol. Med.*, 6, 583, 2002.
21. Kragelund, C. et al., *N*-terminal pro-B-type natriuretic peptide and long-term mortality in stable coronary heart disease, *N. Engl. J. Med.*, 352, 666, 2005.
22. Thiele, H. et al., Functional cardiac MR imaging with steady-state free precession (SSFP) significantly improves endocardial border delineation without contrast agents, *J. Magn. Reson. Imaging*, 14, 362, 2001.
23. Thiele, H. et al., Improved accuracy of quantitative assessment of left ventricular volume and ejection fraction by geometric models with steady-state free precession, *J. Cardiovasc. Magn. Reson.*, 4, 327, 2002.
24. Bellenger, N. et al., Reduction in sample size for studies of remodeling in heart failure by the use of cardiovascular magnetic resonance, *J. Cardiovasc. Magn. Reson.*, 2, 271, 2000.

25. Otterstad, J. E. et al., Accuracy and reproducibility of biplane two-dimensional echocardiographic measurements of left ventricular dimensions and function, *Eur. Heart J.*, 18, 507, 1997.
26. Kaus, M. R. et al., Automated segmentation of the left ventricle in cardiac MRI, *Med. Image Anal.*, 8, 245, 2004.
27. Nagel, E. et al., Stress cardiovascular magnetic resonance: consensus panel report, *J. Cardiovasc. Magn. Reson.*, 3, 267, 2001.
28. Nagel, E. et al., Noninvasive diagnosis of ischemia-induced wall motion abnormalities with the use of high-dose dobutamine stress MRI: comparison with dobutamine stress echocardiography, *Circulation*, 99, 763, 1999.
29. Wahl, A. et al., High-dose dobutamine-atropine stress cardiovascular MR imaging after coronary revascularization in patients with wall motion abnormalities at rest, *Radiology*, 233, 210, 2004.
30. Nagel, E. et al., Influence of image quality on the diagnostic accuracy of dobutamine stress magnetic resonance imaging in comparison with dobutamine stress echocardiography for the noninvasive detection of myocardial ischemia, *Z. Kardiol.*, 88, 622, 1999.
31. Wahl, A. et al., Safety and feasibility of high-dose dobutamine-atropine stress cardiovascular magnetic resonance for diagnosis of myocardial ischaemia: experience in 1000 consecutive cases, *Eur. Heart. J.*, 25, 1230, 2004.
32. Hundley, W. G. et al., Magnetic resonance imaging determination of cardiac prognosis, *Circulation*, 106, 2328, 2002.
33. Castillo, E., Lima, J. A. C., and Bluemke, D. A., Regional myocardial function: advances in MR imaging and analysis, *Radiographics*, 23, 127S, 2003.
34. Garot, J. et al., Fast determination of regional myocardial strain fields from tagged cardiac images using harmonic phase MRI, *Circulation*, 101, 981, 2000.
35. Osman, N. F. et al., Cardiac motion tracking using CINE harmonic phase (HARP) magnetic resonance imaging, *Magn. Reson. Med.*, 42, 1048, 1999.
36. Azevedo, C. F. et al., Persistent diastolic dysfunction despite complete systolic functional recovery after reperfused acute myocardial infarction demonstrated by tagged magnetic resonance imaging, *Eur. Heart J.*, 25, 1419, 2004.
37. Al-Saadi, N. et al., Noninvasive detection of myocardial ischemia from perfusion reserve based on cardiovascular magnetic resonance, *Circulation*, 101, 1379, 2000.
38. Al-Saadi, N. et al., Improvement of myocardial perfusion reserve early after coronary intervention: assessment with cardiac magnetic resonance imaging, *J. Am. Coll. Cardiol.*, 36, 1557, 2000.
39. Schwitter, J. et al., Assessment of myocardial perfusion in coronary artery disease by magnetic resonance: a comparison with positron emission tomography and coronary angiography, *Circulation*, 103, 2230, 2001.
40. Paetsch, I. et al., Cardiac magnetic resonance (CMR) imaging: a noninvasive tool for functional and morphological assessment of coronary artery disease: current clinical applications and potential future concepts, *J. Interv. Cardiol.*, 16, 457, 2003.
41. Wagner, A. et al., Contrast-enhanced MRI and routine single photon emission computed tomography (SPECT) perfusion imaging for detection of subendocardial myocardial infarcts: an imaging study, *Lancet*, 361, 374, 2003.
42. Panting, J. R. et al., Abnormal subendocardial perfusion in cardiac syndrome X detected by cardiovascular magnetic resonance imaging, *N. Engl. J. Med.*, 346, 1948, 2002.
43. Giang, T. H. et al., Detection of coronary artery disease by magnetic resonance myocardial perfusion imaging with various contrast medium doses: first European multi-centre experience, *Eur. Heart J.*, 25, 1657, 2004.
44. Wolff, S. D. et al., Myocardial first-pass perfusion magnetic resonance imaging: a multicenter dose-ranging study, *Circulation*, 110, 732, 2004.
45. Kelle, S. et al., Potential intrinsic error of noninvasive coronary angiography, *J. Cardiovasc. Magn. Reson.*, 7, 1, 2005.
46. Jahnke, C. et al., Coronary MR angiography with steady-state free precession: individually adapted breath-hold technique versus free-breathing technique, *Radiology*, 232, 669, 2004.
47. Kim, W. Y. et al., Coronary magnetic resonance angiography for the detection of coronary stenoses, *N. Engl. J. Med.*, 345, 1863, 2001.

48. Jaffer, F. A. et al., Age and sex distribution of subclinical aortic atherosclerosis: a magnetic resonance imaging examination of the Framingham Heart Study, *Arterioscler. Thromb. Vasc. Biol.*, 22, 849, 2002.
49. Helft, G. et al., Progression and regression of atherosclerotic lesions: monitoring with serial noninvasive magnetic resonance imaging, *Circulation*, 105, 993, 2002.
50. Li, A. E. et al., Using MRI to assess aortic wall thickness in the multiethnic study of atherosclerosis: distribution by race, sex, and age, *Am. J. Roentgenol.*, 182, 593, 2004.
51. Fayad, Z. A. et al., In vivo magnetic resonance evaluation of atherosclerotic plaques in the human thoracic aorta: a comparison with transesophageal echocardiography, *Circulation*, 101, 2503, 2000.
52. Barkhausen, J. et al., Detection of atherosclerotic plaque with gadofluorine-enhanced magnetic resonance imaging, *Circulation*, 108, 605, 2003.
53. Botnar, R. M. et al., In vivo magnetic resonance imaging of coronary thrombosis using a fibrin-binding molecular magnetic resonance contrast agent, *Circulation*, 110, 1463, 2004.
54. Winter, P. M. et al., Molecular imaging of angiogenesis in early-stage atherosclerosis with {alpha}v{beta}3-integrin-targeted nanoparticles, *Circulation*, 108, 2270, 2003.
55. Judd, R. M. et al., Physiological basis of myocardial contrast enhancement in fast magnetic resonance images of 2-day-old reperfused canine infarcts, *Circulation*, 92, 1902, 1995.
56. Kim, R. J. et al., Relationship of MRI delayed contrast enhancement to irreversible injury, infarct age, and contractile function, *Circulation*, 100, 1992, 1999.
57. Klein, C. et al., Assessment of myocardial viability with contrast-enhanced magnetic resonance imaging: comparison with positron emission tomography, *Circulation*, 105, 162, 2002.
58. Kim, R. J. et al., The use of contrast-enhanced magnetic resonance imaging to identify reversible myocardial dysfunction, *N. Engl. J. Med.*, 343, 1445, 2000.
59. Choi, K. M. et al., Transmural extent of acute myocardial infarction predicts long-term improvement in contractile function, *Circulation*, 104, 1101, 2001.
60. Wellnhofer, E. et al., Magnetic resonance low-dose dobutamine test is superior to scar quantification for the prediction of functional recovery, *Circulation*, 109, 2172, 2004.
61. McCrohon, J. A. et al., Differentiation of heart failure related to dilated cardiomyopathy and coronary artery disease using gadolinium-enhanced cardiovascular magnetic resonance, *Circulation*, 108, 54, 2003.
62. Moon, J. C. et al., Toward clinical risk assessment in hypertrophic cardiomyopathy with gadolinium cardiovascular magnetic resonance, *J. Am. Coll. Cardiol.*, 41, 1561, 2003.
63. Choudhury, L. et al., Myocardial scarring in asymptomatic or mildly symptomatic patients with hypertrophic cardiomyopathy, *J. Am. Coll. Cardiol.*, 40, 2156, 2002.
64. Friedrich, M. G. et al., Contrast media-enhanced magnetic resonance imaging visualizes myocardial changes in the course of viral myocarditis, *Circulation*, 97, 1802, 1998.
65. Glagov, S. et al., Compensatory enlargement of human atherosclerotic coronary arteries, *N. Engl. J. Med.*, 316, 1371, 1987.
66. Bellenger, N. G. et al., Effects of carvedilol on left ventricular remodelling in chronic stable heart failure: a cardiovascular magnetic resonance study, *Heart*, 90, 760, 2004.
67. Corti, R. et al., Lipid lowering by simvastatin induces regression of human atherosclerotic lesions: two years' follow-up by high-resolution noninvasive magnetic resonance imaging, *Circulation*, 106, 2884, 2002.
68. Fayad, Z. A. and Fuster, V., Clinical imaging of the high-risk or vulnerable atherosclerotic plaque, *Circ. Res.*, 89, 305, 2001.
69. Weissleder, R. and Ntziachristos, V., Shedding light onto live molecular targets, *Nat. Med.*, 9, 123, 2003.
70. Grothues, F. et al., Comparison of interstudy reproducibility of cardiovascular magnetic resonance with two-dimensional echocardiography in normal subjects and in patients with heart failure or left ventricular hypertrophy, *Am. J. Cardiol.*, 90, 29, 2002.
71. Bellenger, N. G. et al., Quantification of right and left ventricular function by cardiovascular magnetic resonance, *Herz*, 25, 392, 2000.
72. Bellenger, N. G. et al., Reduction in sample size for studies of remodeling in heart failure by the use of cardiovascular magnetic resonance, *J. Cardiovasc. Magn. Reson.*, 2, 271, 2000.

73. Mahrholdt, H. et al., Reproducibility of chronic infarct size measurement by contrast-enhanced magnetic resonance imaging, *Circulation*, 106, 2322, 2002.
74. Westwood, M. A. et al., Interscanner reproducibility of cardiovascular magnetic resonance T_2^* measurements of tissue iron in thalassemia, *J. Magn. Reson. Imaging*, 18, 616, 2003.
75. Grothues, F. et al., Interstudy reproducibility of right ventricular volumes, function, and mass with cardiovascular magnetic resonance, *Am. Heart J.*, 147, 218, 2004.

Editorial Comments

Spirometry is a simple and cheap test which allows for global assessments of human lung function. In small rodents, analysis of broncho-alveolar lavage fluid and histology are used to derive information on, e.g., inflammation, or assessments of airway resistance and whole body plethismography are employed to obtain functional information. With their particular advantages, these methods are limited by the fact that they are invasive and/or that they provide only a global assessment of lung function. Despite its noninvasivenesss, unrestrained plethismography in awake animals provides respiratory measures that are so tenuously linked to respiratory mechanics that it is debatable if they can be considered as meaningful indicators of lung function [1].

Imaging providing information on a regional basis may enhance the understanding of the pathophysiology of respiratory diseases and improve the disease classification. In particular, functional imaging methods could be more sensitive than conventional lung function tests; subtle effects might be masked by the global assessment of lung function since the nondiseased lung may compensate for the functional impairment of the diseased lung. Exactly the detection of such small changes is important for the assessment of early treatment since the course of the disease can be more easily altered and irreversible tissue damage prevented.

Currently computerized tomography is the reference for anatomical imaging of the lung. Nonetheless, it is surprising to verify that up to now few drug studies have been performed using this technique [2–6], perhaps because of issues related to radiation exposure. Chapter 18 and Chapter 19 show that ongoing developments to image the lung might turn MRI into a competitive imaging technique for preclinical and clinical drug testing in the area of respiratory diseases. Of particular interest is the fact that MRI is free of radiation exposure, so that repetitive and frequent follow-up examinations are feasible.

REFERENCES

1. Bates, J. H. and Irvin, C. G., Measuring lung function in mice: The phenotyping uncertainty principle, *J. Appl. Physiol.*, 94, 1297, 2003.
2. Abboud, R. T., Ford, G. T., and Chapman, K. R., Emphysema in alpha1-antitrypsin deficiency: Does replacement therapy affect outcome?, *Treat. Respir. Med.*, 4, 1, 2005.
3. Berger, P. et al., Airway wall thickness in cigarette smokers: Quantitative thin-section CT assessment, *Radiology*, 235, 1055, 2005.

4. Robinson, T. E. et al., Domase alfa reduces air trapping in children with mild cystic fibrosis lung disease: a quantitative analysis, *Chest*, 128, 2327, 2005.
5. Lam, S. et al., A randomized phase IIb trial of Pulmicort Turbuhaler (Budesonide) in people with Dysplasia of the bronchial epithelium, *Clin. Cancer Res.*, 10, 6502, 2004.
6. Robinson, T. E. et al., Composite spirometric-computed tomography outcome measure in early cystic fibrosis lung disease, *Am. J. Respir. Crit. Care Med.*, 168, 588, 2003.

18 Lung MRI in Small Rodents as a Tool for the Evaluation of Drugs in Models of Airways Diseases

Nicolau Beckmann, Yannick Crémillieux, Bruno Tigani, Harry Karmouty Quintana, François-Xavier Blé, and John R. Fozard

CONTENTS

18.1 INTRODUCTION

Diseases of the airways, such as asthma and chronic obstructive pulmonary disease (COPD), involve a complex interplay of many inflammatory and structural cell types, all of which can release inflammatory mediators including cytokines, chemokines, growth factors, and adhesion molecules. Activated eosinophils are considered particularly important in asthma, contributing to epithelial cell damage, bronchial hyperresponsiveness, plasma exudation, and edema of the airway mucosa, as well as smooth muscle hypertrophy and mucus plugging, through the release of enzymes and proteins [1–3]. In COPD, inflammation of the small airways and lung parenchyma with the involvement of neutrophils, macrophages and cytotoxic ($CD8^+$) T-lymphocytes results in chronic obstructive bronchitis, destruction of the lung parenchyma by proteolytic enzymes (emphysema), and mucus hypersecretion leading to severe airflow limitation [4,5].

Although *in vivo* MR techniques have been in use in pharmaceutical research for more than 20 years, it is only recently that they have been applied to preclinical studies in the area of respiratory diseases [6]. Interestingly, a similar time-lag is evident for the clinical applications of lung MRI. Probably the main reasons for this delay are the inherent difficulties imposed by the lung tissue on the MR signal properties and, in the clinical arena, the fact that computerized tomography (CT) is the imaging technique of choice for diagnosis of lung diseases. The aim of this chapter is to illustrate how the flexibility of MRI can be exploited to derive information on lung inflammation and on its functional status in models of airway diseases in rats, and how this information can be ultimately used to profile compounds in these animal models [6].

18.2 MRI OF THE LUNG

18.2.1 Proton Imaging

The living lung is one of the most challenging organs to image by MRI. Because of the low water density of approximately 20 to 30%, the proton density is significantly lower than in other tissues. Moreover, due to the difference in magnetic susceptibilities between lung tissue and the air that comprises about 80% of the pulmonary volume, local inhomogeneities in the magnetic field arise, resulting in very short T_2 and T_2^* relaxation times. Using a gradient-echo sequence, mean T_2^* values of the order of 1.4 msec and 500 μsec have been measured *in vivo* at 1.5 T in normal volunteers [7] and at 4.7 T in normal rat and mouse lungs [8,9], respectively. These values are in agreement with the linear dependency between $1/T_2^*$ and the field strength described for lung parenchymal tissue [10], consistent with the air/water interface model being the major mechanism for the inhomogeneous magnetic field broadening of the water MR signal in the lung [11].

In order to detect a signal from lung parenchyma, especially at high fields, nonstandard techniques need to be used to reduce considerably the echo time (TE) [12]. Different protocols have been developed to overcome some of the inherent difficulties associated with the detection of parenchymal signal. For rodent imaging, the projection reconstruction method with self-refocused radio-frequency (RF) pulses has been used to achieve TE <300 μsec and thus enhance the visibility of lung parenchyma [12,13]. Susceptibility maps and postprocessing corrections were applied to compensate for susceptibility effects in the $x-y$ plane [14]. Projection reconstruction methods are not commonly implemented in MR scanners and hence require a high level of expertise concerning the sampling and reconstruction of the data. An inherent problem of projection methods is the inefficient radial sampling of *k*-space imposed by the acquisition. In order to alleviate this drawback, complicated sampling schemes have been proposed such as *k*-space sampling along spiral trajectories [15] and variable-density spiral trajectories [16].

A further challenge in lung MRI is that cardiac and respiratory movements can cause marked image artefacts. These problems are more evident in small rodents, because of their higher cardiac and respiratory rates. To address this issue, scan-synchronous ventilation has been developed [13,17], in which breathing is restricted to the recovery period after data acquisition, thereby minimizing breathing-related motion artefacts. Breathing rate is controlled by initiating a breath after the appropriate number of pulse sequence repetitions to maintain about 120 breaths/min. In addition, imaging acquisition is triggered by the electrocardiogram. Although the combination of projection reconstruction methods with synchronous ventilation and cardiac gating enables high resolution images to be obtained from the rat lung [13], the acquisition time is long, amounting to about 30 to 40 min per image.

For drug testing *in vivo* in animal models of airway diseases, it is important to keep the acquisition conditions as simple as possible so that repeated measurements interfering minimally with the physiology and the well-being of the animals can be carried out on a routine basis. It has been shown that the gradient-echo sequence produces sharp images from the rat chest, in which potential artefacts caused by cardiac and respiratory movements are suppressed by image averaging

[8,18], despite the fact that neither respiratory nor cardiac gating is applied. Animals respire spontaneously during data collection.

The availability of fast gradients makes short TEs possible without the use of nonstandard RF pulses and spatial encoding techniques, thereby avoiding difficulties associated with them. For instance, signal of lung parenchymal tissue from spontaneously breathing rats and mice can be detected at 4.7 T, a field strength commonly available in animal scanners, with a reasonable signal-to-noise ratio of about 16 using a gradient-echo sequence with TE of the order of 500 μsec within about 1 min measurement time [8]. This approach enables ventilation-related information to be derived exploring the weakly paramagnetic character of molecular oxygen (see Section 18.4.2.2 and Section 18.4.2.4), along the lines of the original proposal by Edelman et al. [19]. Indeed, a highly significant negative correlation was found between the parenchymal signal in the rat lung and the partial pressure of oxygen in the blood, for different amounts of oxygen administered [9]. Following this reasoning, an increased parenchymal signal should be consistent with a reduced oxygen level or vice versa (Figure 18.1).

The magnitude of the signal intensity variations caused by changes in the oxygen concentration is larger than expected solely from the paramagnetic properties of molecular oxygen. Diamagnetic

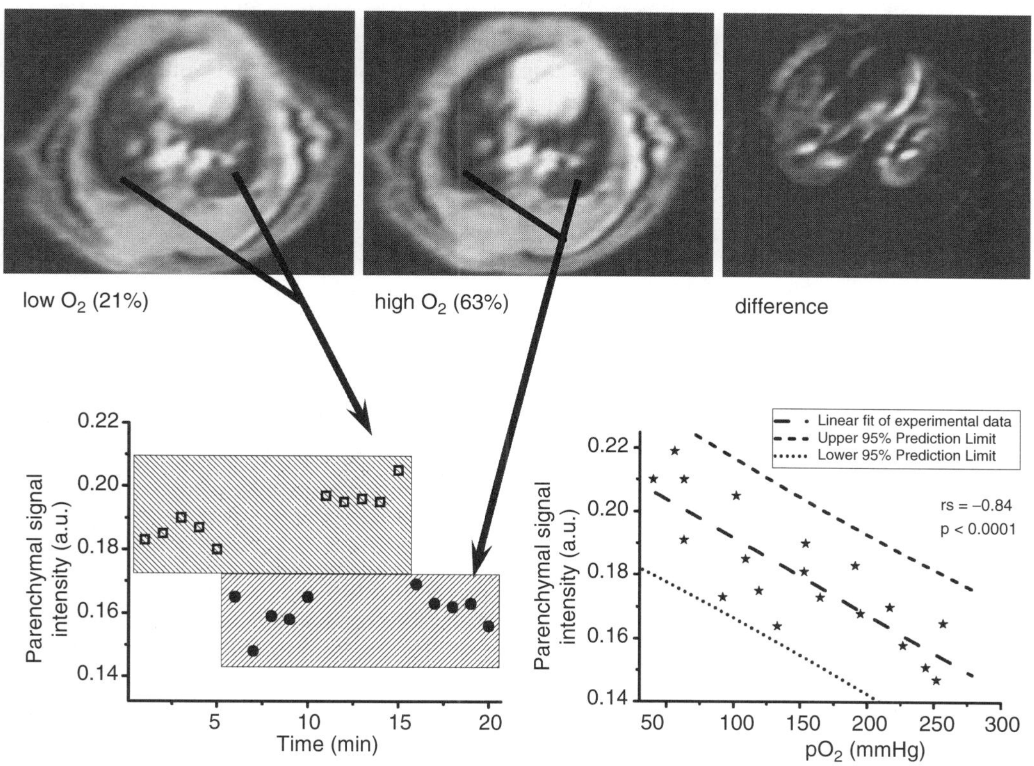

FIGURE 18.1 Axial sections through the chest of a ventilated rat, acquired during administration of a gas mixture having low (21%) or high (63%) oxygen content. Gradient-echo sequence with TR 1.95 msec, TE 545 μsec, field-of-view (FOV) $= 6 \times 6$ cm^2, matrix size $= 36 \times 128$, and slice 2 mm. An image was computed from 40 individual acquisitions with an interval of 500 msec between them, resulting in a total acquisition time of 30 sec for a single slice. No respiratory or cardiac triggering was applied. Change of the oxygen content in the mixture from 21 to 63% led to differences of 17 to 25% in the signal intensity of parenchymal tissue, as illustrated by the difference image. The effect was reversible as shown in the left graph. A significant correlation was found between the proton parenchymal signal and the partial pressure of oxygen in the blood (right graph). (Adapted from Beckmann, N. et al., *Magn. Reson. Med.*, 52, 258, 2004. With permission of John Wiley & Sons, Inc. Copyright 2004.)

effects in the foam-like structure of the inflated lung cause inhomogeneous line broadening (equivalent to a shortened free-induction decay) not found in totally collapsed lung or in other tissues [20,21]. The anomalously short free-induction decay is caused by local perturbations in the magnetic field near air-tissue interfaces [20], which are produced by the differences in magnetic susceptibility of tissue and air. Since lung inflation and oxygenation are intrinsically correlated, it is conceivable that the paramagnetic effects of molecular oxygen and the line broadening caused by an inflated lung add up. Therefore, the effects of changes of the tissue oxygen content upon image contrast become more evident in the lung than in other tissues.

18.2.2 Hyperpolarized Gas Imaging

Compared to conventional water proton imaging, MRI of gases is inherently limited by the much lower spin density (typically three orders of magnitude drop in spin density). Despite this low MR sensitivity, MR ventilation imaging using gaseous fluorinated compounds have been demonstrated in several animal studies [22–24]. However, these techniques suffer from poor spatial resolution and long acquisition times, of the order of 30 min per image.

Another approach for MRI of gases is based on the use of hyperpolarized (HP) or laser-polarized gases. To overcome the low NMR sensitivity of gases, dedicated optical pumping (OP) apparatuses are used. In these polarizing systems, the gases to be polarized are introduced into an OP glass cell illuminated by an appropriately tuned circularly polarized laser beam. The absorption of the circularly polarized light by the gas atoms results in the orientation of the nuclear magnetic moments in a preferential direction. This nuclear spin alignment translates into a large macroscopic magnetization and results subsequently in a large increase of the NMR signal and sensitivity. The efficacy of the OP process is related to the final polarization level, expressed as a percentage of the maximal gas magnetization. Polarization levels can be typically increased by five orders of magnitude, resulting in a similar increase in detectable NMR signal. For detailed description of the principles, design and practical implementation of the OP laser polarization techniques, the reader is referred to the reviews of Goodson [25] and Möller et al. [26].

Following the end of the laser-polarization process, the macroscopic magnetization returns to its original, thermal-equilibrium value with a time constant equal to the longitudinal relaxation time T_1 of the gas nuclei (of the order of hours to days when the gas is kept under appropriate conditions). As a result, the laser-polarization technique requires the use of nuclear spins with long longitudinal relaxation times. The OP techniques have been so far demonstrated on two long-T_1 rare gas 1/2 spin isotopes: He-3 and Xe-129.

Xenon is an inert gas unable to form covalent chemical bonds. However, its large electronic polarizability results in high solubility in apolar solvents and in high affinity for lipids or for hydrophobic sites in proteins. Probably as a consequence of its lipid affinity, xenon has well-known anesthetic properties. Xe-133, one of its radioactive isotopes, is used in clinical lung scintigraphy imaging. Xe-129 is a stable isotope with a natural abundance of 26.4% and a gyromagnetic ratio equal to 11.8 MHz/T. It can be polarized using the so-called spin-exchange OP technique. Typical polarization levels reported in the literature are of the order of 15%.

Helium is an inert gas with very low solubility in body fluids and tissues. He-3 is a stable isotope with a natural abundance of 1.4 ppm. The He-3 nucleus has a gyromagnetic ratio equal to 32.4 MHz/T. It can be polarized by two different OP techniques, the spin-exchange and the metastable OP techniques, with typical polarization levels of 30 and 60%, respectively.

The large NMR signal offered by HP gases allows their distribution in the pulmonary tree and the alveolar spaces to be imaged. The first biomedical application of HP Xe-129 was reported in 1994 and dealt with intrapulmonary imaging of excised mouse lungs [27]. The first *in vivo* animal lung ventilation images obtained using HP He-3 were reported one year later [28]. Due to its larger gyromagnetic ratio and polarization levels, the He-3 sensitivity is about one order of magnitude higher than that obtained with Xe-129. As a result, most of the reported small animal HP gas ventilation studies are based on He-3; for this reason, we will restrict the discussion to HP He-3 investigations. For a recent overview of Xe-129 MRI applications in small animals, the reader is referred to Oros and Shah [29].

The gas polarization can be rapidly destroyed if the gas is allowed to be in contact with or in the vicinity of ferromagnetic materials. Similarly, oscillating and inhomogeneous static magnetic fields are a potential source of gas depolarization. As a result, polarized gas is transported, stored, and distributed using nonmagnetic materials (e.g., plastic syringes, bags, and tubing). Electrical devices such as valves and sensors are generally precluded. Oxygen, as a paramagnetic molecule, represents another important source of He-3 relaxation and subsequently of gas polarization losses. While longitudinal relaxation times of pure He-3 in appropriate reservoirs can exceed hours, He-3 relaxation time drops to 11 sec when mixed with oxygen at a concentration of 21% v/v [30,31]. As a consequence, helium and oxygen mixing should be avoided as much as possible and restricted to the ventilation image acquisition period.

Hyperpolarized He-3 can be introduced into the animal lungs using either tracheal intubation or invasive tracheotomy. The gas delivery to the animal lungs can be performed using a variety of protocols and apparatus. Small animal respirators compatible with polarized He-3 have been developed by several groups [17,31–33]. These respirators allow fine control of the delivered gas volume and of the lung ventilation timing. Triggering and synchronization of the imaging sequence with the gas delivery can be used for performing lung ventilation As an example, CINE-type imaging [34–36] yielding very high spatial and temporal resolution images of the gas intrapulmonary distribution is shown in Figure 18.2. In this type of ventilation imaging experiment, each image is acquired in a short time window (typically a few tens of milliseconds) that is synchronized with the animal's breathing cycle. The completion of the image acquisition is performed over several breaths. The number of breaths required for completing the image depends on the desired final spatial resolution of the image and on the duration of the acquisition window. Typically, 40 to 150 breaths are used to achieve ventilation images with a spatial resolution of a few hundreds of micrometers.

18.2.3 Lung Perfusion

Lung perfusion imaging has been demonstrated in human studies using proton MRI techniques, based on contrast agent enhancement [37] or spin labeling [38,39]. Although contrast-enhanced perfusion imaging studies have been reported in small animals [40,41], these techniques are limited by the low signal-to-noise ratio of lung parenchyma.

He-3 MRI has been suggested as an alternative to proton imaging for probing lung perfusion [42,43]. Ventilation images are acquired during the injection of a contrast agent bolus (a suspension of superparamagnetic iron oxide nanoparticles). The bolus passing through the lung vasculature results in a transient intrapulmonary He-3 signal drop. This signal decrease is due to the magnetic susceptibility difference between the alveoli and the blood vessels containing the magnetic contrast agent. The magnetic field inhomogeneities induced by the iron oxide nanoparticles result in reduced He-3 apparent transverse relaxation times and thus in a decrease in the He-3 signal. The He-3 signal variations are analyzed in a similar way to proton first-pass contrast agent perfusion measurements and pulmonary blood volume maps can be generated [42,44].

Polarized He-3 can also be used as an intravascular contrast agent to highlight the blood vessels. To overcome the low solubility of helium in blood, an appropriate carrier agent is required, for instance phospholipid-based microbubbles of mean diameter of 3 μm which encapsulate He-3 [44,45]. Callot et al. [44] demonstrated in rats that, when such a suspension is administered intravenously, the distribution of helium microbubbles inside the lung vasculature allows the derivation of information on lung perfusion.

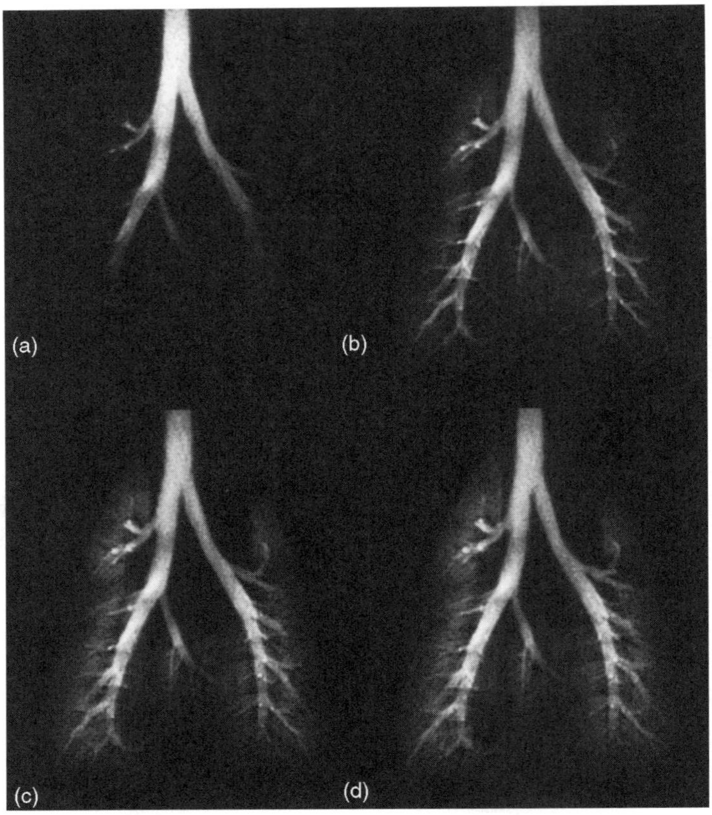

FIGURE 18.2 High resolution CINE ventilation images in rats. The image acquisition window was equal to 36 msec with a FOV of 5 × 5 cm^2 and a slice thickness of 5 mm. (Reproduced from Chen, B. T., Brau, A. C. S., and Johnson, G. A., *Magn. Reson. Med.*, 49, 78, 2003. Courtesy of Prof. G. A. Johnson, Duke University. With permission of John Wiley & Sons, Inc. Copyright 2003.)

18.3 RAT MODELS OF AIRWAYS DISEASES

Many species of animals can be used to provide models for human airways diseases. Unfortunately, there is no animal model that exactly reproduces the human pathology. Nonetheless, these models are useful for the development of novel therapies and to mimic and study specific aspects of human respiratory diseases [46–48].

Actively sensitized Brown Norway (BN) rats exposed to allergen develop airway hyperresponsiveness and eosinophilic inflammation together with an increase in activated T cells ($CD25^+$) in the airways [49–51], hence reflecting key features of asthmatic inflammation. Alternatively, an inflammation similar to that observed in COPD patients can be elicited in rodents by the administration of endotoxin (lipopolysaccharide [LPS]), a bacterial macromolecular cell surface antigen. LPS activates mononuclear phagocytes through a receptor-mediated process, leading to the release of a number of cytokines, including tumor necrosis factor-α (TNF-α) [52,53]. TNF-α increases the adherence of neutrophils to endothelial cells, therefore facilitating a massive infiltration of neutrophils into the lung [54]. Exposure of BN rats to LPS leads to pulmonary neutrophilia [55,56] and induces mucus cell metaplasia [57].

One of the most critical components of COPD is emphysema, which results in the destruction of lung parenchymal tissue by a number of proteases such as neutrophil elastase or matrix metalloproteinases (see also Chapter 19, Section 19.3.2). Destruction of parenchyma leads to an enlargement of air spaces in the lung and consequently to a loss of lung elasticity, ultimately resulting in severe impairment of gas exchange [5]. Experimental emphysema can be induced in rats by the application of a single dose of porcine pancreatic elastase (PPE) [58].

Pulmonary embolism (PE) is a relatively common but still poorly understood disease with high mortality (10% of all cases) [59]. It causes physical obstruction of the pulmonary microvasculature and inflammatory changes following embolic injury of the lung tissue (see also Chapter 19, Section 19.5). A rat model of acute PE consists in the administration of micro air bubbles into, for example, the left femoral vein [60].

The inflammatory status of the lungs in such models is usually inferred from broncho-alveolar lavage (BAL) fluid analysis and/or histology [56,61,62]. For lung function analysis rats are normally tracheotomized and artificially ventilated. To suppress spontaneous respiration animals receive a muscle relaxant. From measurements of airflow and transpulmonary pressure, airway resistance is calculated after each respiratory cycle (see, for example, Ref. [51]). Clearly, the invasive character of these procedures precludes repeated assessments in the same animal. The much less invasive nature of MRI can provide important information in these models, especially concerning chronic aspects, which can contribute significantly to profiling compounds with therapeutic potential.

18.4 APPLICATION OF MRI TO MODELS OF AIRWAYS DISEASES

18.4.1 Lung Inflammation

A characteristic feature of respiratory diseases such as asthma is edema of the airways due to an increase in the permeability of lung microvessels to plasma proteins. The resulting effect is the leakage of fluid from the microvascular circulation into the surrounding tissue. Assessment of this fluid can be important for diagnostic purposes and for planning and guiding treatment.

Proton MRI is the natural candidate for trying to detect inflammatory responses in the lungs in models of airway diseases. As mentioned above, a conventional gradient-echo technique can be used to generate images of the rat thorax in which motion artifacts are suppressed by averaging. Neither respiratory nor cardiac triggering is applied, and the animals are able to respire spontaneously during data collection. Under the conditions chosen for acquisition (TE of the order of 3 msec), the signal from the lung parenchyma itself is too weak to be detected at 4.7 T. However, the absence of any detectable lung parenchymal signal in combination with a background devoid of artifacts, provides high contrast-to-noise ratio for the detection of fluid signals associated with the inflammatory process [18,63].

In rats actively sensitized to ovalbumin (OVA) and challenged with the antigen, an intense, homogeneous fluid signal is detected in the lungs 24 h after challenge (Figure 18.3). By acquiring about 20 images displaced from each other by an amount corresponding to a single slice thickness, the whole thorax of the animal can be scanned and the total volume of the fluid signal determined [18]. The volume of the fluid signal is dependent on the dose of allergen and reaches a maximum 48 h after challenge (Figure 18.3). The MRI signal can be seen for approximately 100 h and is highly significantly correlated with a variety of inflammatory parameters determined in the BAL fluid recovered from the same animals [56]. Of special interest, the strongest correlations are with the eosinophil numbers, eosinophil peroxidase activity (a marker of eosinophil activation), and the total protein content (a marker for plasma extravasation). Importantly, the signal detected by MRI correlates significantly with the perivascular edema assessed by histology [61].

One particularly interesting aspect of the signal detected by MRI is its predominant location on the left side of the animals despite the fact that allergen was administered into the trachea above the carina, i.e., before the bifurcation of the trachea. Near-infrared fluorescence imaging and histology confirmed the anomalous localization of the inflammation as revealed by the fluid signal distribution detected by MRI [64]. This difference in the distribution following intratracheal

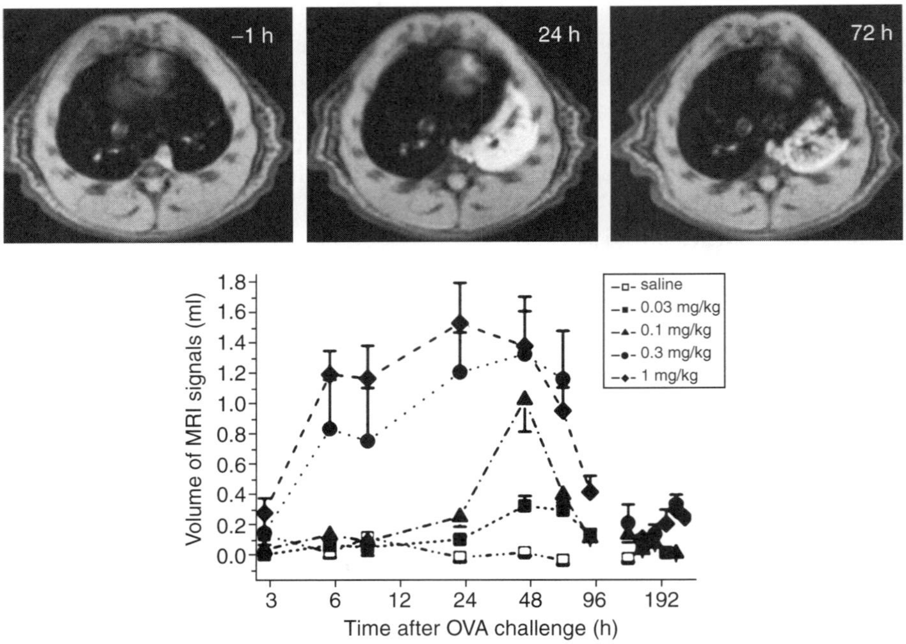

FIGURE 18.3 Images from an actively sensitized BN rat at different time points with respect to an OVA challenge (0.3 mg/kg i.t. at time point 0). Gradient-echo sequence with TR 5.6 msec, TE 2.7 msec, FOV 6×6 cm^2, matrix size 256×128, slice thickness 1.5 mm. An image was computed from 80 individual acquisitions with an interval of 530 msec between them, resulting in a total acquisition time of 100 sec for a single slice. The animal respired spontaneously, and neither respiratory nor cardiac triggering was applied. Course of fluid signal volumes was derived from images acquired at different time points with respect to saline or OVA challenge at the specified dose. The number of animals per experimental group was 6. (Adapted from Beckmann, N. et al., *Magn. Reson. Med.*, 45, 88, 2001. With permission of John Wiley & Sons, Inc. Copyright 2001.)

instillation of allergen may be due to the inherent geometry of the bronchus of each lobe with respect to the left and right primary bronchi. Casting of the rat lung showed that the bronchio-alveolar tree is indeed more developed in the left lobe [65]. Interestingly, an asymmetry in T_2^* relaxation times, possibly related to a more prominent bronchial tree on the left lung [66], has also been observed between the left and right lungs [8,9].

Following challenge of nonsensitized rats with LPS, the signals that appear in the lungs are uneven and significantly less intense than those detected after OVA administration to actively sensitized animals (Figure 18.4). They are of long duration, being detectable 8 days after dosing [63]. The only parameter in the BAL fluid that correlates significantly with the MRI signal is the mucus concentration [56,63]. Histological analysis indicates a substantial and sustained increase in goblet cell number up to 16 days after LPS challenge, and flocculent mucoid material is consistently detected close to the apical surface of epithelial cells [63]. These observations suggest that the long-lasting MRI signal following LPS is due to secreted mucus.

18.4.2 Lung Ventilation

Gas exchange is the major function of the lungs. The regional pulmonary blood flow (perfusion) and the ventilation in the lungs need to be matched for this process to occur efficiently. In diseases of the airways like asthma and COPD, lung ventilation can be compromised. Asthma is a highly prevalent chronic inflammatory disorder of the airways characterized by periodic and reversible

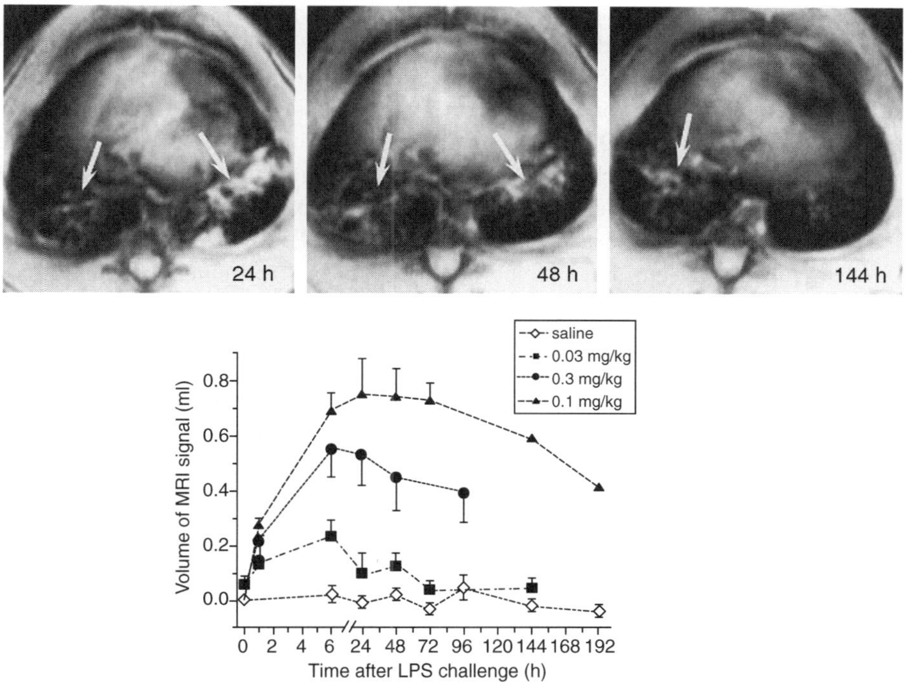

FIGURE 18.4 Images from a naïve BN rat at different time points with respect to an LPS challenge (1.0 mg/kg i.t. at time point 0). Acquisition parameters as described for Figure 18.4. The animal respired spontaneously, and neither respiratory nor cardiac triggering was applied. Notice that the LPS-induced signals are discontinuous and significantly less intense than those detected after OVA. The course of signals, derived from images acquired at different time points with respect to a saline or LPS challenge at the specified dose, reveals that they are of long duration. The number of animals per experimental group was six. (Reproduced from Beckmann, N. et al., *Am. J. Physiol. Lung Cell. Mol. Physiol.*, 283, L22, 2002. With permission from The American Physiological Society 2002.)

narrowing of the airways making breathing difficult. Bronchial hyperresponsiveness to various stimuli such as irritants, infection, exercise, cold air, or allergens is a key feature of asthma and is related to an enhanced sensitivity of the airway smooth muscle to contractile stimuli. In COPD, sustained smoking causes chronic inflammation of the airways responsible for mucosal thickening, airway narrowing, and loss of elastic recoil.

Pulmonary function tests providing global lung function information (such as forced expired volume in one second [FEV_1] or flow-volume pattern) are used to quantify the severity of lung diseases and to evaluate the efficiency of treatment. As mentioned previously, invasive measurements of airflow and transpulmonary pressure following stimulus by agents inducing bronchoconstriction are used to monitor lung function in rats [51]. However, these tests do not provide any regional information. The following subsections address efforts made to obtain regional information about lung function in rat models in a less invasive manner using HP He-3 or proton MRI (see also Chapter 19, Section 19.2.3.1).

18.4.2.1 Elastase-Induced Emphysema Model

At room temperature and atmospheric pressure, the self-diffusion coefficient of He-3 is equal to 2×10^5 cm^2/sec, whereas the diffusion coefficient of free water is about 2 cm^2/sec. However, the apparent diffusion coefficient (ADC) of He-3 in the healthy lung is typically one order of magnitude smaller than that of free water. This decrease in ADC is due to gas mixing effects (dilution of helium in pulmonary gases) and to the restriction of helium diffusion by the broncho-alveolar walls. The diffusion length of helium atoms during typical diffusion sensitizing times (a few milliseconds) exceeds the diameter of alveolar sacks (150 μm for small animals). Hence, in the time scale of MR diffusion acquisition, He-3 diffusion in the alveolar space takes place in a restricted regime.

The dependence of helium ADC values upon the dimensions of the alveolar space has been proposed as a noninvasive approach for probing the lung architecture at a subpixel level. Indeed, He-3 ADC values were shown to be significantly increased in patients with emphysema compared to healthy volunteers [67–69] (see also Chapter 19, Section 19.3.2). These He-3 ADC changes in emphysematous lungs were attributed to morphological changes in alveolar structure and more specifically to the airspace enlargements that characterize emphysema.

Elastase-induced emphysema [58] has been investigated in small rodents [70–72] using He-3 diffusion MRI. Measurements performed at end-expiratory inflation volume demonstrated an increase by 20% of ADC values in the lungs of elastase-treated rats compared to those in healthy control animals [70]. When measurements were carried out at total lung capacity, He-3 ADC values increased from 0.15 cm^2/sec in normal rats to 0.18 cm^2/sec in elastase-challenged animals. Moreover, a significant correlation (Figure 18.5) was found between the He-3 ADC values and the alveolar internal area assessed by histology in lungs fixed with formalin at an airway pressure corresponding to the total lung capacity [71]. Similarly, He-3 ADC values averaged over the entire lung were found to be approximately 25% higher in emphysema mice than in healthy animals [72]. However, mice exposed to cigarette smoke for a 12-month period did not reveal any significant increase in ADC values [72].

18.4.2.2 Airway Smooth Muscle Contraction

Methacholine is a synthetic analogue of the natural neurotransmitter acetylcholine. It can be administrated by inhalation and produces a muscle contraction in airways and parenchyma by stimulating the muscarinic cholinergic receptors. The methacholine challenge test is used routinely in the clinic to assess airway responsiveness. Results of pulmonary function tests (e.g., spirometry, specific conductance) performed before and after inhalation are used to quantify the bronchoconstrictor response.

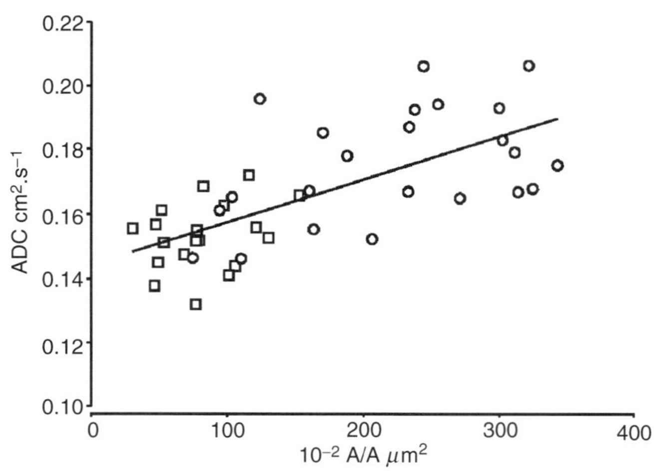

FIGURE 18.5 Correlation between ADC values of He-3 gas and the alveolar internal area determined by histology in elastase-treated (circles) and in control rats (squares). (Reproduced from Peces-Barba, G. et al., *Eur. Respir. J.*, 22, 14, 2003. With permission of European Respiratory Society Journals Ltd. Copyright 2003.)

The potential of He-3 MRI for assessing airway constriction has been investigated in methacholine-induced bronchoconstriction in rats. To allow for the acquisition of images, methacholine was injected i.v. and slowly, over a period of 30 to 60 sec. Using a CINE–MRI approach in which image acquisition (comprising a dynamic series of images over 150 gas breaths) was synchronized with the inhalation of the gas mixture (He-3 with oxygen and nitrogen), Chen and Johnson [73] showed heterogeneously distributed airway constriction resulting in a partition of the lung between ventilated and nonventilated regions (Figure 18.6). Superposition of helium and proton images allowed airway closure leading to air-trapping in the nonventilated lung regions to be observed. The diameter of the main airways decreased by approximately 11% following methacholine (30 μg). However, in some rats (four out of 24 animals) the ventilation images showed a hyperresponsiveness to methacholine, with a large fraction of the inspired gas confined to the major airways. Complete closure of the small airways resulted in hypoventilation of the animals and eventually led to their death. In this hyperreactive pattern, the diameters of the main airways (trachea, right and left major airway branch) increased by an average of 67%. A series of dynamic ventilation images obtained from a single breath were also used to generate parametric pixel-by-pixel maps of gas arrival time, filling time constant, inflation rate and gas volume in distal areas of the lung [74]. An average 12% decrease in inflation rate was measured following the administration of 85 μg methacholine. The inflation rate decreased further after 170 μg methacholine [74].

Proton MRI may also be used to detect the effects of bronchoconstrictor and bronchodilator compounds in spontaneously breathing rats. For instance, a significant increase of the parenchymal signal intensity was observed in the upper airways, from the first minutes following i.v. administration of a compound eliciting bronchoconstriction (Figure 18.7). The long lasting signal increase was reversed by application of a bronchodilator agent, consistent with an increase in oxygenation. Airway resistance measures derived invasively in anesthetized, paralyzed, and

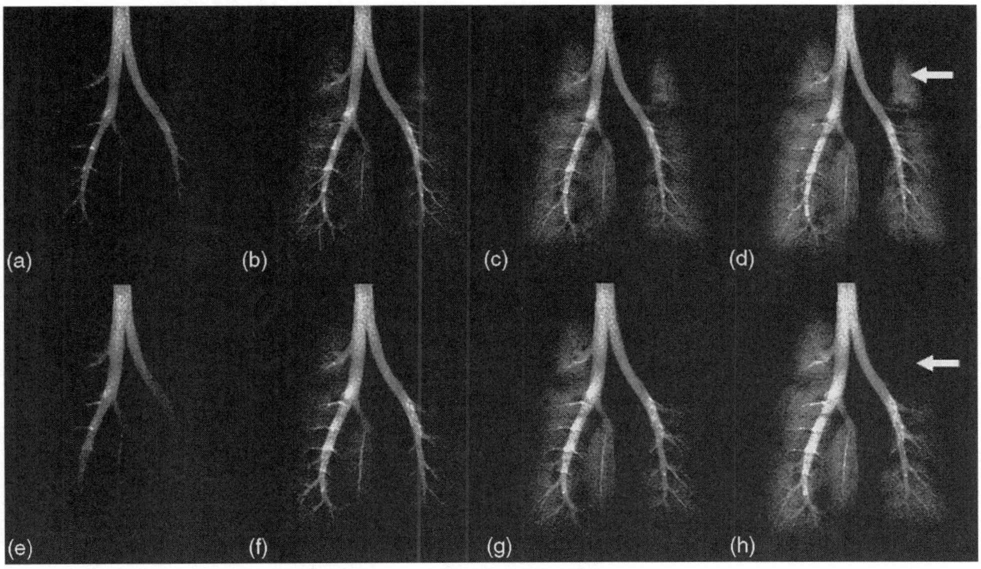

FIGURE 18.6 Bronchoconstriction induced in rats by methacholine administered intravenously. He-3 images were acquired using ventilation synchronized CINE imaging (28 msec acquisition window). Compared with the premethacholine images (a–d), delays of the inspired airflow and increases in the airway size were noticable in the postmethacholine images (e–h). (Reproduced from Chen, B. T. and Johnson, G. A., *Magn. Reson. Med.*, 52, 1080, 2004. Courtesy of Prof. G. A. Johnson, Duke University. With permission of John Wiley & Sons, Inc. Copyright 2004.)

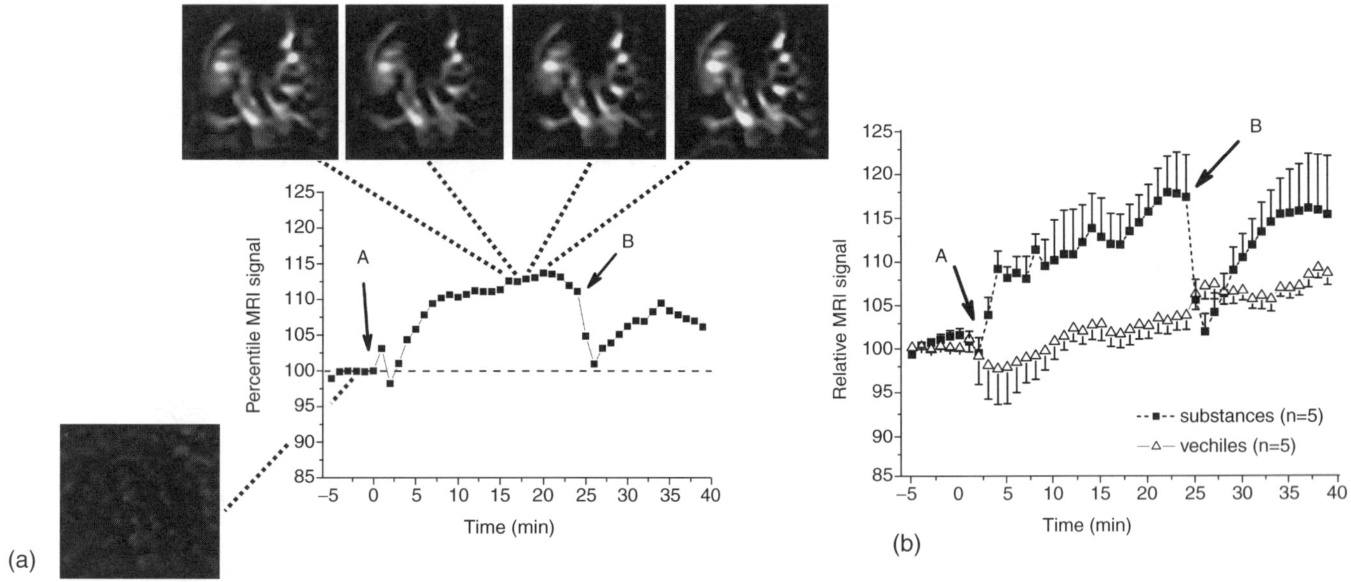

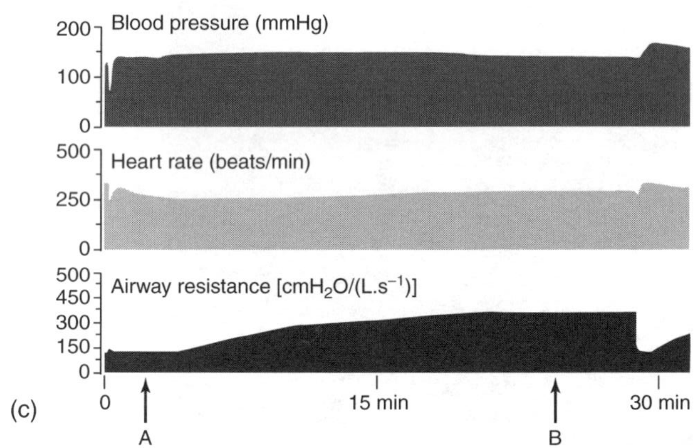

FIGURE 18.7 Bronchoconstriction examined using proton MRI in spontaneously breathing rats. Acquisition parameters as described in Figure 18.1, except for a number of averages 80, resulting in a measurement time of 1 min per image. Neither cardiac nor respiratory gating were applied. A bronchoconstrictor and a bronchorelaxant agent were administered i.v. at time points A and B, respectively. The agents induced significant signal changes as evidenced in the difference images (with respect to baseline images, acquired before time point A) and the course of the signal intensity in the upper airways. Note the similarity between the MRI signal profile and the airway resistance assessed invasively as described in Section 18.3. The compounds did not affect the blood pressure and heart rate. (Pulmonary function data included are a courtesy of Chica Ogueri and Lazzaro Mazzoni.)

artificially ventilated rats showed the same time profile as that of the MRI signal. These observations suggest that the MRI signal changes in the upper airways were due to bronchoconstrictor effects.

18.4.2.3 Pulmonary Embolism

As mentioned above, perfusion and ventilation matching is of crucial importance to maintain an efficient gas exchange in the lung. Regional mismatches between perfusion and ventilation distribution are typical of pulmonary embolism (PE) arising from pulmonary vessel obstruction. However, perfusion defects are not specific to PE and can also be found in neoplasms, infections, and COPD. Ventilation studies are needed to increase the diagnosis accuracy since, in contrast to PE, the latter diseases are also associated with ventilation defects. Usually, pulmonary ventilation and perfusion are estimated using radionuclide techniques such as scintigraphy which is a well-established clinical tool (for reviews, see Refs. [75–77]).

Perfusion measurements using He-3 MRI (see Section 18.2.3) were made in an experimental rat embolism model consisting in the intravascular injection of an air bubble [42,44,78]. Figure 18.8 shows transverse projection He images, obtained using He-3 microbubbles administered i.v. as contrast agent, superimposed on proton images. The left and right images were acquired, respectively, before and after the air bubble injection. Large perfusion defects are clearly visualized.

18.4.2.4 Airway Remodeling and Hyporesponsiveness Induced by Inflammation

Inflammation in the airways leads to pathophysiological changes in the structure of the lung tissue, including thickening of the airway smooth muscle [79], which may influence the responsiveness to bronchospasmogens [80] and alter ventilation. The progressive structural change known as airway remodeling, which is driven by chronic local inflammation, is a fundamental component in the development of airway hyperresponsiveness (for a recent review, see Ref. [81]).

Effects of airway remodeling and hyporesponsiveness following, respectively, allergen or endotoxin challenges can be monitored noninvasively in spontaneously breathing rats with a gradient-echo sequence as described in Beckmann et al. [8]. The basis of the approach consists of detecting modulations of proton signals of lung parenchyma induced by changes in oxygenation levels. As mentioned previously, an increased parenchymal signal should be consistent with a reduced oxygen level and vice versa. This hypothesis has been verified in the allergen and

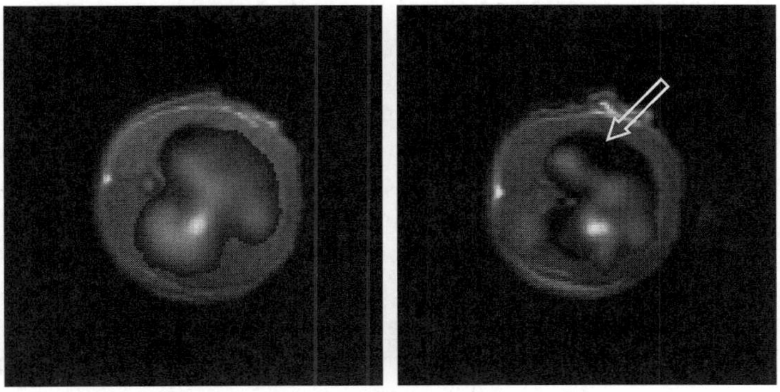

FIGURE 18.8 Combined proton and He-3 images in rats in an experimental rat pulmonary embolism. The helium images correspond to the distribution of He-3 microbubbles inside the lung vasculature. The image on the right was acquired a few minutes following the induction of a gaseous pulmonary embolism as indicated by the white arrow. (Reproduced from Callot, V. et al., *Magn. Reson. Med.*, 46, 535, 2001. With permission of John Wiley & Sons, Inc. Copyright 2001.)

endotoxin models of airways inflammation in the rat [9]. In actively sensitized rats, increased parenchymal signal intensity (in areas devoid of fluid signals) was detected at 6 h and up to 180 h after challenge, at a time when fluid signals reflecting inflammation had completely resolved. Histological analysis revealed airway remodeling in the lungs of OVA-challenged rats characterized as increased bronchial epithelium thickness and smooth muscle area, as well as bronchial goblet cell hyperplasia. Thus, the increased parenchymal signal in lung images of rats treated with allergen was consistent with a significant reduction of air space determined by histology, pointing to an impaired lung ventilation in these animals. The ventilation defect remained even after fluid signals detected by MRI were completely resolved [9].

In a second model, a significantly decreased parenchymal signal intensity was detected 24 h after intratracheal instillation of LPS [9]. The effect was abolished by pretreatment with N^G-nitro-L-arginine methyl ester (L-NAME), an inhibitor of nitric oxide (NO) synthase (NOS). A possible role of NO in the inflammatory response elicited by endotoxin has been demonstrated by Pauwels et al. [82], who showed that a period of significant hyporesponsiveness, characterized by reduced pulmonary resistance due to increased airway caliber, followed from 9 to 12 h after exposure of rats to aerosolized LPS. In the same model, LPS-induced airway hyporesponsiveness was eliminated by L-NAME [83]. Moreover, marked expression of inducible NOS in rat macrophages recovered from the airways has been demonstrated 16 h after local LPS instillation [84]. Therefore, endogenous synthesis of NO, a potent bronchodilator [85], induced by the endotoxin might have been responsible for an increased oxygenation of the lung tissue, thus contributing to a reduction of the parenchymal signal in the gradient-echo images 24 h following LPS administration.

18.5 DRUG TREATMENT ANALYSIS

A variety of new compounds for the treatment of respiratory diseases are in development, many of which are designed as anti-inflammatory therapies [5,86]. Since edema is an integral component of experimental pulmonary inflammation, MRI has the potential to provide a noninvasive means of monitoring the course of the inflammatory response and the consequence of therapy with antiinflammatory drugs.

We consider first the classic approach of analyzing the effects of antiinflammatory drugs administered prior to allergen challenge. A clear dose-related reduction of the fluid signal has been shown for compounds such as the glucocorticosteroids budesonide [18,61] and mometasone [87], and for a mitogen-activated protein kinase inhibitor [87]. The effects correlated with changes in the parameters of inflammation assessed in the BAL fluid [56]. Repeated measurements allowed information on the duration of action to be easily defined.

The MRI technique was also applied to address the effects of drugs administered after the allergic inflammatory response has developed. In one experimental paradigm the drugs are given 24 h after the challenge with OVA, a time point when an extensive MRI signal is present in the rat lung. Treatment with budesonide, mometasone, or with a selective inhibitor of phosphodiesterase type 4 (PDE4), which is also a powerful inhibitor of allergic pulmonary inflammation in the rat [88], accelerated the rate of resolution of the MRI signal [18,61,87]. For these compounds, a clear trend towards a reduction in the fluid signal was observed as early as 3 h after drug administration, and the effect was statistically significant from 6 to 72 h (Figure 18.9). The decline in the fluid signal correlated significantly with the reduction in perivascular edema quantified by histology of the lungs [61]. This suggests that an effect to suppress perivascular edema underlied the decrease in the MRI signal following therapeutic treatment with budesonide, mometasone, or the PDE4 inhibitor. By contrast, BAL fluid markers of inflammation were not affected by either compound 6 h after treatment [61]. It seems, accordingly, that the early resolution of MRI fluid signals by the antiinflammatory drugs did not involve general suppression of the inflammatory response at least as monitored by BAL fluid analysis. At 48 h following treatment with the steroids

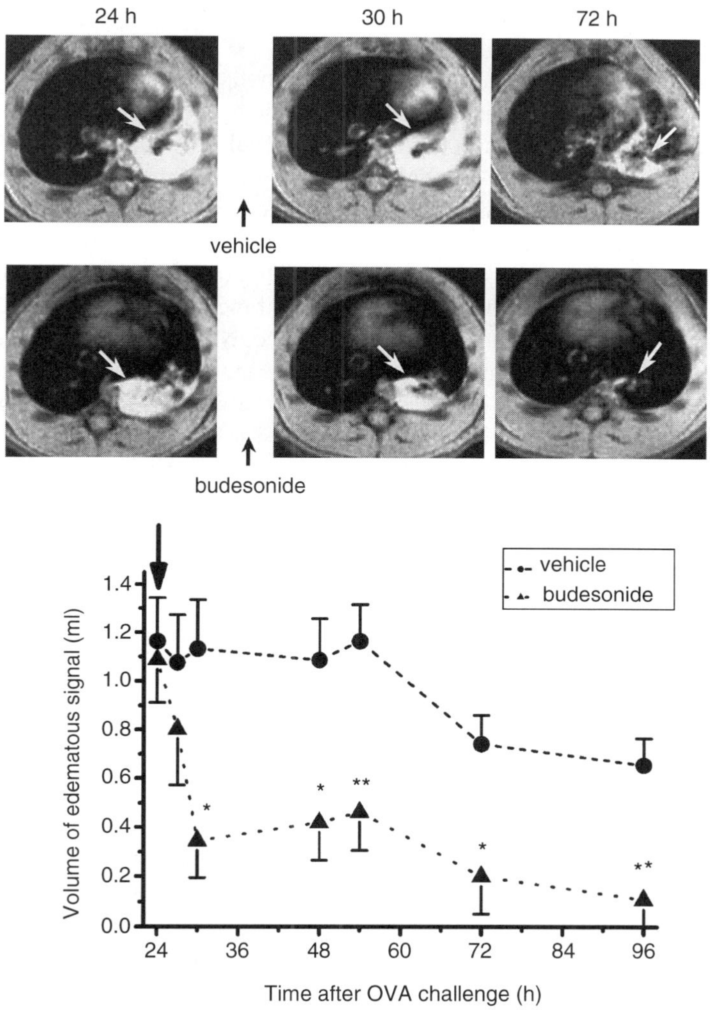

FIGURE 18.9 Assessment of posttreatment effects on established allergic inflammation of a glucocorticosteroid (budesonide). Either budesonide (1 mg/kg i.t.) or its vehicle were applied 24 h after OVA (0.3 mg/kg i.t.) challenge. Images were acquired at several time points with respect to OVA challenge. Acquisition parameters as in Figure 18.3. The animal respired spontaneously and neither respiratory nor cardiac triggering was applied. The number of rats per group was six. The rapid effect of the compound on the established inflammation was translated into a reduction of the fluid signals detected by MRI in the lungs. (Adapted from Beckmann, N. et al., *Magn. Reson. Med.*, 45, 88, 2001 and Tigani, B. et al., *Br. J. Pharmacol.*, 140, 239, 2003. With permission of John Wiley & Sons, Inc. and from the Nature Publishing Group Copyright 2001.)

or with a PDE4 inhibitor, MPO activity and protein concentrations were significantly reduced and, in animals treated with the PDE4 inhibitor, eosinophil number and EPO activity were also significantly diminished [61]. These changes may be the mechanistic basis for the sustained resolution of MRI signals.

The question arises as to the mechanism(s) by which budesonide, mometasone, or a PDE4 inhibitor suppressd perivascular edema and the fluid signal in the absence of any effect on BAL fluid parameters of inflammation at 6 h following drug administration. Postulated mechanisms for changes in permeability would be that the compounds suppressd the ongoing protein extravasation by local vasoconstriction [89] or cAMP-induced relaxation of tight junctions between epithelial and endothelial cells.

In the last two decades, studies of lung liquid transport have provided important new concepts on the cellular mechanisms contributing to lung edema clearance. Fluid transport is believed to be regulated by ion transport through epithelial sodium channels (ENaC), and Na^+-K^+-ATPase, with water movement occuring osmotically (for a review see Ref. [90]). Proposed mechanisms for upregulation of sodium transport proteins by cAMP include augmented channel open probability, enhanced regulation of ENaC channels and stimulated Na^+-K^+-ATPase activity [91]. There is evidence that pharmacological treatment with β_2 adrenoceptor agonists increases fluid clearance [92] and that cAMP is a second messenger for the effects [93]. Another possible mechanism for the prompt resolution of the MRI signals seen at 6 h would be involvement of aquaporins, a family of water membrane channel proteins, which has been suggested to have a potential role in water movement between the vascular, interstitial spaces and airway compartments (for a review see Ref. [94]). The ability of inflammatory cytokines to decrease aquaporin expression might help to explain the relationship between inflammation and edema in the lung [95].

In addition to profiling antiinflammatory compounds, MRI can also be used to address the effects of compounds designed to improve lung function. For instance, the examples discussed in Section 18.4.2.2 suggest that He-3 and proton MRI approaches have the potential to profile bronchodilator compounds in models of airways obstruction.

18.6 DISCUSSION

In the past few years, especially since the introduction of HP approaches, significant developments have been made in imaging the lungs of humans and animals. Such developments are of interest for many aspects of research in the area of respiratory diseases. In this chapter we have discussed how several proton and HP MRI techniques enable one to reliably detect anatomical and functional changes in the lungs of rats in models of airway diseases. This opens the opportunity to noninvasive analyses of drug effects in such models, in which inflammation plays a key role.

In pharmacological studies of pulmonary inflammation at the preclinical level, analysis of BAL fluid or histology are the techniques routinely used to assess the inflammatory status of the lung and the result of drug intervention. Albeit providing comprehensive information at the cellular level, these methods have the drawback of being terminal. Here, we showed how proton MRI can provide complementary information with a fundamental asset: its noninvasive character. Repeated measurements can be carried out on the same animal, and time courses of events become easily assessable. The significant correlation between the proton MRI signals and the perivascular edema determined by histology provides the base for the noninvasive assessment of a key component of inflammation in a rat model of allergic asthma, enabling rapid effects of drugs to be detected *in vivo* by monitoring the rate at which fluid signals resolve. Also, the prospect of using MRI to detect noninvasively a sustained mucus hypersecretory phenotype induced by endotoxin brings an important new perspective to models of COPD in animals. Hence, despite being a macroscopic technique, MRI allows overall assessment of the time-related behavior of compounds in models of lung inflammation in rats. With this information it becomes easier to choose the time point for carrying out BAL fluid or histological analysis in order to obtain more specific information on the drug mechanism. A further important consideration is the fact that proton MRI acquisitions can be carried out on spontaneously breathing animals. Therefore, interference with the pathophysiology should be minimal. The method allows a reasonably high throughput, of about 30 to 40 rats measured per day. Semi-automatic image analysis procedures enable relatively fast data evaluation, so that results are available the same day of measurement.

Besides addressing inflammation, MRI is also able to provide important information on the functional status of the lungs. For sensitivity reasons, HP techniques are extremely attractive in this context. Regional information on ventilation and gas diffusion are the primary readouts. For instance, HP He-3 MRI allows detection of bronchoconstriction at high spatial and temporal resolution. This is of great interest when testing bronchodilator compounds and their sites of action. The routine application of HP gas MRI in the context of pharmaceutical research is, however, not trivial:

1. Systems for the generation of HP gases are currently not commercially available.
2. Complex instrumentation is required for controlling the respiration and delivering the gas. Animals are ventilated and sometimes tracheotomized, which in many respects may hamper repetitive measurements, reduce throughput, and influence the pathophysiology. Measurements in spontaneously breathing animals would require the use of more gas and further diminish throughput because of the limited amount of HP gas that can be generated per day (about 1 to 2 L with a polarization of up to 30% using the spin-exchange OP technique; with the more involved metastable OP approach, higher quantities of gas with a polarization of up to 60% can be produced).
3. Nonstandard acquisition schemes are necessary to generate the images.

It is clear that the sensitivity and spatial resolution achieved using this approach are tremendous. It still needs to be shown, however, that the better quality of He-3 compared to proton images translates into meaningful advantages within the realm of pharmaceutical research. Some of the examples presented above illustrate the fact that proton MRI also provides important information on lung function. Of particular interest is its potential to map bronchoconstriction in spontaneously breathing animals, as shown in Figure 18.7. Comparative studies for the same models are required to establish the pros and cons of each approach.

Several developments are to be expected in the area of lung imaging in small rodents. Several studies have demonstrated the usefulness of lung MRI in mice [8,33,72,96–98]. This is a very important development in view of the use of wildtype and transgenic mice in pharmaceutical research, since a large number of models is available in such animals. Furthermore, a new generation of imaging devices, part of a collective effort known as molecular imaging, provides the potential to generate both structural and functional images for the study of lung biology in small rodents (see Ref. [99] for a review). In addition to MRI, micro x-ray computed tomography (micro-CT) and positron emission tomography scanners, highly sensitive cooled charge coupled device cameras for bioluminescence and fluorescence imaging, and recent advances in ultrasound system technology can be used to study such diverse processes as ventilation, perfusion, pulmonary hypertension, lung inflammation, and gene transfer, among others. The idea is to fuse images from more than one imaging modality, allowing structure-function relationships to be studied on a regional basis.

Let us consider micro-CT as an example. This modality is important since CT is the imaging modality of choice for diagnosis of lung diseases in the clinics. Commercially available micro-CT devices are able to perform respiratory gated *in vivo* acquisitions suitable for thoracic imaging [100,101]. The radiation dose is approximately 0.15 Gy for a respiratory-gated micro-CT imaging protocol. The combination of high-resolution CT imaging and respiratory-gated acquisitions appears to be well suited for serial *in vivo* scanning. In a recent *ex vivo* study, Langheinrich et al. [102] showed that micro-CT is feasible for structural evaluation of the lung fine structure and its alterations during endotoxin-induced lung injury in the rat. Systemic application of endotoxin led to a significant increase in the soft-tissue volume of the lungs (i.e., tissue edema) and significant thickening of the alveolar walls at micro-CT.

Overall, we are confident that MRI and other imaging techniques will play an increasingly important role in preclinical research on small rodents in the area of airway diseases. The noninvasive character of the approaches should facilitate not only drug assessments in animal models, but also provide relevant data for the transition into clinical trials.

ACKNOWLEDGMENTS

Dr. Lazzaro Mazzoni is gratefully acknowledged for important insights into the areas of lung physiology and pharmacology. We thank Catherine Cannet for the excellent histological support. NB acknowledges the receipt of an award from the 3R Research Foundation, Münsingen, Switzerland (Project No. 82/02).

REFERENCES

1. Kroegel, C. et al., Pulmonary immune cells in health and disease: the eosinophil leucocyte (Part I), *Eur. Respir. J.*, 7, 519, 1994.
2. Barnes, P. J., Pathophysiology of asthma, *Br. J. Clin. Pharmacol.*, 42, 3, 1996.
3. Moqbel, R., Eosinophil-derived cytokines in allergic inflammation and asthma, *Ann. N.Y. Acad. Sci.*, 796, 209, 1996.
4. Sethi, S., Pathogenesis and treatment of acute exacerbations of chronic obstructive pulmonary disease, *Semin. Respir. Crit. Care Med.*, 26, 192, 2005.
5. Barnes, P. J., New treatments for COPD, *Nat. Rev. Drug Discov.*, 1, 437, 2002.
6. Beckmann, N. et al., Magnetic resonance imaging of the lung provides potential for non-invasive preclinical evaluation of drugs, *Trends Pharmacol. Sci.*, 24, 550, 2003.
7. Hatabu, H. et al., T_2^* and proton density measurement of normal human lung parenchyma using submillisecond echo time gradient echo magnetic resonance imaging, *Eur. J. Radiol.*, 29, 245, 1999.
8. Beckmann, N. et al., MRI of lung parenchyma in rats and mice using a gradient-echo sequence, *NMR Biomed.*, 14, 297, 2001.
9. Beckmann, N. et al., Proton MRI of lung parenchyma reflects allergen-induced airway remodeling and endotoxin-aroused hyporesponsiveness: a step towards ventilation studies in spontaneously breathing rats, *Magn. Reson. Med.*, 52, 258, 2004.
10. Kveder, M. et al., Water proton relaxation mechanisms in lung tissue, *Magn. Reson. Med.*, 7, 432, 1988.
11. Burney, C. H., Bertolina, J., and Ailion, D. C., Calculation and interpretation of inhomogeneous line broadening in models of lung and other heterogeneous structures, *J. Magn. Reson.*, 85, 554, 1989.
12. Bergin, C. J., Pauly, J. M., and Macovski, A., Lung parenchyma: projection reconstruction MR imaging, *Radiology*, 179, 777, 1991.
13. Gewalt, S. L. et al., MR microscopy of the rat lung using projection reconstruction, *Magn. Reson. Med.*, 29, 99, 1993.
14. Bergin, C. J. et al., MR imaging of lung parenchyma: a solution to susceptibility, *Radiology*, 183, 673, 1992.
15. Ahn, C. B., Kim, J. H., and Cho, Z. H., High speed spiral-scan echo planar NMR imaging, *IEEE MI-5*, 1, 2, 1986.
16. Liao, J. R. et al., Reduction of motion artifacts in cine MRI using variable-density spiral trajectories, *Magn. Reson. Med.*, 37, 569, 1997.
17. Hedlund, L. W. et al., MR-compatible ventilator for small animals: computer-controlled ventilation for proton and noble gas imaging, *Magn. Reson. Imaging*, 18, 753, 2000.
18. Beckmann, N. et al., Pulmonary edema induced by allergen challenge in the rat: noninvasive assessment by magnetic resonance imaging, *Magn. Reson. Med.*, 45, 88, 2001.
19. Edelman, R. R. et al., Noninvasive assessment of regional ventilation in the human lung using oxygen-enhanced magnetic resonance imaging, *Nature Med.*, 2, 1236, 1996.
20. Morris, A. H. et al., A new nuclear magnetic resonance property of lung, *J. Appl. Physiol.*, 58, 759, 1985.

21. Case, T. A. et al., A mathematical model of diamagnetic line broadening in lung tissue and similar heterogeneous systems: calculations and measurements, *J. Magn. Reson.*, 73, 304, 1987.
22. Kuethe, D. O. et al., Imaging lungs using inert fluorinated gases, *Magn. Reson. Med.*, 39, 85, 1998.
23. Kuethe, D. O. et al., Imaging obstructed ventilation with NMR using inert fluorinated gases, *J. Appl. Physiol.*, 88, 2279, 2000.
24. Kuethe, D. O., Behr, V. C., and Begay, S., Volume of rat lungs measured throughout the respiratory cycle using 19F NMR of the inert gas SF6, *Magn. Reson. Med.*, 48, 547, 2002.
25. Goodson, B. M., Nuclear magnetic resonance of laser-polarized noble gases in molecules, materials, and organisms, *J. Magn. Reson.*, 155, 157, 2002.
26. Möller, H. E. et al., MRI of the lungs using hyperpolarized noble gases, *Magn. Reson. Med.*, 47, 1029, 2002.
27. Albert, M. S. et al., Biological magnetic resonance imaging using laser-polarized 129Xe, *Nature*, 370, 199, 1994.
28. Middleton, H. et al., MR imaging with hyperpolarized 3He gas, *Magn. Reson. Med.*, 33, 271, 1995.
29. Oros, A. M. and Shah, N. J., Hyperpolarized xenon in NMR and MRI, *Phys. Med. Biol.*, 49, R105, 2004.
30. Kauczor, H.-U., Surkau, R., and Roberts, T., MRI using hyperpolarized noble gases, *Eur. Radiol.*, 8, 820, 1998.
31. Hedlund, L. W. et al., Mixing oxygen with hyperpolarized (3)He for small-animal lung studies, *NMR Biomed.*, 13, 202, 2000.
32. Ramirez, M. P. et al., Physiological response of rats to delivery of helium and xenon: implications for hyperpolarized noble gas imaging, *NMR Biomed.*, 13, 253, 2000.
33. Chen, B. T., Yordanov, A. T., and Johnson, G. A., Ventilation-synchronous magnetic resonance microscopy of pulmonary structure and ventilation in mice, *Magn. Reson. Med.*, 53, 69, 2005.
34. Viallon, M. et al., Functional MR microscopy of the lung with hyperpolarized ^{3}He, *Magn. Reson. Med.*, 41, 787, 1999.
35. Viallon, M. et al., Dynamic imaging of hyperpolarized (3)He distribution in rat lungs using interleaved-spiral scans, *NMR Biomed.*, 13, 207, 2000.
36. Chen, B. T., Brau, A. C. S., and Johnson, G. A., Measurement of regional lung function in rats using hyperpolarized 3Helium dynamic MRI, *Magn. Reson. Med.*, 49, 78, 2003.
37. Hatabu, H. et al., Pulmonary perfusion: qualitative assessment with dynamic contrast-enhanced MRI using ultra-short TE and inversion recovery Turbo FLASH, *Magn. Reson. Med.*, 36, 503, 1996.
38. Mai, V. M. et al., Ventilation-perfusion ratio of signal intensity in human lung using oxygen-enhanced and arterial spin labeling techniques, *Magn. Reson Med.*, 48, 341, 2002.
39. Lipson, D. A. et al., Pulmonary ventilation and perfusion scanning using hyperpolarized helium-3 MRI and arterial spin tagging in healthy normal subjects and in pulmonary embolism and orthotopic lung transplant patients, *Magn. Reson. Med.*, 47, 1073, 2002.
40. Berthezène, Y. et al., Contrast-enhanced MR imaging of the lung: assessments of ventilation and perfusion, *Radiology*, 183, 667, 1992.
41. Crémillieux, Y. et al., A combined ^{1}H perfusion/^{3}He ventilation NMR study in rat lungs, *Magn. Reson. Med.*, 41, 645, 1999.
42. Viallon, M. et al., Laser-polarized 3He as a probe for dynamic regional measurements of lung perfusion and ventilation using magnetic resonance imaging, *Magn. Reson. Med.*, 44, 1, 2000.
43. Stupar, V. et al., Helium3 polarization using spin exchange technique: application to simultaneous pulmonary ventilation/perfusion imaging in small animals, *Invest. Radiol.*, 38, 334, 2003.
44. Callot, V. et al., Vascular and perfusion imaging using encapsulated laser-polarized helium, *MAGMA*, 12, 16, 2001.
45. Callot, V. et al., Hyperpolarized helium3 encapsulated in microbubbles: a new class of blood pool MRI contrast agent, *Acad. Radiol.*, 9(Suppl. 2), S501, 2002.
46. Dawkins, P. A. and Stockley, R. A., Animal models of chronic obstructive pulmonary disease, *Thorax*, 56, 972, 2001.

47. Canning, B. J., Modeling asthma and COPD in animals: a pointless exercise?, *Curr. Op. Pharmacol.*, 3, 244, 2003.
48. Isenberg-Feig, H., Justice, J. P., and Keane-Myers, A., Animal models of allergic asthma, *Curr. Allergy Asthma Rep.*, 3, 70, 2003.
49. Renzi, P. M., Olivenstein, R., and Martin, J. G., Inflammatory cell populations in the airways and parenchyma after antigen challenge in the rat, *Am. Rev. Resp. Dis.*, 147, 967, 1993.
50. Haczku, A. et al., Adoptive transfer of allergen-specific $CD4^{+}T$ cells induces airway inflammation and hyperresponsiveness in brown-Norway rats, *Immunology*, 91, 176, 1997.
51. Hannon, J. P. et al., Mechanism of airway hyperresponsiveness to adenoside induced by allergen challenge in actively sensitized Brown Norway rats, *Br. J. Pharmacol.*, 132, 1509, 2001.
52. Watson, R. W., Redmond, H. P., and Bouchier-Hayes, D., Role of endotoxin in mononuclear phagocyte-mediated inflammatory responses, *J. Leukoc. Biol.*, 56, 95, 1994.
53. Yang, R. B. et al., Toll-like receptor-2 mediates lipopolysaccharide-induced cellular signalling, *Nature*, 395, 284, 1998.
54. Albelda, S. M., Smith, C. W., and Ward, P. A., Adhesion molecules and inflammatory injury, *FASEB J.*, 8, 504, 1994.
55. Tesfaigzi, Y. et al., Bcl-2 in LPS- and allergen-induced hyperplastic mucous cells in airway epithelia of Brown Norway rats, *Am. J. Physiol. Lung Cell Mol. Physiol.*, 279, L1210, 2000.
56. Tigani, B. et al., Pulmonary inflammation monitored non-invasively by MRI in freely breathing rats, *Biochem. Biophys. Res. Commun.*, 292, 216, 2002.
57. Harkema, J. R. and Hotchkiss, J. A., In vivo effects of endotoxin on intraepithelial mucosubstances in rat pulmonary airways. Quantitative histochemistry, *Am. J. Pathol.*, 141, 307, 1992.
58. Busch, R. H. et al., Experimental pulmonary emphysema induced in the rat by intratracheally administered elastase: morphogenesis, *Environ. Res.*, 33, 497, 1984.
59. Riedel, M., Venous thromboembolic disease; acute pulmonary embolism 1: pathophysiology, clinical presentation, and diagnosis, *Heart*, 1, 229, 2001.
60. Ayach, B. et al., Effects of a selective endothelin A receptor antagonist, ABT-627, in healthy normotensive anaesthetized rats developing acute pulmonary air embolism, *Clin. Sci. (Lond.)*, 103(Suppl. 48), 371S, 2002.
61. Tigani, B. et al., Resolution of the oedema associated with allergic pulmonary inflammation in rats, *Br. J. Pharmacol.*, 140, 239, 2003.
62. Jansson, A. H., Eriksson, C., and Wang, X., Lung inflammatory responses and hyperinflation induced by an intratracheal exposure to lipopolysaccharide in rats, *Lung*, 182, 163, 2004.
63. Beckmann, N. et al., Non-invasive detection of endotoxin induced mucus hypersecretion in rat lung by magnetic resonance imaging, *Am. J. Physiol. Lung Cell. Mol. Physiol.*, 283, L22, 2002.
64. Tigani, B. et al., Near-infrared fluorescence imaging and histology confirm anomalous edematous signal distribution detected in the rat lung by MRI after allergen challenge, *J. Magn. Reson. Imaging*, 20, 967, 2004.
65. Yeh, H. C., Schum, G. M., and Duggan, M. T., Anatomic models of the tracheobronchial and pulmonary regions of the rat, *Anat. Rec.*, 195, 483, 1979.
66. Burri, P. A., Dhaly, J., and Weibel, E. R., The post-natal growth of the rat lung: I Morphometry, *Anat. Rec.*, 178, 711, 1973.
67. Saam, B. T. et al., MR imaging of diffusion of (3)He gas in healthy and diseased lungs, *Magn. Reson. Med.*, 44, 174, 2000.
68. Salerno, M. et al., Emphysema: hyperpolarized helium 3 diffusion MR imaging of the lungs compared with spirometric indexes — initial experience, *Radiology*, 222, 252, 2002.
69. Salerno, M. et al., Rapid hyperpolarized 3He diffusion MRI of healthy and emphysematous human lungs using an optimized interleaved-spiral pulse sequence, *J. Magn. Reson. Imaging*, 17, 581, 2003.
70. Chen, X. J. et al., Detection of emphysema in rat lungs by using magnetic resonance measurements of ^{3}He diffusion, *Proc. Natl. Acad. Sci. USA*, 97, 11478, 2000.
71. Peces-Barba, G., et al., Helium-3, M R I diffusion coefficient: correlation to morphometry in a model of mild emphysema, *Eur. Respir. J.*, 22, 14, 2003.
72. Dugas, J. P. et al., Hyperpolarized (3)He MRI of mouse lung, *Magn. Reson. Med.*, 52, 1310, 2004.

73. Chen, B. T. and Johnson, G. A., Dynamic lung morphology of methacholine-induced heterogeneous bronchoconstriction, *Magn. Reson. Med.*, 52, 1080, 2004.
74. Dupuich, D. et al., Dynamic 3He imaging for quantification of regional lung ventilation parameters, *Magn. Reson. Med.*, 50, 777, 2003.
75. Schumichen, C., V/Q-scanning/SPECT for the diagnosis of pulmonary embolism, *Respiration*, 70, 329, 2003.
76. Worsley, D. F. and Alavi, A., Radionuclide imaging of acute pulmonary embolism, *Semin. Nucl. Med.*, 33, 259, 2003.
77. Khan, A., Cann, A. D., and Shah, R. D., Imaging of acute pulmonary emboli, *Thorac. Surg. Clin.*, 14, 113, 2004.
78. Callot, V. et al., MR perfusion imaging using encapsulated polarized He3, *Magn. Reson. Med.*, 46, 535, 2001.
79. Ebina, M. et al., Cellular hypertrophy and hyperplasia of airway smooth muscles underlying bronchial asthma: A 3-D morphometric study, *Am. Rev. Respir. Dis.*, 148, 720, 1993.
80. Martin, J. G., Duguet, A., and Eidelman, D. H., The contribution of airway smooth muscle to airway narrowing and airway hyperresponsiveness in disease, *Eur. Respir. J.*, 16, 349, 2000.
81. Halayko, A. J. and Amrani, Y., Mechanisms of inflammation-mediated airway smooth muscle plasticity and airways remodeling in asthma, *Respir. Physiol. Neurobiol.*, 137, 209, 2003.
82. Pauwels, R. A. et al., The effect of endotoxin inhalation on airway responsiveness and cellular influx in rats, *Am. Rev. Respir. Dis.*, 141, 540, 1990.
83. Kips, J. C. et al., The effect of a nitric oxide synthase inhibitor on the modulation of airway responsiveness in rats, *Am. J. Respir. Crit. Care Med.*, 151, 1165, 1995.
84. Kobzik, L. et al., Nitric oxide synthase in human and rat lung: immunocytochemical and histochemical localization, *Am. J. Respir. Cell. Mol. Biol.*, 9, 371, 1993.
85. Abderrahmane, A. et al., Direct activation of K_{Ca} channel in airway smooth muscle by nitric oxide: involvement of a nitrothiosylation mechanism?, *Am. J. Respir. Cell. Mol. Biol.*, 19, 485, 1998.
86. Barnes, P. J., New drugs for asthma, *Nat. Rev. Drug Discov.*, 3, 831, 2004.
87. Tigani, B. et al., Effects of a mitogen-activated protein kinase inhibitor on allergic airways inflammation in the rat studied by magnetic resonance imaging, *Eur. J. Pharmacol.*, 482, 319, 2003.
88. Trifilieff, A. et al., Pharmacological profile of a novel phosphodiesterase 4 inhibitor, 4-(8-benzo[1,2,5]oxadiazol-5-yl-[1,7]naphthyridin-6-yl)-benzoic acid (NVP-ABE171), a 1,7-naphthyridine derivative, with anti-inflammatory activities, *J. Pharmacol. Exp. Ther.*, 301, 241, 2002.
89. Acuna, A. A. et al., Fluticasone propionate attenuates platelet-activating factor-induced gas exchange defects in mild asthma, *Eur. Respir. J.*, 19, 872, 2002.
90. Matthay, M. A., Folkesson, H. G., and Clerici, C., Lung epithelial fluid transport and the resolution of pulmonary edema, *Physiol. Rev.*, 82, 569, 2002.
91. Chen, X.-J., Eaton, D. C., and Jain, L., β-Adrenergic regulation of amiloride-sensitive lung sodium channels, *Am. J. Physiol. Lung Cell. Mol. Physiol.*, 282, L609, 2002.
92. Charron, P. D., Fawley, J. P., and Maron, M. B., Effect of epinephrine on alveolar liquid clearance in the rat, *J. Appl. Physiol.*, 87, 611, 1999.
93. Goodman, B. E., Anderson, J. L., and Clemens, J. W., Evidence for regulation of sodium transport from airspace to vascular space by cAMP, *Am. J. Physiol. Lung Cell. Mol. Physiol.*, 257, L86, 1989.
94. Beitz, E. and Schultz, J. E., The mammalian aquaporin water channel family: a promising new drug target, *Curr. Med. Chem.*, 6, 457, 1999.
95. Towne, J. E. et al., Tumor necrosis factor-a inhibits aquaporin 5 expression in mouse lung epithelial cells, *J. Biol. Chem.*, 276, 18657, 2001.
96. Garbow, J. R., Zhang, Z., and You, M., Detection of primary lung tumors in rodents by magnetic resonance imaging, *Cancer Res.*, 64, 2740, 2004.
97. Heverhagen, J. T. et al., Volumetric analysis of mice lungs in a clinical magnetic resonance imaging scanner, *MAGMA*, 17, 80, 2004.
98. Huang, M. Q. et al., MRI detection of tumor in mouse lung using partial liquid ventilation with a perfluorocarbon-in-water emulsion, *Magn. Reson. Imaging*, 22, 645, 2004.

99. Schuster, D. P. et al., Recent advances in imaging the lungs of intact small animals, *Am. J. Respir. Cell. Mol. Biol.*, 30, 129, 2004.
100. Cavanaugh, D. et al., In vivo respiratory-gated micro-CT imaging in small-animal oncology models, *Mol. Imaging*, 3, 55, 2004.
101. Hu, J. et al., Dynamic small animal lung imaging via a postacquisition respiratory gating technique using micro-cone beam computed tomography, *Acad. Radiol.*, 11, 961, 2004.
102. Langheinrich, A. C. et al., Acute rat lung injury: feasibility of assessment with micro-CT, *Radiology*, 233, 165, 2004.

19 Clinical Applications of MRI in Respiratory Diseases

Christian Fink and Hans-Ulrich Kauczor

CONTENTS

19.1 INTRODUCTION

During recent years, magnetic resonance imaging (MRI) has been established as a first-line imaging modality for a number of indications in various parts of the body. In the lungs, however, MRI has not gained the importance of computed tomography (CT) for the radiological evaluation of respiratory disease, and has only been considered as an alternative imaging modality when findings were inconclusive or in the case of contraindication to iodinated contrast media. On the other hand, MRI offers potential advantages over CT for the assessment of respiratory disease. In addition to the lower toxicity of the used MR contrast media and the lack of ionizing radiation, MRI provides a much better soft tissue contrast than CT and offers a variety of contrast options (e.g., T_1-weighting, T_2-weighting, fat saturation) [1]. One of the most important advantages of MRI, however, is the ability of functional measurements allowing for an evaluation of lung function on a regional basis. This chapter will discuss the various technical aspects of clinical pulmonary MRI, as well as its clinical application to different kinds of respiratory diseases.

19.2 LUNG MRI

19.2.1 MORPHOLOGICAL MRI

Using conventional spin-echo (SE) MRI, the normal lung is barely visible. Apart from the low proton density of lung tissue, the signal is further corrupted by flow, motion, and the high magnetic susceptibility of lung tissue [2]. The latter is caused by multiple air-tissue interfaces in the lungs which induce many local gradients leading to signal loss from intravoxel phase dispersion. The result is a complex spectrum of frequencies spread across up to 9 ppm and a very short T_2^* relaxation time of approximately 7 ms at 1.5 T *in vitro* and *in vivo* [3]. While this may hamper the visualization of normal lung parenchyma or emphysematous lung, the low signal intensity of the normal lung makes it quite easy to visualize consolidations within the lung. This is because the loss of air and concomitant increase of tissue, cells, or fluid significantly reduces the number of air–tissue interfaces and thus the susceptibility of the lung with an increase of the T_2^*-relaxation time at 1.5 T to 35 ms in atelectatic lung and to more than 140 ms in lung tumor [1].

Technically, the signal of normal lung can be increased by reducing the effects of the short T_2^*. For T_1-weighted MRI, gradient echo pulse sequences such as fast low-angle shot (FLASH) with short echo times (TE) have been proposed [4]. An additional advantage of gradient echo MRI is that due to the short acquisition times, imaging can be performed during breath-hold, thereby minimizing the amount of artifacts from respiratory motion. With the availability of high-performance gradient hardware, 3D gradient echo MRI with short TE and repetition time (TR) has become feasible. Using this technique, the thorax can be visualized with high spatial resolution during a single breath-hold. In comparison to 2D techniques, 3D MRI such as volumetric interpolated breathhold examination (VIBE) additionally results in a significantly better through-plane resolution and thus improved visibility of pulmonary lesions such as subtle infiltrates and pulmonary nodules [5].

For T_2-weighted MRI of the lung, turbo-spin-echo (TSE) sequences with short TE and high turbo factors are favorable, since the multiple 180° radio-frequency refocusing pulses minimize susceptibility artifacts. Furthermore, short echo spacing improves the signal of lung parenchyma. In half-Fourier single-shot turbo-spin-echo (HASTE) the central portion of *k*-space is acquired immediately after the radiofrequency pulse, which contributes to acquiring high signal from lung parenchyma [6]. As the acquisition time of HASTE is well below 1 sec, even nonbreath-hold acquisitions can be performed with a low level of artifacts from respiratory or cardiac motion. A well-known drawback of single-shot MRI, however, is a blurring of small structures with short T_2 components, particularly in the phase-encoding direction [7]. Parallel imaging, which has recently become available, enables an elegant and significant reduction in imaging time by using the spatial information inherent in a multiple receiver coil array. This can be used to reduce the effects of signal attenuation in single-shot imaging, resulting in images with increased spatial resolution in a reduced imaging time [7]. Moreover, breath-hold time can be further reduced in dyspnoeic patients without trade-offs regarding the spatial resolution.

19.2.2 Pulmonary MRA

In addition to morphologic imaging of the lung parenchyma pulmonary magnetic resonance angiography (MRA) has been developed as a noninvasive imaging tool for the assessment of pulmonary vascular diseases. While early development of pulmonary MRA focused on black blood and time-of-flight approaches, contrast-enhanced MRA is now considered the method of choice for pulmonary MRA. Technically, contrast-enhanced MRA consists of heavily T_1 weighted gradient echo MRI after intravenous injection of a paramagnetic MR contrast agent [8]. The combination of heavy T_1 weighting and the T_1 shortening effect of the MR contrast agent on the blood, results in a high contrast between the pulmonary vasculature and the surrounding tissue.

Since the pulmonary transit time of the contrast bolus and therefore the time gap between opacification of pulmonary arteries and veins is very short (~3 to 5 sec), selective visualization of the pulmonary arterial tree is difficult. To guarantee an optimal bolus profile, administration of the contrast agent by an automatic power injector with flow rates between 2 and 5 ml/sec is mandatory. The Gd concentration should be optimal at the time of central *k*-space acquisition, as this will determine the vascular signal intensity. Since a quite significant number of patients referred for

MRA of the pulmonary arteries presents with right heart compromise and/or pulmonary hypertension, the scan delay should be individually adjusted using a test or care bolus examination.

Due to the high susceptibility for motion artifacts, another prerequisite for high quality of pulmonary MRA is data acquisition during sustained breathing. With the development of strong gradient hardware (>20 mT/m) short TR (<5 msec) can be achieved allowing for high-resolution 3D pulmonary MRA acquired within breath-hold (20 to 30 sec). However, in patients with respiratory disease the required breath-hold duration often may exceed the patient's ability for breath-hold. As an alternative to conventional MRA protocols which acquire a single 3D data set during one breath-hold, time-resolved multiphasic MRA protocols have been developed [9,10].

In time-resolved MRA the scan time for an individual 3D data set is reduced to below 10 sec. As a consequence this approach even allows for the investigation of severely breathless patients. Further advantages of time-resolved MRA protocols are the independence of a bolus timing examination and the improved arterial-venous discrimination. A potential drawback of time-resolved MRA, however, is the reduction of spatial resolution which might limit the diagnostic accuracy.

19.2.3 Functional MRI

Finally, several functional MRI techniques have been developed allowing for an estimation of the functional relevance of the respiratory disease. Functional MRI techniques include ventilation MRI, perfusion MRI, and MRI of respiratory mechanics.

19.2.3.1 Ventilation Imaging

Two different approaches of ventilation MRI have been proposed (see also Chapter 18, Section 18.4.2). The first uses hyperpolarized noble gases as inhalative contrast agents to overcome the limitations of the low spin density of ventilated air spaces. Hyperpolarization, i.e., the artificial enrichment of the spin density of noble gases by optical pumping, has been applied to two noble gases, He-3 and Xe-129. The nonequilibrium polarization of He-3 compensates for the 2500 times lower density of He-3 as compared with tissue concentrations of hydrogen used for proton imaging [11]. After inhalation the helium can be detected with high signal intensity in airways and ventilated airspaces. Imaging can be performed with commercially available MR scanners using a Larmor frequency of approximately 48.4 MHz at 1.5 T [12]. Basically, four different imaging techniques for He-3 MRI have been developed: spin density (static ventilation distribution), diffusion imaging (pulmonary microstructure), dynamic ventilation imaging (gas in- and outflow), and oxygen partial pressure imaging (oxygen uptake or ventilation/perfusion [V/Q] matching). In spin density He-3 MRI low flip angle pulse sequences that use multiple excitation RF pulses such as 2D FLASH have been adopted as the clinical gold standard [12]. With this technique a considerably higher spatial resolution can be achieved than with lung scintigraphy. By applying ultrafast pulse sequences, the respiratory cycle, i.e., the in- and outflow of the helium gas can be imaged [12]. An important property of 3-He is its extremely high self-diffusion coefficient which enables an indirect assessment of the microstructure of the lung by measurement of the movement of the 3-He atoms (Figure 19.1). Finally, the paramagnetic effect of oxygen on the polarization of 3-He can be used to estimate the intrapulmonary pO_2 [13].

The second approach for ventilation imaging by MRI is based on proton MRI in combination with inhalation of gadolinium (Gd) aerosols or molecular oxygen. Gd-aerosolization was investigated with different gadolinium formulations in animal experiments [14,15] and volunteer studies [16]. In pharmacokinetic studies, complete renal excretion and no acute toxicity of aerosolized Gd was shown [15]. Although administration of aerosolized gadolinium chelates produces a relatively homogeneous enhancement of the lungs, the achievable signal intensity is low. Clinical studies using aerosolized gadolinium chelates in patients with respiratory disease are still pending.

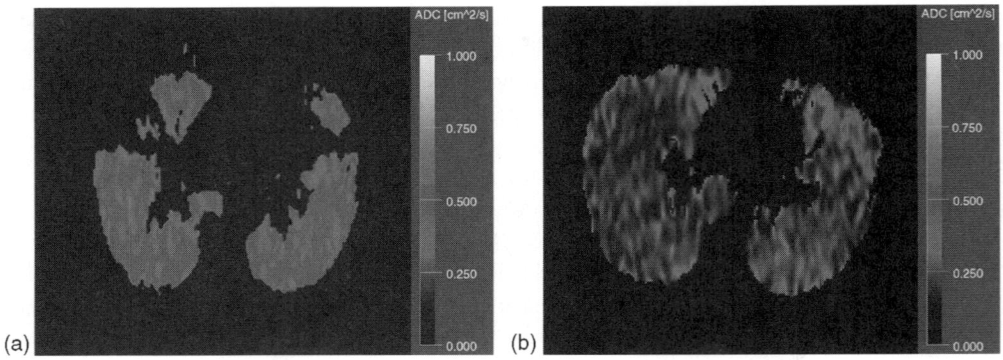

FIGURE 19.1 (See color insert following page 328.) Color-coded parametric maps of the apparent diffusion coefficient (ADC) obtained from diffusion-weighted 3-He MRI in a patient with emphysema (a) and a healthy volunteer (b). In the patient with emphysema ventilated air spaces show higher ADC values (red) indicating structural lung changes with enlarged air spaces. In addition, nonventilated lung regions can be observed (arrows).

Oxygen-enhanced MRI uses the paramagnetic property of molecular oxygen. The signal changes in the lung are explained by T_1-shortening in lung tissue and blood due to the paramagnetic properties of dissolved molecular oxygen [17]. Therefore, oxygen-enhanced MRI represents a mixture of ventilation, perfusion, and diffusion. The technique is most commonly carried out using T_1-weighted inversion-recovery single-shot turbo spin-echo (IR-HASTE) MRI, which is performed with the subject alternately inhaling room air and 100% oxygen. The optimal inversion time (T_1) to achieve the maximal signal intensity difference between MR images obtained during breathing room air and pure oxygen is in the range of 900 to 1300 msec [18]. Both cardiac and respiratory triggering significantly improve the achievable SNR of oxygen-enhanced MRI [18,19]. In clinical studies in patients with different respiratory diseases oxygen-enhanced MRI showed a high agreement with ventilation scintigraphy. In combination with contrast-enhanced pulmonary perfusion MRI oxygen-enhanced MRI could further differentiate diseases with V/Q mismatch (e.g., pulmonary embolism) and matched V/Q abnormalities [20].

19.2.3.2 Perfusion Imaging

MR perfusion imaging has been accomplished using either contrast-enhanced perfusion MRI or nonenhanced pulmonary arterial spin labeling (ASL) based on spin tagging.

The basic principle of contrast-enhanced perfusion MRI is a dynamic MR image acquisition following an intravenous bolus injection of a paramagnetic contrast agent. Perfusion MRI of the lung requires a high temporal resolution in order to visualize the peak enhancement of the lung parenchyma. Consequently, contrast-enhanced perfusion MRI uses T_1-weighted ultrashort TR and TE gradient echo MRI [21]. Depending on the spatial resolution, gradient hardware, and pulse sequence design, both two-dimensional (2D) and three-dimensional (3D) perfusion MRI have been described [22–30].

The advantage of 2D perfusion MRI is the excellent temporal resolution of up to 0.3 sec per image [31]; however, limited anatomic coverage and insufficient spatial resolution in the z-axis limit its clinical value (e.g., for the assessment of pulmonary embolism). With the introduction of parallel imaging techniques 3D perfusion imaging with a high spatial and temporal resolution, as well as an improved anatomic coverage and z-axis resolution could be achieved. Various studies have demonstrated the feasibility of quantification of pulmonary perfusion MRI by applying the indicator dilution theory [23,24,30–32].

Besides contrast-enhanced pulmonary perfusion MRI, nonenhanced perfusion MRI has also been evaluated. ASL uses the moving blood cells as magnetic particles. Thus, the inflowing blood cells can be visualized, providing information of lung perfusion. Although the effectiveness of ASL for the assessment of pulmonary perfusion has been demonstrated in a number of studies, this technique has not entered the stage of a clinical application in patients with respiratory diseases. Among the reasons for this are the more complex MRI technique, higher artifact susceptibility and lower SNR compared to contrast-enhanced pulmonary perfusion MRI [33,34].

19.2.3.3 Imaging of Respiratory Mechanics

With the continuous improvement of MR gradient hardware and the development of real-time MR pulse sequences (e.g., trueFISP), visualization of respiratory motion of the chest wall and diaphragm with high spatial and temporal resolution has recently become feasible [35,36]. Using dynamic MRI lung volumes (e.g., vital capacity) can also be calculated which show a high correlation to conventional spirometry [36]. In addition to the assessment of chest wall and diaphragmatic respiratory motion, dynamic MRI also allows for a simultaneous assessment of the respiratory motion of intrapulmonary pathology, such as lung tumors. This information is receiving increasing attention for radiotherapy planning of lung cancer [37].

19.3 MRI FOR THE ASSESSMENT OF AIRWAYS DISEASES

19.3.1 Diseases Affecting Large Airways

A common disease of the upper airway system which has been approached by MRI is obstructive sleep apnea (OSA). OSA affects up to 4% of middle-aged men and 2% of postmenopausal women and is characterized by a periodic cessation of airway flow caused by relaxation of the pharyngeal dilators (e.g., tensor veli palatini) and anatomic features causing inspiratory collapse of the upper airway (e.g., nasopharyngeal adenoidal tissues). Although OSA is usually diagnosed by combining clinical assessments and polysomnography, numerous studies have indicated that static and dynamic MRI may provide an improved diagnosis [38]. Static T_1- and T_2-weighted MRI is useful to detect predisposing anatomic factors in OSA and to outline the anatomy of the upper airways for a potential surgical intervention [39,40]. Besides static and dynamic volumetric imaging, image segmentation was used to quantify these predisposing anatomic factors of OSA [41,42]. Using dynamic axial or sagittal gradient echo MRI, several groups could further demonstrate significant differences in the patterns of dynamic airway motion between subjects with and without OSA [43,44]. Regarding the diagnosis of persistent OSA, a combination of static and dynamic MRI helps to identify different anatomical reasons for obstruction of the upper airways [45].

Increased collapsibility and saber sheath trachea are frequent tracheal abnormalities in patients with chronic obstructive pulmonary disease (COPD) [38]. MRI has the advantage not only to visualize the tracheal anatomy in arbitrary planes with a high soft tissue contrast, but also allows for a functional assessment of the tracheal collapsibility using dynamic MRI [46]. Frequent tracheal abnormalities are tracheomalacia and tracheal stenosis. Tracheomalacia is defined as tracheal wall softening due to an abnormality of the cartilaginous ring and hypotonia of the myoelastic elements, causing expiratory collapse of the trachea [47]. Cine MRI is helpful for the functional assessment of airway obstruction and stability in these patients [48]. Furthermore, MRI is helpful to elucidate the reason for tracheal pathology such as compression by vascular rings and slings [49,50] or mediastinal masses such as goiter or bronchogenic cysts [47].

19.3.2 Diseases Affecting Small Airways

Also small airway diseases have been approached by MRI. Although small airways usually cannot be visualized by current MRI techniques, functional MRI may pick up signs of small airways disease.

Several studies have evaluated 3-He MRI for the functional assessment of emphysema (see also Chapter 18, Section 18.4.2.1). MRI proved to be superior to high resolution computerized tomography (HRCT) for the assessment of ventilated lung areas, showing a better agreement with pulmonary function tests than HRCT (Figure 19.1) [51,52]. Dynamic 3-He MRI can be used to assess the temporal dynamics of ventilation [53]. Using the paramagnetic effect of oxygen on the 3-He polarization, inhomogeneous pO_2 distribution was found in patients with emphysema indicating severe alterations of ventilation/perfusion matching [13]. Also oxygen-enhanced MRI has been used for the assessment of emphysema. Compared to normal subjects patients with emphysema not only revealed a lower but also a slower increase of the signal intensity following oxygen inhalation [54]. Moreover, dynamic oxygen-enhanced MRI was proposed to visualize the spatial distribution of the diffusing capacity [55].

Using contrast-enhanced perfusion MRI, hypoperfused regions due to hypoxic vasoconstriction and tissue loss can be visualized in the lung [25,27] (Figure 19.2). Concerning the detection of perfusion abnormalities, perfusion MRI agrees well with conventional radionuclide scintigraphy. This information can be used for the planning of invasive therapy such as lung volume reduction surgery [27,28]. Using dynamic MRI, impaired respiratory mechanics including paradoxical diaphragmatic motion can be visualized in patients with emphysema [56]. A study used this technique to monitor the effect of theophylline treatment on the diaphragmatic excursion. MRI demonstrated an increase of 48% in diaphragmatic contractility following theophylline medication which correlated with pulmonary function tests and clinical status [57].

Due to the lack of radiation exposure, MRI is also a very attractive imaging modality in young patients with cystic fibrosis (CF). As earlier diagnosis and supportive therapy have improved the survival of CF patients beyond the age of 30, they usually undergo multiple follow-up studies over a long time period. Thus, MRI has been used to evaluate bronchiectasis, bronchial wall thickening, and mucus plugging in CF (Figure 19.3) (see also Chapter 18, Section 18.4.1). MRI with short TE (7 msec) was found to be comparable to CT regarding the extent of bronchiectasis [58]; however, it is inferior to CT for the direct visualization of bronchial wall thickness. In addition to morphology the

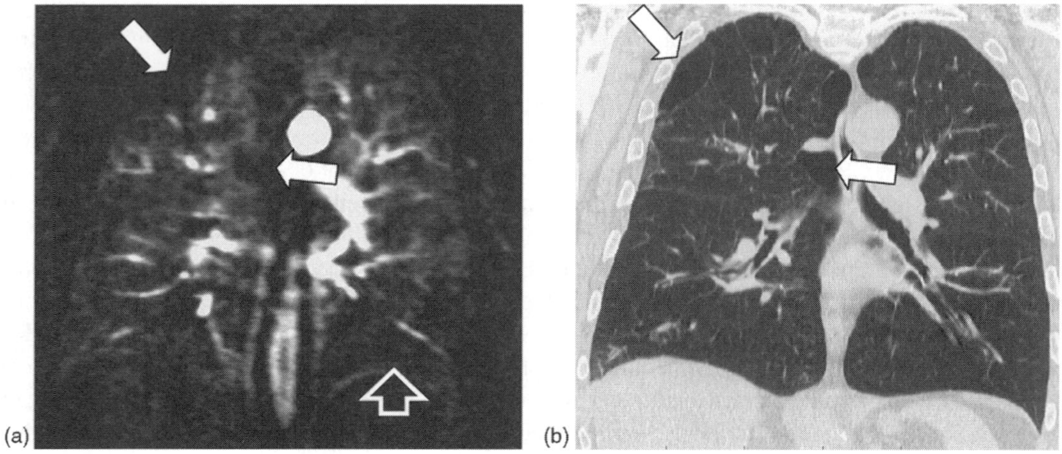

FIGURE 19.2 Perfusion MRI in a patient with COPD (a). Perfusion impairment (arrow) partly corresponds to tissue loss (arrow), as revealed by HRCT (b). In other regions, such as in the basal left lower lobe, perfusion loss may be explained by hypoxic vasoconstriction (open arrow).

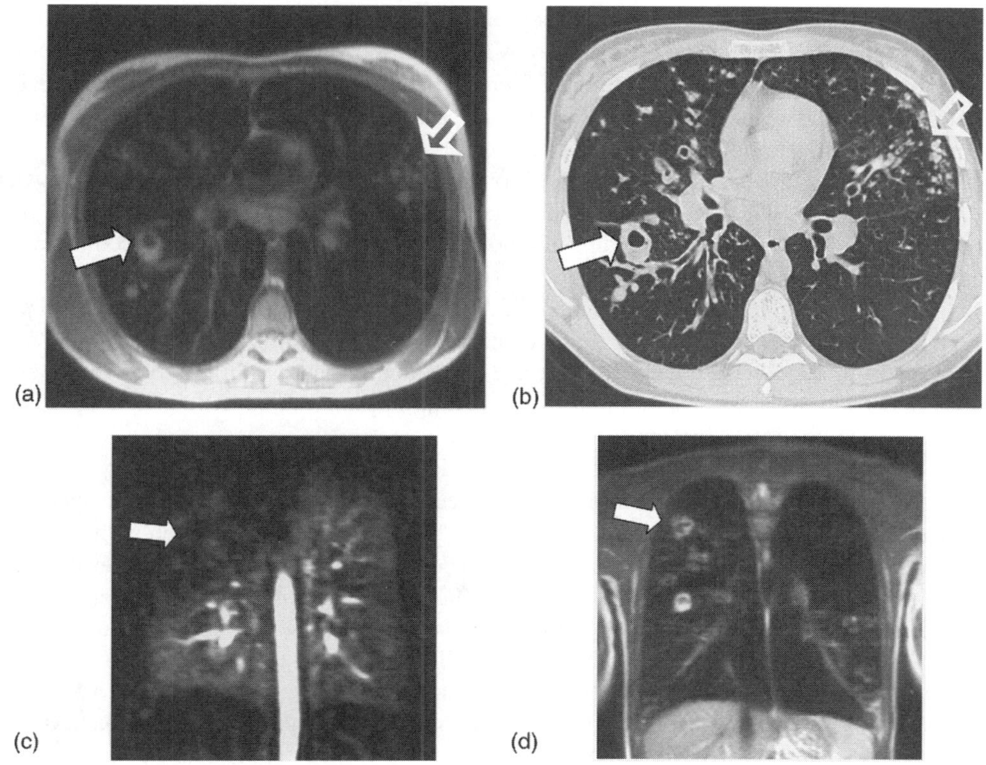

FIGURE 19.3 MRI of a patient with cystic fibrosis. HASTE MRI (a) similarly to HRCT (b) reveals bronchiectasis with mucus plugging of the segmental bronchi (closed arrows) as well as a tree in bud sign in the lung periphery (open arrows). Perfusion MRI (c) shows perfusion impairment of the right upper lobe (arrow), which corresponds to morphologic changes in the coronal HASTE (d) (arrow).

functional impairment of CF may also be investigated by MRI [59–61]. Ventilation defects demonstrated by He-3 MRI tend to be more severe than morphologic changes revealed by proton MRI [59]. Using T_1-mapping of oxygen-enhanced MRI, the oxygen transfer function was compared between patients with CF and healthy volunteers. Areas with a low oxygen transfer function correlated well with hypoperfused, diseased lung areas [61]. In a recent study correlating morphologic MRI with perfusion MRI, a high correlation between areas with severe morphologic changes (e.g., bronchiectasis) and areas with impaired perfusion could be demonstrated [62] (Figure 19.3).

Also the use of MRI for the investigation of patients with asthma has been evaluated. 3-He MRI could demonstrate varying degrees and locations of ventilation defects in asthmatics over time without conclusively defining the severity of asthma. Nevertheless, good correlation was demonstrated between MRI and spirometry indicating that objective findings are not directly linked to subjective symptoms [63]. The capability of evaluating response of both broncholysis and bronchial provocation by ventilation MRI has been shown [64]. Furthermore, a recent study in moderate and severe asthmatics demonstrated a high correlation between 3-He MRI and spirometry findings following albuterol inhalation [65].

19.4 MRI FOR THE ASSESSMENT OF PARENCHYMAL DISEASE

In addition to airway disease, MRI has also been proposed for the assessment of respiratory diseases affecting the alveoli and lung parenchyma. In patients with chronic infiltrative lung disease, a common pulmonary disease which progresses at varying rates from inflammatory alveolitis to interstitial fibrosis, a good correlation between the MRI signal intensity and the clinical disease severity, as well as a potential response to therapy has been shown [66]. Although CT is superior in the anatomic assessment and visualization of fibrosis, a high rate of agreement between MRI and CT with regard to parenchymal opacification and ground-glass opacities has been observed, allowing for visualization of areas with active alveolitis [67] (Figure 19.4).

In patients receiving radiation therapy for bronchogenic carcinoma, MRI was used to evaluate the temporal dynamics of radiation-induced lung tissue changes. After a steady increase of the signal intensity of the tumor surrounding pulmonary parenchyma over several months, a slow decrease of the signal intensities of T_1- and T_2-weighted images was demonstrated. These signal changes reflect the pathologic changes of the lung parenchyma following radiation. An initial phase of interstitial edema (weeks 1 to 3 following radiation) is followed by an exudative phase with high protein content in the alveoli (weeks 3 to 8), and pneumonitic phase with progressive septal and alveolar edema with mononuclear and fibroblastic cell infiltration (6 months). Finally, fibrosis may be observed 6 months following lung irradiation [68].

MRI has also been used for the detection and characterization of inflammatory respiratory disease (see also Chapter 18, Section 18.4.1). In pediatric patients with suspected pneumonia, steady-state free precession projection MRI generally achieved a high correlation with findings of chest x-ray, and could visualize effusions and small pneumonic infiltrates even better than x-ray [69]. The assessment of pulmonary infiltrates by MRI in immunocompromized patients has also been evaluated. Invasive aspergillosis belongs to the most dangerous complications in these patients. Typical image patterns of invasive aspergillosis are a target sign, which characterizes central necrotizing infiltrates with a peripheral rim enhancement on contrast-enhanced T_1-weighted MRI, as well as hyperintense areas on plain T_1-weighted images indicating hemorrhagic infarcts due to vascular invasion [70]. In a prospective study in immunocompromized patients, MRI confirmed round infiltrates already seen on conventional chest x-ray in all cases. While a specific diagnosis with regard to the pathogen of the infiltrates could not be established at this early stage of disease, further follow-up with the visualization of specific target signs on contrast-enhanced T_1-weighted images and so-called reverse target signs on T_2-weighted images allowed for the specific diagnosis of invasive aspergillosis [71]. Another study addressed the use of T_2-weighted MRI in the diagnosis of different types of pneumonia. While the visualization of infiltrations was as good as with CT, MRI was more accurate than CT for revealing necrotizing lesions [72]. In children with CF an open MRI system was used for follow-up examinations of pneumonic infiltrates and atelectasis [73]. MRI proved suitable to monitor the pulmonary complications of CF in all cases,

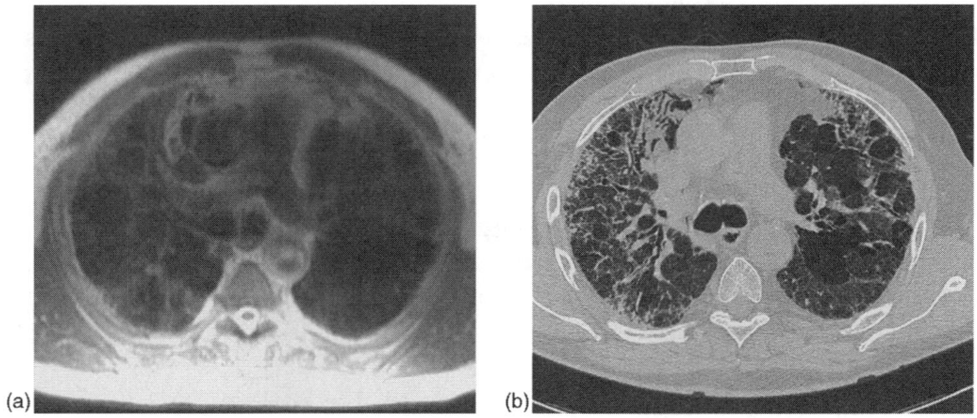

FIGURE 19.4 MRI (HASTE) in a patient with lung fibrosis (a). Although HRCT (b), due to the better spatial resolution, offers a superior visualization of fibrosis, a high rate of agreement between MRI and CT with regard to parenchymal opacification and ground-glass opacities can be observed.

thus avoiding additional chest x-ray or CT scans. MRI was also helpful for therapeutic decisions such as duration of antibiotic treatment or bronchoscopy [73].

MRI has also been applied for the detection of pulmonary nodules. Despite a lower spatial resolution, the high contrast between nodules and underlying parenchyma in MR images is a potential advantage of MRI with regard to CT [74]. Various MR techniques have been proposed for the assessment of lung nodules by MRI. A high contrast between lung nodules and underlying parenchyma at a low rate of artifacts has been obtained with T_2-weighted TSE MRI [75]. Using this technique, pulmonary metastases were detected with an overall sensitivity of 84% compared with CT as the gold standard. In different studies, either a combination of nonenhanced T_1-weighted and T_2^*-weighted turbo FLASH sequences or short inversion time inversion recovery (STIR) yielded a similar sensitivity of 82% for the detection of pulmonary nodules [4,76]. Two studies using FLASH or TrueFISP MRI at an open 0.2 T system also showed a high accuracy of MRI for the detection of pulmonary nodules compared to CT or conventional chest x-ray [77,78]. In more recent studies, the application of T_1-weighted 3D VIBE and HASTE also achieved a high sensitivity for pulmonary nodules with a size below 10 mm [79,80]. With the introduction of parallel imaging techniques and the improvement of spatial resolution, an improved accuracy of MRI for the detection of lung nodules can be expected [74]. In addition to their detection, MRI has also been proposed for the characterization of lung nodules. Several studies using dynamic contrast-enhanced MRI have shown that malignant nodules are characterized by a faster and stronger enhancement when compared to benign lesions [81–84]. However, an overlap with inflammatory lesions, which may also show a rapid and strong enhancement, can be observed [82].

19.5 MRI FOR THE ASSESSMENT OF PULMONARY VASCULAR DISEASE

Although CT and ventilation-perfusion scintigraphy remain the clinically accepted imaging modalities for the evaluation of patients with suspected pulmonary embolism, MRI is an interesting alternative for various reasons. In addition to the use in patients with contraindication to iodinated contrast media, MRI can be used for a comprehensive evaluation of patients with suspected pulmonary embolism (see also Chapter 18, Section 18.4.2.3). Using a combination of high-resolution MRA and contrast-enhanced pulmonary perfusion MRI, the diagnostic information of CT and perfusion scintigraphy can be combined in a single MR examination. Using MR phlebography, the entire venous system might be assessed for thrombosis in the same imaging session without using ionizing radiation [85] (Figure 19.5). Whereas in indirect MR phlebography the venous system is imaged after the contrast agent bolus has passed the arterial system and capillary bed, direct or ascending MR phlebography refers to an enhancement of the veins of the lower extremity after peripheral injection into the veins of the foot. Additionally, ventilation MRI might be used allowing for a differentiation of perfusion changes caused by hypoxic vasoconstriction. Finally, the right heart function which is important for the patient prognosis, may be assessed by CINE MRI and phase-contrast MR flow measurements.

Various groups have evaluated the accuracy of MRA for the diagnosis of acute pulmonary embolism. In a study with 30 patients, a mean sensitivity of 87%, a specificity of 95%, a positive predictive value of 87%, and a negative predictive value of 100% were obtained for the diagnosis of pulmonary embolism [86]. Similarly, MRA in patients with intermediate- or low-probability V/Q scans and a high clinical suspicion for pulmonary embolism achieved a sensitivity of 85%, a specificity of 96%, a positive predictive value of 92%, and a negative predictive value of 92% [87]. In a more recent study in 118 patients with clinical suspicion of pulmonary embolism and an abnormal radionuclide perfusion lung scan were examined by a double contrast injection MRA protocol comprising acquisition of two sagittal 3D MRA data sets for both lungs. Despite an improved spatial resolution, the sensitivity for isolated subsegmental was low (40%), thus resulting in a lower overall sensitivity (77%) [88].

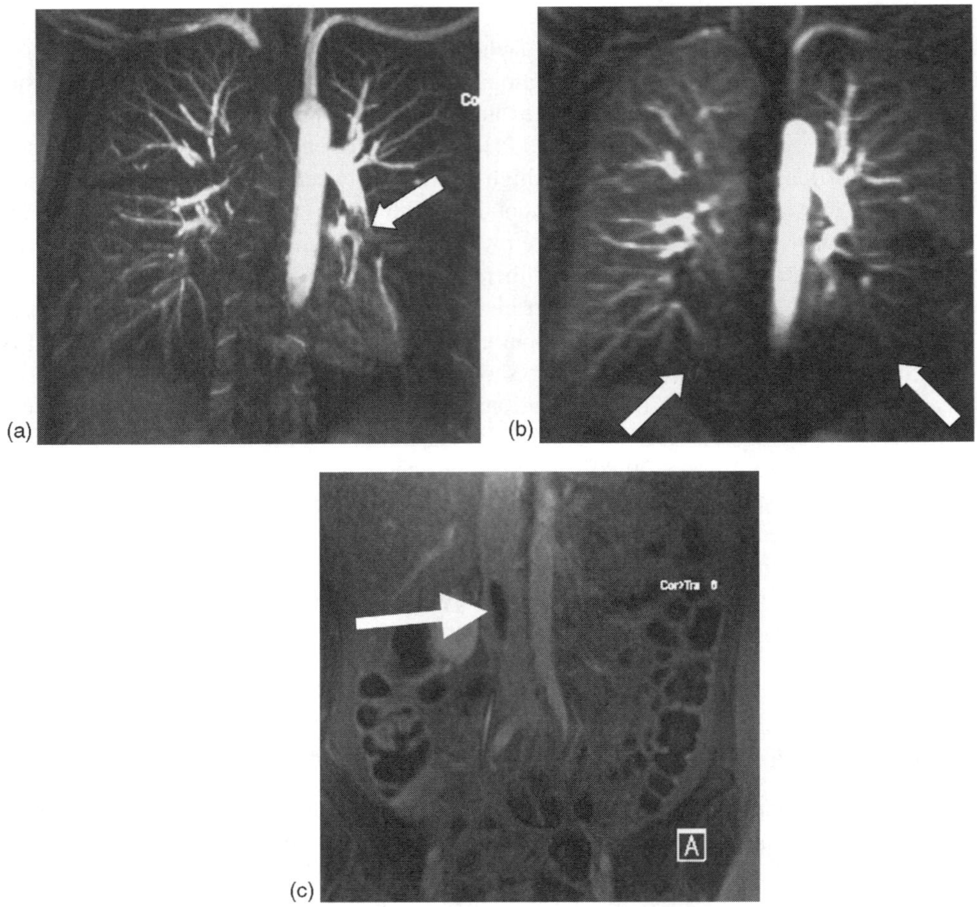

FIGURE 19.5 Comprehensive MRI of a patient with pulmonary embolism. High-resolution pulmonary MRA (a) shows thrombotic material in the pulmonary artery of the left lower lobe (arrow). Perfusion MRI (b) correspondingly demonstrates a perfusion defect in the left lower lobe as well as in the right lower lobe (arrows). Indirect MR phlebography (c) reveals thromboembolism in the inferior vena cava (arrow).

In addition to acute pulmonary embolism, also chronic thromboembolic pulmonary hypertension (CTEPH), a form of pulmonary hypertension which is believed to result from recurrent pulmonary thromboemboli, has been approached by MRI. Typical MRA findings of CTEPH include dilation of the central pulmonary arteries, direct visualization of wall-adherent thrombotic material, intraluminal webs, cut-off of segmental vessels, abnormal proximal-to-distal tapering, and heterogeneous lung perfusion. Several studies have shown a high accuracy of MRA for the visualization of thrombotic material in CTEPH compared to conventional angiography or CT [89–91]. MRA is also useful to differentiate between CTEPH and primary or idiopathic primary pulmonary hypertension [92] (Figure 19.6). In a recent study evaluating MRA with parallel imaging in patients with CTEPH, a sagittal data acquisition was superior with regard to image quality, vessel coverage, depiction of patent peripheral arteries, and pathological findings when compared to standard coronal MRA [93].

Using CINE MRI and phase-contrast MR flow measurements, MRI is able to demonstrate the postoperative improvement of hemodynamics following pulmonary thromboendarterectomy, a surgical procedure in which the fibrous material of chronic thromboembolism is removed, thus restoring pulmonary arterial blood flow [91].

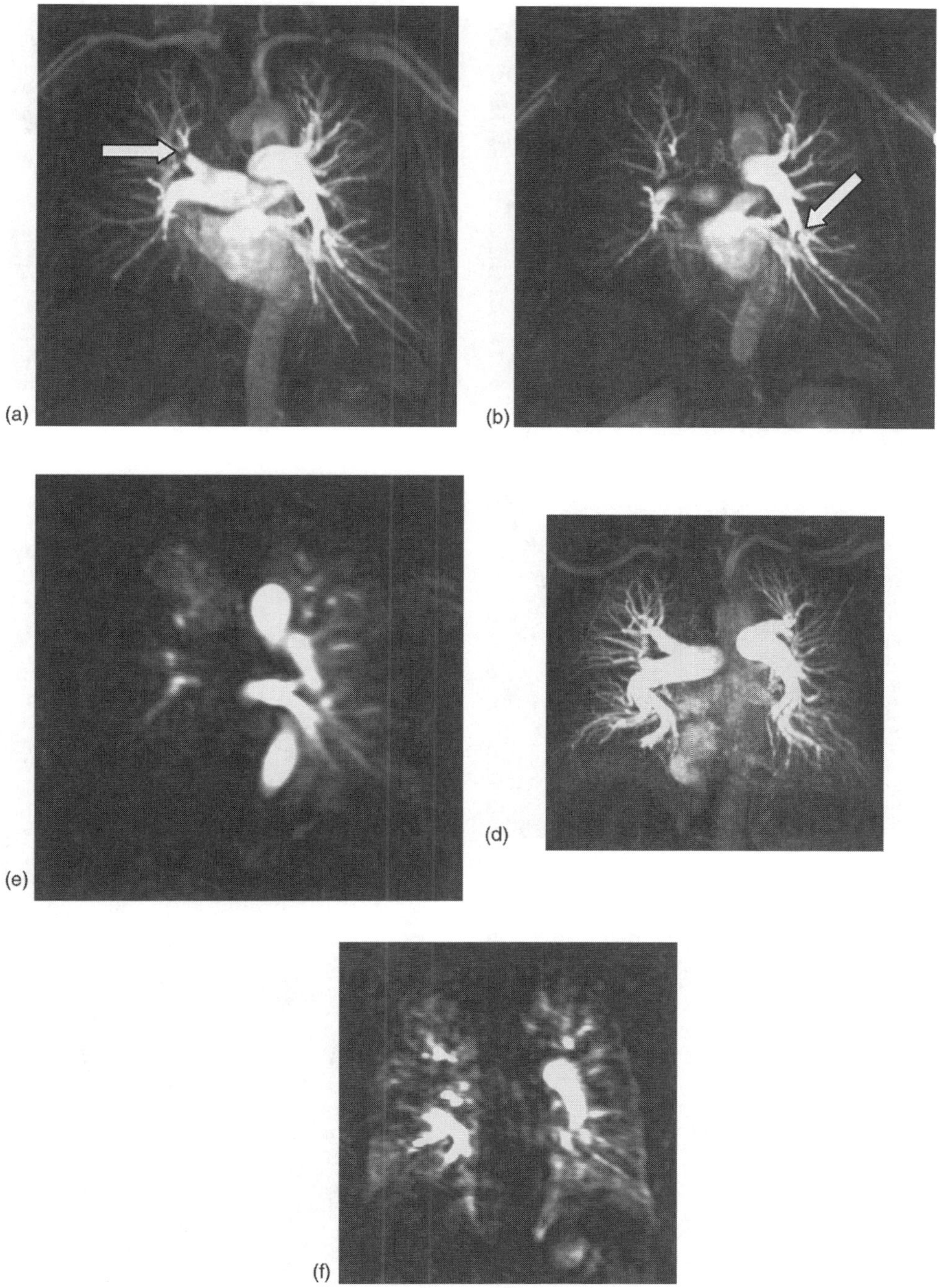

FIGURE 19.6 Differentiation of different forms of pulmonary hypertension using MRA and perfusion MRI. In patients with chronic thromboembolic pulmonary hypertension (CTEPH) (a–c) MRA (a,b) shows abnormal proximal-to-distal tapering with cut-off of segmental vessels. Furthermore, intraluminal webs can be observed (arrows). Perfusion MRI (c) shows segmental perfusion defects in both lungs. In patients with primary pulmonary hypertension (e,d) no signs of thromboembolism are observed. At MRA (d) the pulmonary arterial tree is visualized up to the subpleural space. Perfusion MRI (e) shows a decreased and patchy lung perfusion without segmental perfusion defects.

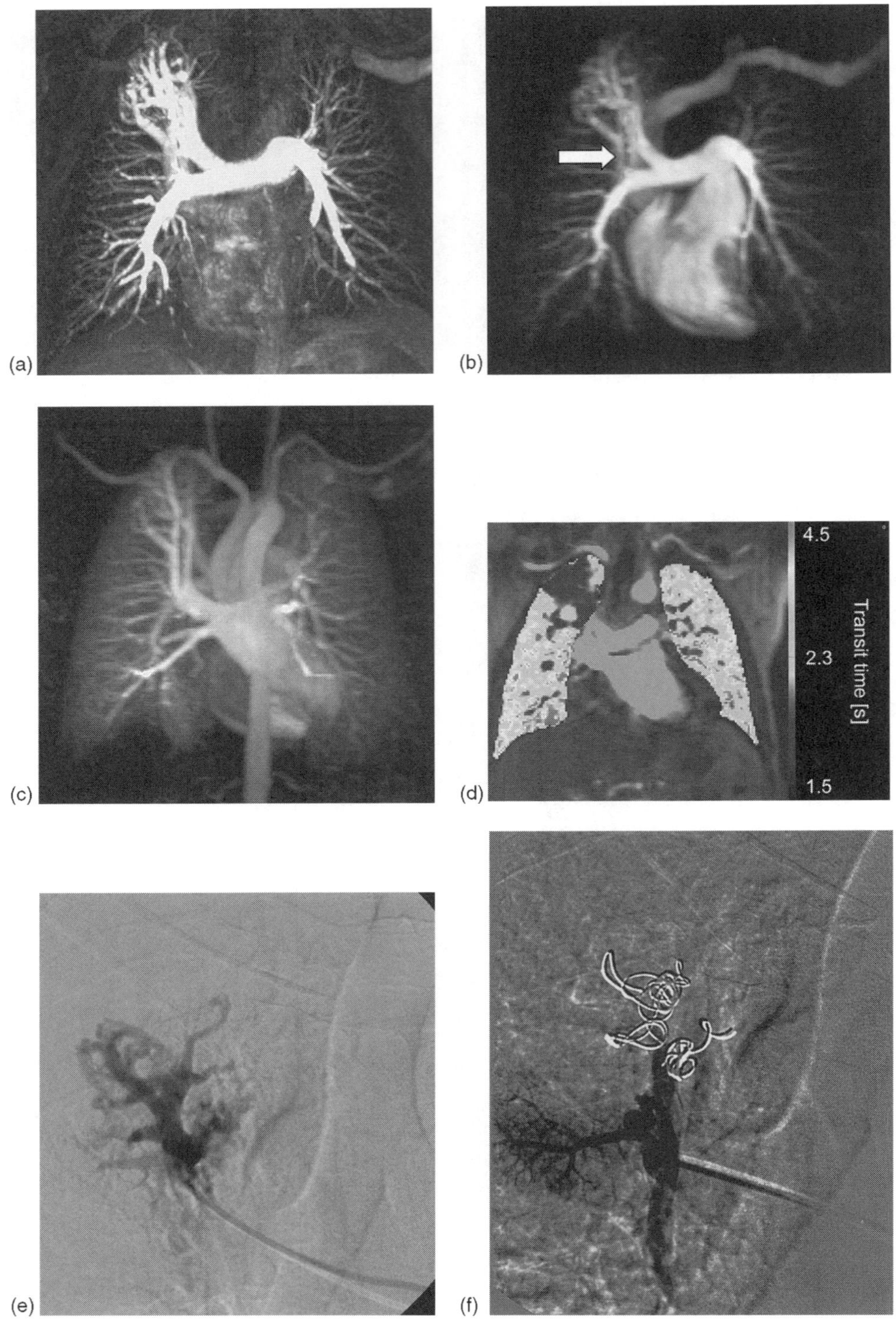

FIGURE 19.7 (See color insert for (d) following page 328.) MRI in a patient with a pulmonary arteriovenous malformation (AVM). High-resolution MRA (a) shows a large AVM of the right upper lobe. Time-resolved MRA (b,c) shows an early venous filling of the pulmonary vein of the right upper lobe (arrow). Color-coded map of pulmonary transit time (d) calculated from time-resolved MRA shows decreased transit time in that area compared to the rest of the lung. Findings of MRI were confirmed by catheter angiography (e), which was performed for embolization (f).

A rare, but important differential diagnosis for chronic thromboembolism is primary and metastatic tumor involving the pulmonary arteries. Sarcomas of or metastases to the pulmonary artery are depicted as filling defects at MRA. Dynamic or delayed imaging may be used to demonstrate enhancement indicating neoplasms instead of pulmonary embolism. However, neoplasms may also have low vascularity, and may be associated with secondary thrombus formation [94,95].

MRI can also be used for the evaluation of central pulmonary arterial and venous involvement in lung cancer. Besides conventional SE and TSE MRI, which have the advantage of a high contrast between the vascular lumen, wall, and surrounding tissue, contrast-enhanced 3D MRA has been demonstrated to be effective for the evaluation of bronchogenic carcinoma [74,96]. Due to its poorer spatial resolution, MRA is still inferior to CT for the assessment of segmental or subsegmental lung vessels; however, the accuracy for the assessment of the mediastinal vessels is similar for both techniques.

MRI can also be applied for imaging congenital anomalies of the pulmonary arteries. One example is pulmonary arteriovenous malformation which may appear as pulmonary nodules but can be differentiated by the visualization of feeding arteries and draining veins [97]. MRA and pulmonary perfusion MRI can be used for the management of pulmonary arteriovenous malformations including planning of embolotherapy and follow-up [98] (Figure 19.7).

19.6 MRI IN CLINICAL TRIALS

Direct or indirect quantitative and regional measurements of lung function as provided by MRI seem to be highly attractive for clinical drug testing. Although currently there is no scientific evidence proving MRI to be superior to conventional methods (i.e., V/Q scintigraphy, spirometry) for the functional assessment of respiratory disease, a broader application of MRI in clinical drug testing may be justified in the future.

Unlike conventional lung function tests, which allow only for a global assessment of lung function, MRI is able to visualize lung function on a regional basis. This might be advantageous for several reasons. The regional correlation of lung function with morphologic changes allows for a better understanding of the pathophysiology of respiratory diseases and improves the disease classification. Even more important, potential treatment effects of drugs may be directly visualized. By the direct correlation of lung function and morphology, MRI may be more specific than conventional lung function tests. Moreover, functional MRI methods may be more sensitive than conventional lung function tests: subtle treatment effects may be masked by the global assessment of lung function since the nondiseased lung may compensate for the functional impairment of the diseased lung. In this context it was recently shown that in patients with CF, despite evidence of small airway obstruction as shown by surfactant analysis, the overall lung function was not compromised [99]. However, although not influencing the lung function and not causing symptoms, these changes may be an ideal target for early treatment eventually altering the course of the disease and preventing irreversible tissue damage.

Although CT might be still considered to be superior to MRI for the morphologic assessment of lung disease, the ongoing development of functional MRI methods might make MRI a more suitable imaging technique for the application in clinical drug trials. This is especially the case as MRI is free of radiation-exposure, thus allowing frequent follow-up exams in benign disease.

Although MRI examinations *per se* are more expensive than conventional lung function tests, assuming a higher sensitivity and specificity for the assessment of therapeutic effects, the costs of clinical trials might even be reduced by limiting the required number of subjects and allowing for earlier end points in clinical drug trials. Even if not used for the monitoring of therapeutic effects in drug trials, MRI might also be used to improve the selection of patients approaching therapeutic trials, thereby having the potential to reduce the overall costs of trials.

REFERENCES

1. Kauczor, H. U. and Kreitner, K. F., MRI of the pulmonary parenchyma, *Eur. Radiol.*, 9, 1755, 1999.
2. Bergin, C. J., Glover, G. M., and Pauly, J., Magnetic resonance imaging of lung parenchyma, *J. Thorac. Imaging*, 8, 12, 1993.
3. Bergin, C. J., Glover, G. H., and Pauly, J. M., Lung parenchyma: magnetic susceptibility in MR imaging, *Radiology*, 180, 845, 1991.
4. Knopp, M. V. et al., MR-Tomographie von Lungenmetastasen mit schnellen Gradientenechosequenzen, *Radiologe*, 34, 581, 1994.
5. Bader, T. R. et al., Magnetic resonance imaging of pulmonary parenchymal disease using a modified breath-hold 3D gradient-echo technique: initial observations, *J. Magn. Reson. Imaging*, 15, 31, 2002.
6. Hatabu, H. et al., MR imaging of pulmonary parenchyma with a half-Fourier single-shot turbo spin-echo (HASTE) sequence, *Eur. J. Radiol.*, 29, 152, 1999.
7. Heidemann, R. M. et al., Resolution enhancement in lung 1H imaging using parallel imaging methods, *Magn. Reson. Med.*, 49, 391, 2003.
8. Prince, M. R., Gadolinium-enhanced MR aortography, *Radiology*, 191, 155, 1994.
9. Goyen, M. et al., Dynamic 3D MR angiography of the pulmonary arteries in under four seconds, *J. Magn. Reson. Imaging*, 13, 372, 2001.
10. Schoenberg, S. O. et al., High-resolution pulmonary arterio- and venography using multiple-bolus multiphase 3D-Gd-mRA, *J. Magn. Reson. Imaging*, 10, 339, 1999.
11. Kauczor, H., Surkau, R., and Roberts, T., MRI using hyperpolarized noble gases, *Eur. Radiol.*, 8, 820, 1998.
12. van Beek, E. J. et al., Functional MRI of the lung using hyperpolarized 3-helium gas, *J. Magn. Reson. Imaging*, 20, 540, 2004.
13. Kauczor, H. U., Hanke, A., and van Beek, E. J., Assessment of lung ventilation by MR imaging: current status and future perspectives, *Eur. Radiol.*, 12, 1962, 2002.
14. Haage, P. et al., Gadolinium containing contrast agents for pulmonary ventilation magnetic resonance imaging: preliminary results, *Invest. Radiol.*, 37, 120, 2002.
15. Berthezene, Y. et al., Safety aspects and pharmacokinetics of inhaled aerosolized gadolinium, *J. Magn. Reson. Imaging*, 3, 125, 1993.
16. Haage, P. et al., MR-Bildgebung der Lungenventilation mittels aerosolierter Gadolinium-Chelate, *Rofo*, 175, 187, 2003.
17. Edelman, R. R. et al., Noninvasive assessment of regional ventilation in the human lung using oxygen-enhanced magnetic resonance imaging, *Nat. Med.*, 2, 1236, 1996.
18. Loffler, R. et al., Optimization and evaluation of the signal intensity change in multisection oxygen-enhanced MR lung imaging, *Magn. Reson. Med.*, 43, 860, 2000.
19. Vaninbroukx, J. et al., The use of ECG and respiratory triggering to improve the sensitivity of oxygen-enhanced proton MRI of lung ventilation, *Eur. Radiol.*, 13, 1260, 2003.
20. Nakagawa, T. et al., Pulmonary ventilation-perfusion MR imaging in clinical patients, *J. Magn. Reson. Imaging*, 14, 419, 2001.
21. Hatabu, H. et al., Pulmonary perfusion: qualitative assessment with dynamic contrast-enhanced MRI using ultra-short TE and inversion recovery turbo FLASH, *Magn. Reson. Med.*, 36, 503, 1996.
22. Berthezene, Y. et al., Prospective comparison of MR lung perfusion and lung scintigraphy, *J. Magn. Reson. Imaging*, 9, 61, 1999.
23. Ohno, Y. et al., Quantitative assessment of regional pulmonary perfusion in the entire lung using three-dimensional ultrafast dynamic contrast-enhanced magnetic resonance imaging: preliminary experience in 40 subjects, *J. Magn. Reson. Imaging*, 20, 353, 2004.
24. Nikolaou, K. et al., Quantification of pulmonary blood flow and volume in healthy volunteers by dynamic contrast-enhanced magnetic resonance imaging using a parallel imaging technique, *Invest. Radiol.*, 39, 537, 2004.
25. Fink, C. et al., Partially parallel three-dimensional magnetic resonance imaging for the assessment of lung perfusion — Initial results, *Invest. Radiol.*, 38, 482, 2003.
26. Amundsen, T. et al., Perfusion abnormalities in pulmonary embolism studied with perfusion MRI and ventilation-perfusion scintigraphy: an intra-modality and inter-modality agreement study, *J. Magn. Reson. Imaging*, 15, 386, 2002.

27. Amundsen, T. et al., Perfusion magnetic resonance imaging of the lung: characterization of pneumonia and chronic obstructive pulmonary disease. A feasibility study, *J. Magn. Reson. Imaging*, 12, 224, 2000.
28. Johkoh, T. et al., Scintigraphic and MR perfusion imaging in preoperative evaluation for lung volume reduction surgery: pilot study results, *Radiat. Med.*, 18, 277, 2000.
29. Fink, C. et al., Regional lung perfusion: assessment with partially parallel three-dimensional MR imaging, *Radiology*, 231, 175, 2004.
30. Fink, C. et al., Quantitative analysis of pulmonary perfusion using time-resolved parallel 3D MRI — Initial results, *Rofo*, 176, 170, 2004.
31. Levin, D. L. et al., Evaluation of regional pulmonary perfusion using ultrafast magnetic resonance imaging, *Magn. Reson. Med.*, 46, 166, 2001.
32. Hatabu, H. et al., Quantitative assessment of pulmonary perfusion with dynamic contrast-enhanced MRI, *Magn. Reson. Med.*, 42, 1033, 1999.
33. Keilholz, S. D. et al., Comparison of first-pass Gd-DOTA and FAIRER MR perfusion imaging in a rabbit model of pulmonary embolism, *J. Magn. Reson. Imaging*, 16, 168, 2002.
34. Kauczor, H. U., *Functional Imaging of the Chest*, Springer, Berlin, 2004.
35. Suga, K. et al., Impaired respiratory mechanics in pulmonary emphysema: evaluation with dynamic breathing MRI, *J. Magn. Reson. Imaging*, 10, 510, 1999.
36. Plathow, C. et al., Evaluation of chest motion and volumetry during the breathing cycle by dynamic MRI in healthy subjects: comparison with pulmonary function tests, *Invest. Radiol.*, 39, 202, 2004.
37. Plathow, C. et al., Analysis of intrathoracic tumor mobility during whole breathing cycle by dynamic MRI, *Int. J. Radiat. Oncol. Biol. Phys.*, 59, 952, 2004.
38. Stark, P. and Norbash, A., Imaging of the trachea and upper airways in patients with chronic obstructive airway disease, *Radiol. Clin. North Am.*, 36, 91, 1998.
39. Arens, R. et al., Upper airway size analysis by magnetic resonance imaging of children with obstructive sleep apnea syndrome, *Am. J. Respir. Crit. Care Med.*, 167, 65, 2003.
40. Arens, R. et al., Magnetic resonance imaging of the upper airway structure of children with obstructive sleep apnea syndrome, *Am. J. Respir. Crit. Care Med.*, 164, 698, 2001.
41. Abbott, M. B., Dardzinski, B. J., and Donnelly, L. F., Using volume segmentation of cine MR data to evaluate dynamic motion of the airway in pediatric patients, *Am. J. Roentgenol.*, 181, 857, 2003.
42. Schwab, R. J. et al., Identification of upper airway anatomic risk factors for obstructive sleep apnea with volumetric magnetic resonance imaging, *Am. J. Respir. Crit. Care Med.*, 168, 522, 2003.
43. Donnelly, L. F. et al., Upper airway motion depicted at cine MR imaging performed during sleep: comparison between young patients with and those without obstructive sleep apnea, *Radiology*, 227, 239, 2003.
44. Schoenberg, S. O. et al., Combined assessment of obstructive sleep apnea syndrome with dynamic MRI and parallel EEG registration: initial results, *Invest. Radiol.*, 35, 267, 2000.
45. Donnelly, L. F. et al., Causes of persistent obstructive sleep apnea despite previous tonsillectomy and adenoidectomy in children with down syndrome as depicted on static and dynamic cine MRI, *Am. J. Roentgenol.*, 183, 175, 2004.
46. Heussel, C. P. et al., Respiratory lumenal change of the pharynx and trachea in normal subjects and COPD patients: assessment by cine-MRI, *Eur. Radiol.*, 14, 2188, 2004.
47. Berrocal, T. et al., Congenital anomalies of the tracheobronchial tree, lung, and mediastinum: embryology, radiology, and pathology, *Radiographics*, 24, e17, 2004.
48. Faust, R. A., Rimell, F. L., and Remley, K. B., Cine magnetic resonance imaging for evaluation of focal tracheomalacia: innominate artery compression syndrome, *Int. J. Pediatr. Otorhinolaryngol.*, 65, 27, 2002.
49. Eichhorn, J. et al., Rings, slings and other vascular abnormalities. Ultrafast computed tomography and magnetic resonance angiography in pediatric cardiology, *Z. Kardiol.*, 93, 201, 2004.
50. Simoneaux, S. F. et al., MR imaging of the pediatric airway, *Radiographics*, 15, 287, 1995.
51. Ley, S. et al., Functional evaluation of emphysema using diffusion-weighted 3Helium-magnetic resonance imaging, high-resolution computed tomography, and lung function tests, *Invest. Radiol.*, 39, 427, 2004.
52. Zaporozhan, J. et al., Functional analysis in single-lung transplant recipients: a comparative study of high-resolution CT, 3He-MRI, and pulmonary function tests, *Chest*, 125, 173, 2004.

53. Gast, K. K. et al., Distribution of ventilation in lung transplant recipients: evaluation by dynamic 3He-MRI with lung motion correction, *Invest. Radiol.*, 38, 341, 2003.
54. Ohno, Y. et al., Oxygen-enhanced MR ventilation imaging of the lung: preliminary clinical experience in 25 subjects, *Am. J. Roentgenol.*, 177, 185, 2001.
55. Ohno, Y. et al., Dynamic oxygen-enhanced MRI reflects diffusing capacity of the lung, *Magn. Reson. Med.*, 47, 1139, 2002.
56. Iwasawa, T. et al., Paradoxical motion of the hemidiaphragm in patients with emphysema, *J. Thorac. Imaging*, 15, 191, 2000.
57. Etlik, O. et al., Demonstrating the effect of theophylline treatment on diaphragmatic movement in chronic obstructive pulmonary disease patients by MR-fluoroscopy, *Eur. J. Radiol.*, 51, 150, 2004.
58. Carr, D. H. et al., Magnetic resonance scanning in cystic fibrosis: comparison with computed tomography, *Clin. Radiol.*, 50, 84, 1995.
59. Donnelly, L. F. et al., Cystic fibrosis: combined hyperpolarized 3He-enhanced and conventional proton MR imaging in the lung-preliminary observations, *Radiology*, 212, 885, 1999.
60. Puderbach, M. et al., Visualisation of parenchymal lung changes in patients with cystic fibrosis (CF): MRI versus HRCT, *J. Cyst. Fibros.*, 3, 54, 2004.
61. Jakob, P. M. et al., Assessment of human pulmonary function using oxygen-enhanced T(1) imaging in patients with cystic fibrosis, *Magn. Reson. Med.*, 51, 1009, 2004.
62. Eichinger, M. et al., Contrast-enhanced 3D MRI of lung perfusion in children with cystic fibrosis, *J. Cyst. Fibros.*, 3, 52, 2004.
63. Altes, T. A. et al., Hyperpolarized 3He MR lung ventilation imaging in asthmatics: preliminary findings, *J. Magn. Reson. Imaging*, 13, 378, 2001.
64. Altes, T. A. and de Lange, E. E., Applications of hyperpolarized helium-3 gas magnetic resonance imaging in pediatric lung disease, *Top. Magn. Reson. Imaging*, 14, 231, 2003.
65. Gaare, J. et al., *Hyperpolarized Helium-3 MR (H3-HeMR) Imaging of the Lung in Asthmatics: ventilation Changes Following Treatment with Albuterol, RSNA, Chicago*, 2004.
66. McFadden, R. G., Carr, T. J., and Wood, T. E., Proton magnetic resonance imaging to stage activity of interstitial lung disease, *Chest*, 92, 31, 1987.
67. Muller, N. L., Mayo, J. R., and Zwirewich, C. V., Value of MR imaging in the evaluation of chronic infiltrative lung diseases: comparison with CT, *Am. J. Roentgenol.*, 158, 1205, 1992.
68. Yankelevitz, D. F. et al., Lung cancer: evaluation with MR imaging during and after irradiation, *J. Thorac. Imaging*, 9, 41, 1994.
69. Rupprecht, T. et al., Steady-state free precession projection MRI as a potential alternative to the conventional chest X-ray in pediatric patients with suspected pneumonia, *Eur. Radiol.*, 12, 2752, 2002.
70. Herold, C. J. et al., Invasive pulmonary aspergillosis: evaluation with MR imaging, *Radiology*, 173, 717, 1989.
71. Blum, U. et al., Invasive pulmonary aspergillosis. MRI, CT, and plain radiographic findings and their contribution for early diagnosis, *Chest*, 106, 1156, 1994.
72. Leutner, C. C. et al., MR imaging of pneumonia in immunocompromised patients: comparison with helical CT, *Am. J. Roentgenol.*, 175, 391, 2000.
73. Hebestreit, A. et al., Follow-up of acute pulmonary complications in cystic fibrosis by magnetic resonance imaging: a pilot study, *Acta Paediatr.*, 93, 414, 2004.
74. Fink, C. et al., MRT des Bronchialkarzinoms, *Radiologe*, 44, 435, 2004.
75. Kersjes, W. et al., Diagnosis of pulmonary metastases with turbo-SE MR imaging, *Eur. Radiol.*, 7, 1190, 1997.
76. Feuerstein, I. M. et al., Pulmonary metastases: MR imaging with surgical correlation — a prospective study, *Radiology*, 182, 123, 1992.
77. Schafer, J. F. et al., Bildgebende Diagnostik solitärer Lungenrundherde am offenen Niederfeld-MRT — Ein Vergleich zweier MR-Sequenzen mit der Spiral-CT, *Rofo*, 174, 1107, 2002.
78. Heussel, C. P. et al., Prospektive Machbarkeitsstudie zum Vergleich von Röntgenübersichtsaufnahme und Thorax-MRT in Atemanhaltetechnik am offenen Niederfeldgerät, *Rofo*, 174, 854, 2002.
79. Vogt, F. M. et al., HASTE MRI versus chest radiography in the detection of pulmonary nodules: Comparison with MDCT, *Am. J. Roentgenol.*, 183, 71, 2004.
80. Biederer, J. et al., Lung morphology: fast MR imaging assessment with a volumetric interpolated breath-hold technique: initial experience with patients, *Radiology*, 226, 242, 2003.

81. Schaefer, J. F. et al., Solitary pulmonary nodules: dynamic contrast-enhanced MR imaging — perfusion differences in malignant and benign lesions, *Radiology*, 232, 544, 2004.
82. Ohno, Y. et al., Solitary pulmonary nodules: potential role of dynamic MR imaging in management initial experience, *Radiology*, 224, 503, 2002.
83. Guckel, C. et al., Solitary pulmonary nodules: MR evaluation of enhancement patterns with contrast-enhanced dynamic snapshot gradient-echo imaging, *Radiology*, 200, 681, 1996.
84. Hittmair, K. et al., Evaluation of solitary pulmonary nodules with dynamic contrast-enhanced MR imaging — A promising technique, *Magn. Reson. Imaging*, 13, 923, 1995.
85. Ruehm, S. G., MR venography, *Eur. Radiol.*, 13, 229, 2003.
86. Meaney, J. F. et al., Diagnosis of pulmonary embolism with magnetic resonance angiography, *N. Engl. J. Med.*, 336, 1422, 1997.
87. Gupta, A. et al., Acute pulmonary embolism: diagnosis with MR angiography, *Radiology*, 210, 353, 1999.
88. Oudkerk, M. et al., Comparison of contrast-enhanced magnetic resonance angiography and conventional pulmonary angiography for the diagnosis of pulmonary embolism: a prospective study, *Lancet*, 359, 1643, 2002.
89. Kreitner, K. F. et al., Kontrastmittelverstärkte dreidimensionale MR-Angiographie der Lungenarterien bei Patienten mit chronisch-rezidivierender Lungenembolie — Vergleich mit der selektiven intraarteriellen DSA, *Rofo*, 172, 122, 2000.
90. Ley, S. et al., Value of contrast-enhanced MR angiography and helical CT angiography in chronic thromboembolic pulmonary hypertension, *Eur. Radiol.*, 13, 2365, 2003.
91. Kreitner, K. F. et al., Chronic thromboembolic pulmonary hypertension: pre- and postoperative assessment with breath-hold MR imaging techniques, *Radiology*, 232, 535, 2004.
92. Ley, S. et al., Assessment of pulmonary hypertension by CT and MR imaging, *Eur. Radiol.*, 14, 359, 2004.
93. Oberholzer, K. et al., Kontrastmittelverstärkte 3D-MRA der Pulmonalarterien mit integrierter paralleler Akquisitionstechnik (iPAT) bei Patienten mit CTEPH — sagittale oder koronare Datenaufnahme?, *Rofo*, 176, 605, 2004.
94. Fasse, A. et al., Das Pulmonalarteriensarkom — Prä- und postoperative radiologische Befunde bei der Tumorerstmanifestation und beim Rezidiv, *Rofo*, 170, 112, 1999.
95. Mader, M. T. et al., Malignant tumors of the heart and great vessels: MR imaging appearance, *Radiographics*, 17, 145, 1997.
96. Ohno, Y. et al., Multiphase ECG-triggered 3D contrast-enhanced MR angiography: utility for evaluation of hilar and mediastinal invasion of bronchogenic carcinoma, *J. Magn. Reson. Imaging*, 13, 215, 2001.
97. Fink, C. et al., Zeitlich aufgelöste multiphasische 3D-MR-Angiographie zur Diagnostik des Lungengefäßsystems bei Kindern, *Rofo*, 175, 929, 2003.
98. Ohno, Y. et al., Contrast-enhanced MR perfusion imaging and MR angiography: utility for management of pulmonary arteriovenous malformations for embolotherapy, *Eur. J. Radiol.*, 41, 136, 2002.
99. Griese, M. et al., Pulmonary surfactant, lung function, and endobronchial inflammation in cystic fibrosis, *Am. J. Respir. Crit. Care Med.*, 170, 1000, 2004.

Editorial Comments

Most research on human glucose metabolism has been centered around using tracer methodologies detecting what is going on in the blood. Despite its importance, this approach is limited by the fact that it does not address directly what is happening in the tissues. Information on tissue metabolism can be obtained by analyzing fat or muscle biopsies. However, this is not ideal. Biopsies involve the removal of tissue under local anesthesia, which is not something one would volunteer for too many times. On the other hand, a biopsy provides only punctual information.

Magnetic resonance spectroscopy (MRS) allows the determination of the levels of biochemical substrates in different organs of the body in a noninvasive manner. Metabolic fluxes and intracellular metabolites can be monitored continuously in the tissues. In particular, ^{13}C, ^{31}P, and ^{1}H MRS techniques have been used to follow glucose metabolism in the muscle, the liver, and the brain. They are thus especially suited to the study of diabetes, which is characterized by a chronically raised blood glucose concentration (hyperglycemia) due to a relative or absolute lack of the pancreatic hormone, insulin.

The use of MRS in preclinical and clinical diabetes research is detailed in Chapter 20 and Chapter 21.Because of their nature and costs, MRS studies in this area do not account for a high throughput. They are rather designed as explorative studies in small groups of individuals. This is not necessarily a limitation, since deriving information at the tissue level contributes to improvement in the knowledge of the yet poorly understood underlying disease mechanisms, and may finally shed light on new therapeutic approaches.

20 MR in Preclinical Diabetes and Obesity Drug Discovery

Beat M. Jucker and Didier Laurent

CONTENTS

20.1 INTRODUCTION

20.1.1 Diabetes

At least 170 million people worldwide suffered from diabetes in 2000 and this figure is likely to double by 2030 [1]. Approximately 4 million deaths every year are attributable to complications related to diabetes. The prevalence of diabetes is unusually high in the U.S. ($\sim$8%), and many go undiagnosed and are at major risk of health complications. The majority of diabetics may be categorized as type 1 or type 2 diabetics. Type 1 diabetes results from the failure of the pancreas to secrete insulin. It is estimated that $<$ 10% of all diabetics have type 1 diabetes with a high incidence rate among children and adolescents. Type 2 diabetes, also referred to as noninsulin dependent diabetes mellitus (NIDDM), accounts for the vast majority of diabetes cases. The type 2 diabetes condition results from peripheral tissue insulin resistance and usually occurs later in life (i.e., "adult onset diabetes"). Most people with diabetes present with co-risk factors such as high blood pressure and cholesterol that increase one's risk for heart disease and stroke. These additional risk factors result in more than 65% of people with diabetes dying from heart disease or stroke.

20.1.2 Obesity

Obesity is becoming increasingly prevalent in the West as a consequence of a shift toward increased caloric consumption and a sedentary lifestyle [2]. Obesity, defined as a body mass index (BMI) $>$ 30, is known to be a major risk factor for both coronary heart disease and type 2 diabetes [3]. It is a serious medical condition that affects over 300 million obese adults worldwide, and is becoming increasingly more prevalent in children and adolescents [4]. The prevalence of obesity in industrialized and developing countries is estimated to be between 40 and 60% of the population [5]. The health risks associated with obesity are far reaching including cardiovascular disease risk due to its effect on blood lipid levels, type 2 diabetes, hypertension, renal dysfunction, stroke, arthritis, among others.

20.1.3 MRI/S vs. Conventional Methodologies to Assess Metabolism

Insulin-stimulated uptake of plasma glucose and its storage as glycogen by muscle are the chief mechanisms of postprandial glucose disposal [6–8]. Although glycogen concentration can be readily measured in muscles of preclinical species using biochemical methodology [9], the temporal nature of glycogen synthesis is not captured in this static assessment. Additionally, ^{3}H or ^{14}C glucose tracer techniques have been used to assess glycogen synthesis [9,10]. Unfortunately, even this measurement is arguably an interpolation of the final tracer detection in the glycogen molecule. By comparison, ^{13}C NMR spectroscopic applications allow for true kinetic information to be obtained on glycogen synthesis in animal and man as serial measurements of the glycogen molecule (natural abundance or ^{13}C-labeled) can be made [11,12].

Recently, *in vivo* ^{13}C MRS methods have been developed to directly measure rates of glycolysis and glycogen synthesis simultaneously in skeletal muscle of awake rats [13–15]. In addition to glycogen synthesis, ^{13}C-labeled glucose turnover through glycolysis can be measured by examining the turnover of ^{13}C label in lactate and alanine pools which are in equilibrium with the glycolytic pyruvate pool. This method represents an advancement over traditional measurements of whole body glycolysis which suffer from the inability to reflect tissue-specific glycolytic measurements. Currently, whole body glucose oxidation can be assessed by indirect calorimetry [16] or by measurements of tritiated water production from 3-^{3}H glucose [17]. The significant advantage of the MRS technique for glycolytic flux measurements is that it provides a direct assessment of intramuscular glycolytic metabolism. The necessity for an *in vivo*, noninvasive measurement of both glycogen synthesis and glycolysis becomes increasingly apparent in the presence of differing results with regard to the glucose metabolic fate as measured, for example, *ex vivo* in thiazolidinedione (TDZ)-treated muscle strips [18] or *in vivo* in TDZ-treated animals [19,20].

Studies which are designed to address the control of metabolic pathways are of particular importance in drug studies as the pharmacological agent being investigated may have pleitropic effects on metabolism. Traditional enzymatic studies do not fully capture the complex distribution of control over the entire system of enzymes comprising a metabolic pathway [21]. However, by using ^{13}C MRS to measure glucose disposal and associated pathways (glycogen synthesis and glycolysis) and ^{31}P MRS to measure glucose 6-phosphate [14,22], metabolic control analysis can be performed to assign metabolic control to multiple metabolic pathways [15,23]. Therefore, metabolic control analysis may be particularly useful in understanding how pharmacological agents targeting a specific metabolic pathway may be studied and the pharmacokinetic/pharmacodynamic (PK/PD) relationship on the control of these pathways further explored.

Mitochondrial uncoupling proteins (UCPs) play an integral role in regulating cellular energy consumption via nonshivering thermogenesis [24]. This regulation is accomplished by diminishing the proton motive force across the inner mitochondrial membrane, which results in uncoupling of respiration from ATP synthesis. Unlike UCP1, which is expressed exclusively in brown adipose tissue, the recently discovered homolog UCP3 [25,26] is expressed primarily in muscle. Because quiescent skeletal muscle accounts for 33% of whole-body oxygen consumption, much attention has been given to the control and function of UCP3 as a means of regulating energy expenditure and body weight. However, investigation into the regulation of uncoupling protein has been hampered by the inability to assess its activity in intact tissue. By combining ^{13}C MRS to measure rates of mitochondrial substrate oxidation with ^{31}P MRS measurements of rates of unidirectional ATP synthesis, one may assess a decrease in mitochondrial energy coupling (i.e., ratio of ATP synthesis to substrate oxidation) resulting from increased uncoupling protein function and/or other thermogenic processes [27].

One of the most extensive uses of MRS for preclinical application to diabetes drug discovery is the intramyocellular lipid (IMCL) content measurement. It is well documented that skeletal muscle triglyceride, long chain acyl-coenzyme A, or diacylglycerol content is negatively correlated with insulin-stimulated glucose uptake [28,29]. Traditionally, biochemical or gas chromatographic methods are used to analyze lipid metabolites in tissue biopsy extracts. The inherent limitation to measuring the metabolically active lipid pool in gross skeletal muscle tissue is the inability to discriminate between intramyocellular (within muscle fibers) and extramyocellular (between muscle fibers, typically in adipocytes) pools of triglyceride. *In vivo* ^{1}H MRS, by virtue of different magnetic field environments associated with the different lipid pools when oriented along the magnetic field, allows for discrimination of IMCL from extramyocellular lipid (EMCL) at magnetic fields as low as 1.5 T [30]. Due to the high sensitivity of this measurement, and with excellent spatial resolution (down to 4 mm^3) [31], the IMCL measurement represents an excellent technique to serially assess the effects of pharmacological agents which modulate muscle lipid content and consequently muscle insulin sensitivity in preclinical animal models.

Examination of the relationship between whole body fat distribution and disease risk by MRI is a topic of great interest. Body or tissue specific fat composition has been measured indirectly using anthropometric techniques [32], or directly using dual energy x-ray absorptiometry (DEXA) [33], computed tomography (CT) [34], or MRI [35]. Although DEXA is relatively inexpensive and has been used routinely in the clinic, its limitation is that it only provides a measure of whole body fat content, whereas MRI and CT allow for compartmental fat distribution to be determined. Both cross-sectional and longitudinal studies have related visceral fat to type 2 diabetes mellitus and cardiovascular disease, independently of BMI [36]. Therefore, the need to probe differences in fat distribution for drug discovery is clear. With the advent of rapid imaging sequences, whole body imaging of rodent obesity models may be performed within minutes. However one should realize that the *in vivo* assessment of fat distribution suffers from the significant time required for image segmentation, hence limiting the use of MRI for high throughput analysis.

20.1.4 Applications to Drug Discovery

In an industrial environment, the application of preclinical MRI/S to diabetes and obesity drug discovery is diverse. Often, model development or target validation is of paramount importance before any pharmacology may be examined. For example, a particular high fat feeding regimen may be required in a rodent to achieve a specific phenotype, or genetically altered mice expressing a particular genotype with relevance to a drug target may need to be assessed in order to generate confidence in the target. MRI/S applications may also be applied to the lead optimization stage of drug development so that an understanding of how blood levels of a particular drug candidate correspond to the phenotypic readout required (i.e., establish a PK/PD relationship). In some instances where perhaps the throughput for MRI/S studies is not very high (e.g., ^{13}C glucose infusion studies), a differentiation study between two or three quality, late stage drug candidates may provide valuable insight as to the selection of a final molecule to go into clinical development. It is essential that there is iterative communication with clinical colleagues within the organization so that experimental medicine studies may be initiated in the clinic before or while phase II studies are ongoing. Perhaps MRI/S support of clinical trials at this point are more suited to phase IIa or IIb studies, rather than phase III unless pre-established MRI/S biomarkers are accepted by the drug registration agencies (e.g., Food and Drug Administration [FDA]).

20.2 METABOLIC DISEASE TARGETS

20.2.1 Diabetes: Current Therapies and Targets

Anti-diabetic therapy, including insulin injection, has been used for over 80 years, and oral administration of therapeutic agents has been in existence for nearly 5 decades. These agents are divided into classes with varying therapeutic targets, but all having glucose-lowering effects. At present, marketed oral drugs include: (1) sulfonylureas, such as glipizide (brand names Glucotrol® and Glucotrol XL®), glyburide (Micronase®, Glynase®, and Diabeta®), and glimepiride (Amaryl®), are drugs that stimulate the beta cells of the pancreas to release more insulin; (2) meglitinides, such as repaglinide (Prandin®) and nateglinide (Starlix®), are drugs that also stimulate the beta cells to release insulin only by a different mechanism from sulfonylureas; (3) biguanides, such as metformin (Glucophage®), are drugs that lower blood glucose levels primarily by decreasing the amount of glucose produced by the liver. An added benefit of metformin therapy is its ability to increase peripheral insulin sensitivity; (4) thiazolidinediones (TZDs), such as rosiglitazone (Avandia®) and pioglitazone (ACTOS®), are peroxisome proliferator activator receptor-γ (PPAR-γ) agonists that improve insulin sensitivity in peripheral tissue (i.e., skeletal muscle and adipose tissue); and (5) alpha-glucosidase inhibitors, such as acarbose (Precose®) and meglitol (Glyset®), help the body to lower blood glucose levels by blocking the breakdown of starches in the intestines. Investigational new drug therapeutic targets include agonists of glucagons-like-peptide 1 (GLP-1) which would enhance insulin secretion, antagonists of dipeptidylpeptidase IV (DPP-IV inhibitor) which would functionally antagonize the breakdown of incretins like GLP-1, and combined PPAR agonists (e.g., PPAR-α/γ) to treat metabolic syndrome.

20.2.1.1 MR Applications to Diabetes Drug Discovery

Rosiglitazone, an oral antihyperglycemic agent used to treat type 2 diabetes, is a potent PPAR-γ agonist (see also Chapter 21, Section 21.6.2.2). Studies in animal models of type 2 diabetes showed that rosiglitazone improves glycemic control by enhancing insulin-stimulated whole-body glucose disposal [37,38]. The increase in whole-body insulin sensitivity is the result of increased insulin action in skeletal muscle [29,37], liver [29,37], and adipose tissue [39]. Skeletal muscle accounts for the largest proportion of insulin-stimulated, whole-body glucose uptake.

Therefore, much of the focus on the insulin-sensitizing benefits of TZDs has been targeted to this tissue [29,37,40]. Despite the fact that skeletal muscle expresses low levels of PPAR-γ, direct actions of TZDs on muscle glucose metabolism *in vitro* have been reported [39]. However, the precise mechanism of action of TZDs in skeletal muscle remains unclear. Evidence exists to suggest that the improvement in muscle insulin sensitivity may be an indirect consequence of activation of PPAR-γ in fat, a tissue in which the receptor is abundantly expressed [29,37].

Combined ^{13}C MRS to assess glucose and its distributed fluxes (glycogen synthesis and glycolysis) and ^{31}P MRS to determine glucose-6-phosphate modulation has been used to examine the effect of rosiglitazone treatment on the control of these fluxes in skeletal muscle or Zucker fatty rats [41]. A number of preclinical studies [31,42,43] further examined the effect of TZDs in lowering the IMCL pool in rodent skeletal muscle by ^{1}H MRS. It was shown that rosiglitazone treatment resulted in a rapid (days) and sustained (weeks) reduction in IMCL in the tibialis anterior muscle of Zucker fatty rats [42]. Differences in regional adipose physiology are implicated as potential factors involved in the pathogenesis of insulin resistance. In animal studies, TZDs increase body weight due largely to increases in fat pad mass [44,45] and alteration of adipocyte size and number [46,47]. MRI has been used to examine the redistribution of fat from the metabolically deleterious visceral adipose tissue to the more inert subcutaneous fat depots following TZD treatment in both animals [48] and humans [49].

Metformin reduces fasting plasma glucose by reducing the rate of its production [50]. However, its effect on the relative contribution of glycogenolysis vs. gluconeogenesis is controversial and was only recently studied using ^{13}C MRS techniques [51] (see also Chapter 21, Section 21.6.1.2). Because of limitations in traditional methods in assessing these metabolic fluxes, ^{13}C MRS may be used to directly assess glycogenolysis, as well as to indirectly calculate gluconeogenic rates if the endogenous glucose production rate is known. In this manner, Hundal et al. [51] showed that metformin reduced endogenous glucose production in poorly controlled type 2 diabetics by decreasing gluconeogenesis [51].

20.2.2 Obesity: Current Therapies and Targets

Antiobesity drug therapy treatments are multifarious in their mechanisms of action. These mechanisms include reduction in food intake, inhibition of fat absorption, and increase of thermogenesis. At present, marketed oral drugs include (1) Sibutramine (brand names are Meridia® and Reductil®), which is an inhibitor of norepinephrine, dopamine and serotonin reuptake, reduces food consumption, and increases thermogenesis; and (2) Orlistat (Xenical®), an inhibitor of pancreatic lipase, which is capable of blocking the absorption of 30% of ingested fat. Investigational antiobesity compounds comprise: (a) central nervous system agents that affect neurotransmitters or neural ion channels; (b) leptin/insulin/central nervous system pathway agents, including leptin analogues, leptin transport and/or leptin receptor promoters, neuropeptide Y, melanocortin-4 receptor agonists; and (c) agents aimed at increasing resting metabolic rate (beta-3 agonists, UCP homologues, and thyroid receptor agonists) [52].

20.2.2.1 MR Applications to Obesity Drug Studies

Pharmacological agents which have been evaluated by *in vivo* MR include Sibutramine whose effects on whole body tissue water and fat were assessed in rats by MR relaxometry [53]. This rapid acquisition technique was performed in awake rats and allowed for high throughput testing (>30 animals per hour) with excellent reproducibility. Exendin-4, a peptide with homology to the glucagon-like peptide-1, was shown in Zucker rats to successfully reduce food intake, weight gain, and fat deposition as assessed by MRI [54]. MRI was also used to analyze lipid in muscle and subcutaneous regions of the thigh following PPPAR-α activation with fenofibrate in Otsuka Long-Evans Tokushima Fatty rats [55]. Finally, MRI proved particularly useful in examining the effects of UCP3 overexpression in mice where a striking reduction in adipose tissue mass was observed [56]. It should be noted that antiobesity agents targeting UCP expression/function may be analyzed using both MRS techniques to probe mitochondrial function and MRI to assess regulation of fat distribution.

20.3 PRECLINICAL ANIMAL MODELS OF DIABETES AND OBESITY

20.3.1 Rodents

The discovery of the *ob* gene [57] and its product, leptin, revealed that the latter is an adipocyte-derived satiety factor involved not only in the regulation of food intake but also of energy expenditure. Leptin, while secreted into the circulation, is abundantly expressed in abdominal white adipose among other tissues [57]. Animals in which the *ob* gene is defective (e.g., ob/ob mouse) or which lack the leptin receptor (e.g., db/db mouse, *fa*/*fa* Zucker rat) develop an obesity-like syndrome [57]. Therefore these rodent models are routinely used for pharmacological investigation of obesity and insulin resistance.

The Zucker diabetic fatty (ZDF) rat is a rodent model commonly used for the study of type II diabetes [58,59]. While nondiabetic *fa*/*fa* Zucker rats exhibit initial signs of glucose intolerance by 7 to 8 weeks of age and maximum glucose intolerance by 12 to 13 weeks of age [60], they remain normoglycemic. However, the transition to an overt type 2 diabetic condition with hyperglycemia in ZDF rats occurs at 7 to 8 weeks of age [61]. This is due in part to a decrease in insulin production, concomitant with a loss of β-cell mass [62]. Interestingly, it appears that early treatment with TZDs may be able to prevent the increase in net β-cell death that normally occurs in these relatively young animals [63]. However, the continuous decline in plasma insulin concentration may not be sufficient on its own to explain the reduction in glucose uptake as it is well established that ZDF rats exhibit peripheral insulin resistance [61].

Insulin resistance and conditions that mimic metabolic syndrome is often generated in rodents in the context of dietary manipulation (e.g., carbohydrate-enriched diets, high fat, varying fatty acid chain length, degree of saturation, etc.) [64–67]. In essence, these models aim to mimic some of the risk factors associated with obesity and the development of type 2 diabetes. Indeed, it is now well accepted that the central adiposity resulting from high-fat feeding of rodents predisposes them to insulin resistance. Accumulation of visceral rather than subcutaneous fat is thought to constitute the link between glucose intolerance and IMCL stores [68]. However, in transgenic fatless mice, a model for lipodystrophy, insulin resistance is developed due to an increase in muscle triglyceride content independent of visceral adiposity [69].

Glucocorticoids and their synthetic analogues are known to modulate a wide range of physiological processes through a variety of mechanisms involving the endocrine, renal, immune, and vascular systems, and also to exert a direct impact on substrate metabolism. Thus, dexamethasone has been used as a diabetogenic agent because of its potent effects on lipid and glucose metabolism. In Sprague-Dawley and in hyperinsulinemic Zucker rats, dexamethasone is able to counteract the antilipolytic effects of insulin [70] by contributing to the release of fatty acids from adipose tissue. At the same time, proliferation of new adipocytes may be limited and their endocrine function impaired. Recently, Korach-Andre et al. [71] showed using MRS that both the muscle glucose uptake and the glycolytic flux are lowered by dexamethasone, while glycogen stores increase through inhibition of glycogen breakdown. Dexamethasone offers the advantage of inducing muscle insulin resistance in an acute fashion, which allows performance of drug profiling studies in a relatively short time period.

The wealth of potential metabolic targets to treat insulin resistance has triggered the development of various genetic mouse models that provide new insights into the physiopathological mechanism of type 2 diabetes. Not surprisingly, a number of these models are directed to the insulin signaling pathways. Among these recent transgenic developments, a model has been developed in which the phosphorylation of the insulin receptor substrate-1 (IRS-1) is increased on specific serine residues [Ser (P)-302 and Ser (P)-307], a condition that leads to insulin resistance seemingly through a JNK1-mediated inhibition of the IRS-1 interaction [72]. Interestingly, genetically obese ob/ob mice, diet-induced obese animals, and hyperinsulinemic mice display a similar defect, providing further evidence for the effect of such phosphorylation on the inhibition of glucose utilization. In line with this, heterozygous knockout of the IRS-1 gene in mice increases insulin resistance, especially in the presence of obesity [73]. Indeed, IRS-1-deficient mice are well recognized as a nonobese animal model of insulin resistance [74]. The deletion of the muscle glucose transport (GLUT) protein 4 or the abrogation of the insulin-like growth factor I (IGF-1) receptor are other possible conditions mimicked in genetically engineered mice which may lead to severe insulin resistance (see review by Le Roith et al [75]). Knowing that GLUT4 translocation itself is regulated by syntaxin 4, researchers developed a heterozygous knockout mouse model lacking the gene Syn4(+/−) which manifests impaired glucose tolerance due in part to a reduction in muscle glucose uptake [76]. Given the growing interest in lipid-associated insulin resistance and obesity, mouse models such as transgenic mice overexpressing leptin [77] or apolipoprotein A-II [78] are also appealing as they may reflect the central role of adipose tissue in insulin resistance with circulating lipids most likely contributing upstream to the accumulation of fat in ectopic regions.

Transgenic and gene knockout rodent models engineered to share common features with human insulin resistance will aid in the design of new antidiabetic drugs targeting specific pathways. However, an in-depth characterization and/or validation of these models is often necessary as these models do not always display an apparent phenotype. *In vivo* MR techniques may prove very useful to better define these models with regard to metabolic disorders.

20.3.2 Nonhuman Primates

Nonhuman primate models of insulin resistance are also of significant relevance for the development of new antidiabetic agents. Because the pathophysiology in spontaneously obese rhesus monkeys closely resembles that of humans, the etiology and mechanisms of obesity-associated type 2 diabetes has been examined in rhesus monkeys for over 2 decades [79]. Fasting hyperglycemia, which is typically observed in these animals as well as in humans, results from an increase in hepatic glucose production [79,80]. In addition, defects in peripheral insulin sensitivity exist prior to the development of overt diabetes in these obese monkeys [81], similarly to type 2 diabetic patients [82,83]. It should be noted though that peripheral insulin resistance may actually develop concurrently with an impairment of insulin action on glycogen synthase in skeletal muscles and adipose tissue [84,85], but not in the liver of prediabetic obese rhesus monkeys [86].

Despite the appeal of using nonhuman primate models of type 2 diabetes, several issues have contributed to the lack of development of antidiabetic drugs in these models. The long-term expense may be prohibitive as it takes years to breed these animals. In addition, ethical standards and recommendations by the institutional animal care and use committees are usually such that experiments on nonhuman primates, in particular those aimed at testing new therapeutic agents, may only be done under careful scrutiny which by definition can limit the final impact on the drug development process. In this respect, noninvasive techniques, such as MRS and MRI, may offer a reasonable alternative as animals can serve as their own controls, allowing for improved statistical power and reduction of the number of animals tested.

20.4 MRI/S TECHNIQUES

A variety of MRI and MRS methodologies has been used to assess aspects of lipid and carbohydrate metabolism in tissues of relevancy for diabetes and obesity preclinical research. A number of these preclinical methodologies with technical aspects are discussed below.

20.4.1 ^{1}H MRS

20.4.1.1 Intramyocellular Lipid Spectroscopy

The ^{1}H MRS measurement of intramyocellular lipid (IMCL) content has made some of the most profound impact on drug discovery programs in part due to the fact that it is a validated and established technique, used in both preclinical and clinical studies. This technique offers the unique opportunity to noninvasively discriminate between the IMCL and extramyocellular lipid (EMCL) content. Thus, a number of pharmaceutical companies have employed this technology to assess pharmacology around targets which alter lipid metabolism [31,71,87–89].

The relationship between dyslipidemia and insulin resistance in animals [28,88] and man [90,91] is well documented (see also Chapter 21, Section 21.4.5). Because skeletal muscle tissue accounts for the majority of whole body insulin-stimulated glucose disposal in man, significant interest in examining the relationship between skeletal muscle lipid metabolite concentrations and insulin sensitivity exists. Spatially localized measurements of IMCL and EMCL have been performed using a variety of ^{1}H sequences including PRESS, STEAM, and chemical shift imaging with or without water suppression (e.g., CHESS). By acquiring short- and long-axis scout images, the spectroscopic region-of-interest (ROI) may be placed in specific muscle beds (e.g., soleus, tibialis anterior) which must be oriented such that the fibers are aligned with the static magnetic field [31,71,87,88]. The RF hardware typically comprises of a transmit/receive surface coil or a volume transmit with actively decoupled receive surface coil for increased sensitivity. Prominent ^{1}H peaks include Creatine (Cr) and Phosphocreatine (PCr) collectively referred to as total creatine (tCr), EMCL (methylene), IMCL (methylene), EMCL (methyl), and IMCL (methyl) appearing at 3.0, 1.5, 1.3, 1.1, and 0.9 ppm, respectively (Figure 20.1a). By decreasing the voxel size, the EMCL peak may be significantly diminished (Figure 20.1b). In Zucker fatty rats treated with rosiglitazone, the IMCL peak was rapidly (within days) reduced in the tibialis anterior muscle (Figure 20.2).

20.4.1.2 Hepatic Lipid Spectroscopy

Similarly to the IMCL measurement, hepatic lipid content may be assessed using ^{1}H MRS in conjunction with respiratory gating to minimize motion artifacts (see also Chapter 21, Section 21.5.4). Image-guided voxel placement in the liver must be scrutinized such that the voxel is distant from the portal vein, the surface of the liver and any fatty deposits (Figure 20.3) [43].

20.4.2 ^{1}H MRI

20.4.2.1 Whole Body Lipid Distribution Imaging

Although the whole body lipid content may be rapidly measured in animals using ^{1}H MRS [42] or relaxometry [53], due to the significant ^{1}H aliphatic lipid signal that is afforded by the concentrated lipid pools in adipocyte depot areas (i.e., subcutaneous or visceral fat depots), it may be advantageous to simultaneously assess lipid stores in different regions of the body using MRI.

^{1}H MRI is well grounded as a technology that can rapidly provide whole body as well as spatially distinct fat depot measurements (Figure 20.4) [48]. Generally, a rapid imaging sequence (e.g., turbo-spin echo) with short echo and repetition times is used to allow for signal suppression from tissues other than fat. Contiguous, two-dimensional transverse images covering the animal's

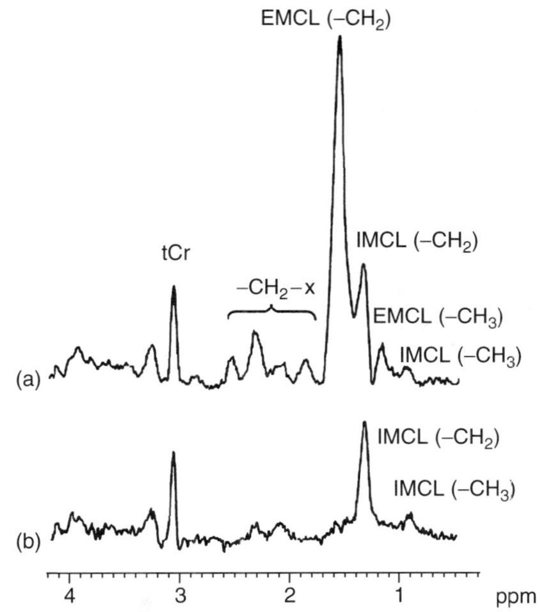

FIGURE 20.1 ^{1}H-spectra in the rat M. soleus (muscle fibers oriented parallel to the magnetic field B_0) from a VOI of (a) 18 mm^3 and (b) 8 mm^3. In (a) signals due to IMCL and EMCL are present, while in (b) the EMCL signals are no longer detectable. Resonances were assigned to tCr, to the methyl and methylene groups of IMCL and EMCL ($-CH_3$ or $-CH_2$), and to the several methylene groups next to a carbonyl group or double bond (labeled with $-CH_2-x$). These last resonances are a combination of EMCL and IMCL. In (a) they are quite intense, while in (b) they are strongly reduced, in line with the absence of EMCL signals. (Reproduced from Neumann-Haefelin, C., et al., *Magn. Res. Med.*, 50, 242, 2003. With permission of John Wiley & Sons, Inc. Copyright 2003.)

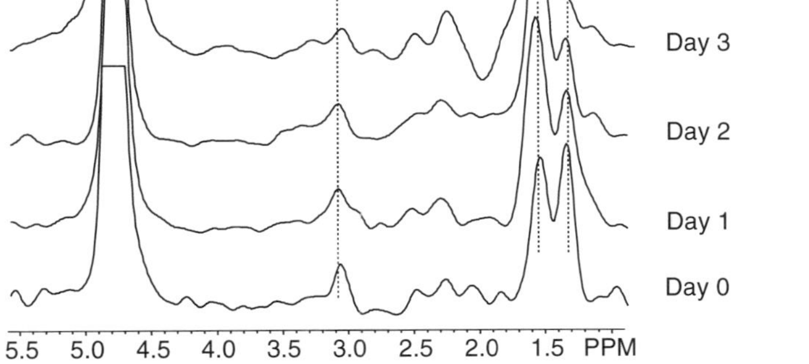

FIGURE 20.2 Serial ^{1}H spectra acquired in the tibialis anterior muscle of a Zucker fatty rat following rosiglitazone administration (3 mg/kg/day p.o.). Volume-selective ^{1}H NMR spectra taken from a $3 \times 3 \times 3$ mm voxel in the tibialis anterior muscle. The temporal decrease in IMCL (1.3 ppm) over the 4-day treatment period can be observed. (Reproduced from Jucker, B. M., et al., *Metabolism*, 52, 218, 2003. With permission of Elsevier Science. Copyright 2003.)

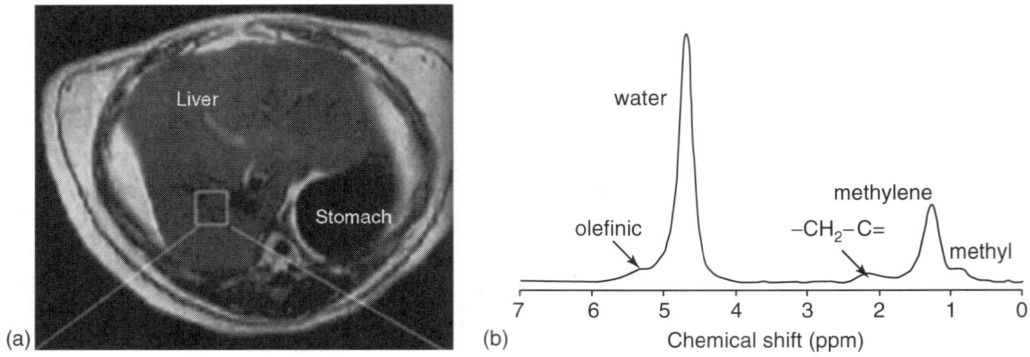

FIGURE 20.3 (a) Axial spin-echo image through the liver of a 28-week-old Fatty Zucker rat showing placement of the localized 5 × 5 × 5 mm cube spectroscopy voxel, and (b) typical resultant *in vivo* localized ^{1}H spectrum. (Reproduced from Hockings, P. D., et al., *Diabetes Obes. Metab.*, 5, 234, 2003. With permission of Blackwell Publishing. Copyright 2003.)

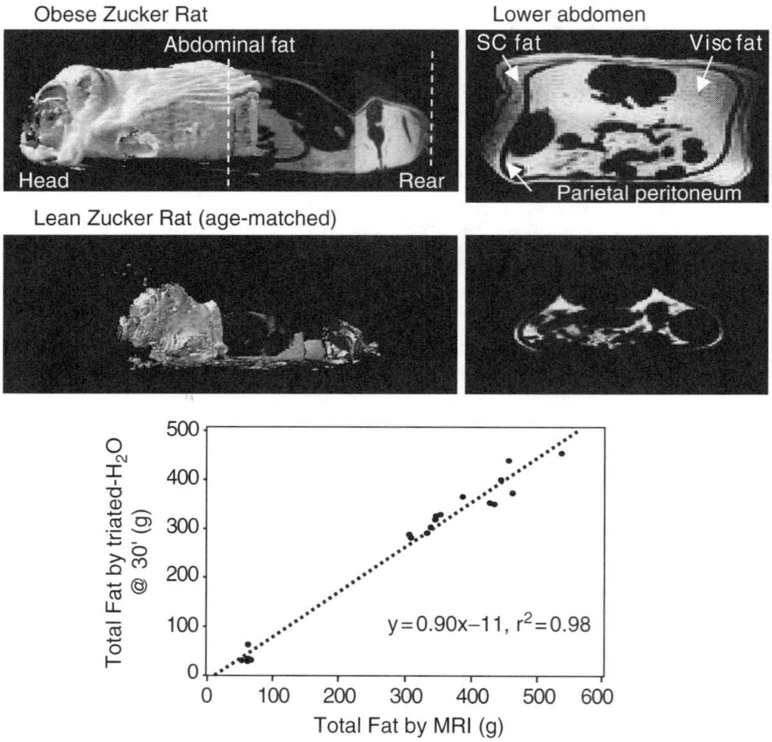

FIGURE 20.4 3-D surface rendered images and corresponding transverse MRI sections from the abdominal region of a lean (bottom) and an obese Zucker rat (top) delineating the subcutaneous (SC) and visceral (Visc) fat mass. The MRI technique for determining total body fat mass has been validated by comparison of data from both the MRI and a tritiated-water dilution technique in lean and obese *fa/fa* Zucker rats (bottom panel).

torso (typically 70 to 90 slices at 2-mm slice thickness) may be acquired in <45 min total acquisition time [48]. As discussed earlier, a number of studies examining the role of visceral vs. subcutaneous fat and its link to insulin resistance in the presence of pharmacological intervention have been performed [48,49].

20.4.3 ^{13}C MRS

20.4.3.1 Carbohydrate Metabolism: Glycogen Synthesis and Glycolysis

Although technically more challenging, ^{13}C MRS can be used to assess aspects of both carbohydrate (glycolysis and glycogen synthesis) and lipid metabolism *in vivo* (see also Chapter 21, Section 21.4 and Section 21.5). These experiments typically require ^{13}C precursor (e.g., 1-^{13}C glucose, 1,6-$^{13}C_2$ glucose, or 2-^{13}C acetate) administration over a period of time necessary to acquire kinetic data reflecting the ^{13}C label transfer to downstream metabolites (e.g., glycogen, lactate, alanine, and glutamate). Although most commercial spectrometer systems are equipped with broadband synthesizers and preamplifiers, allowing for multinuclear experiments, due to technical limitations including animal surgery, infusion and blood sampling in the magnet, as well as post-experiment *ex situ* tissue measurements (e.g., metabolite concentration and ^{13}C enrichment), there may be reluctance to use these techniques in the lead optimization phase of a drug discovery program. However, they may certainly be beneficial in late stage preclinical development of a compound before endorsement for first time in man studies (see Chapter 21).

^{13}C observe/^{1}H decouple MRS is typically performed using dual concentric surface coils which allow for high ^{13}C sensitivity and ^{1}H decoupling. Composite broadband ^{1}H decoupling (e.g., Waltz-16) should be applied during acquisition, and additional nuclear Overhauser enhancement may be achieved using low power decoupling during the relaxation delay. Animals are required to be catheterized, so that the ^{13}C-labeled precursor (e.g., 1-^{13}C glucose, 1,6-$^{13}C_2$ glucose for greater sensitivity, or 2-^{13}C acetate) may be administered. If a glucose–insulin clamp is performed, frequent blood sampling will be required. Spectra acquired from the hindlimb of a Sprague-Dawley rat to which 1-^{13}C glucose had been administered are shown in Figure 20.5. The C-1 glucose peak appears at 96.8 ppm (β-anomer) and 93.0 ppm (α-anomer), whereas the temporal increase in the C-1 glycogen peak can be seen at 100.5 ppm (Figure 20.5(a) Turnover of C-3 lactate (21.0 ppm) and C-3 alanine (16.9 ppm) may be clearly resolved following baseline subtraction (Figure 20.5(b).

20.4.3.2 Tri-Carboxylic Acid Cycle Turnover

Because the tri-carboxylic acid (TCA) cycle activity is coupled to O_2 consumption via a stoichiometric relationship with substrate use, the flux through the TCA cycle may be used as an index of substrate oxidation at steady state. Previously, ^{13}C MRS measurements of TCA cycle activity *in vivo* have been performed by observation of ^{13}C label turnover in glutamate, which reflects TCA cycle activity as a result of its equilibration with α-ketoglutarate [92–94]. An example of rat hindlimb TCA cycle turnover assessment using 2-^{13}C acetate as a precursor is shown in Figure 20.6.

20.4.3.3 Relative Fat vs. Glucose Oxidation: Isotope Analysis

Following *in vivo* ^{13}C glucose label incorporation into various tissues, *in vitro* NMR analysis can be performed to determine the skeletal muscle 3-^{13}C lactate, 3-^{13}C alanine, and 4-^{13}C glutamate enrichments for determining the relative contribution of flux entering the TCA cycle originating from glycolysis vs. free fatty acid (FFA)/ketone oxidation [14,88]. The 4-^{13}C glutamate pool is diluted to the degree by which unlabeled FFA/ketone oxidation vs. glycolysis is present during the clamp.

20.4.4 ^{31}P MRS

20.4.4.1 Glucose-6-Phosphate

Metabolic flux control may be assessed with the knowledge of changes in whole body glucose disposal, glycogen synthesis, glycolysis, and glucose-6-phosphate following metabolic

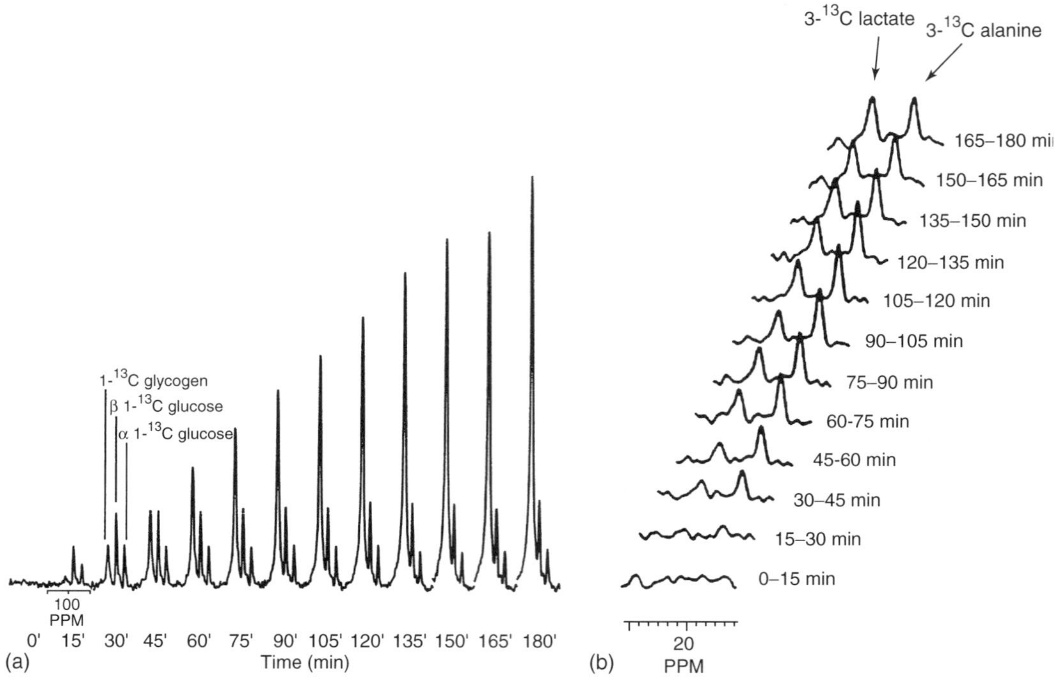

FIGURE 20.5 (a) *In vivo* ^{13}C spectra of 1-^{13}C glucose and 1-^{13}C glycogen. A series of 15-min acquired ^{13}C spectra from the hindlimb during a euglycemic-hyperinsulinemic clamp in a Sprague-Dawley rat (TR = 0.5 sec, SW = 20 KHz, 4 K data). At 0 min before infusion, no basal glycogen is detected at 100.5 ppm in the 24-h fasted rats. At 15 min, 1-^{13}C glucose appears at 96.8 ppm (β-anomer) and 93.0 ppm (α-anomer). 1-^{13}C Glycogen also appears at 15 min and continues to increase at a constant rate throughout the clamp experiment as 1-^{13}C glucose remains approximately constant. (b) *In vivo* ^{13}C spectra of 3-^{13}C lactate and 3-^{13}C alanine. 15 min acquired baseline subtracted ^{13}C spectra of the hindlimb during a euglycemic-hyperinsulinemic clamp in a Sprague-Dawley rat are staggered to illustrate the ^{13}C label turnover in 3-^{13}C lactate (21.0 ppm) and 3-^{13}C alanine (16.9 ppm). Spectra were baseline subtracted to minimize lipid distortion in measurements of the peaks. (Reproduced from Jucker, B. M., et al., *J. Biol. Chem.*, 272, 10464, 1997. With permission of The American Society for Biochemistry and Molecular Biology, Inc. Copyright 1997.)

perturbation (e.g., elevated FFA or hyperglycemia). Because pharmacological agents may target glucose transport (directly or indirectly), glycogen synthesis or glycolysis, it can be advantageous to assign control to these pathways for compound differentiation purposes. An example of glucose-6-phosphate perturbation during a hyperinsulinemic, euglycemic to hyperglycemic clamp is presented in Figure 20.7. Using metabolic control analysis and ^{13}C MRS to measure the flux through these metabolic pathways, in combination with ^{31}P NMR measurements of glucose-6-phosphate, it was determined that the majority of control for glucose uptake in rat skeletal muscle resides at the glucose transport/phosphorylation step [15,23]. In order to determine which of the two metabolic steps, transport or phosphorylation, is rate controlling, one may assess the intracellular glucose concentration *in vivo* by ^{13}C MRS combined with a spectroscopic marker of the extracellular space [95].

20.4.4.2 ATP Synthesis Flux

Unidirectional ATP production may be assessed noninvasively in rat skeletal muscle (see Figure 20.8) by using a ^{31}P saturation transfer method as initially described for measurements

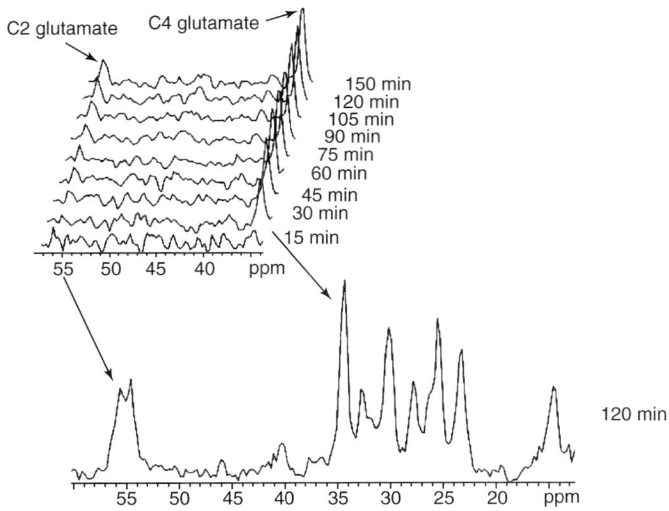

FIGURE 20.6 ^{13}C spectra acquired from the hindlimb of a Sprague-Dawley rat during infusion of 2-^{13}C acetate. The 2-^{13}C glutamate peak appears at 55.5 ppm on the shoulder of the creatine/phosphocreatine peak (54.4 ppm), and the 4-^{13}C glutamate peak obscured by a co-resonating aliphatic lipid peak appears at 34.4 ppm. Therefore, all spectra were baseline-subtracted before peak integration. 3-^{13}C glutamate (27.9 ppm) and 2-^{13}C acetate (24.2 ppm) were not observed, since they reside in the frequency bandwidth that was partially suppressed due to the aliphatic lipid suppression pulse sequence used. Turnover of the 2-^{13}C- and 4-^{13}C-labeled glutamate peaks in the hindlimb muscles of a fed rat is illustrated in the baseline-subtracted spectra shown above. 2-^{13}C acetate label incorporates rapidly into 4-^{13}C glutamate and more slowly into 2-^{13}C glutamate (second turn of the tricarboxylic acid cycle). (Reproduced from Jucker, B. M., et al., *J. Biol. Chem.*, 275, 39283, 2000. With permission of The American Society for Biochemistry and Molecular Biology, Inc. Copyright 2000.)

in *Escherichia coli* [96] and later in skeletal muscle [97]. A saturation transfer experiment provides unique information with regard to unidirectional metabolic flux (see Alger and Shulman [98] for a review). In this procedure, the γ-ATP peak is nulled with a saturating radio frequency pulse, and the reduction of the P_i peak as a result of the transfer of the saturated spins between γ-ATP and the P_i pool via F_1F_0 ATP_{ase} and other $P_i \rightarrow$ ATP pathways (e.g., GAPDH and PGK reactions) is monitored. This decrease in magnetization of P_i (ΔM) may be used to determine the kinetics of ATP_{ase} activity once the glycolytic contributions of coupled GAPDH and PGK are accounted for. Although the net glycolytic contribution to the production of ATP (via GAPDH and PGK) vs. that of oxidative phosphorylation is small, these enzymes are nearly at equilibrium, and consequently, the unidirectional production of ATP (measured with the ^{31}P saturation transfer experiment) via these enzymes can be high. However, one may account for this contribution by examining U-^{2}H glucose turnover in glycolytic intermediates [27]. The rate constant (k) for $P_i \rightarrow$ ATP is defined by

$$k = 1/T_{1app} \times \Delta M/M_0 \tag{20.1}$$

where T_{1app} is the longitudinal relaxation time of P_i during γ-ATP saturation and $\Delta M/M_0$ is the fractional change of the P_i magnetization during the saturation transfer experiment. Therefore, k may be calculated after acquiring spectra from the saturation transfer and inversion recovery experiments. The unidirectional ATP synthesis flux ($P_i \rightarrow$ ATP) may be calculated as $k \times [P_i]$.

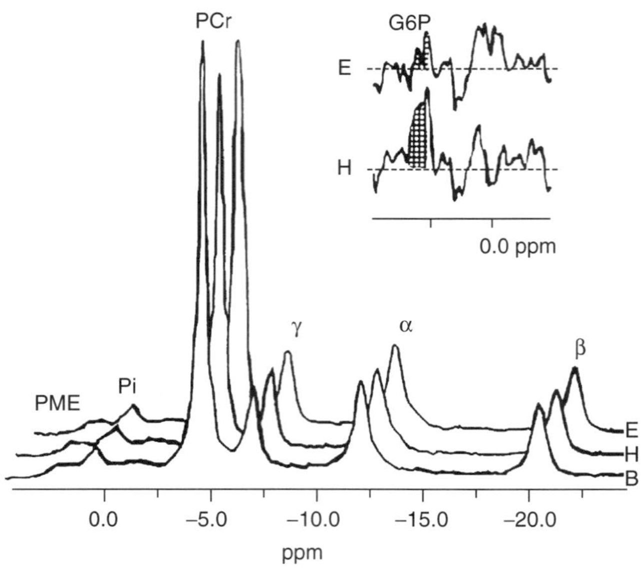

FIGURE 20.7 Sample ^{31}P spectra acquired in a Sprague–Dawley rat during a glucose insulin clamp, with the characteristic phosphomonoester peaks (left to right): inorganic phosphate (P_i), phosphocreatine (PCr), γ-ATP, α-ATP, and β-ATP. Inset: × 10 magnification of the glucose 6-phosphate (G-6-*P*) peak (crosshatched) from difference spectra for hyperglycemia (H) [H to baseline (B)] and for euglycemia (E) [E to B]. (Reproduced from Chase, J. R., Rothman, D. L., and Shulman, R. G., *Am. J. Physiol. Endocrinol. Metab.*, 280, E598, 2001. With permission of The American Society for Biochemistry and Molecular Biology, Inc. Copyright 2001.)

20.4.4.3 Mitochondrial Energetic Coupling

The ratio of the measured unidirectional ATP synthesis flux to TCA cycle flux may be used as a qualitative index of the degree of coupling between mitochondrial substrate oxidation and ATP synthesis (if the measured unidirectional ATP synthesis flux and the glycolytic contribution to this measurement are equal in all groups). The limitation of this analysis is that, if the measured ATP synthesis flux or glycolytic contribution to this flux were different between groups, then the glycolytic contribution would have to be subtracted from the overall ATP synthesis flux to obtain accurate ratios. Since we do not know the extent of basal mitochondrial uncoupling present as a result of combined proton transport and leaks across the inner mitochondrial membrane, this ratio should be normalized to the vehicle-treated group.

20.5 EXPERIMENTAL LIMITATIONS

When designing *in vivo* obesity or diabetes pharmacology studies using some of the spectroscopic techniques discussed earlier in this chapter, one must be aware of the technical challenges facing the investigator, which are discussed as follows.

20.5.1 Sensitivity

The field strength of the magnet is a practical issue to consider when designing a spectroscopic experiment. Due to the inherently low sensitivity of ^{13}C MRS, these studies are typically performed at higher magnetic field strength. The investigator must consider the spectroscopic SNR required for a given study and balance the tissue mass necessary for observation with the

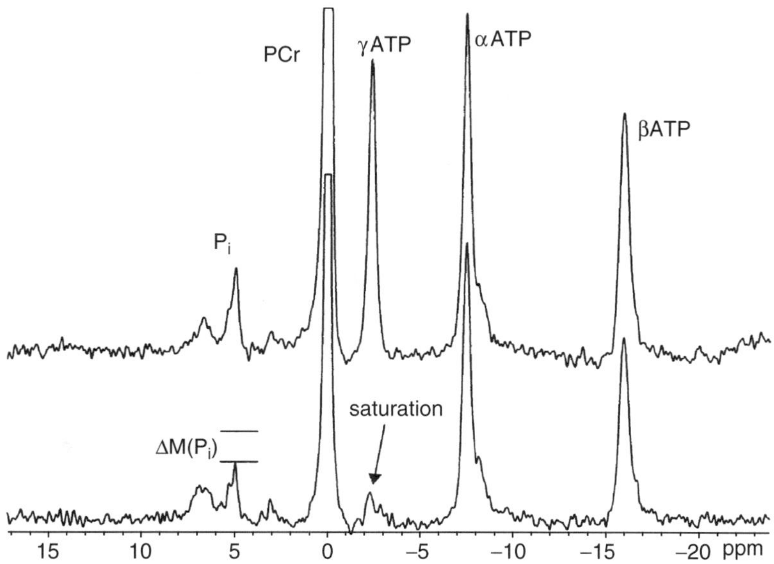

FIGURE 20.8 ^{31}P NMR saturation transfer study. The spectra shown were obtained from a saturation transfer experiment performed in the hindlimb muscles of an awake rat. In the bottom spectrum, a continuous wave radio frequency pulse was used to saturate the γ-ATP resonance (2.4 ppm). In the upper spectrum (no γ-ATP saturation), the continuous wave pulse frequency was placed symmetrically to the down-field side of P_i (4.9 ppm). The resulting loss in magnetization of P_i (ΔM) was due to the exchange of saturated γ-ATP nuclei with nonsaturated P_i nuclei. (Reproduced from Jucker, B. M., et al., *Proc. Natl. Acad. Sci. U.S.A*, 97, 6880, 2000. With permission of The National Academy of Sciences. Copyright 2000.)

magnet field strength required as there is a trade off between the two. To illustrate this point, while an *in vivo* ^{13}C spectroscopic study assessing TCA cycle turnover in rat liver (~5 to 15 g) was performed at 7 T [99], similar ^{13}C spectroscopic studies in the liver of obese monkeys (~400 to 600 g) can only be performed in scanners with a relatively large bore diameter (>40 cm) generally at 1.5 to 3 T. Therefore, the trade off between tissue size and magnet field strength may be sufficient in this respect to perform these studies. Indeed, a number of clinical ^{13}C spectroscopic studies in liver have been performed at 1.5 T or greater fields [12,51,100,101]. While extrapolating spectroscopic studies to larger animals is feasible, spectroscopic studies in mouse skeletal muscle or liver have been limited to ^{1}H and ^{31}P MRS. However, with the recent advances in magnet technology, there may be opportunity for such studies to be routinely performed in the future. Finally, the use of surface RF coils will significantly enhance the SNR achieved during the spectroscopic studies. However, standard surface RF coils provided by the magnet vendor may not be adequate with respect to coil architecture or multinuclear capabilities. Therefore RF coils with the necessary features for a specific study may have to be custom built or purchased from an independent RF coil manufacturer.

20.5.2 Animal Handling and Preparation

Because anesthetic agents can induce insulin resistance not only in the liver, but also in peripheral tissues, experiments should ideally be conducted in the awake animal. However, in most cases this is not feasible, so that a possible effect of anesthesia on data interpretation must be documented. If glucose/insulin clamps are to be performed or if ^{13}C labeled precursors are to be administered to rodents, animals will generally require having a cannula inserted up to 1 week prior to the study. While chronic cannulation can be routinely performed in rats, this may be technically challenging in mice. Logistical concerns following surgery include careful monitoring for possible infection at the surgical site, maintaining catheter patency, and minimal animal handling (e.g., oral dosing) to minimize animal stress prior to the MR experiment. Additional resources should also be considered during the scanning session such that the glucose/insulin clamp and MR data acquisition are handled by different investigators. One should also be aware that the throughput of such experiments is low, generally not exceeding two to three animals a day.

20.5.3 Administration of ^{13}C-Labeled Compounds

Due to the inherent low sensitivity of ^{13}C MRS, it is necessary to administer ^{13}C-labeled glucose to allow for the detection of glycogen and/or downstream glycolytic and TCA cycle intermediates in rodent liver or muscle. In addition, in order to calculate absolute glycogen synthesis or glycolytic rates, the animal will have to be sacrificed at the end of the experiment [13–15,41]. Consequently for a longitudinal study, each animal cannot be used as its own control, which will reduce the statistical power of the study. The cost of ^{13}C-labeled precursor substrates may also be of concern, especially if the number of studies or animal size (e.g., nonhuman primate) is large. Generally speaking, if a hyperinsulinemic/glycemic clamp is performed in a 300-g rat, the whole body glucose disposal rate may be ~30 to 50 mg/kg/min. Therefore, a study conducted for 200 min would require up to 3 g of ^{13}C-labeled glucose. At a cost of ~$40 to 50 per g of 1-^{13}C glucose, the cost of the experiment may be ~$150/rat. However, if increased sensitivity is required for glycolytic or TCA cycle intermediate enrichment, 1,6-$^{13}C_2^-$labeled glucose may be considered, but at a cost of ~$600/g, these experiments may be prohibitively expensive even in rodents.

20.5.4 Safety

The use of properly optimized MR pulse sequences will contribute to optimal signal sensitivity for a number of applications. In the case of ^{13}C MRS, ^{1}H decoupling is often necessary to increase sensitivity and resolution. However, this poses an inherent problem as ^{1}H decoupling can lead to substantial power deposition and heat generation in the animal. There are ways to minimize power deposition such that institutional limits are not exceeded (e.g., <4 Watt/kg in humans). Therefore, pulse sequences need to be carefully optimized prior to drug study and physiological monitoring should be present for the safety and well-being of the animal.

20.6 TRANSLATION TO CLINICAL STUDIES

The ultimate goal for preclinical MRI and/or MRS studies is to be translated to the clinic. This factor may be a limitation for spectroscopy studies as ^{1}H is typically the only nucleus routinely used in the clinic. However, many academic centers which have experimental clinical scanners capable of multinuclear studies at high field strength are generally in close proximity of a hospital. Therefore, small-scale clinical studies designed to be of "experimental medicine" nature, or even proof-of-concept studies examining the potential for a positive drug indication in a small cohort of patients, may ultimately be performed in an academic facility. The design and questions asked in the preclinical study will provide guidance for clinical colleagues in the design of their study. It is important to be realistic in achieving clinical goals given the patient population, disease area, and instrumentation available.

Another aspect of translational MRI is the necessity to develop novel ways to address unique aspects of a drug target. For example, in order to examine insulin sensitivity in skeletal muscle following TZD treatment, one might want to examine whether the IMCL content in the muscle correlates with insulin sensitivity. MRS provides a means of measuring specific IMCL pools noninvasively. This technology means that analyzing lipid content nonspecifically in tissue biopsies can be avoided. This is an example of how MRS can be translated into the clinic to provide key insight as to the PK/PD relationship of an antidiabetic compound. Clinical MRI may be used as well to provide accurate and rapid assessment as to the distribution of fat stores throughout the body (e.g., visceral vs. subcutaneous) [35]. Examples of clinical pharmacology experiments using some of the techniques discussed for the preclinical setting will be addressed in the following chapter.

REFERENCES

1. Wild, S. et al., Global prevalence of diabetes: estimates for the year 2000 and projections for 2030, *Diabetes Care*, 27, 1047, 2004.
2. Flegal, K. M. et al., Overweight and obesity in the United States: prevalence and trends, 1960–1994, *Int. J. Obes. Relat. Metab. Disord.*, 22, 39, 1998.
3. James, W. P., What are the health risks? The medical consequences of obesity and its health risks, *Exp. Clin. Endocrinol. Diabetes*, 106, S1, 1998.
4. James, P. T., Obesity: the worldwide epidemic, *Clin. Dermatol.*, 22, 276, 2004.
5. Scaglione, R. et al., Obesity and cardiovascular risk: the new public health problem of worldwide proportions, *Expert Rev. Cardiovasc. Ther.*, 2, 203, 2004.
6. Cline, G. W. et al., Mechanism of impaired insulin-stimulated muscle glucose metabolism in subjects with insulin-dependent diabetes mellitus, *J. Clin. Invest.*, 99, 2219, 1997.
7. DeFronzo, R. A., The triumvirate: beta-cell, muscle, liver: a collusion responsible for NIDDM, *Diabetes*, 37, 667, 1988.
8. DeFronzo, R. A. et al., The effect of insulin on the disposal of intravenous glucose: results from indirect calorimetry and hepatic and femoral venous catheterization, *Diabetes*, 30, 1000, 1981.
9. Kim, J. K., Wi, J. K., and Youn, J. H., Plasma free fatty acids decrease insulin-stimulated skeletal muscle glucose uptake by suppressing glycolysis in conscious rats, *Diabetes*, 45, 446, 1996.
10. Nolte, L. A. et al., Elevated free fatty acid levels inhibit glucose phosphorylation in slow-twitch rat skeletal muscle, *Acta. Physiol. Scand.*, 151, 51, 1994.
11. Gruetter, R. et al., Validation of ^{13}C NMR measurements of liver glycogen in vivo, *Magn. Reson. Med.*, 31, 583, 1994.
12. Jue, T. et al., Direct observation of glycogen synthesis in human muscle with ^{13}C NMR, *Proc. Natl. Acad. Sci. U S A.*, 86, 4489, 1989.
13. Jucker, B. M. et al., In vivo NMR investigation of intramuscular glucose metabolism in conscious rats, *Am. J. Physiol.*, 273, E139, 1997.
14. Jucker, B. M. et al., ^{13}C and ^{31}P NMR studies on the effects of increased plasma free fatty acids on intramuscular glucose metabolism in the awake rat, *J. Biol. Chem.*, 272, 10464, 1997.
15. Jucker, B. M., Barucci, N., and Shulman, G. I., Metabolic control analysis of insulin stimulated glucose disposal in skeletal muscle, *Am. J. Physiol.*, 277, E505, 1999.
16. Frayn, K., Calculation of substrate oxidation rates in vivo from gaseous exchange, *J. Appl. Physiol.*, 55, 628, 1983.
17. Rossetti, L. et al., Quantitation of glycolysis and skeletal muscle glycogen synthesis in humans, *Am. J. Physiol.*, 265, E761, 1993.
18. Furnsinn, C. et al., Acute non-insulin-like stimulation of rat muscle glucose metabolism by troglitazone *in vitro*, *Br. J. Pharmacol.*, 122, 1367, 1997.
19. Stevenson, R. W. et al., Actions of novel antidiabetic agent englitazone in hyperglycaemic hyperinsulinemic ob/ob mice, *Diabetes*, 39, 1218, 1990.
20. Sreenan, S. et al., Effects of troglitazone on substrate storage and utilization in insulin-resistant rats, *Am. J. Physiol.*, 276, E1119, 1999.
21. Kacser, H. and Burns, J. A., The control of flux, *Symp. Soc. Exp. Biol.*, 27, 65, 1973.
22. Bloch, G. et al., In vivo ^{31}P NMR measurement of glucose-6-phosphate in the rat muscle after exercise, *Magn. Reson. Med.*, 30, 347, 1993.

23. Chase, J. R., Rothman, D. L., and Shulman, R. G., Flux control in the rat gastrocnemius glycogen synthesis pathway by in vivo $^{13}C/^{31}P$ NMR spectroscopy, *Am. J. Physiol. Endocrinol. Metab.*, 280, E598, 2001.
24. Himms-Hagen, J., Brown adipose tissue thermogenesis and obesity, *Prog. Lipid Res.*, 28, 67, 1989.
25. Boss, O. et al., Uncoupling protein-3: a new member of the mitochondrial carrier family with tissue-specific expression, *FEBS Lett.*, 408, 39, 1997.
26. Vidal-Puig, A. et al., UCP3: an uncoupling protein homologue expressed preferentially and abundantly in skeletal muscle and brown adipose tissue, *Biochem. Biophys. Res. Commun.*, 235, 79, 1997.
27. Jucker, B. M. et al., Assessment of mitochondrial energy coupling *in vivo* by $^{13}C/^{31}P$ NMR, *Proc. Natl. Acad. Sci. U.S.A.*, 97, 6880, 2000.
28. Storlien, L. H. et al., Influence of dietary fat composition on development of insulin resistance in rats. Relationship to muscle triglyceride and omega-3 fatty acids in muscle phospholipids, *Diabetes*, 40, 280, 1991.
29. Oakes, N. D. et al., The insulin sensitizer, BRL 49653, reduces systemic fatty acid supply and utilization and tissue lipid availability in the rat, *Metabolism*, 46, 935, 1997.
30. Schick, F. et al., Comparison of localized proton NMR signals of skeletal muscle and fat tissue in vivo: two lipid compartments in muscle tissue, *Magn. Reson. Med.*, 29, 158, 1993.
31. Kuhlmann, J. et al., Intramyocellular lipid and insulin resistance. A longitudinal in vivo ^{1}H-spectroscopic study in Zucker diabetic fatty rats, *Diabetes*, 52, 138, 2003.
32. Mateigka, J., The testing of physical efficiency, *Am. J. Phys., Anthropol.*, 4, 223, 1921.
33. Mazess, R. B. et al., Dual-energy x-ray absoptiometry for total-body and regional bone-mineral and soft-tissue composition, *Am. J. Clin. Nutr.*, 51, 1106, 1990.
34. Thaete, F. L. et al., Reproducibility of computed tomography measurement of visceral adipose tissue area, *Int. J. Obes. Relat. Metab. Disord.*, 19, 464, 1995.
35. Seidell, J. C., Bakker, C. J., and van der Kooy, K., Imaging techniques for measuring adipose-tissue distribution: a comparison between computed tomography and 1.5 T magnetic resonance, *Am. J. Clin. Nutr.*, 51, 953, 1990.
36. Pi-Sunyer, F. X., The epidemiology of central fat distribution in relation to disease, *Nutr. Rev.*, 62, S120, 2004.
37. Oakes, N. D. et al., A new antidiabetic agent, BRL 49653, reduces lipid availability and improves insulin action and glucoregulation in the rat, *Diabetes*, 43, 1203, 1994.
38. Young, P. W. et al., Repeat treatment of obese mice with BRL 49653, a new potent insulin sensitizer, enhances insulin action in white adipocytes: association with increased insulin binding and cell surface GLUT4 as measured by photoaffinity labeling, *Diabetes*, 44, 1087, 1995.
39. Kanoh, Y. et al., Rosiglitazone, insulin treatment, and fasting correct defective activation of protein kinase C-zeta/lambda by insulin in vastus lateralis muscles and adipocytes of diabetic rats, *Endocrinology*, 142, 1595, 2001.
40. Petersen, K. F. et al., Mechanism of troglitazone action in type 2 diabetes, *Diabetes*, 49, 827, 2000.
41. Jucker, B. M. et al., Normalization of skeletal muscle glycogen synthesis and glycolysis in rosiglitazone-treated Zucker fatty rats: an *in vivo* nuclear magnetic resonance study, *Diabetes*, 51, 2066, 2002.
42. Jucker, B. M. et al., Reduction of intramyocellular lipid following short-term rosiglitazone treatment in Zucker fatty rats: an *in vivo* nuclear magnetic resonance Study, *Metabolism*, 52, 218, 2003.
43. Hockings, P. D. et al., Rapid reversal of hepatic steatosis, and reduction of muscle triglyceride, by rosiglitazone: MRI/S studies in Zucker fatty rats, *Diabetes Obes. Metab.*, 5, 234, 2003.
44. Burkey, B. F. et al., Pioglitazone promotes energy storage and not expenditure in brown adipose tissue of obese fa/fa Zucker rats: comparison with CL 316,243, *Metabolism*, 49, 1301, 2000.
45. Wang, Q. et al., Increased feeding in fatty Zucker rats by the thiazolidinedione BRL 49653 (rosiglitazone) and the possible involvement of leptin and hypothalmic neuropeptide Y, *Br. J. Pharm.*, 122, 1405, 1997.
46. Okuno, A. et al., Troglitazone increases the number of small adipocytes without the change of white adipose tissue mass in obese Zucker rats, *J. Clin. Invest.*, 101, 1354, 1998.
47. Hallakou, S. et al., Pioglitazone induces *in vivo* adipocyte differentiation in the obese Zucker *fa/fa* rat, *Diabetes*, 46, 1393, 1997.

48. de Souza, C. J. et al., Effects of pioglitizone on adipose tissue remodeling within the setting of obesity and insulin resistance, *Diabetes*, 50, 1863, 2001.
49. Kelly, I. E. et al., Effects of a thiazolidinedione compound on body fat and fat distribution of patients with type 2 diabetes, *Diabetes Care*, 22, 288, 1999.
50. Bailey, C. J., Metformin, *N. Engl. J. Med.*, 334, 574, 1996.
51. Hundal, R. S. et al., Mechanism by which metformin reduces glucose production in Type 2 diabetics, *Diabetes*, 49, 2063, 2000.
52. Bays, H. E., Current and investigational antiobesity agents and obesity therapeutic treatment targets, *Obes. Res*, 12, 1197, 2004.
53. Kunnecke, B. et al., Quantitative body composition analysis in awake mice and rats by magnetic resonance relaxometry, *Obes. Res.*, 12, 1604, 2004.
54. Szayna, M. et al., Exendin-4 decelerates food intake, weight gain, and fat deposition in Zucker rats, *Endocrinol.*, 141, 1936, 2000.
55. Lee, H. J. et al., Fenofibrate lowers abdominal and skeletal adiposity and improves insulin sensitivity in OLETF rats, *Biochem. Biophys. Res. Commun.*, 296, 293, 2002.
56. Clapham, J. C. et al., Mice overexpressing human uncoupling protein-3 in skeletal muscle are hyperphagic and lean, *Nature*, 406, 415, 2000.
57. Ogawa, Y. et al., Molecular cloning of rat obese cDNA and augmented gene expression in genetically obese Zucker fatty (fa/fa) rats, *J. Clin. Invest.*, 96, 1647, 1995.
58. Corsetti, J. P. et al., Effects of dietary fat on the development of non-insulin dependent diabetes mellitus in obese Zucker diabetic fatty male and female rats, *Atherosclerosis*, 148, 231, 2000.
59. Phillips, M. S. et al., Leptin receptor missense mutation in the fatty Zucker rat (Letter), *Nat. Genet.*, 13, 18, 1996.
60. Apweiler, R. and Freund, P., Development of glucose intolerance in obese (*fa/fa*) Zucker rats, *Horm. Metab. Res.*, 25, 521, 1993.
61. Etgen, G. J. and Oldham, B. A., Profiling of Zucker diabetic fatty rats in their progression to the overt diabetic state, *Metabolism*, 49, 684, 2000.
62. Pick, A. et al., Role of apoptosis in failure of beta-cell mass compensation for insulin resistance and beta-cell defects in the male Zucker diabetic fatty rat, *Diabetes*, 47, 358, 1998.
63. Finegood, D. T. et al., β-cell mass dynamics in Zucker diabetic fatty rats. Rosiglitazone prevents the rise in net cell death, *Diabetes*, 50, 1021, 2001.
64. Storlien, L. H. et al., Influence of dietary fat composition on development of insulin resistance in rats. Relationship to muscle triglyceride and omega-3 fatty acids in muscle phospholipids, *Diabetes*, 40, 280, 1991.
65. Wake, S. A. et al., Effects of exercise training and dietary manipulation on insulin-regulatable glucose-transporter mRNA in rat muscle, *Diabetes*, 40, 275, 1991.
66. Kraegen, E. W. et al., Triglycerides, fatty acids and insulin resistance-hyperinsulinemia, *Exp. Clin. Endocrinol. Diabetes*, 109, S516, 2001.
67. D'Alessandro, M. E. et al., Role of skeletal muscle on impaired insulin sensitivity in rats fed a sucrose-rich diet: effect of moderate levels of dietary fish oil, *J. Nutr. Biochem.*, 11, 273, 2000.
68. Sinha, R. et al., Assessment of skeletal muscle triglyceride content by (1)H nuclear magnetic resonance spectroscopy in lean and obese adolescents: relationships to insulin sensitivity, total body fat, and central adiposity, *Diabetes*, 51, 1022, 2002.
69. Kim, J. K. et al., Mechanism of insulin resistance in A-ZIP/F-1 fatless mice, *J. Biol. Chem.*, 275, 8456, 2000.
70. Bagdade, J. D. et al., Glucocorticoids and triglyceride transport: effects on triglyceride secretion rates, lipoprotein lipase, and plasma lipoproteins in the rat, *Metabolism*, 25, 533, 1976.
71. Korach-Andre, M. et al., Relationship between visceral adiposity and intramyocellular lipid content in two rat models of insulin resistance, *Am. J. Physiol. Endocrinol. Metab.*, 288, E106, 2005.
72. Werner, E. D. et al., Insulin resistance due to phosphorylation of insulin receptor substrate-1 at serine 302, *J. Biol. Chem.*, 279, 35298, 2004.
73. Shirakami, A. et al., Heterozygous knockout of the IRS-1 gene in mice enhances obesity-linked insulin resistance: a possible model for the development of type 2 diabetes, *J. Endocrinol.*, 174, 309, 2002.

74. Abe, H. and Yamada, N., Animal models for hyperinsulinemia and insulin resistance, *Ann. NY Acad. Sci.*, 902, 134, 2000.
75. Le Roith, D. et al., Inactivation of muscle insulin and IGF-1 receptors and insulin responsiveness, *Curr. Opin. Clin. Nutr. Metab. Care*, 5, 371, 2002.
76. Yang, C. et al., Syntaxin 4 heterozygous knockout mice develop muscle insulin resistance, *J. Clin. Invest.*, 107, 1311, 2001.
77. Chehab, F. F., Qiu, J., and Ogus, S., The use of animal models to dissect the biology of leptin, *Recent Prog. Horm. Res.*, 59, 245, 2004.
78. Castellani, L. W. et al., Mechanisms mediating insulin resistance in transgenic mice overexpressing mouse apolipoprotein A-II, *J. Lipid Res.*, 45, 2377, 2003.
79. Hansen, B. C. and Bodkin, N. L., Heterogeneity of insulin responses; phases in the continuum leading to non-insulin-dependent diabetes mellitus, *Diabetologia*, 29, 713, 1986.
80. Bogardus, C. et al., Relationships between insulin secretion, insulin action and fasting plasma glucose concentration in nondiabetic and noninsulin-dependent diabetic subjects, *J. Clin. Invest.*, 74, 1238, 1984.
81. Bodkin, N. L., Metger, B. L., and Hansen, B. C., Hepatic glucose production and insulin sensitivity preceding diabetes in monkeys, *Am. J. Physiol.*, 256, E676, 1989, Endocrinol. Metab. 19.
82. DeFronzo, R. A. and Ferrannini, E., The pathogenesis of non-insulin-dependent diabetes, *Medicine*, 61, 313, 1982.
83. Baron, A. D. et al., Role of hyperglucagonemia in maintenance of increased rates of hepatic glucose output in type II diabetes, *Diabetes*, 36, 274, 1987.
84. Ortmeyer, H. K., Bodkin, N. L., and Hansen, B. C., Adipose tissue glycogen synthase activation by in vivo insulin in spontaneously insulin-resistant and non-insulin-dependent diabetic rhesus monkeys, *Diabetologia*, 36, 200, 1993.
85. Ortmeyer, H. K., Bodkin, N. L., and Hansen, B. C., Insulin-mediated glycogen synthase activity in muscle of spontaneously insulin-resistant and diabetic rhesus monkeys, *Am. J. Physiol.*, 265, R552, 1993, Regul. Integr. Comp. Physiol. 34.
86. Ortmeyer, H. K. and Bodkin, N. L., Lack of defect in insulin action on hepatic glycogen synthase and phosphorylase in insulin-resistant monkeys, *Am. J. Physiol.*, 274, G1005, 1998, Gastr. L. Physiol. 37.
87. Neumann-Haefelin, C. et al., Determinants of intramyocellular lipid concentrations in rat hindleg muscle, *Magn. Res. Med.*, 50, 242, 2003.
88. Jucker, B. M. et al., Differential effects of safflower oil versus fish oil feeding on insulin-stimulated glycogen synthesis, glycolysis, and pyruvate dehydrogenase flux in skeletal muscle: a ^{13}C nuclear magnetic resonance study, *Diabetes*, 48, 134, 1999.
89. Korach-André, M., et al., Age and muscle-type modulated role of intramyocellular lipids (IMCL) in the progression of insulin resistance in nondiabetic Zucker rats, *Metabolism*, 54, 522, 2005.
90. Kolterman, O. G., Reaven, G. M., and Olefsky, J. M., Relationship between in vivo insulin resistance and decreased insulin receptors in obese man, *J. Clin. Endocrinol. Metab.*, 48, 487, 1979.
91. Yki-Jarvinen, H. and Kiovisto, V. A., Effects of body composition on insulin sensitivity, *Diabetes*, 32, 965, 1983.
92. Fitzpatrick, S. M. et al., The flux from glucose to glutamate in the rat brain in vivo as determined by ^{1}H-observed, ^{13}C-edited NMR spectroscopy, *J. Cereb. Blood Flow Metab.*, 10, 170, 1990.
93. Mason, G. F. et al., NMR determination of the TCA cycle rate and alpha-ketoglutarate/glutamate exchange rate in rat brain, *J. Cereb. Blood Flow Metab.*, 12, 434, 1992.
94. Yu, X. et al., Kinetic analysis of dynamic ^{13}C NMR spectra: metabolic flux, regulation, and compartmentation in hearts, *Biophys. J.*, 69, 2090, 1995.
95. Cline, G. W. et al., A novel ^{13}C NMR method to assess intracellular glucose concentration in muscle, in vivo, *Am. J. Physiol.*, 274, E381, 1998.
96. Brown, T. R., Ugurbil, K., and Shulman, R. G., ^{31}P nuclear magnetic resonance measurements of ATPase kinetics in aerobic Escherichia coli cells, *Proc. Natl. Acad. Sci. U.S.A*, 74, 5551, 1977.
97. Brindle, K. M. et al., ^{31}P NMR magnetization-transfer measurements of ATP turnover during steady-state isometric muscle contraction in the rat hind limb in vivo, *Biochemistry*, 28, 4887, 1989.
98. Alger, J. R. and Shulman, R. G., NMR studies of enzymatic rates in vitro and in vivo by magnetization transfer, *Q. Rev. Biophys.*, 17, 83, 1984.

99. Jucker, B. M., Lee, J. Y., and Shulman, R. G., In vivo ^{13}C NMR measurements of hepatocellular tricarboxylic acid cycle flux, *J. Biol. Chem.*, 273, 12187, 1998.
100. Krssak, M. et al., Alterations in postprandial hepatic glycogen metabolism in type 2 diabetes, *Diabetes*, 53, 3048, 2004.
101. Flück, C. E. et al., Normal hepatic glycogen storage after fasting and feeding in children and adolescents with type 1 diabetes, *Ped. Diabetes*, 4, 70, 2003.

21 MR in Clinical Diabetes Research and Drug Trials

Michael Roden

CONTENTS

21.1 BACKGROUND

Diabetes mellitus is defined by increased blood glucose (hyperglycemia) in the fasted and/or in the postprandial state [1]. Hyperglycemia is a consequence of inappropriate insulin secretion by pancreatic β cells due to autoimmune destruction in type 1 diabetes mellitus (T1DM) or rare inherited defects in maturity onset diabetes of the young (MODY). The most frequent diabetes type, type 2 diabetes mellitus (T2DM), is primarily due to impaired insulin action, i.e., insulin resistance, at its target tissues such as skeletal muscle, liver, and adipose tissue [1]. Insulin resistance is usually linked to increased visceral fat mass, arterial hypertension, hyperuricemia, dyslipidemia, and endothelial dysfunction, which are summarized as term pluri or dysmetabolic syndrome [2]. These abnormalities are also found in women who develop glucose intolerance during pregnancy, i.e., gestational or type 4 diabetes mellitus (T4DM). The dysbalance of energy homeostasis with caloric intake exceeding energy expenditure is currently held responsible for the epidemic spread of obesity and diabetes [3,4]. Abnormalities of fat distribution such as lipodystrophy also lead to severe insulin resistance and diabetes [5]. With *in vivo* MRS, clinical studies became feasible for the detailed investigation of the pathophysiology and therapeutic options in human diabetes mellitus.

21.2 NON-MRS METHODS FOR METABOLIC RESEARCH IN HUMANS

Glucose metabolism can be studied in humans using the insulin clamp technique by measuring whole-body glucose disposal during fasting or for various degrees of glycemia and plasma insulin concentrations [1]. While this approach is considered the gold standard for assessment of insulin-sensitive glucose disposal, it does not allow examination of intracellular glucose fluxes in different tissues. Other approaches including the frequent sampling oral and intravenous glucose tolerance tests rather provide information on the body's integrated response to a glucose challenge but not on tissue metabolism. Thus, prior to the advent of *in vivo* MRS additional invasive or noninvasive techniques were needed to gain more information on intracellular glucose and lipid metabolism in humans (Table 21.1). These techniques include direct measurement of intracellular metabolites or enzyme activities involved in metabolic processes requires taking biopsies from the tissues of interest [6,7]. In addition, arteriovenous balance techniques can be performed for the assessment of substrate exchange across tissues or organs of interest following catheterization of the local arteries and veins. Less invasive techniques include the oral or intravenous administration of isotopically labeled substrates for tracing their absorption, disposal, and production using the isotope dilution method. These techniques have many limitations which are briefly summarized in Table 21.1.

21.3 MRS FOR METABOLIC RESEARCH IN HUMANS

MRS avoids invasive procedures, radiolabeled compounds, and offers the possibility of real-time monitoring of metabolic reactions and thereby to trace fluxes through metabolic pathways under *in vivo* conditions. The main limitation of MRS is that subjects need to fit into and to lie still within the magnet for prolonged periods of time. Careful screening is therefore mandatory to exclude subjects with paramagnetic metal implants, body circumferences exceeding the dimensions of the magnet, and claustrophobia.

Compared with experiments in isolated tissues and cells, MRS studies in humans generally have limited sensitivity and require measures for improving the signal-to-noise ratio [6–8] such as the use of high field (1.5 to 7 T) magnets. At present, clinical MRS studies mostly use the ^{1}H, ^{31}P, and ^{13}C nuclei to examine metabolism in humans.

TABLE 21.1
Limitations of Methods to Assess Glucose Metabolism in Humans

Technique	Measured Parameter	Limitation	References
Biopsy		Invasive	
	Metabolite concentration		
	e.g., ADP, G6P	Artifactual high concentrations	7,9
	e.g., muscle fat	Insufficient discrimination intra/extracellular concentrations	
	Metabolic flux	Limited time resolution	
	Enzyme activity, e.g., glycogen synthase	Artifactual low or high acitivities due to subcellular compartmentization	
Arteriovenous substrate balance		Invasive	
	Net production/uptake, e.g., gluconeogenesis	Not quanitative, not accounting for substrate exchange within tissue	52,88
Isotope dilution techniques (including mass isotopomer analysis)		Restrictions of use of radioactive isotopes (except for stable isotopes)	
	Metabolic fluxes		
	e.g., glucose production	Loss of tracer during metabolism	6,7,89
	e.g., gluconeogenesis, glycogen metabolism	Unknown tissue concentrations, extensive assuamptions needed	

21.3.1 ^{1}H MRS

Protons (^{1}H) have a natural abundance of ~100% and offer the highest sensitivity for MRS observation. The relatively high triglyceride concentrations allow the use of ^{1}H MRS for quantification of intracellular lipids in the liver (hepatocellular lipids, HCL) and in skeletal muscle, mostly soleus muscle (IMCL-S) and tibialis anterior muscle (IMCL-T), already at 1.5 T [9–11] (Figure 21.1). Different physical properties of triglycerides in the extra and intramyocellular space, further allow resolution of signals from extramyocellular (EMCL) and intramyocellular lipids (IMCL) localized ^{1}H MRS spectra [11–15] (see also Chapter 20, Section 20.4.1.1).

21.3.2 ^{31}P MRS

Phosphorus-31 (^{31}P) occurs 100% in nature and allows quantification of intracellular adenosine-triphosphate (ATP), adenosine-diphosphate (ADP), inorganic phosphate (P_i), pH in the liver and skeletal muscle. In addition, phosphocreatine (PCr) and glucose-6-phosphate (G6P) can be measured in skeletal muscle [16–18] (Figure 21.1). Recently, ATP synthesis was assessed in humans by employing saturation transfer ^{31}P MRS [19,20] (see also Chapter 20, Section 20.4.4).

21.3.3 ^{13}C MRS

Carbon-13 (^{13}C) has a natural abundance of 1.1% and therefore an overall low sensitivity, but can be used to study metabolites occurring in millimolar concentrations such as glycogen in the liver and skeletal muscle [21–24], and triglycerides in the liver [25] (Figure 21.1). Administration of ^{13}C-enriched isotopes, e.g., [1-^{13}C]glucose, enhances the sensitivity by approximately two orders of magnitude and makes monitoring of intracellular metabolite fluxes, such as glycogen synthesis, possible [23,26] (see also Chapter 20, Section 20.4.3). The [1-^{13}C]/[^{12}C]glucose pulse chase

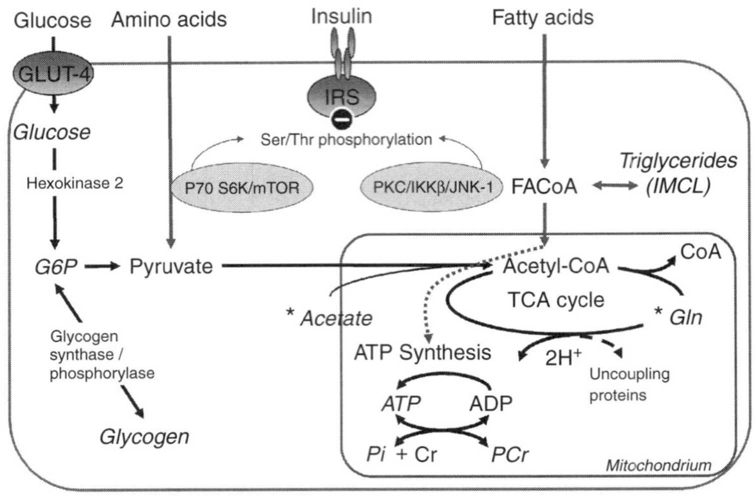

FIGURE 21.1 Intracellular glucose fluxes and mechanisms of insulin resistance in human skeletal muscle. ADP = adenosine diphosphate, ATP = adenosine triphosphate, G6P = glucose-6-phosphate, Gln = glutamine, IKKβ = IkappaB kinase β, IMCL = intramyocellular lipids, IRS = insulin receptor substrates, JNK = Jun N-terminal kinase, mTOR = mammalian target of rapamycin, P70 S6K = P70 S6 kinase, PKC = protein kinase C, Ser/Thr = serine/threonin, TCA = tricarboxylic acid.

technique enables the determination of relative fluxes through glycogen synthase and phosphorylase for assessment of glycogen turnover [27–29]. Intracellular concentration of free glucose in skeletal muscle can be assessed by measuring total muscle glucose, mannitol, and creatine with ^{13}C MRS during intravenous infusion of [1-^{13}C]glucose and [1-^{13}C]mannitol [30,31]. The calculation is based on the knowledge of the ratio of the volumes of the intracellular to the extracellular space as determined by the relative ^{13}C signal intensities for extracellular mannitol and intracellular total creatine, i.e., creatine + PCr. Finally, the rate of tricarboxylic acid (TCA) cycle flux can be assessed by monitoring the rate of appearance of ^{13}C label into the carbon atoms at positions 2 and 4 of muscle glutamate by ^{13}C MRS during intravenous infusion of [2-^{13}C]acetate [19,20] (Figure 21.1). From combined ^{13}C/^{31}P MRS, mitochondrial energy coupling can then be determined as the ratio of ATP synthesis to TCA cycle oxidation.

21.4 CLINICAL STUDIES ON SKELETAL MUSCLE METABOLISM

Skeletal muscle represents the major tissue responsible for insulin-stimulated glucose uptake in the body [1]. When the combination of ^{13}C MRS with administration of [1-^{13}C]glucose was employed for the first time to study the metabolic effects of insulin in healthy volunteers [23], muscle glycogen formation was found to account for ~90% of insulin-stimulated whole-body glucose disposal and for all nonoxidative glucose disposal. After ingestion of a mixed meal, the maximum increment in glycogen of ~17 mM as measured with natural abundance ^{13}C MRS indicated that at least 25% of the absorbed carbohydrates were stored as muscle glycogen [32,33] (see also Chapter 20, Section 20.4.3).

21.4.1 DEFECTS IN TYPE 2 DIABETIC PATIENTS

T2DM individuals are typically insulin resistant as defined by a reduction in insulin-stimulated whole-body glucose disposal during insulin clamp tests [1]. *In vivo* ^{13}C MRS demonstrated that glycogen synthesis is ~60% lower in T2DM than in nondiabetic volunteers serving as controls

($\sim$0.08 vs. $\sim$0.18 mmol/kg muscle/min) under hyperglycemic ($\sim$10 mM) hyperinsulinemic ($\sim$400 pM) conditions [23]. After ingestion of mixed meals, the increase in glycogen synthesis was $\sim$32% lower in diet-controlled T2DM despite twofold greater serum insulin concentrations than in nondiabetic subjects serving as controls ($\sim$0.1 mmol/l/min at plasma glucose of $\sim$7.3 mM and serum insulin of $\sim$900 pM) [33].

The decreased flux through glycogen synthase could result from a defect in this enzyme or from defects in glucose transport (GLUT4) or phosphorylation (hexokinase II, HKII) (Figure 21.1). As a result of its location between GLUT4/HKII and glycogen synthase enzymes, the intramyocellular G6P concentration is sensitive to the relative activities of these enzymes and to the rate of glycolysis [7]. A defect in glycogen synthase activity would not affect the initial rate of glucose entering the G6P pool, but then a slower removal of G6P would increase G6P in T2DM during stimulation by insulin. In contrast, a defect in GLUT4/HKII would result in identical or lower increments in G6P. The flux controlling steps of muscle glycogen synthesis became accessible by monitoring the time course of G6P with ^{31}P MRS [17]. Insulin-stimulated G6P levels were $\sim$29% lower in T2DM ($\sim$0.17 vs. $\sim$0.24 mM) suggesting that a defect located at GLUT4 and/or HKII is responsible for the reduced flux through glycogen synthase in T2DM. To delineate the flux controlling steps further, intramyocellular free glucose concentration was assessed with ^{13}C MRS. In analogy to G6P, the concentration of free glucose reflects the relative activities of GLUT4 and of HKII (Figure 21.1). A reduction in HKII relative to GLUT4 fluxes would increase free glucose, whereas a primary defect in GLUT4 would result in proportional changes of free glucose and G6P. The observation of very low free glucose concentrations is in line with the contention that glucose transport primarily controls the flux through glycogen synthase in T2DM [31], at least during hyperinsulinemic clamps when glycogen synthesis completely accounts for nonoxidative glucose disposal (Figure 21.2a).

21.4.2 Defects in Type 1 Diabetic Patients

Poorly controlled T1DM patients are also insulin resistant, a situation which resolves after normalization of their glycemic control. To examine the underlying mechanism of their insulin resistance, poorly controlled (glycosylated hemoglobin A1, HbA1 $\sim$13.6%) T1DM subjects were studied using ^{13}C/^{31}P MRS during hyperglycemic hyperinsulinemia [29]. Reduction of the whole-body nonoxidative glucose disposal by $\sim$40% and of the muscle glycogen synthesis ($\sim$0.11 mmol/l/min) by $\sim$50% showed that these patients were insulin resistant. The [1-^{13}C]/[^{12}C]glucose pulse chase technique showed that glycogen turnover was also lower in T2DM individuals ($\sim$16 vs. $\sim$33% in controls) so that glycogen breakdown cannot explain the lower rates of glycogen synthesis [28]. Insulin-stimulated G6P was also $\sim$40% lower in T1DM subjects ($\sim$0.18 mM) so that decreased glucose transport/phosphorylation was responsible for their insulin resistance [28], which most probably resulted from chronic hyperglycemia (glucose toxicity) [34].

21.4.3 Defects in Offspring of Type 2 Diabetic Patients

It has been suggested that hyperglycemia might increase muscle glycogen stores and thereby limit glycogen synthesis, but fasting muscle glycogen levels were even lower in T2DM patients ($\sim$39 to 57 mM vs. 69 to 73 mM in controls) [23,32]. In order to exclude that the observed defects in T2DM could be attributed to glucose toxicity [33], lean normoglycemic offsprings of T2DM individuals were studied under similar hyperglycemic hyperinsulinemic conditions [35]. These offsprings already featured the same defects as overt T2DM including reductions by $\sim$50, $\sim$70, and $\sim$40% in insulin-stimulated whole-body glucose disposal, glycogen synthesis, and G6P, respectively. Interestingly, 6 weeks of aerobic exercise training completely normalized insulin-stimulated G6P and improved glycogen synthesis by $\sim$70%, suggesting that training unmasks an additional abnormality of glycogen synthase [36].

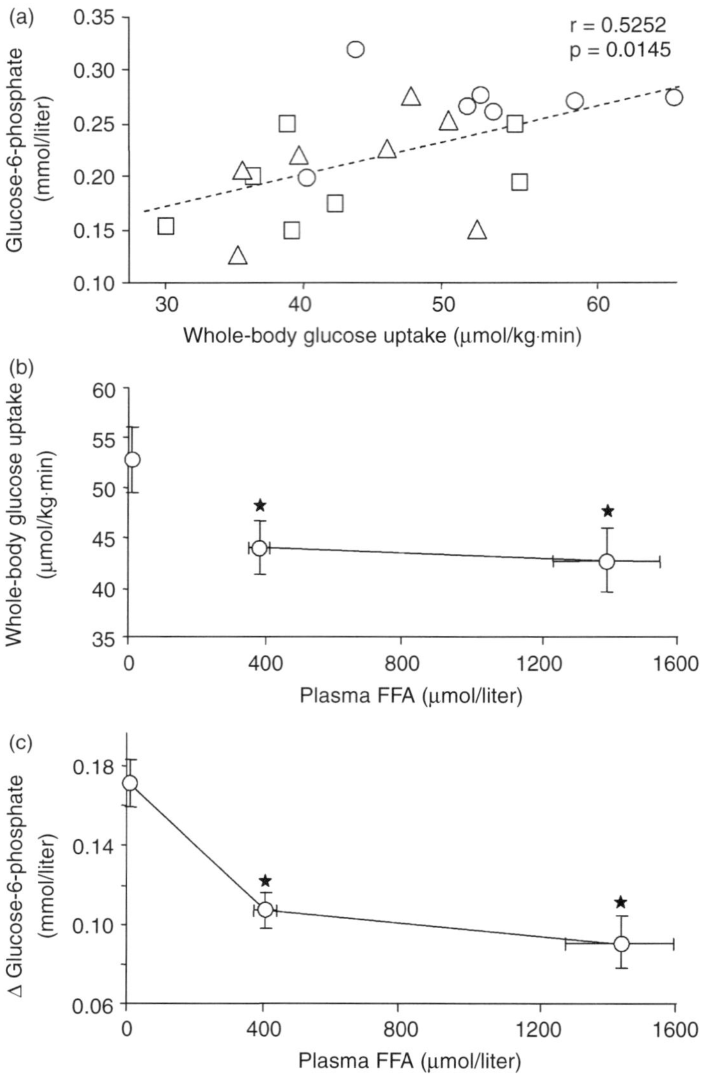

FIGURE 21.2 Insulin-stimulated glucose transport/phosphorylation as shown (a) by the correlation between whole-body glucose disposal and intramyocellular glucose-6-phosphate (G6P) concentrations during hyperinsulinemic–euglycemia in the presence suppressed (○), fasting (Δ), and postprandial (□) plasma free fatty acid (FFA) concentrations. Plasma FFA elevation concentration dependently inhibits (b) whole-body glucose disposal and (c) the rise in G6P over baseline (ΔG6P). (Reproduced from Roden, M. et al., *Diabetes*, 48, 358, 1999. With permission of the American Diabetes Association. © 1999.)

21.4.4 Nutrient-Induced Insulin Resistance and Obesity

Although inherited factors are involved, acquired factors such as hypercaloric diet and lack of physical activity are mainly responsible for the rise in the metabolic syndrome. $^{13}C/^{31}P$ MRS studies showed that severely obese humans exhibit a ~70% lower insulin-stimulated glycogen synthesis and blunted incremental G6P, suggesting a common defect in muscle glucose transport/phosphorylation in acquired and inherited insulin resistance [37].

Obesity is characterized by adipose tissue mass, disbalance of the release of adipocytokines, storage of triglycerides and lipolysis, all of which result in increased plasma concentrations of free fatty acids (FFA) [4,9]. For a long time, a hypothetical mechanism based on rat muscle experiments has served to explain how FFA compete with glucose for mitochondrial oxidation and inhibit glucose uptake (glucose FFA cycle) [38]. According to this hypothesis, FFA oxidation first alters intramitochondrial metabolite concentrations, thus inhibiting the activities of glycolytic key enzymes and the flux through glycolysis. This would increase G6P and thereby allosterically inhibit glucose phosphorylation by HKII.

In order to test this hypothesis, we intravenously infused healthy humans with lipid/heparin to increase plasma FFA to ~2 mM and measured glucose metabolism in calf muscles with $^{13}C/^{31}P$ MRS while infusing [1-^{13}C]glucose during euglycemic hyperinsulinemia [26]. Plasma FFA elevation decreased whole-body glucose disposal and glycogen synthesis by ~50%, which was preceded by a ~60% inhibition of insulin-stimulated G6P. Another study showed that FFA elevation also results in ~80% lower free glucose concentrations [30], indicating that the glucose FFA cycle does not play a role under these conditions.

Nevertheless, these studies could not rule out that the glucose FFA cycle is operative at lower plasma FFA and insulin concentrations. By employing ^{31}P MRS with increased time resolution, we found that plasma FFA elevation blunts the insulin-stimulated rise in G6P by ~25% already at 45 min [18]. Furthermore, FFA concentration dependently inhibits both insulin-stimulated whole-body glucose disposal and G6P (Figure 21.2b and Figure 21.2c). The current hypothesis for the molecular interaction between FFA and insulin action postulates that intracellular long chain fatty acyl–CoA (FACoA) stimulates atypical isoforms of protein kinase C (PKC), nuclear factor κB (NFκB), and JNK which impair insulin signaling by phosphorylation of serine/threonin residues of insulin receptor substrates (IRS-1) [4] (Figure 21.1).

To examine whether FFA can also affect glucose metabolism independently of interfering with insulin signaling, we monitored G6P during variable glycemia and constant fasting insulinemia. These conditions may favor FFA flux into mitochondria and stimulate substrate competition with glucose [39]. Again, plasma FFA elevation decreased whole-body glucose disposal but did not affect G6P, indicating that FFA also interferes with glucose-dependent glucose transport/phosphorylation.

Nutrient excess not only of fat but also of protein has been associated with alterations of insulin action and glucose metabolism. We therefore examined the effect of an amino acid infusion on skeletal muscle metabolism with $^{31}P/^{13}C$ MRS [40]. Doubling the plasma amino acid concentrations decreased insulin-stimulated whole-body glucose disposal by ~25% which was preceded by an impaired rise in G6P and followed by a ~64% reduction in glycogen synthesis. Recent studies provided evidence that amino acids stimulate the mammalian target of rapamycin (mTOR)/p70 S60 kinase pathway which inhibits insulin signaling (Figure 21.1).

Taken together, these studies indicate that glucose transport becomes flux controlling during increased availability of nutrients such as glucose, FFA, and amino acids (gluco-lipo-proteo toxicity). Moreover, the observed abnormalities in muscle glucose transport are identical to the metabolic changes typically occurring in T2DM patients and their insulin-resistant offsprings.

21.4.5 The Role of Intramyocellular Fat

Histological and biochemical analysis of human muscle biopsies provided evidence for a relationship between muscle lipids and insulin resistance [9] (see also Chapter 20, Section 20.4.1.1). ^{1}H MRS overcomes the limitations of these semiquantitative methods and can now be easily applied in the MR systems of many hospitals. We reported that IMCL-S negatively correlates ($r = -0.69$, $p < .002$) with insulin-stimulated whole-body glucose disposal in healthy humans [12]. Further studies demonstrated increased IMCL in various insulin-resistant groups such as offsprings of T2DM patients [14,15], overt T2DM subjects [41,42], T1DM individuals [42], women with previous T4DM [43], obese glucose intolerant adolescents [44,45], and in inherited [46] and acquired lipodystrophy [47]. IMCL is higher in soleus muscle containing predominantly slow twitch oxidative type I fibres, and lower in tibialis anterior muscle (IMCL-T) containing predominantly fast twitch glycolytic type II fibres [14,15,41,43]. These studies also suggested that IMCL-S relates rather to whole-body adiposity, whereas IMCL-T correlates better with skeletal muscle insulin resistance in sedentary humans. IMCL levels are elevated in endurance-trained populations which raised the question of whether increased IMCL are the cause of insulin resistance or rather the result of impaired oxidative capacity of skeletal muscle [9].

To examine this question, the interaction between IMCL and insulin resistance was studied under various metabolic conditions. Elevation of plasma FFA [48] and amino acid concentrations [40] resulted in a parallel increase of IMCL and insulin resistance. However, plasma FFA elevation without simultaneous insulin stimulation decreased glucose transport and/or phosphorylation but did not affect IMCL, which also remained unchanged despite diet-induced improvement of the insulin sensitivity [49]. Moreover, endurance training further augmented the IMCL stores despite an obvious increase in insulin sensitivity [50]. Thus, variations in mitochondrial oxidative and phosphorylation capacity could also contribute to insulin resistance and increased IMCL (Figure 21.1).

The relationship between insulin resistance, intracellular lipids, and mitochondrial metabolism was recently studied by combining $^{1}H/^{31}P$ MRS with [6,6-$^{2}H_2$]glucose and [5-^{2}H]glycerol in lean insulin-resistant elderly humans [20]. Impairment by ~35% of insulin-stimulated glucose disposal was associated with an increase in IMCL-S and HCL by ~45 and ~229%, respectively. Mitochondrial fluxes through the TCA cycle and ATP synthesis were ~35 and ~46% lower in the elderly than in controls. Likewise, lean offspring of T2DM patients with ~60% lower insulin-stimulated glucose disposal and ~80% higher IMCL-S presented reductions in ATP synthesis and in the P_i/PCr ratio of ~30 and ~20%, respectively [51].

Taken together, increased IMCL in untrained individuals seems to be a result of lipid oversupply and defective lipid oxidation rather than a direct cause of insulin resistance.

21.5 LIVER

The liver is the only organ that can rapidly switch from producing to storing glucose as glycogen during the transition from the fasted to the fed state [1,52]. MRS studies elucidated the intracellular fate of glucose within the liver which was not directly accessible with previously applied techniques. First, combination of ^{13}C MRS with [3-^{3}H]glucose was used to monitor the time course of hepatic glycogen concentrations and EGP in healthy volunteers [24]. The linear decrease of the liver glycogen signal during fasting allowed quantifying net glycogenolysis which contributed only ~36% to EGP during the first 22 h. Glycogenolysis maximally contributes ~45% to EGP after 5 to 12 h, indicating that gluconeogenesis accounts for the majority of glucose metabolism even in the early postabsorptive state [53].

Determination of gluconeogenesis by ^{13}C MRS as the difference between rates of glycogen breakdown and EGP yielded a higher contribution of gluconeogenesis to EGP than earlier techniques [52], but similar results as assessed using the $^{2}H_2O$ method [54,55]. The $^{2}H_2O$ method circumvents limitations of the earlier techniques by measuring ^{2}H enrichments in plasma glucose with gas chromatography–mass spectrometry (GCMS) [54,56] or *in vitro* deuterium NMR [55] upon ingestion of $^{2}H_2O$. These methods found that the contribution of gluconeogenesis to EGP is between 47 and 56% at 14 to 16 h and between 51 and 73% at 18 h of fasting [52,54–56].

In the postprandial state, liver glycogen concentrations were shown to rise from ~250 to 350 mM within the first ~4 to 5 h following ingestion of a mixed meal [57–59] (Figure 21.3a). Several studies revealed that 19 to 26% of the glucose derived from a meal is deposited as glycogen in the liver [57–61] due primarily to changes in the portal vein insulin/glucagon ratio (Figure 21.4). Glycogen turnover is markedly higher in the fed state than after 12 to 14 h of fasting (~60 vs. ~30%) [27]. It is conceivable that the higher liver glycogen content in the fed state may itself stimulate glycogen breakdown according to the concept of hepatic autoregulation of glycogen

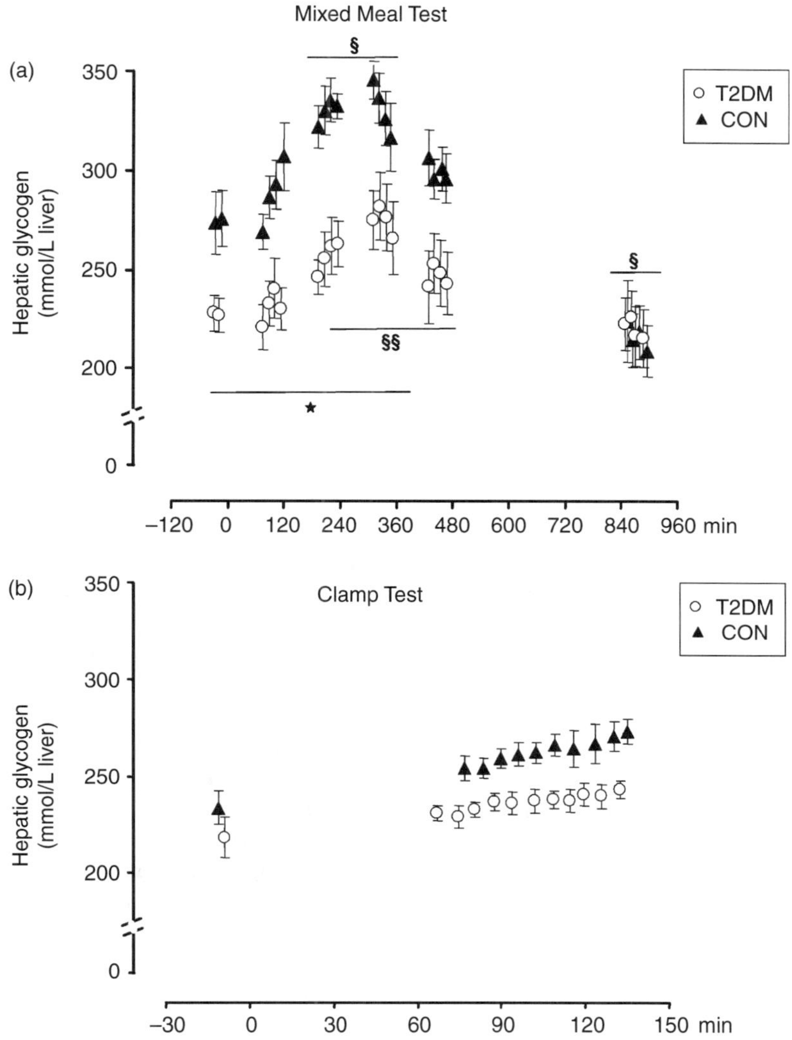

FIGURE 21.3 Time course hepatic glycogen concentrations (a) during mixed meal ingestion and (b) during the pulse period of [1-^{13}C]/[^{12}C] glucose pulse chase studies in nondiabetic humans (CON, full triangles) and in type 2 diabetic (T2DM, empty circles). (Reproduced from Krssak, M. et al., *Diabetes*, 53, 3048, 2004. With permission of the American Diabetes Association. © 2004.)

stores. Likewise, elevation of plasma FFA and triglycerides reduced net glycogenolysis by ~84% and increased gluconeogenesis by ~40% but did not affect EGP, suggesting that lipids partcipate in hepatic autoregulation of liver glycogen pools [62].

Studies simulating conditions of normal eating behavior demonstrated that liver glycogen concentrations continuously rise during the daytime [57,59]. This indicates negligible hepatic glycogenolysis during the daytime so that glucose absorption from meals and gluconeogenesis account for the major part of whole-body glucose appearance during the day, while net hepatic glycogenolysis contributes to whole-body glucose production only during the night.

21.5.1 Defects in Type 1 Diabetic Patients

Excessive rates of fasting EGP in T1DM correlate with the degree of fasting hyperglycemia and could result from decreased glycogenolysis and/or increased gluconeogenesis [52]. After ingestion

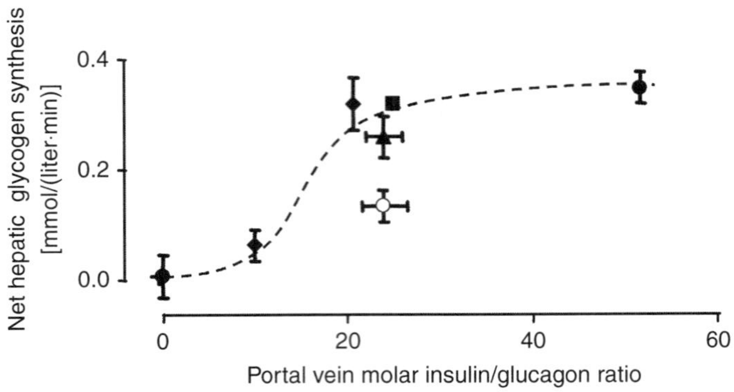

FIGURE 21.4 Rates of net hepatic glycogen synthesis depending on the prevailing portal vein insulin/glucagon ratio in nondiabetic humans (CON, filled symbols) and in type 2 diabetic (T2DM, empty circles). (Reproduced from Roden, M. et al., *J. Clin. Invest.*, and Krssak, M. et al., *Diabetes*, 53, 3048, 2004. With permission of the American Diabetes Association. © 2004.)

of three mixed meals, poorly controlled T1DM patients on conventional insulin therapy synthesize only 25 to 30% liver glycogen compared with controls [57,61]. Glycogenolysis during the subsequent overnight fast is also ~50% lower than in controls. These results help to explain why T1DM individuals exhibit normal fasting liver glycogen concentrations despite marked defects in glycogen synthesis and glycogenolysis [57,60,61].

21.5.2 Defects in Patients with other Pancreas Disorders

While complete agenesis of the pancreas is not compatible with life, partial pancreas agenesis can be detected in some diabetic patients. A rare form of familiar agenesis of the dorsal pancreas provided the opportunity to examine the effects of different degrees of insulin secretion on glucose fluxes after mixed meal ingestion by using ^{13}C MRS [63]. The diabetic mother and both nondiabetic sons featured reductions by ~55 and ~40% in glycogen synthesis and glycogenolysis, respectively. Gluconeogenesis was ~60% higher and contributed more to the slightly elevated fasting EGP than in nondiabetic humans (~70 vs. ~50%).

Mutations of the glucokinase gene on chromosome 7 are the cause of the autosomal dominant inherited MODY-2. Glucokinase deficiency leads to glucose-dependent insulin secretion and moderate postprandial hyperglycemia in these patients. *In vivo* ^{13}C MRS revealed that MODY-2 patients feature impaired hepatic glycogen synthesis and augmented contribution of the gluconeogenic pathway to glycogen synthesis [64]. Interestingly, the lower portal vein insulin/glucagon ratio could not entirely explain the reduction of glycogen synthesis suggesting that a decreased flux through hepatic glucokinase, at least in part, accounts for impaired glycogen storage in MODY-2.

21.5.3 Defects in Type 2 Diabetic Patients

As in T1DM, fasting hyperglycemia correlates with fasting EGP, which was therefore held responsible for the rise in plasma glucose also in T2DM subjects [52]. On the other hand, rates of fasting EGP in T2DM range from normal to markedly increased depending on the method of quantification, the experimental design, and other factors rather than the degree of glycemia (Bernoider).

The mechanism of defective glucose production in poorly controlled T2DM was elucidated by ^{13}C MRS [65]. Net hepatic glycogenolysis was lower so that gluconeogenesis accounted for 89% of EGP in T2DM patients vs. 70% in controls [65]. Further studies compared *in vivo* ^{13}C MRS with the

^2H_2O method using either GCMS [54] or deuterium NMR [55]. Contribution of gluconeogenesis to EGP (between 10 and 15 h after dinner) was higher as assessed by ^{13}C MRS than by GCMS (84 vs. 59%) in poorly controlled (glycosylated Hb ~14.1%) T2DM individuals; however, both techniques rendered similar results in controls (60 vs. 56%) [54]. In well-controlled (HbA1c ~7.1%) T2DM, contribution of gluconeogenesis to EGP (between 14 and 16 h after dinner) was again higher when determined by ^{13}C MRS than by GCMS and deuterium NMR (85 vs. 63 and 75%), while the results were comparable for controls (65 vs. 51 and 63%) [55]. Measurement of gluconeogenesis by deuterium NMR correlated linearly with ^{13}C MRS and GCMS assessments (both $r = 0.76$, $p = .0007$). These studies suggest that substantial glycogen cycling occurs in T2DM irrespective of their long-term glycemic control.

During mixed meal ingestion, T2DM subjects exhibit excessive and prolonged hyperglycemia which has been attributed to decreased glucose-induced insulin secretion, to insufficient suppression of glucagon and of FFA, and to hyperglycemia *per se* [1,52]. Quantification of EGP by labeled glucose becomes even more complicated because of rapid changes in the tracer/tracee ratios. Recently, we addressed this issue by combing oral [1-^{13}C]glucose to trace glucose absorption, a variable intravenous [6,6-$^2H_2$]glucose infusion to calculate EGP and ^{13}C MRS to measure hepatic glycogen metabolism in overweight (BMI <27 kg/m^2), well-controlled (HbA1c <7.5%) T2DM individuals [59]. Before dinner hepatic glycogen was lower in T2DM patients (~227 vs. controls ~273 mM) (Figure 21.3a). After meal ingestion glycogen synthesis was ~44% lower (~0.8 mg/kg/min) and EGP was temporarily ~44% higher in T2DM. Gluconeogenesis contributed similarly to glycogen synthesis in T2DM subjects and in controls (~60 vs. ~56%). Rates of net glycogenolysis were ~50% lower in T2DM (~0.4 mg/kg/min) resulting in similar fasting hepatic glycogen concentrations of ~215 mM in both groups the next morning.

21.5.4 The Role of Intrahepatic Fat

In analogy to IMCL, HCL represent another lipid pool which affects carbohydrate metabolism and can be quantified by localized ^1H MRS [9,10]. HCL was found to be increased and associated with various measures of insulin resistance in T2DM [41,66,67], in women with previous T4DM [68], in obese [69], and in insulin-resistant lipodystrophic patients [70,71]. HCL is tightly correlated with hepatic insulin resistance as measured by suppression of EGP during hyperinsulinemic clamps [41]. In this context it is of note that excessive increases in HCL result in nonalcoholic fatty liver disease and nonalcoholic steatohepatitis, which are now grouped among the features of the metabolic syndrome [72].

21.6 CLINICAL DRUG TRIALS IN METABOLIC DISEASES

21.6.1 Insulin Treatment in Diabetes Mellitus

21.6.1.1 Type 1 Diabetes

When poorly controlled (HbA1c ~8.8%) T1DM subjects were studied during a variable insulin infusion resulting in near-normoglycemia for 24 h, hepatic glycogen synthesis was found to nearly double, but was still ~50% lower than in controls after mixed meal ingestion [60]. Likewise, glycogenolysis during the night remained ~25% lower than in controls indicating that short-term near-normoglycemia improves but does not normalize hepatic glycogen metabolism in T1DM.

In order to examine the impact of long-term near-normoglycemia, we studied seven intensively treated T1DM patients (HbA1c (7% for more than one year) [61]. During mixed meal ingestion, glycemic profiles were again normalized by variable insulin infusion. By these means, glycogen synthesis, breakdown, and EGP were identical in T1DM and in controls: ~7.3 vs. ~7.1, 4.2 vs. ~3.8, and ~8.7 vs ~8.4 μmol/kg/min, respectively. Although the portal vein insulin concentrations were doubled, the flux through the indirect pathway of glycogen synthesis was higher in T1DM (~70 vs ~50%). These findings suggest that optimized long- and short-term metabolic control of T1DM reverses the defects in hepatic glycogen synthesis only in the face of higher portal vein insulinemia and flux through gluconeogenic pathways compared with controls. However, even conditions of hyperglycemia and portal vein insulin/glucagon ratios leading to normalized glycogen synthesis did not abolish the increased gluconeogenic flux to glycogen (~65 vs. ~40%) and decreased pyruvate oxidation in T1DM [73]. These residual defects could be due to impaired glucokinase activity, increased phosphoenolpyruvate carboxykinase activity, or muscle insulin resistance resulting in increased flux of gluconeogenic precursors to the liver [52].

Taken together, the clinical relevance of these studies resides in the finding that long-term excellent metabolic control ensures sufficient glycogen storage despite the nonphysiologic, but usual, peripheral route of exogenous insulin delivery [52]. Restoring hepatic glycogen synthesis in T1DM can help improve postprandial blood glucose excursions and glucagon-dependent hypoglycemia counterregulation which critically depends on sufficient liver glycogen stores.

21.6.1.2 Type 2 Diabetes

As described before, T2DM subjects exhibit severely reduced hepatic glycogen synthesis after mixed meal ingestion [59]. This abnormality is accompanied by up to ~69% higher plasma glucose, ~55% impaired suppression of plasma FFA, ~61% lower rise in plasma insulin, ~32% higher plasma glucagon resulting in an ~50% lower portal vein insulin/glucagon ratio in T2DM than in controls [59]. To address the question to what extent short-term insulin treatment ameliorates the metabolic defects, we examined hepatic glycogen metabolism in the same T2DM individuals [59] with $^{1}H/^{13}C$ MRS and the [1-^{13}C]/[^{12}C]glucose pulse chase technique during hyperglycemic hyperinsulinemic–somatostatin clamps [29]. T2DM patients still featured ~54% lower hepatic glycogen synthesis and ~0.5 mg/kg/min higher EGP. HCL was three times higher in T2DM and negatively correlated with rates of glycogen synthesis ($r = -0.60$, $p < .05$) and whole-body glucose disposal ($r = -0.58$, $p < .05$) (Figure 21.3b). Thus, impaired hepatic insulin sensitivity due to either intrinsic insulin resistance or chronic glucolipotoxicity in addition to altered insulin/glucagon ratio can explain the defective hepatic glycogen metabolism in well-controlled T2DM (Figure 21.4).

As these findings did not exclude the possibility that a longer duration of insulin treatment could further improve glucose metabolism, we performed stepped hyperinsulinemic–euglycemic clamps in eight T2DM patients at baseline and again after 12 and 67 h of insulin-mediated near-normoglycemia (~120 mg/dl) [41]. At baseline, T2DM subjects were insulin resistant and had higher HCL (~18.3 vs. controls ~5.8%). IMCL–TA negatively correlated with insulin sensitivity ($r = -0.97$, $p < .001$). After 67-h insulin infusion, fasting EGP decreased by ~10%, whilse IMCL-S and HCL increased by ~36 and ~18%, respectively, and now correlated positively with insulin sensitivity ($r = 0.98$, $p < .0005$ and $r = 0.87$, $p < .03$, respectively). These results indicate that insulin-mediated near-normoglycemia for ~3 d improves EGP, but stimulates lipid accumulation in liver and skeletal muscle. Whether this increase in ectopic fat deposition continues or ceases during long-term insulin treatment is presently unknown.

Glucose metabolism and fat deposition might also depend on the use of different insulin regimens in T2DM. Regimens with a single injection of bedtime NPH insulin and oral antidiabetic drugs, particularly with metformin, may be advantageous with respect to glycemic control and insulin requirements which determine weight gain and frequency of hypoglycemic events [74] (see also Chapter 20, Section 20.2.1.1). Thus, another study examined 20 mostly overweight (BMI ~29 kg/m^2) T2DM individuals who were reasonably well-controlled (HbA1c ~7.6%) with bedtime NPH insulin and metformin [67]. Insulin action on FFA and glucose disposal correlated with insulin dosage and absorption. Of all measures of adiposity, HCL was the best parameter to explain the daily insulin dose ($r = 0.76$) and also related to insulin-mediated suppression of EGP ($r = 0.72$). Thus, the authors concluded that the insulin action determines interindividual variation in insulin requirements, which may be influenced by HCL via effects on insulin-mediated suppression of EGP.

21.6.1.3 Gestational Diabetes

At present, no clinical drug trial employing MRS is available in women with T4DM. One study analyzed the role of IMCL for antidiabetic treatment during pregnancy in women with previous T4DM [43]. Nearly all (88%) these women (compared with only 50% of insulin-sensitive women) had required insulin therapy during pregnancy. Women with previous T4DM treated before with insulin had higher IMCL-S and IMCL-T than diet-treated patients despite no difference in metabolic or anthropometric parameters (Figure 21.5). IMCL also inversely related to the gestational week of diabetes diagnosis. Thus, IMCL may serve to predict the requirement of insulin treatment during pregnancy in T4DM.

21.6.2 Oral Antidiabetic Drugs

21.6.2.1 Metformin

International guidelines recommend metformin as the first-line drug for monotherapy in overweight and obese T2DM patients, because it has proved more effective than insulin or sulfonylurea in reducing severe complications of diabetes including mortality and stroke [75]. Whether the glucose lowering effects of metformin occur from reducing gluconeogenesis or hepatic glycogenolysis remained controversial for a long time [76]. Hepatic glucose metabolism was studied by combining ^{13}C MRS with [6,6-$^2H_2$]glucose and ^2H_2O in overweight (BMI ~29 kg/m^2) poorly controlled (glycosylated Hb ~14.1%) T2DM subjects [54]. Metformin treatment for 3 months reduced fasting plasma glucose by ~30%, EGP by ~24%, and gluconeogenesis by ~35% indicating that

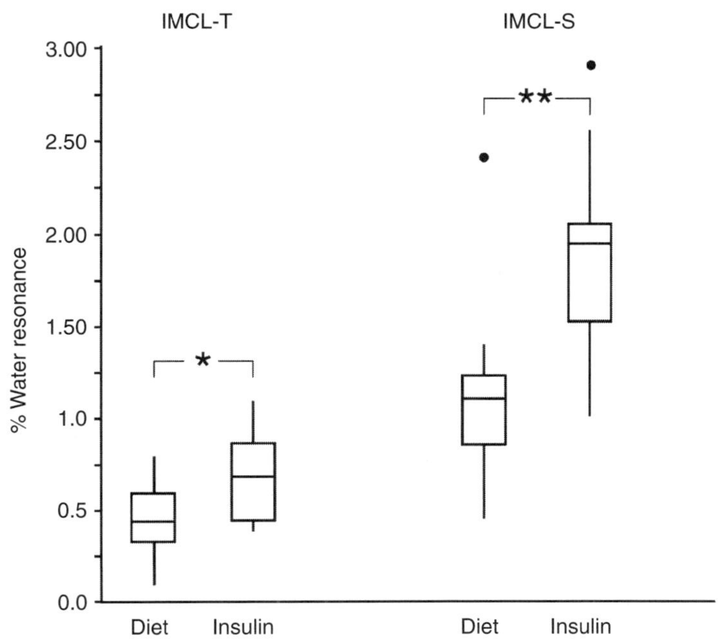

FIGURE 21.5 Intramyocellular lipids in soleus (IMCL-S) and tibialis anterior muscle (IMCL-T) in women with prior gestational diabetes who had been treated by diet or insulin during pregnancy. (Reproduced from Kautzky-Willer, A. et al., *Diabetes*, 52, 244, 2003. With permission of the American Diabetes Association. © 2003.)

metformin lowers EGP primarily through reduction in gluconeogenesis (see also Chapter 20, Section 20.2.1.1).

21.6.2.2 Insulin Sensitizer

Thiazolidinediones (TZDs, known also as glitazones) effectively decrease blood glucose concentrations in T2DM [77]. There is evidence that TZDs enhance insulin sensitivity by activating the transcription peroxisome proliferator activated receptor γ (PPARγ), thereby controlling adipocyte differentiation [78]. This modulates the release of adipocytokines such as adiponectin and of FFA which are important signals for adipocyte–myocyte communication (see also Chapter 20, Section 20.2.1.1).

Troglitazone was the first widely used TZD, but it was withdrawn because of hepatoxicity [77]. The mechanism by which troglitazone improves insulin resistance was studied with $^{13}C/^{31}P$ MRS in the calf muscle of seven T2DM subjects before and after three months of troglitazone (400 mg/d) therapy [78]. Troglitazone increased insulin-stimulated whole-body glucose disposal by ~58%, and glucose oxidation and glycogen synthesis by factors of ~3 and ~2, respectively. G6P rose by ~0.083 mM whereas free glucose remained >50-fold lower (<0.1 mmol/l) than what would be expected if HKII was rate controlling. It was concluded that troglitazone improves muscular insulin responsiveness in T2DM by facilitating glucose transport activity.

As PPARγ receptors are rare in myocytes [77], the insulin sensitizing effect of TZDs is unlikely to result from a direct action on skeletal muscle but rather from altered adipocyte-myocyte communication such as reduced FFA flux and redistribution of triglycerides from liver and muscle to peripheral adipocytes (see also Chapter 20, Section 20.2.1.1). This hypothesis was tested by studying, in nine obese (BMI ~31 kg/m^2), well-controlled (HbA1c ~6.7%) T2DM subjects, the effects of a three-month rosiglitazone treatment (4 mg bid.) on whole-body insulin sensitivity and peripheral adipocyte insulin sensitivity using a two-step hyperinsulinemic–euglycemic clamp and glycerol release through microdialysis from subcutaneous fat [66]. Rosiglitazone treatment resulted in 68 and 20% increased insulin stimulated glucose disposal during the low- and high-dose insulin clamps, respectively. This was accompanied by an ~40% reduction in plasma FFA and an ~52% rise in the sensitivity of peripheral adipocytes to insulin-mediated inhibition of lipolysis. In parallel, both HCL and EMCL-S decreased by ~40%, whereas IMCL-S did not change. These data were in favor of the hypothesis that TZDs enhance insulin sensitivity by promoting insulin sensitivity in peripheral adipocytes, which results in lower plasma FFA and redistribution of triglycerides from the liver into peripheral adipocytes.

These findings were extended by a similarly designed study comparing the effects of a three-month treatment with rosiglitazone (8 mg/d, bid.) vs. placebo on insulin sensitivity and regional adiposity in 33 obese (BMI ~31 kg/m^2), well-controlled (HbA1c ~7.1%) T2DM patients [79]. Rosiglitazone increased glycemic control by ~10% and glucose disposal by ~86%. Total body weight and fat mass increased, with 95% of the increase in adiposity occurring in nonabdominal regions. Rosiglitazone slightly increased subcutaneous fat and did not affect the intraabdominal fat area, but reduced HCL by 45%, further supporting the hypothesis that TZDs cause fat redistribution.

To analyze whether the decrease in HCL is linked to splanchnic glucose uptake (SGU), which contributes to the control of EGP, the effects of a four-month treatment with pioglitazone (45 mg/d) on the relationships between SGU, EGP, and HCL were studied in 14 overweight (BMI ~29 kg/m^2) moderately controlled (HbA1c ~7.8%) T2DM subjects [80]. Despite a rise in body weight by ~3 kg, pioglitazone improved glycemic control by ~14%, insulin-mediated glucose disposal by ~33%, and suppression of EGP by ~71%. In parallel, SGU as calculated from oral glucose load-insulin clamps with [3-^{3}H]glucose increased by ~32%, whereas HCL decreased from ~20 to ~10%. These studies underlined that TZDs primarily increase hepatic insulin sensitivity and HCL.

Subsequent studies analyzed the effect of an identical pioglitazone regimen on the relationships between adipocytokines and HCL in similar T2DM populations. Reduction of HCL from ~21 to ~11% was accompanied by a rise of plasma adiponectin from ~7 to ~21 mg/l, which correlated negatively with HCL before ($r = -0.60, p < .05$) and after treatment ($r = -0.65, p < .03$) [81]. A comparable decrease of HCL was observed in parallel with a decrease of plasma resistin from ~5.3 to ~3.5 μg/l which correlated positively with HCL before ($r = 0.58$) and after ($r = 0.55$) treatment [82].

Recently, the effect of metformin (1 g bid.) and rosiglitazone (4 mg bid.) treatment for four months were compared in 20 obese (BMI ~31 kg/m^2) drug-naive (HbA1c ~7%) T2DM individuals [68]. In the face of similar reduction of HbA1c, plasma insulin, and FFA, metformin but not rosiglitazone decreased body weight by ~2 kg. Only rosiglitazone increased insulin clearance and insulin-stimulated glucose uptake and decreased HCL from ~15 to ~7%. Basal hepatic insulin sensitivity increased similarly in both groups but only rosiglitazone led to an increase in serum adiponectin by ~120% (from ~5.6 to ~12.5 mg/l). The increase in serum adiponectin correlated with the decrease in HCL ($r = -0.74$, $p < .001$). Expression of PPARγ, adiponectin, and lipoprotein lipase increased in adipose tissue.

Taken together, these studies provided compelling evidence that TZDs ameliorate hyperglycemia and increase hepatic insulin sensitivity by modulating the release of adipocytokines and FFA which ultimately leads to decreased liver triglyceride accumulation. Of note, this is distinct from the hepatic effects of metformin and insulin treatments which do not change [68] or even increase [41] HCL.

21.6.2.3 Insulin Secretagogues

Sulfonylurea drugs are currently recommended as the first-line treatment for nonobese T2DM [75, 83]. Most probably, insulin secretagogues such as sulfonylurea drugs and glinides (repaglinide, nateglinide) primarily act at the pancreatic β cell and stimulate insulin secretion. However, there is evidence that the second-generation sulfonyurea, glimepiride, also exerts direct peripheral effects and increases insulin sensitivity [77]. These possible effects were recently addressed by comparing glimepiride (3 mg/d) + placebo with pioglitazone (30 mg/d) + nateglinide (60 mg/d, tid.) treatment for 12 weeks in overweight, well-controlled T2DM patients [84]. Preliminary data of this ^{31}P/^{1}H MRS study suggest that insulin-stimulated whole-body glucose disposal and G6P do not change, whereas HCL tends to decrease after glimepiride and effectively decreases after pioglitazone + nateglinide. When glibenclamide instead of glimeperide was compared with troglitazone (400 mg/d) treatment for 6 months, only troglitazone decreased insulin resistance as well as fat accumulation in the liver, muscle, and visceral as assessed from computed tomography scans [85]. Taken together, these data suggest that sulfonylurea drugs administered without insulin sensitizing agents, such as glibenclamide, could lead to fat accumulation which can be reversed by TZDs in T2DM.

21.6.3 Treatment of Lipodystrophy

Lipodystrophies comprise acquired or inherited disorders characterized by heterogenous forms of selective loss of adipose tissue along with insulin resistance, dyslipidemia, and hepatic steatosis [5]. When diabetes develops, insulin or oral antidiabetic drugs are used to treat hyperglycemia, but other therapeutic regimens addressing the metabolic alterations have been investigated and examined in detail using MRS.

21.6.3.1 Leptin

Patients with severe generalized lipodystrophy present very low fasting plasma leptin concentrations. In one study, three diabetic (HbA1c ~8.5%) patients with acquired or inherited lipodystrophy (BMI ~19 kg/m^2) underwent subcutaneous replacement with methionyl human leptin for three to five months [70]. Leptin treatment improved hepatic and peripheral insulin resistance resulting in withdrawal of their antidiabetic therapy. Likewise, HCL and IMCL fell by ~86 and ~33%, respectively, as measured with ^{1}H MRS. These data were confirmed in two patients with acquired and one patient with congenital generalized lipodystrophy during leptin treatment for eight to ten months [46]. Leptin therapy improved glycemic control, serum lipoproteins, and insulin sensitivity, which was accompanied by ~80 and ~42% reductions in HCL and IMCL, respectively.

21.6.3.2 Insulin Sensitizers

Lipodystrophy, which is characterized by atrophy of subcutaneous fat and accumulation of intraabdominal fat and insulin resistance, commonly complicates highly active antiretroviral therapy (HAART) of HIV-1 infected patients [86]. As TZDs promote subcutaneous fat deposition in congenital lipodystrophy and can prevent HAART toxicity in adipocytes *in vitro*, 30 patients with HAART-associated lipodystrophy received rosiglitazone (8 mg/d) or placebo for 6 months [71]. Rosiglitazone did not affect body fat mass or its distribution, but decreased HCL, serum insulin, and liver function tests, and increased serum triglycerides and cholesterol. Rosiglitazone further increased serum adiponectin and the expression of adiponectin, PPARγ and its coactivator, and decreased interleukin-6 expression [87]. These studies showed that increased expression of adiponectin mediates the favorable insulin-sensitizing effects of rosiglitazone. However, these effects did not suffice to improve the alterations of body fat distribution in these patients. This was supported by a large randomized, double-blind, placebo-controlled trial demonstrating that 12 months of rosiglitazone treatment did not improve lipoatrophy in a similar group [86]. Thus, the clinical benefit of TZDs in these patients is still uncertain and requires further studies.

21.7 CONCLUSIONS

Application of *in vivo* MRS overcame many limitations of previous approaches to study metabolism in humans. The main advantages are its noninvasive nature and the absence of artifactual alterations of metabolite concentrations which are typical for tissue biopsies. MRS provided new insights into cellular metabolism in humans under both physiological and pathological conditions by showing that conclusions drawn from animal studies and cell culture experiments not necessarily hold true for humans *in vivo*.

Nevertheless, *in vivo* MRS studies generally require expensive hardware and infrastructure as well as a team of trained experts. While some of the techniques, such as measurement of ectopic fat content in the liver and skeletal muscle, can be performed using clinical magnets on a larger scale, others such as assessment of metabolic fluxes require high field magnets, custom-designed radiofrequency coils, and special infusion protocols. The costs of MRS studies are mostly defined by the amount of stable isotopes and manpower needed so that one experiment's costs range from hundreds up to thousands of euros or dollars.

Thus, MRS studies are generally designed as explorative studies in smaller groups of individuals in order to examine (patho)physiological mechanisms and to provide proofs-of-concept and/or mechanisms of new therapeutic principles.

ACKNOWLEDGMENTS

The author's studies are and/or have been supported by the Austrian Science Fund (Fonds zur Förderung der wissenschaftlichen Forschung, FWF), the Austrian National Bank (Österreichische Nationalbank, ÖNB), the Herzfelder Family Trust (Herzfelder'sche Familienstiftung), the European Foundation for the Study of Diabetes (EFSD), and institutional grants by Novo-Nordisk and Aventis.

REFERENCES

1. DeFronzo, R. A., Pathogenesis of type 2 diabetes: metabolic and molecular implications for identifying diabetes genes, *Diabetes Rev.*, 5, 177, 1997.
2. Reaven, G. M., Banting lecture role of insulin resistance in human disease, *Diabetes*, 37, 1595, 1988.
3. Kahn, B. B. and Flier, J. S., Obesity and insulin resistance, *J. Clin. Invest.*, 106, 473, 2000.
4. Roden, M., How free fatty acids inhibit glucose utilization in human skeletal muscle, *News Physiol. Soc.*, 19, 92, 2004.
5. Garg, A., Acquired and inherited lipodystrophies, *N. Engl. J. Med.*, 350, 1220, 2004.
6. Roden, M., Petersen, K. F., and Shulman, G. I., Nuclear magnetic resonance studies of hepatic glucose metabolism in humans, *Recent Prog. Horm. Res.*, 56, 219, 2001.
7. Roden, M., Non-invasive studies of glycogen metabolism in human skeletal muscle using magnetic resonance spectroscopy, *Curr. Opin. Clin. Nutr. Metab. Care*, 4, 26, 2001.
8. Beckmann, N., *Carbon-13 NMR Spectroscopy of Biological Systems*, Academic Press, San Diego, p. 269, chap. 6, 1995.
9. Krssak, M. and Roden, M., The role of lipid accumulation in liver and muscle for insulin resistance and type 2 diabetes mellitus in humans, *Rev. Endocr. Metab. Dis.*, 5, 127, 2004.
10. Thomsen, C. et al., Quantification of liver fat using magnetic resonance spectroscopy, *Magn. Reson. Imaging*, 12, 487, 1994.
11. Krssak, M. et al., Intramyocellular lipid concentrations are correlated with insulin sensitivity in humans: a ^{1}H NMR spectroscopy study, *Diabetologia*, 42, 113, 1999.
12. Schick, F. et al., Comparison of localized proton NMR signals of skeletal muscle and fat tissue in vivo: two lipid compartments in muscle tissue, *Magn. Reson. Med.*, 29, 158, 1993.
13. Szczepaniak, L. S. et al., Measurement of intracellular triglyceride stores by H spectroscopy: validation in vivo, *Am. J. Physiol.*, 276, E977, 1999.
14. Perseghin, G. et al., Intramyocellular triglyceride content is a determinant of in vivo insulin resistance in humans: a ^{1}H-^{13}C nuclear magnetic resonance spectroscopy assessment in offspring of type 2 diabetic parents, *Diabetes*, 48, 1600, 1999.
15. Jacob, S. et al., Association of increased intramyocellular lipid content with insulin resistance in lean nondiabetic offspring of type 2 diabetic subjects, *Diabetes*, 48, 1113, 1999.
16. Radda, G. K., Control, bioenergetics, and adaptation in health and disease: noninvasive biochemistry from nuclear magnetic resonance, *FASEB J.*, 6, 3032, 1992.
17. Rothman, D. L., Shulman, R. G., and Shulman, G. I., ^{31}P nuclear magnetic resonance measurements of muscle glucose-6-phosphate. Evidence for reduced insulin-dependent muscle glucose transport or phosphorylation activity in non-insulin-dependent diabetes mellitus, *J. Clin. Invest.*, 89, 1069, 1992.
18. Roden, M. et al., Rapid impairment of skeletal muscle glucose transport/phosphorylation by free fatty acids in humans, *Diabetes*, 48, 358, 1999.
19. Lebon, V. et al., Effect of triiodothyronine on mitochondrial energy coupling in human skeletal muscle, *J. Clin. Invest.*, 108, 733, 2001.
20. Petersen, K. F. et al., Mitochondrial dysfunction in the elderly: possible role in insulin resistance, *Science*, 300, 1140, 2003.
21. Beckmann, N., Seelig, J., and Wick, H., Analysis of glycogen storage disease by in vivo ^{13}C NMR: comparison of normal volunteers with a patient, *Magn. Reson. Med.*, 16, 150, 1990.
22. Jue, T. et al., Natural abundance ^{13}C NMR spectrum of glycogen in humans, *Magn. Reson. Med.*, 5, 377, 1987.
23. Shulman, G. I. et al., Quantitation of muscle glycogen synthesis in normal subjects and subjects with non-insulin-dependent diabetes by ^{13}C nuclear magnetic resonance spectroscopy, *N. Engl. J. Med.*, 322, 223, 1990.
24. Rothman, D. L. et al., Quantitation of hepatic glycogenolysis and gluconeogenesis in fasting humans with ^{13}C NMR, *Science*, 254, 573, 1991.
25. Petersen, K. F. et al., Noninvasive assessment of hepatic triglyceride content in humans with ^{13}C nuclear magnetic resonance spectroscopy, *Hepatology*, 24, 114, 1996.
26. Roden, M. et al., Mechanism of free fatty acid-induced insulin resistance in humans, *J. Clin. Invest.*, 97, 2859, 1996.

27. Magnusson, I. et al., Liver glycogen turnover in fed and fasted humans, *Am. J. Physiol.*, 266, E796, 1994.
28. Cline, G. W. et al., ^{13}C-nuclear magnetic resonance spectroscopy studies of hepatic glucose metabolism in normal subjects and subjects with insulin-dependent diabetes mellitus, *J. Clin. Invest.*, 94, 2369, 1994.
29. Roden, M. et al., The roles of insulin and glucagon in the regulation of hepatic glycogen synthesis and turnover in humans, *J. Clin. Invest.*, 97, 642, 1996.
30. Dresner, A. et al., Effects of free fatty acids on glucose transport and IRS-1-associated phosphatidylinositol 3-kinase activity, *J. Clin. Invest.*, 103, 253, 1999.
31. Cline, G. W. et al., Impaired glucose transport as a cause of decreased insulin stimulated muscle glycogen synthersis in type 2 diabetes, *N. Engl. J. Med.*, 341, 240, 1999.
32. Taylor, R. et al., Direct measurements of change in muscle glycogen concentrations after a mixed meal in normal subjects, *Am. J. Physiol.*, 265, E224, 1993.
33. Carey, P. E. et al., Direct assessment of muscle glycogen storage after mixed meals in normal and type 2 diabetic subjects, *Am. J. Physiol.*, 284, E688, 2003.
34. Rossetti, L., Giaccari, A., and DeFronzo, R. A., Glucose toxicity, *Diabetes Care*, 13, 610, 1990.
35. Rothman, D. L. et al., Decreased muscle glucose transport/phosphorylation is an early defect in the pathogenesis of non-insulin-dependent diabetes mellitus, *Proc. Natl Acad. Sci. USA*, 92, 983, 1995.
36. Perseghin, G. et al., Increased glucose transport-phosphorylation and muscle glycogen synthesis after exercise training in insulin-resistant subjects, *N. Engl. J. Med.*, 335, 1357, 1996.
37. Petersen, K. F. et al., ^{13}C/^{31}P NMR studies on the mechanism of insulin resistance in obesity, *Diabetes*, 47, 381, 1998.
38. Randle, P. J., Regulatory interactions between lipids and carbohydrates: the glucose fatty acid cycle after 35 years, *Diabetes Metab. Rev.*, 14, 263, 1998.
39. Krebs, M. et al., Free fatty acids inhibit the glucose-stimulated increase of intramuscular glucose-6-phosphate concentration in humans, *J. Clin. Endocrinol. Metab.*, 86, 2153, 2001.
40. Krebs, M. et al., Mechanism of amino acid-induced skeletal muscle insulin resistance in humans, *Diabetes*, 51, 599, 2002.
41. Anderwald, C. et al., Effects of insulin treatment in type 2 diabetic patients on intracellular lipid content in liver and skeletal muscle, *Diabetes*, 51, 3025, 2002.
42. Perseghin, G. et al., Insulin resistance, intramyocellular lipid content and plasma adiponectin in patients with type 1 diabetes, *Am. J. Physiol.*, 285, E1174, 2003.
43. Kautzky-Willer, A. et al., Increased intramyocellular lipid concentration identifies impaired glucose metabolism in women with previous gestational diabetes, *Diabetes*, 52, 244, 2003.
44. Sinha, R. et al., Assessment of skeletal muscle triglyceride content by (1)H nuclear magnetic resonance spectroscopy in lean and obese adolescents: relationships to insulin sensitivity, total body fat, and central adiposity, *Diabetes*, 51, 1022, 2002.
45. Weiss, R. et al., Prediabetes in obese youth: a syndrome of impaired glucose tolerance, severe insulin resistance, and altered myocellular and abdominal fat partitioning, *Lancet*, 362, 951, 2003.
46. Simha, V. et al., Effect of leptin replacement on intrahepatic and intramyocellular lipid content in patients with generalized lipodystrophy, *Diabetes Care*, 26, 30, 2003.
47. Luzi, L. et al., Intramyocellular lipid accumulation and reduced whole body lipid oxidation in HIV lipodystrophy, *Am. J. Physiol.*, 284, E274, 2003.
48. Bachmann, O. P. et al., Effects of intravenous and dietary lipid challenge on intramyocellular lipid content and the relation with insulin sensitivity in humans, *Diabetes*, 50, 2579, 2001.
49. Frost, G. S. et al., Carbohydrate-induced manipulation of insulin sensitivity independently of intramyocellular lipids, *Br. J. Nutr.*, 89, 365, 2003.
50. Schrauwen-Hinderling, V. B. et al., The increase in intramyocellular lipid content is a very early response to training, *J. Clin. Endocrinol. Metab.*, 88, 1610, 2003.
51. Petersen, K. F. et al., Impaired mitochondrial activity in the insulin-resistant offspring of patients with type 2 diabetes, *N. Engl. J. Med*, 350, 664, 2004.
52. Roden, M. and Bernroider, E., Hepatic glucose metabolism — its role in health and disease, *Best Pract. Res. Clin.*, 17, 365, 2003.
53. Petersen, K. F. et al., Contribution of net hepatic glycogenolysis to glucose production during the early postprandial period, *Am. J. Physiol.*, 270, E186, 1996.

54. Hundal, R. S. et al., Mechanism by which metformin reduces glucose production in type 2 diabetes, *Diabetes*, 49, 2063, 2000.
55. Kunert, O. et al., Measurement of fractional whole-body gluconeogenesis in humans from blood samples using ^{2}H nuclear magnetic resonance spectroscopy, *Diabetes*, 52, 2475, 2003.
56. Landau, B. R. et al., Use of $^{2}H_2O$ for estimating rates of gluconeogenesis. Application to the fasted state, *J. Clin. Invest.*, 95, 172, 1995.
57. Hwang, J. H. et al., Impaired net hepatic glycogen synthesis in insulin-dependent diabetic subjects during mixed meal ingestion. A ^{13}C nuclear magnetic resonance spectroscopy study, *J. Clin. Invest.*, 95, 783, 1995.
58. Taylor, R. et al., Direct assessment of liver glycogen storage by ^{13}C nuclear magnetic resonance spectroscopy and regulation of glucose homeostasis after a mixed meal in normal subjects, *J. Clin. Invest.*, 97, 126, 1996.
59. Krssak, M. et al., Postprandial hepatic glycogen metabolism in type 2 diabetes, *Diabetes*, 53, 3048, 2004.
60. Bischof, M. G. et al., Intensive insulin therapy does not normalise all defects of hepatic carbohydrate metabolism in type 1 diabetes mellitus, *Diabetes*, 50, 392, 2001.
61. Bischof, M. G. et al., Hepatic glycogen metabolism in type 1 diabetes mellitus after long-term near normoglycemia, *Diabetes*, 51, 49, 2002.
62. Stingl, H. et al., Lipid-dependent control of hepatic glycogen stores in healthy man, *Diabetologia*, 44, 48, 2001.
63. Stingl, H. et al., Reduction of hepatic glycogen synthesis and breakdown in patients with agenesis of the dorsal pancreas, *J. Clin. Endocrinol. Metab.*, 87, 4678, 2002.
64. Velho, G. et al., Impaired hepatic glycogen synthesis in glucokinase-deficient (MODY-2) subjects, *J. Clin. Invest.*, 98, 1755, 1996.
65. Magnusson, I. et al., Increased rate of gluconeogenesis in type II diabetes mellitus. A ^{13}C nuclear magnetic resonance study, *J. Clin. Invest.*, 90, 1323, 1992.
66. Mayerson, A. B. et al., The effects of rosiglitazone on insulin sensitivity, lipolysis, and hepatic and skeletal muscle triglyceride content in patients with type 2 diabetes, *Diabetes*, 51, 797, 2002.
67. Ryysy, L. et al., Hepatic fat content and insulin action on free fatty acids and glucose metabolism rather than insulin absorption are associated with insulin requirements during insulin therapy in type 2 diabetic patients, *Diabetes*, 49, 749, 2000.
68. Tiikkainen, M. et al., Liver-fat accumulation and insulin resistance in obese women with previous gestational diabetes, *Obes. Res.*, 10, 859, 2002.
69. Seppala-Lindroos, A. et al., Fat accumulation in the liver is associated with defects in insulin suppression of glucose production and serum free fatty acids independent of obesity in normal men, *J. Clin. Endocrinol. Metab.*, 87, 3023, 2002.
70. Petersen, K. F. et al., Leptin reverses insulin resistance and hepatic steatosis in patients with severe lipodystrophy, *J. Clin. Invest.*, 109, 1345, 2002.
71. Sutinen, J. et al., Increased fat accumulation in the liver in HIV-infected patients with antiretroviral therapy-associated lipodystrophy, *Aids*, 16, 2183, 2002.
72. Marchesini, G. et al., Nonalcoholic fatty liver disease: a feature of the metabolic syndrome, *Diabetes*, 50, 1844, 2001.
73. Cline, G. W. et al., Mechanism of impaired insulin-stimulated muscle glucose metabolism in subjects with insulin-dependent diabetes mellitus, *J. Clin. Invest.*, 99, 2219, 1997.
74. Yki-Jarvinen, H. et al., Comparison of bedtime insulin regimens in patients with type 2 diabetes mellitus: a randomized, controlled trial, *Ann. Intern. Med.*, 130, 389, 1999.
75. UK Prospective Diabetes Study (UKPDS) Group, Effect of intensive blood–glucose control with metformin on complications inoverweight patients with type 2 diabetes (UKPDS 34), *Lancet*, 352, 854, 1998.
76. Cusi, K. and DeFronzo, R. A., Metformin: a review of its metabolic effects, *Diabetes Rev.*, 6, 89, 1998.
77. Stingl, H. and Roden, M., Future targets in the treatment of type 2 diabetes, *Wien. Klin. Wschr.*, 116, 217, 2004.
78. Petersen, K. F. et al., Mechanism of troglitazone action in type 2 diabetes type 2 diabetes, *Diabetes*, 49, 827, 2000.

79. Carey, D. G. et al., Effect of rosiglitazone on insulin sensitivity and body composition in type 2 diabetic patients [corrected], *Obes. Res.*, 10, 1008, 2002.
80. Bajaj, M. et al., Pioglitazone reduces hepatic fat content and augments splanchnic glucose uptake in patients with type 2 diabetes, *Diabetes*, 52, 1364, 2003.
81. Bajaj, M. et al., Decreased plasma adiponectin concentrations are closely related to hepatic fat content and hepatic insulin resistance in pioglitazone-treated type 2 diabetic patients, *J. Clin. Endocrinol. Metab.*, 89, 200, 2004.
82. Bajaj, M. et al., Plasma resistin concentration, hepatic fat content, and hepatic and peripheral insulin resistance in pioglitazone-treated type II diabetic patients, *Int. J. Obes.*, 28, 783, 2004.
83. Gaede, P. et al., Multifactorial intervention and cardiovascular disease in patients with type 2 diabetes, *N. Engl. J. Med.*, 348, 383, 2003.
84. Bernroider, E. et al., Effekte oraler Antidiabetika auf die Insulinsensitivität bei guteingestellten Typ 2 Diabetikern, *Acta Medica Austriaca*, 31(Suppl. 64), 2, 2004, abstract.
85. Katoh, S. et al., Troglitazone prevents the rise in visceral adiposity and improves fatty liver associated with sulfonylurea therapy-a randomized controlled trial, *Metabolism*, 50, 414, 2001.
86. Carr, A. et al., Rosey investigators. No effect of rosiglitazone for treatment of HIV-1 lipoatrophy: randomised, double-blind, placebo-controlled trial, *Lancet*, 363, 429, 2004.
87. Sutinen, J. et al., Effects of rosiglitazone on gene expression in subcutaneous adipose tissue in highly active antiretroviral therapy-associated lipodystrophy, *Am. J. Physiol.*, 286, E941, 2004.
88. Björkman, O. et al., Gut exchange of glucose and lactate in basal state and after oral glucose ingestion in postoperative patients, *Diabetes*, 39, 747, 1990.
89. Landau, B. R. et al., Methods for measuring glycogen cycling, *Am. J. Physiol.*, 281, E413, 2001.

Editorial Comments

Usually, initial treatment of patients suffering from rheumatoid arthritis is based on nonsteroidal antiinflammatory drugs, which display no disease-modifying effects. Therapy is changed to more toxic disease-modifying antirheumatic drugs only when radiographic damage has been detected. Although some of these compounds improve outcomes in rheumatoid arthritis, in particular by slowing the rate of radiographic progression, there is a clear need to reduce the toxic effects caused by the therapies. A particular challenge consists in differentiating early rheumatoid arthritis from other forms of inflammatory arthritis in order to target therapy in a timely manner. In this context, development of disease-modifying compounds causing fewer side-effects is an urgent matter.

New therapeutic strategies are also being pursued to correct, prevent, or slow the progression of osteoarthritis. Importantly, the ability to evaluate the efficacy of these therapies, or to determine the cases in which they might be most useful, critically depends on diagnostic measures that not only provide information on the present state of cartilage, but also that may allow prediction of its development. Promising MRI tools developed over the past years have shown technical validity in probing the morphologic and molecular state of cartilage.

In Chapter 23, Manish Kothari and Charles Peterfy discuss how MRI can assist in the early diagnosis of rheumatoid and osteoarthritis and aid in the monitoring of response to therapy aiming to decrease the rate of structural damage. The use of MRI techniques in preclinical studies involving animal models of arthritis is extensively addressed in Chapter 22. Overall, the efforts in this domain constitute an appropriate example of a paradigm shift in which therapeutic strategies are developed hand-in-hand with diagnostic approaches. This shift holds the promise of speeding the development of effective disease-modifying therapies.

22 Rheumatoid and Osteoarthritis: Preclinical Applications of *In Vivo* MR

Didier Laurent and Nicolau Beckmann

CONTENTS

22.1 INTRODUCTION

With aging of the population, chronic diseases affecting the joints, such as rheumatoid arthritis (RA) and osteoarthritis (OA), are a major medical challenge. The pharmaceutical industry is eager to develop new drugs that would not only treat for the pain caused by these diseases, but also restore joint function and overall mobility. Hence, the identification of new drug targets that are involved in the etiology of the diseases is of high relevance for the development of structure-modifying therapies.

Clinically, RA is a chronic deforming disease characterized mainly by joint swelling and destruction. Although synovial inflammation and bone erosion are the hallmarks of this disease, the presentation of various features between patients is clearly heterogenous, suggesting that there are several variants of RA. OA is a degenerative disease caused in part by prolonged wear -and tear of the joints. At an early stage, the disease is characterized by failure of the solid (i.e., macromolecular) phase within the cartilage matrix. Eventually the joint produces fluid in an attempt to improve lubrication. This latter process, also called synovitis or inflammation of the synovial membrane which develops in response to the effusion of cartilage degradation products in adjacent tissues, is the major source of debilitating pain. Unlike RA then, OA at an early stage is a noninflammatory condition characterized by an initial cartilage damage that sets off the destructive process, ultimately affecting adjacent bones, muscles, and tissues. The main pathological features of OA comprise loss of articular cartilage, osteophytes (i.e., bony outgrowths) around the joint and sclerosis of the subchondral bone.

MRI has become the method of choice in the diagnosis of joint diseases in humans and also in animal models of RA and OA because of its ability to differentiate bone, cartilage, tendons, synovium, muscle, and adipose tissue. Three-dimensional (3D) imaging protocols provide the high spatial resolution required and allow for proper image co-registration, thus enabling reproducible monitoring of the complex joint architecture in longitudinal studies.

In spite of considerable efforts by the pharmaceutical industry, it has proved very difficult to develop new classes of therapeutic agents for arthritis. With MRI, the ability to noninvasively assess the effects of treatment in animal models can only benefit the development of therapies. Along with morphological and functional assessments, MRI can potentially offer qualitative readouts which may be considered as useful surrogate markers. In the present chapter, we address possible roles of MRI in drug testing at the preclinical level in arthritis research. In order to better judge the challenges and advantages of using an imaging technique as MRI, we first describe current models of RA and OA, and have a look at nonMRI methods currently applied. We then proceed to examine which MRI methods and readouts can be routinely employed in noninvasive drug testing in animals. Although some of the techniques are limited to preclinical studies, clearly translational aspects are a key element to be taken into account when evaluating the usefulness of MRI in pharmaceutical research.

22.2 ANIMAL MODELS OF ARTHRITIS

The development of an animal model that has all of the elements of human RA has remained elusive. Nevertheless, a variety of models have provided substantial insights into basic pathogenic mechanisms of chronic inflammatory arthritis and autoimmune diseases in general. These models revealed the complex nature of the balance between T-cell cytokines and the chronic inflammatory processes.

Of the proposed models, collagen-induced arthritis (CIA) is the most characterized in terms of both pathogenesis and underlying immunological basis [1–3]. CIA is also considered to be the model of choice in terms of validating therapeutic targets and testing potential new therapeutic agents for the treatment of human RA. The pathology can be induced in mice or rats by immunization with autologous or heterologous type II collagen in adjuvant. Susceptibility to CIA is strongly associated with major histocompatibility complex class II genes. A pronounced T- and B-cell response to type II collagen is observed. Major pathological features of CIA include proliferative synovitis with infiltration of polymorphonuclear and mononuclear cells, pannus formation, cartilage degradation, bone erosion, and fibrosis. Similarly to RA, proinflammatory cytokines, such as tumor necrosis factor alpha (TNFα) and interleukin (IL)-1β, are abundantly expressed in the arthritic joints. Blockade of these molecules results in a reduction of disease severity [4].

One of the major clinical features of RA is its chronic course. It has been suggested that the chronicity of RA might be due to a local immune response to a renewable articular autoantigen. Chronic arthritis induced by intraarticular injection of antigen into previously immunized animals is used to study the mechanisms responsible for the maintenance of chronic inflammation. Experimental antigen-induced arthritis (AIA) is induced after previous systemic immunization with antigen in Freund's complete adjuvant followed by intraarticular injections of the same soluble antigen (e.g., fibrin, ovalbumin, methylated bovine serum albumin [mBSA], ferritin, or horseradish peroxidase). Rats, mice, and rabbits are susceptible to RA. A few hours after intraarticular injection of the antigen, severe, acute joint swelling with exudation develops. The swelling usually decreases over 2 weeks. About one third of the animals develop a thickened synovium lasting for 8 to 24 weeks. Invasive pannus and cartilage erosions occur after 4 to 6 weeks. The acute phase is characterized by intense infiltration of the tissues with polymorphonuclear lymphocytes. As the arthritis progresses, infiltration by macrophages is prominent [5].

Animal models of OA include mouse and guinea pig spontaneous OA, meniscectomy and ligament transection in guinea pigs, meniscectomy in rabbits [6], and meniscectomy and cruciate transection in dogs [7]. Another model is the surgical goat model, in which joint instability results from medial meniscal transection and disruption of the cartilage surface [8]. Anterior cruciate ligament transection and meniscectomy usually produce only mild pathology in the knee joint. Therefore, the surgical procedure includes unilateral, medial, meniscal transection coupled with multiple partial thickness incisions in the articular cartilage of the medial tibial plateau. These models are slow, rendering longitudinal studies difficult to manage. Acute models involving intraarticular injections of papain [9–12], a proteolytic enzyme, of collagenase [13] or of monosodium iodoacetate [14], an inhibitor of glycolysis, promote loss of articular cartilage similar to that noted in human OA. However, none of these models has a proven track record of predictability in human disease. In fact, no agent has been shown to provide anything other than symptomatic relief in human OA.

The advent of transgenic technology has allowed researchers to study individual gene contributions to the pathogenesis of arthritis. This has been done both in standard inflammatory disease models applied to transgenics and in transgenic animal models associated with spontaneous generation of the disease. Thanks to these activities, advances have been made in the understanding of RA [15] and OA [16].

22.3 MONITORING DISEASE PROGRESSION IN ANIMAL MODELS

The simplest way to analyze the inflammatory response in arthritis models is to assess the joint swelling externally using a caliper. It is obvious that such a procedure is prone to significant error and is very operator-dependent.

Other approaches include analysis of synovial fluid, which is a plasma transudate supplemented with high-molecular-weight, saccharide-rich molecules, notably hyaluronans. Formation of synovial fluid is balanced by its removal via synovial lymphatics. Although the chemical nature of synovial fluid is poorly understood and complex, variation in its volume and composition reflects pathologic processes within the joint. Chemically mediated events, such as inflammation and enzyme-mediated degradation within the synovium and cartilage, are reflected by changes in the chemical composition of synovial fluid. These changes include the production of factors responsible for the accumulation of different cell types within the fluid. Some of the biochemical markers of disease being investigated in the synovial fluid, which is usually extracted *postmortem* by aspiration or lavage, include eicosanoids, cytokines, and proteases as markers of inflammation, type II collagen products and proteoglycan (PG) epitopes as signs of cartilage degradation, or collagen type II propeptides as markers of cartilage synthesis.

Histology continues to be an essential readout in the study of arthritis models. Despite its obvious advantages concerning spatial resolution and staining capabilities, histology is a terminal readout.

22.4 NON-MRI IMAGING READOUTS IN ANIMAL MODELS OF ARTHRITIS

Near-infrared fluorescence (NIRF) imaging is more and more playing an important role in visualizing biological processes under *in vivo* conditions at the cellular and molecular levels (see also Chapter 23, Section 23.2). The method is based on targeting proteins, enzymes, or antigens with fluorochrome-labeled carriers [17]. The near-infrared spectral range (650–950 nm) forms an optical window for cells or tissues, with satisfactory light travel within biologic tissue due to a relative lack of these endogenous absorbers [18]. The main advantages of NIRF are very short acquisition times and, compared with scintigraphic methods, no need for radioactive agents. Using a cathepsin B activatable near-infrared fluorescent probe, OA could be detected at an early stage in a murine model involving intraarticular collagenase injection [19]. Early signs of experimental arthritis have also been measured in a murine model of AIA, in which the target of NIRF was the F4/80 antigen present on the surface of macrophages infiltrating the inflamed synovial membrane [20]. Imaging performed using anti-F4/80 monoclonal antibodies (mAb) labeled with Cy5.5 fluorochrome administered intravenously revealed an accumulation of fluorochrome probes in inflamed knee joints and, to a lesser extent, in contralateral (nonarthritic) knee joints. NIRF in conjunction with protease-activated probes has also been shown to be a sensitive means for imaging the presence of target enzymes in arthritic joints, thereby providing the potential for early monitoring of treatment response to antirheumatic drugs [21]. The rationale for the approach lies in the fact that different proteases are highly upregulated in RA and contribute significantly to joint destruction. Thus, proteases that target the Lys–Lys cleavage site, including cathepsin B, activate the fluorescence of the probe administered intravenously.

Quantitative computed tomography (QCT), an established technique for the determination of bone mineral density (BMD) in the axial and appendicular skeleton, is able to provide separate estimates of trabecular and cortical BMD as a true volumetric density value. Furthermore, QCT can measure geometric properties of cortical bone with great accuracy and predict mechanical properties at high precision [22]. Peripheral QCT (pQCT) is a special type of computed tomography in which scans of the appendicular skeleton are performed at a low radiation dose, enabling noninvasive assessment of bone and muscle development at peripheral sites in rats and mice [23]. Thus, the technique facilitates studies of bone development and loss in experimental models as well as effectiveness of therapeutic interventions.

Microcomputed tomography (micro-CT) provides morphological and architectural 3D information at high resolution from the joints of small rodents under *in vivo* conditions, offering the potential to evaluate bone- and joint-related changes in arthritis models. For instance, the technique has been used to quantify cortical bone loss and periosteal new bone formation for therapeutic evaluation in a murine model of collagen-induced arthritis [24] or to detect progressive changes over time to the subchondral bone (femorotibial joint) of Wistar rats in an OA model [25]. These data demonstrate that *in vivo* micro-CT represents a valuable tool for investigating bone remodeling and has the potential to be used for routine, high-throughput analysis and screening of new therapeutics. Nevertheless, the radiation dose, which affects the image resolution, needs to be applied with caution for safety reasons. Short-term, potentially lethal, effects of ionizing radiation limit high-resolution imaging in live animals [26]. Approaching the lethal dose will affect the way micro-CT experiments are planned, and may reduce opportunities for experiments involving imaging the same animal over time.

22.5 MRI READOUTS IN ANIMAL MODELS OF RA

Animal studies, especially in small rodents, demand high spatial resolution and reproducibility of joint positioning in different imaging sessions (see also Chapter 23, Section 23.2). Three-dimensional (3D) imaging protocols allow reproducible monitoring of the complex joint architecture necessary for longitudinal studies. Proper co-registration of the images is feasible by postprocessing. In addition, 3D images are less affected by partial volume artifacts due to the smaller slice thickness achieved, improving the anatomical definition in the images. Pixel sizes obtained *in vivo* with a 3D gradient-echo sequence at 4.7 or 7 T and using specially built RF probes, designed to be as close as possible to the region of interest, have been of the order of $90 \times 80 \times 60\ \mu m^3$ (rat paw) and $220 \times 220 \times 250\ \mu m^3$ (rabbit knee joint), for measurement times ranging between 30 and 50 min [27–30].

The measures that MRI provides are manifold and dependent on the severity of the disease model, the species, and the region analyzed. In the following subsections, we examine parameters that have been addressed in the literature and that could be potentially used to describe, quantitatively or qualitatively, the development of the disease process and the result of drug intervention in longitudinal studies.

22.5.1 Qualitative Analysis of Soft Tissue and Bony Changes

Because of the complicated joint structures, qualitative analyses of MR images based on scores concerning soft tissue changes and bone destruction have been used to characterize the disease process and the effects of compounds in animal models of arthritis (see also Chapter 23, Section 23.2.1). In an elegant study, Jacobson et al. [31] validated the use of MRI to follow *in vivo* disease progression in an adjuvant arthritis (AA) model in the rat. MRI indices (scores), derived from 2D spin-echo images acquired before and after injection of gadolinium-containing contrast material, were given to characterize soft tissue (edema, joint separation, cysts) and bony changes in the hindpaw (new bone formation in the tibia and the calcaneous, internal changes in the tibia, the talus, and the calcaneous) following subcutaneous administration of *Mycobacterium butyricum*. The MRI parameters were correlated with classic inflammatory parameters (hindpaw volumes assessed with a microcaliper, circulating leukocytes, acute-phase reactants, urinary collagen crosslinks) and histologic evaluation. MRI of arthritic tibiotarsal joints of the uninjected left hindpaws from AA rats, which displayed a typical secondary inflammation, demonstrated two distinct phases of disease activity. The first phase, apparent between days 10 and 18, was characterized by periarticular inflammation with marked synovitis, synovial fibroplasia, and distension of the joint capsule into the surrounding tissue. The secondary phase, occurring between days 18 and 30, was marked by continued soft tissue inflammation, periostitis with osteolysis, and periosteal new bone formation progressing to a state of near complete ankylosis by day 30. The two phases of disease activity observed by MRI paralleled biochemical, cellular, and histologic markers of disease progression [31]. This MRI approach has been employed to show that ABT-963, a highly selective COX-2 inhibitor that may have utility in the treatment of the pain and inflammation associated with arthritis, significantly reduced bone loss and soft tissue destruction in the same AA model [32] (Figure 22.1). Also, protective effects on joint integrity have been found for SB 242235 [33], a potent and selective inhibitor of p38 mitogen-activated protein kinase, and for SB 273005 [34], a potent, orally active nonpeptide antagonist of the integrin $a_v beta_3$ vibronectin receptor. The MRI observations were in agreement with measurements of paw inflammation, with bone mineral density assessments by dual-energy x-ray absorptiometry, and with histologic evaluation.

High resolution, 3D gradient-echo MRI with gadolinium contrast agent enhancement was applied to investigate both soft and hard tissue changes at the knee joint during the time course of rabbit AIA, comparing images to the final histological outcome [29]. At day 7 following antigen challenge, synovial tissue swelling was seen especially at the back of the joint, which was

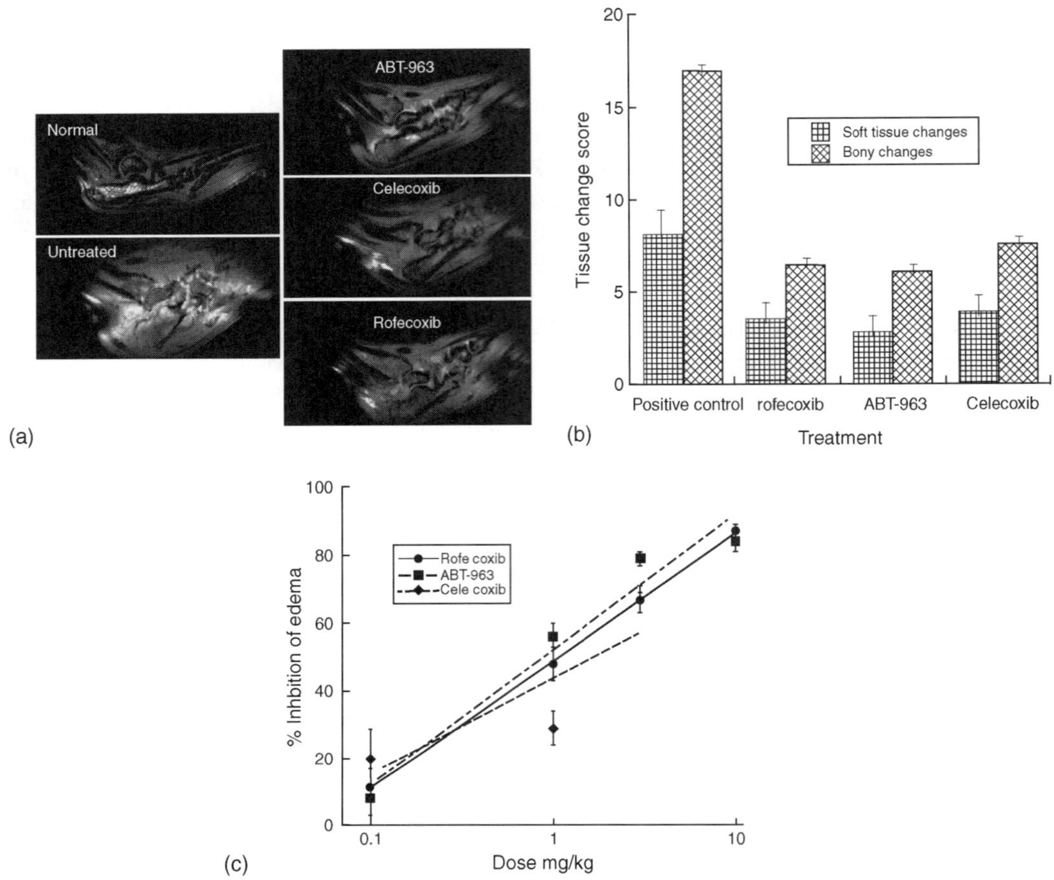

FIGURE 22.1 Dose responses of ABT-963 and celecoxib in established adjuvant arthritis. Rats were injected on day 0 with 0.1 ml of Freund's complete adjuvant. On day 16, rats were again weighed and both hind paws remeasured. Animals demonstrating a typical secondary inflammation as evidenced by swelling of the left paw were randomized into groups of eight to 10 animals. The animals were then dosed with ABT-963, rolecoxib, or celecoxib daily for 14 days. At the end of the treatment period paw volumes were again determined and MRI imaging was conducted. (a) Typical MRI images of the paws; (b) graded scores of the MRI images; (c) effects on edema. The MRI images were scored blind using a standard scoring form. Ten images per treatment group were scored. Data are average $\pm$ S.E.M. Control paw swelling 2.25 $\pm$ 0.11 ml ED for ABT-963 was 0.9 mg/kg (confidence limits of 0.7 to 1.3), the ED_{50} for rofecoxib was 1 mg/kg (confidence limits of 0.7 to 1.3), and the ED_{50} for celecoxib[50] was 0.6 mg/kg (confidence limits of 0.2 to 0.9). (Reproduced from Harris, R. et al., *J. Pharmacol. Exp. Ther.*, 311, 904, 2004. With permission of American Society for Pharmacology and Experimental Therapeutics. Copyright 2004.)

highlighted by the contrast agent, indicative of a highly vascularized tissue. By day 16, a synovial fluid effusion had developed at the back of the joint, which resolved over time into two distinct pockets behind the femur and the tibia. On day 31, there was evidence of hard tissue erosion around the insertion of the anterior cruciate ligament into the tibia, as well as erosion at the back of the femur and tibia by day 60 which was confirmed by joint histology. The active synovial tissue swelling at the back of the knee was also much reduced by day 60, and histologically was characterized by a chronic inflammatory cell infiltrate with a very distinct intimal layer particularly around the fluid effusions. In this example, 3D imaging was essential to examine the complex knee architecture and also because the sites in which changes were detected slightly differed from animal to animal.

22.5.2 Quantitative Analyses

Although scores are useful in providing a global view of the joint status, they are subjective measures. In drug testing it is important to reduce the bias of the person performing the data analysis. Several quantitative parameters extracted from the MR images might be used to study the effects of compounds in the different RA models.

22.5.2.1 Joint Inflammation

MRI in combination with the intravenous administration of gadolinium-containing contrast agents is an established tool for demonstrating inflammatory synovial proliferation in human RA [35] (see also Chapter 23, Section 23.2.1). The rate of contrast enhancement has been shown to correlate with the inflammatory activity of the proliferating synovium [35,36], and is significantly reduced after intraarticular glucocorticoid instillation [37]. The technique has also been proposed as being superior to clinical or radiographic techniques for evaluating disease progression and may have prognostic value with regard to the future development of bone destruction [38].

Inflammation is characterized by increased tissue perfusion and capillary permeability. Synovial uptake of Gd-containing contrast material is dependent on local tissue perfusion and microvascular permeability, resulting in leakage of intravenously injected contrast medium into the interstitial space. This is manifested as an increase in signal intensity (brightness) on T1-weighted MR images. Gaffney et al. [35] described a method for defining the synovium-only phase of Gd-DTPA uptake in the synovium of patients with RA. These authors demonstrated a significant correlation between rate of synovial membrane enhancement and certain histopathological features of synovitis, i.e., polymorphonuclear leukocyte infiltration, hyperemia, and fibrin deposition. This led them to suggest that this technique be used to grade the vascularity of proliferative synovitis, and hence differentiate active hypervascular, pathologically permeable, inflammatory synovial proliferation from noninflammatory, inactive fibrous tissue [39].

This approach can also be applied to animal studies, as exemplified by the AIA model in which mBSA is injected into the knee of presensitized rats. Figure 22.2a shows images acquired 1 day after saline or mBSA challenge, corresponding to tracer uptake experiments in which Gd-DTPA was administered intravenously as a bolus. The insert presents the mean signal intensities in a region-of-interest near the knee where synovial fluid exudation occurred, for images acquired sequentially. The permeability surface-area product (Figure 22.2b) can be estimated from the initial slope of the tracer uptake curves [40]. By day 1, the permeability was increased in antigen-, as compared to saline-challenged knees. This increase was even more pronounced at day 7. In rats treated for 7 days with the glucocorticosteroid dexamethasone (0.3 mg/kg/day p.o.), permeability was reduced as compared to vehicle-treated animals, an observation that is consistent with the antiinflammatory effects of this compound in experimental arthritis [41,42].

22.5.2.2 Angiogenesis

One of the earliest features of rheumatoid synovitis is the development of a new vascular network, which serves to promote the delivery of cells and nutrients to the invading pannus. Vascular endothelial growth factor (VEGF), the main mediator of angiogenesis, is found in the synovial fluid and serum of patients with RA, its expression being correlated with disease severity. Compelling evidence that VEGF is involved in synovitis has been obtained from experimental models of RA. Assessing vascularity using imaging approaches may prove useful for evaluating or even predicting bone destruction [43]. Furthermore, inhibition of angiogenesis may prove useful as an adjunct to current antiinflammatory treatments [44].

Perfusion assessments via bolus tracking MRI using an intravascular contrast agent is a potential means to noninvasively estimate angiogenesis in RA models. This is illustrated for the

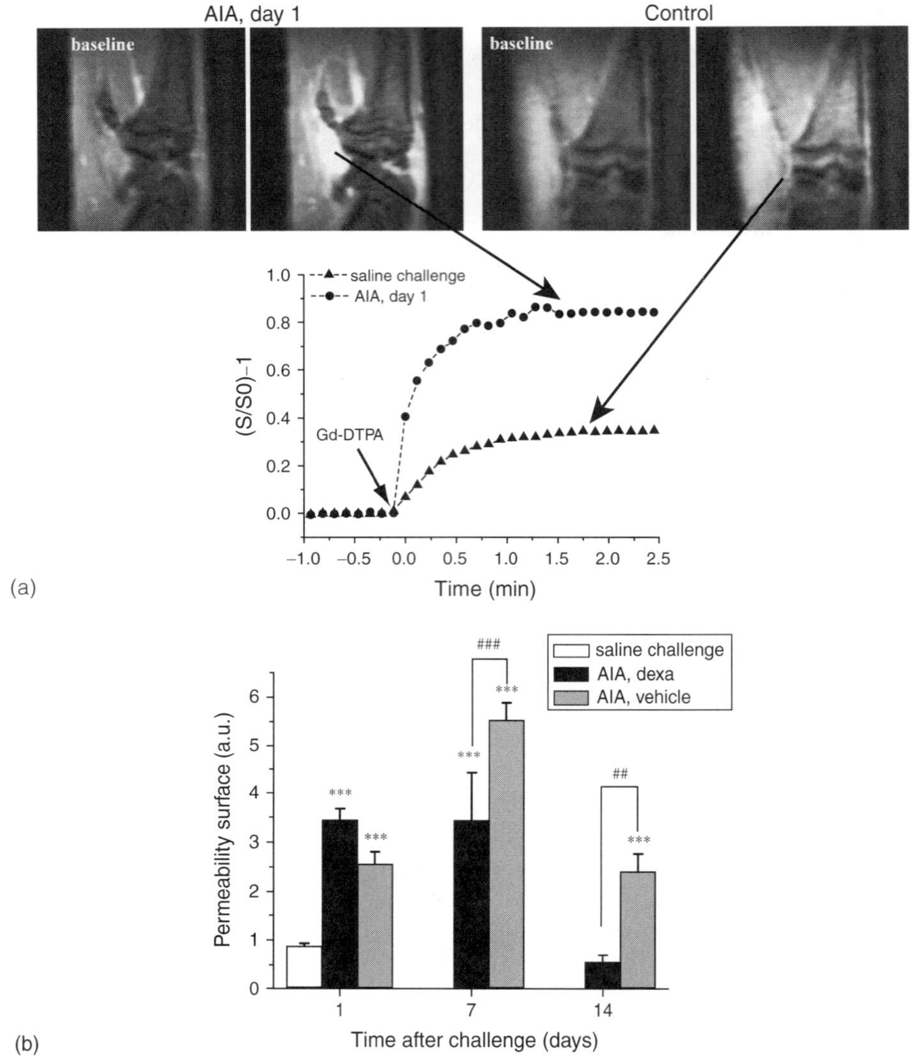

FIGURE 22.2 Vascular permeability and leakage space at the site where synovial fluid exudation takes place in an mBSA-challenged knee. (a) Images acquired before and after administration of Gd–DTPA (Dotarem, 0.5 ml/kg i.v.) as a bolus, with corresponding mean signal intensities of the tracer uptake curves (calculated as $S_i/S_0 - 1$, where S_0 is the mean signal intensity before tracer administration, and S_i the signal intensity for the *i*th image) for an mBSA (AIA) and a saline-challenged control knee. Images were acquired sequentially with a temporal resolution of 7 sec/image. (b) Permeability surface (in arbitrary units, a.u.) assessed from the initial slope of the tracer uptake curves. mBSA-challenged rats were treated with either dexamethasone (0.3 mg/kg/day p.o.) or its vehicle (saline). The significance levels ***$p < .001$ refer to ANOVA comparisons to saline-challenged knees, whereas ## $.001 < p < .01$, ### $p < .001$ refer to ANOVA comparisons with respect to mBSA-challenged knees of vehicle-treated rats.

AIA model consisting of intraarticular injection of mBSA into the knee of presensitized rats. Figure 22.3a presents the course of signal intensity near the knee, for images acquired sequentially during a bolus tracking experiment in which Endorem® was administered intravenously as a bolus, in animals challenged with either antigen or saline. A perfusion index (Figure 22.3b) can be determined from the surface under the tracer uptake curve, for the initial points following the contrast agent bolus. Perfusion was increased at day 7 after the mBSA challenge, suggesting that

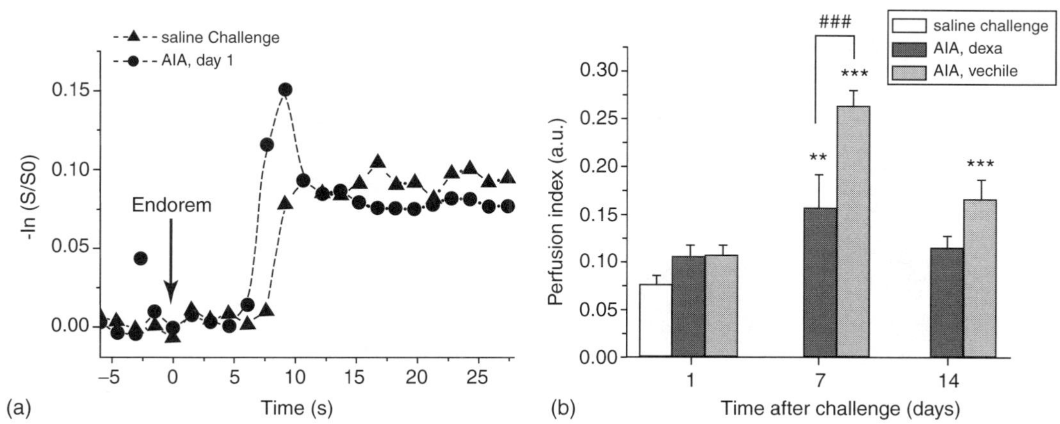

FIGURE 22.3 Perfusion at the site where synovial fluid exudation takes place in a challenged knee. (a) Mean signal intensities of the bolus tracking curves [calculated as $-\ln(S_i/S_0)$], where S_0 is the mean signal intensity before contrast agent (Endorem, 1 ml/kg i.v.) administration, and S_i the signal intensity for the *i*th image. Data were obtained 1 day after challenge with either saline or mBSA. (b) Perfusion indexes determined from the area under the tracer uptake curves for the six points following injection of contrast agent. Data represent means ± S.E.M. for 12 animals in each group. AIA animals were treated with either 0.3 mg/kg/day dexamethasone or its vehicle (saline) administered p.o. The significance levels ** $.001 < p < .01$, *** $p < .001$ refer to ANOVA comparisons to saline-challenged knees, whereas ### $p < .001$ refer to ANOVA comparisons with respect to mBSA-challenged knees of placebo-treated, control rats.

angiogenesis took place. The increase in perfusion was less pronounced in rats treated with dexamethasone (0.3 mg/kg/day p.o.). These observations are in agreement with recently reported data showing the ability of dexamethasone to decrease angiogenesis *in vivo* [45].

22.5.2.3 Macrophage Infiltration

Macrophages possess widespread proinflammatory, destructive, and remodeling capabilities that critically contribute to the acute and chronic phases of RA [46]. Therefore, monitoring the macrophage infiltration into sites of inflammation noninvasively may play an important role in the study of RA models.

While contrast agents, such as Gd–DOTA, are cleared from the vascular system shortly after injection and eventually accumulate in the extravascular extracellular space, superparamagnetic iron oxide (SPIO) particles, of a mean diameter up to 150 nm, are eliminated from the blood by cells of the mononuclear phagocytotic system through absorptive endocytosis [47]. This property has been exploited in murine [48], rat [49], and rabbit [50] models of RA to follow, *in vivo*, the infiltration of macrophages into inflamed areas by administering SPIO or USPIO (particles mean diameter of about 30 nm).

In the same rat AIA model described above, significant negative correlation was found between the MRI signal intensity in the knee and the histologically determined iron content in macrophages located in the same region of animals that had received SPIO (Endorem®) 24 h before image acquisition [49]. Starting 2 days postantigen injection, images from arthritic knees exhibited distinctive signal attenuation in the synovium (Figure 22.4). This signal attenuation was significantly smaller in knees from animals treated with dexamethasone (0.3 mg/kg/day p.o.) and completely absent in contralateral knees that had been challenged with vehicle. These results suggest the feasibility of detecting macrophage infiltration into the knee synovium in this model of AIA by cell labeling with SPIO. This readout may have an impact in preclinical drug studies by shortening the duration of the experimental period and by facilitating the investigation of novel

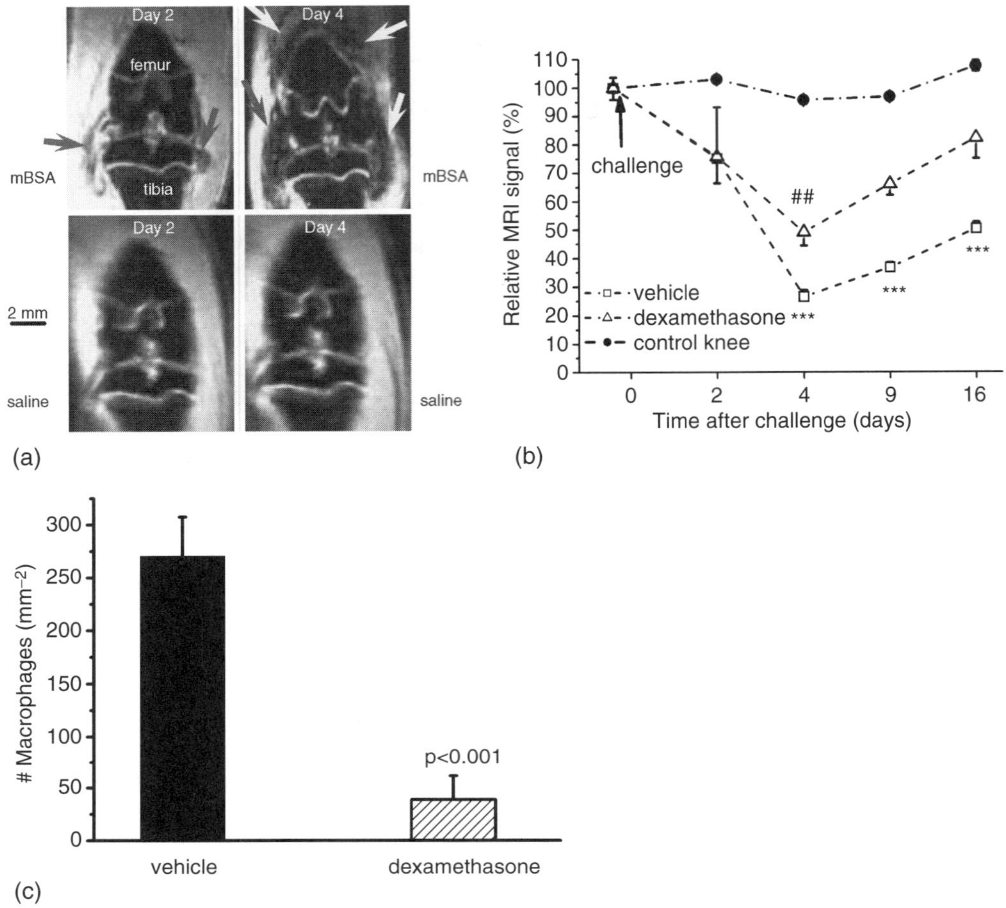

FIGURE 22.4 Macrophage infiltration into the region where synovial fluid exudation takes place in an antigen-challenged knee. (a) Coronal sections through the right, albumin-challenged knee (upper row) and the left, saline-challenged knee (lower row) of a placebo-treated rat, from 3D data sets acquired at 2 and 4 days after challenge. Endorem® (0.7 ml/300 g body weight) was administered i.v. 24 h before each image session. (b) Course of MRI signal intensities (mean ± S.E.M., $n = 5$ for each group of knees) relative to prechallenge values. Control knees refer to contralateral, saline-challenged knees, from the same rats that had received antigen on the ipsilateral joints. The levels of significance, *** $p < .001$, and # $.01 < p < .05$, ## $.001 < p < .01$, correspond to ANOVA comparisons carried out for antigen-challenged knees from vehicle- and dexamethasone (0.3 mg/kg/day p.o.)-treated animals, respectively. (c) Macrophage numbers (mean ± S.E.M., $n = 5$) determined by histology on day 16 after challenge, in mBSA-challenged knees from vehicle- and dexamethasone-treated rats. The level of significance refers to a *t*-test comparison between both groups of animals. A fraction of these macrophages was loaded with iron from the contrast agent. (Reproduced from Beckmann, N. et al., *Magn. Reson. Med.*, 49, 1047, 2003. With permission of John Wiley & Sons, Inc. Copyright 2003.)

immunomodulatory therapies acting on macrophages. The great advantage of this model is that the contralateral, unchallenged knee, can serve as a reference in the same animal.

22.5.2.4 Bony Changes

In addition to the previous readouts which provide early markers of disease progression, before more aggressive changes like cartilage and bone erosion take place, it is fundamental to be able to quantify bony changes, in order to detect if compounds may also interfere at the late phase.

In a rat adjuvant model, 3D gradient-echo MRI detected trabecular bone damage at an early stage (from day 11 after induction onwards), namely a loss of bone density and bone resorption, as well as bone transformations (endostosis and exostosis). In the metaphysis and epiphysis, punched-out lesions formed and progressed to the trabecular bone alveoli [30]. There was also a rupture of the cortical epiphysis from days 11 to 14. From a practical point of view, assessment of trabecular density could be a useful parameter to follow disease progression in a quantitative manner. For the same model, reductions in apparent cartilage thickness between femur and patella have been reported [30]. Despite these encouraging results, a more systematic examination needs to be carried out in order to verify if cartilage thickness is a reliable parameter to be followed in a longitudinal study.

Space volumes of metatarsophalangeal and proximal interphalangeal joints of the midtoes of the hind paw were used as a marker to assess quantitatively the course of CIA in Dark Agouti rats [27]. Thereby pathomorphological changes associated with the CIA process, e.g., increase of joint space and cartilage and bone erosion, could be observed *in vivo*, and they correlated well with histological findings [28]. Paw swelling assessed by a microcaliper was receding before significant changes were detected in the images, pointing to the fact that high resolution MRI is an useful tool to follow the chronic phase of the disease. Using this approach, no significant changes in the joint architecture were observed in cyclosporin- (Sandimmune Neoral®) treated rats.

22.6 MRI READOUTS IN OA: APPLICATIONS TO ANIMALS STUDIES

MRI is not only exquisitely suited to look at the knee as an organ, but also to specifically probe OA-induced macromolecular changes in articular cartilage as early indicators of disease progression. This is also true given the fact that 75% of the weight of the cartilage is water. As described below, several MRI techniques have been developed to probe the integrity of the cartilage matrix, based on its biomolecular structure. In this section, we dwell first on the cartilage properties before discussing the parameters that can be assessed noninvasively by MRI in animal models of the disease and in the preclinical analysis of therapy regimens (see also Chapter 23, Section 23.3).

22.6.1 Biomechanical Properties of Cartilage in Relation to Its Composition

Tensile properties of articular cartilage depend on the composition and ultrastructural organization of the macromolecular network and so may the MR appearance of the tissue be as well. Collagen, which constitutes up to 50 to 60% of the dry weight of adult articular cartilage [51], is aimed at protecting chondrocytes by resisting compression forces, at providing a restraint for entrapped proteoglycan-induced interstitial osmotic swelling pressure, and finally at anchoring cartilage to the subchondral bone. The roughening of the articular surface, as typically observed in OA patients, results of cartilage fibrillation, a process involving denaturation of the collagen fibril structure. In animal models of OA, regions of pathologically softened cartilage are also characterized by a fragmentation of the collagen network, leading to a release of cross-link peptides and collagen fragments in the synovial fluid.

Proteoglycans (PG), another major constituent of the cartilage matrix accounting for about 40% of the tissue dry weight [52], contribute to the stiffness of cartilage. Being entangled in the collagen network, their major function is hydration of the cellular matrix, which in turn provides much of the cartilage resiliency through electrostatic repulsion. Due to abundant negative charges on glycosaminoglycan side chains, a fixed charge density (FCD) has been reported in adult articular cartilage [53]. Mobile cations, such as sodium, potassium, and calcium, are attracted by PG negative charges. As a result of water pouring into collagen interstices, the osmotic pressure induces resistance to the loss of fluid under compression, accounting for the tensile strength of cartilage. In other words, if water from the interstitial space is displaced by a compressive load, proteoglycans can draw the water back when the load is removed. This implies that a decrease in FCD, that is likely to expose cartilage to dehydration and softening [54], will predispose the joint to OA. As an antecedent to the gross destruction of cartilage during the early stage of OA, PGs are lost leading to impaired biomechanical support function of cartilage, which in turn contributes to its further degradation [53].

22.6.2 Cartilage Thickness and Volume

MRI-determined cartilage volume in humans provides a direct measure of tissue growth, adaptation, and tissue loss [55]. Although 3D MRI is less prone to errors resulting from malpositioning and more specific information can be obtained on disease status such as differentiation between femoral vs. tibial loss [56], determination of cartilage loss is often inaccurate, since both weight-bearing and nonweight-bearing regions are considered in the assessments. In this respect, cartilage thickness maps may therefore provide better insights into the location of cartilage lesions and damage progression [57].

In animal studies, spatial resolution is one the main hurdles to overcome since articular cartilage thickness rarely exceeds 1 mm, even in rabbits or dogs. Thus, macroscopic signs of cartilage degeneration may not be visible during preclinical investigations on the early stage of OA. Only in rare occasions has *in vivo* MRI been used to quantify the loss of cartilage volume in conjunction with disease progression in animals. For instance, Tessier et al. [58] were able to successfully segment knee cartilage from 3D MR images in a guinea pig model of chronic OA. In this model, thanks to high-resolution MRI acquisitions within a reasonable time, more than 30% reduction in cartilage volume could be reported over a 3-month period. In another study, *in vivo* MRI was applied to measure cartilage swelling in the rabbit knee at an early stage of experimental OA [59].

Generally speaking, such imaging approaches have difficulty in demonstrating subtle changes of cartilage thickness and consequently beneficial effects of novel therapies in animals. Therefore, methods not limited to inspection of the cartilage surface need to be considered. Again, more promising avenues are imaging techniques addressing functional properties of cartilage in relation to its macromolecular content and interstitial water content.

22.6.3 Functional Properties of Cartilage

Early cartilage lesions are primarily characterized by a depletion of PGs and loosening of the collagen framework [60]. The common assumption is that a reduced osmotic pressure due to the loss of water associated with PG depletion impairs the collagen network, which in turn affects the compressive and tensile strength of cartilage [61]. Methods by which both macromolecules could be followed noninvasively and in parallel may prove ideal to quantify the severity of cartilage degeneration as the disease progresses.

22.6.3.1 Water Content

The water content which determines the cartilage MRI properties is linked to its macromolecular composition. Unfortunately, proton relaxation and density maps have been inconclusive as to measuring regional variations in macromolecules at an early stage of cartilage degeneration. There is, for instance, no correlation between proton T_1 and T_2 relaxation and PG distribution across cartilage [62,63].

Diffusion of small solutes in cartilage is another variable that generated some interest in pioneer studies on cartilage MRI. In their studies, Burstein et al. [64] have shown that diffusivity (or self-diffusion resulting from molecular collisions) of small solutes (water, Na^+, Li^+, and $CF_3CO_2^-$) in cartilage was about 60% of the value found in a free solution and was independent of the net matrix charge. In fact, macromolecules of the cartilage matrix represent the primary barriers to water diffusion. When cartilage was compressed or subjected to various enzymatic treatments (to remove proteoglycans for example), a decrease or an increase, respectively, in water diffusion could then be measured *in vitro* [64]. These studies may have important implications in pharmaceutical research. A better understanding of tissue water movements could potentially help improving drug delivery within the cartilage especially because cartilage is avascular and substrate transport can only occur by diffusive mechanisms. Unfortunately up to now, very few if any *in vivo* MRI applications — at least as far as animal models are concerned — took advantage of the fact that an increase in water diffusion can result from matrix degeneration. One reason may be that the diffusion phenomenon is in fact a little more complex than just explained, involving for instance a dispersion component due to the concentration gradient fading over time. Although likely more relevant in terms of measuring the actual transport into cartilage, this process, also called mutual diffusion, is technically difficult to study by MRI. Like in any diffusion MRI experiment, high field systems (>7 T) equipped with strong gradients are usually required to compensate for the lack of spatial resolution. In addition, a perfect stabilization of the knee is necessary to correct motions that might cause distortion from eddy current and artifacts in diffusion map parameters. This inherently limits *in vivo* applications of diffusion-weighted MRI.

22.6.3.2 Proteoglycan Content

The pivotal role played by proteoglycans in cartilage function contributed to the development of multiple technical solutions to assess the PG content. In addition to reducing the FCD, another consequence associated with the loss of the negatively charged PGs is a concomitant loss of Na^+ counterions. Signal intensity in ^{23}Na MRI can be used to measure the Na^+ concentration in articular cartilage. Subsequently, the Na^+ concentration can be used to calculate FCD [65]. ^{23}Na MRI protocols have been developed to quantify FCD of articular cartilage of human volunteers *in vivo* [66]. Undoubtedly sodium MRI proved to be both sensitive and specific in detecting small changes in PG concentration [63]. However, a lack of spatial and temporal resolution due to hardware limitations, especially the gradient system, still makes this technique difficult to apply for routine MRI applications in humans and animals.

Another approach to monitor PG using proton MRI is based on spin lattice relaxation in a rotating frame, $T_{1\rho}$, of spins under the influence of a radiofrequency field. The idea is that PG depletion induces changes in $T_{1\rho}$-relaxation and dispersion in articular cartilage [67]. It is worth noting that $T_{1\rho}$-weighted images usually depict better signal difference/noise ratios than T_2-weighted images of the knee joint. It has been shown that the hyperintense lamina at the articular surface of trypsin-digested cartilage in $T_{1\rho}$-weighted images was due to PG loss, in agreement with histological analysis [68]. Thus, $T_{1\rho}$ relaxation and dispersion have the potential to detect cartilage abnormalities. However, animal studies that compare MRI with biochemical and histological data are still needed to validate $T_{1\rho}$ as a surrogate to follow cartilage regeneration in an efficacy study.

The delayed gadolinium-enhanced MRI of cartilage (dGEMRIC) technique has been proposed as a method capable of detecting PG loss in the osteoarthritic tissue [69]. Due to its minimal invasiveness, the approach is highly attractive for the evaluation of new drug therapies aimed at protecting and/or replenishing glycosaminoglycans (GAGs) in the cartilage matrix, in particular in the context of longitudinal preclinical and clinical studies. In principle, this contrast-enhanced imaging method allows measurement of the FCD of cartilage, reflecting the negatively charged GAG side chain concentration. The hypothesis, as illustrated in Figure 22.5, is that following intravenous administration, the negatively charged gadolinium complex $Gd(DTPA)^{2-}$ penetrates the interstitial fluid of cartilage to reach an equilibrium concentration that is governed by (1) the $Gd(DTPA)^{2-}$-concentration gradient and (2) electrostatic interactions (inversely proportional to the FCD). Articular $Gd(DTPA)^{2-}$ uptake, due to the paramagnetic properties of the contrast agent, leads to a decrease of the T_1 relaxation time of tissue water, the extent of which depending on the local concentration of the contrast agent. The distribution of $Gd(DTPA)^{2-}$ in degraded cartilage is

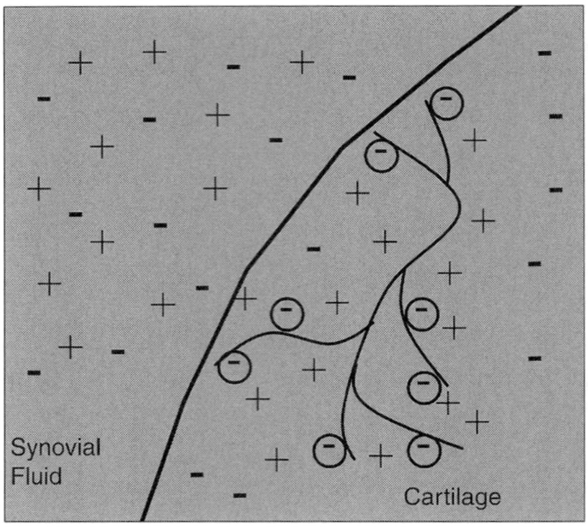

FIGURE 22.5 Principle of the delayed gadolinium-enhanced MRI of cartilage (dGEMRIC) technique. Molecules of Gd(DTPA)$^{2-}$ (blue negative signs) penetrate cartilage to an equilibrium concentration inversely proportional to the charge density that is governed by negatively charged glycosaminoglycan side chains (in bright yellow). A low fixed charge density due to a loss of proteoglycans as encountered in osteoarthritic cartilage will allow more molecules of Gd(DTPA)$^{2-}$ to diffuse in the tissue, which will result in a decrease in T_1 relaxation and hence a brighter signal in T_1-weighted images.

reflected by lower T_1 values, especially where tissue PGs are depleted. In theory, under steady-state conditions, the local Gd(DTPA)$^{2-}$ concentration and the related FCD can be derived from Gd(DTPA)$^{2-}$-T_1 maps [70] as long as the Gd(DTPA)$^{2-}$ relaxivity is tissue independent [71]. As alternatives to Gd(DTPA)$^{2-}$, solutions of manganese ions [72] or nitroxide free radicals [73] have been used as positively charged contrast agents to map the presence of GAGs. However, due to their toxic nature, such agents can only be applied to *ex vivo* or nonsurvival studies. More practical details about dGEMRIC can be found in Appendix 22.1.

We explored the capability of this method to quantitatively assess cartilage degeneration in a goat model of OA, in which proteoglycan depletion was induced by an intraarticular injection of papain the day prior to MRI to mimic the progressive nature of cartilage changes in OA [11]. Papain is known to induce release of both nonhelico–amino–carboxyl ends of collagen type II. A close correlation was found between the extent of proteoglycan loss and the Gd(DTPA)$^{2-}$-induced decrease of the longitudinal relaxation time T_1. Papain injections induced PG depletion ranging from zero to almost 100% in a dose-dependent manner (see Figure 22.6) as confirmed with *postmortem* biochemistry and histology (see Figure 22.7). A 2-h period without passive exercise was determined to be an optimal delay after i.v. Gd(DTPA)$^{2-}$ injection for accurate quantitation of the cartilage defect. As long as a preinjection T_1 map was obtained, the Gd(DTPA)$^{2-}$-enhanced MRI technique revealed good sensitivity in detecting partial loss of PGs in articular cartilage of the goat knee [11]. Of note, experimental procedures were optimized to address aspects such as the influence of joint exercise on contrast agent penetration into cartilage. Performing a series of knee flexions postadministration facilitated the penetration of the contrast agent into the weight-bearing region of articular cartilage. However, the T_1 changes observed in cartilage of exercised goat knees were not affected either by papain or IL1β pretreatment, suggesting that detection of PG loss may be impeded by performing passive flexions post-Gd(DTPA)$^{2-}$ injection.

The feasibility of *in vivo* high-resolution MRI assessments probing PG content was also explored in articular cartilage of the rabbit knee [12]. In line with the goat data, the

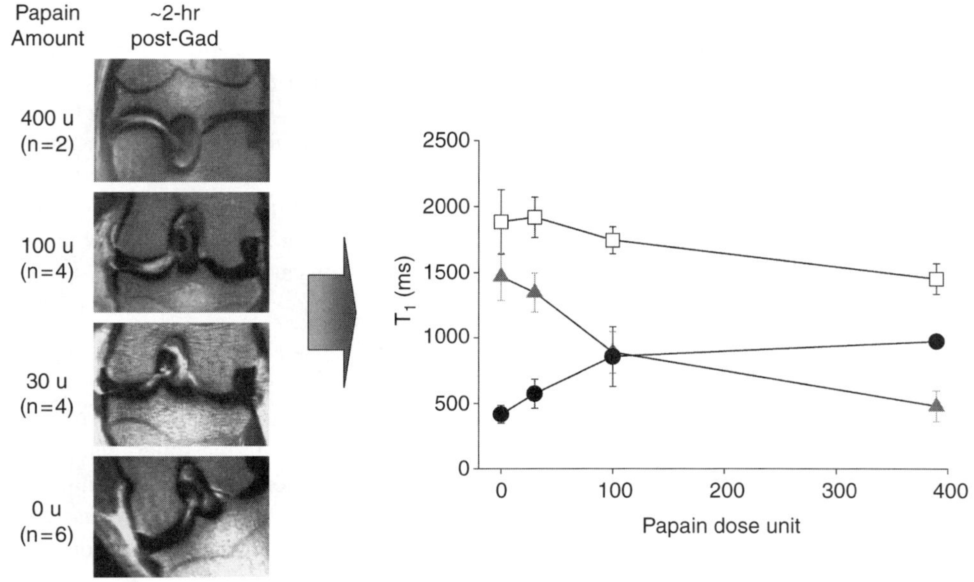

FIGURE 22.6 Dose-dependent effect of papain on proteoglycan content in goat knee cartilage as assessed by $Gd(DTPA)^{2-}$ MRI approximately 2-h postinfusion. Filled circle represent the difference in T_1 relaxation between precontrast (open squares) and ~2-h postcontrast (gray triangles) measurements. (Reproduced from Laurent, D. et al., *Magn. Reson. Med.*, 49, 1037, 2003. With permission of John Wiley & Sons, Inc. Copyright 2003.)

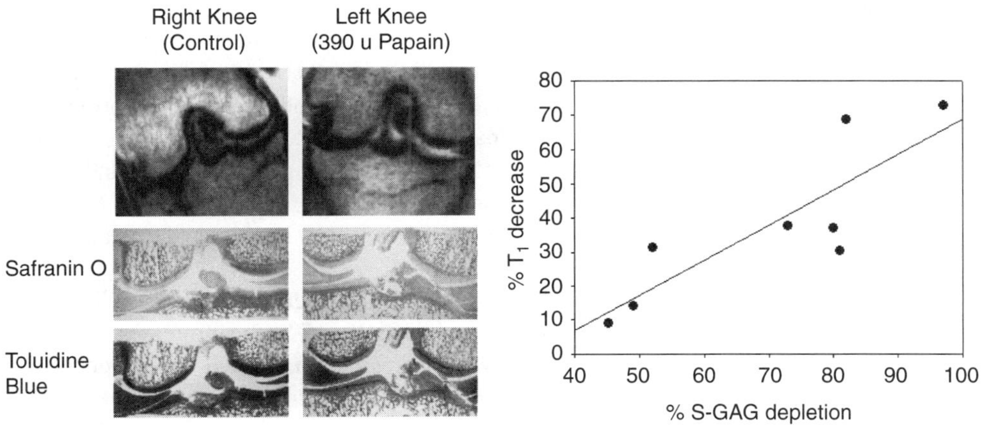

FIGURE 22.7 Validation of the $Gd(DTPA)^{2-}$-MRI technique against histology and biochemistry. On the left panel, a good correlation can be observed between inversion-recovery post$Gd(DTPA)^{2-}$ images and matched histological sections using safranin O and toluidine blue staining. This particular goat was treated with 390 units of papain in the left knee, and the absence of proteoglycans is reflected as an intense bright signal in the cartilage region of the corresponding MRI section. In line with this, while darkness in the gray scale indicates the presence of proteoglycans in cartilage of the control knee (i.e., right knee) from respective histological sections, no such staining was observed in the papain-treated knee. In addition, note that the relative change in T_1 correlates nicely with the glycosaminoglycan (S-GAG) concentration as measured *postmortem* in the articular cartilage (right panel). (Reproduced from Laurent, D. et al., *Magn. Reson. Med.*, 49, 1037, 2003. With permission of John Wiley & Sons, Inc. Copyright 2003.)

$Gd(DTPA)^{2-}$-induced decrease in T_1 relaxation time was approximately twofold higher when papain was injected 1 day prior to the MRI session, indicative of macromolecular alterations in papain-treated rabbits. The two-point method was used as an alternative to the more time-consuming multipoint method typically used to measure T_1 changes (see Appendix 22.1), allowing the kinetics of $Gd(DTPA)^{2-}$ uptake to be followed with a 10-min time resolution. The diffusive transport of $Gd(DTPA)^{2-}$ was characterized by a T_1 decrease approximately two times faster in papain-treated knees. Altogether, these data suggest that both the kinetics of tracer diffusion and the amplitude of T_1 variation may be used as informative markers of PG loss. These parameters are of interest for the identification of new active compounds during efficacy studies on cartilage protection.

22.6.3.3 Collagen Integrity

The measurement of the short transverse relaxation time T_2 may reveal collagen ultrastructure and hydration which depends on collagen content. A significant increase in the superficial T_2 may be observed in the presence of cartilage degeneration [74]. The problem with this technique is that proteoglycan content is also an important contributor to the T_2-weighted hyperintense cartilage signal. This lack of specificity makes difficult the efforts to select the best predictor and most selective marker of tissue integrity [75].

Cartilage is known to display significant magnetization transfer (MT) effects with respect to its high content of collagen, a property which can be exploited for improved contrast and consequently for a better delineation of articular structures [76,77]. More importantly, MT imaging may in addition provide information on the chemical/structural status of cartilage. In fact, several *in vitro* studies have demonstrated that the MT effect in cartilage is dominated by the contribution of collagen, while the influence of PGs is significantly smaller [10,76,78]. The observed changes in MT ratios (MTRs) are likely to reflect changes in collagen structure rather than changes in collagen concentration [10]. The foundations of this technique applied to the *in vivo* assessment of articular cartilage are described in more detail in the Appendix 22.2.

For the articular cartilage of a normal goat, almost 40% signal attenuation was achieved in the MT experiment, resulting in a remarkably improved contrast between meniscus and cartilage structures [10]. Assuming a two-site exchange model, this corresponds to a magnetization exchange rate k of 3.7 per sec. When applied to the papain-damaged knee, MT imaging showed an approximately 30% decrease in the exchange rate, suggesting collagen destruction and/or changes in its structure in the former knee. In a rabbit model of OA using papain as well, MT data also revealed a 22% decrease in the exchange rate between free and macromolecule (collagen)-bound water 24 h after the papain injection [12].

A combination of methods to noninvasively follow both collagen and PG in parallel may prove ideal to quantify the severity of cartilage degeneration as the disease progresses, especially as anatomic signs of cartilage breakdown are not always detected. In a surgical goat model of OA, we applied MT–MRI and dGEMRIC to examine periodically (presurgery, 2-, 6-, 10-, and 14 weeks postsurgery) the effects of the surgery in the weight-bearing articular cartilage (Figure 22.8). Delayed $Gd(DTPA)^{2-}$-enhanced MRI revealed that PG loss in menisectomized goats was early and sustained. Whether this reflected an early increase in aggrecanase activity still remains to be determined. The increase in the MT rate observed at 2 weeks postsurgery may be explained by cartilage swelling, i.e., disrupted collagen structure and influx of water (not inflammation), a normal sequel to surgically induced lesions. The lower MT rates at later intervals may indicate more permanent changes in the collagen structure, i.e., collagen matrix disruption. Preliminary histological observations support these data. In conclusion, for the first time this study demonstrated noninvasively early cartilage degeneration at the macromolecular level in a relevant model of OA. Of note, the MRI procedures were sensitive enough to detect mild/moderate cartilage damage in the region of interest. Furthermore, the irreversibility of damage, for the investigated period, may be

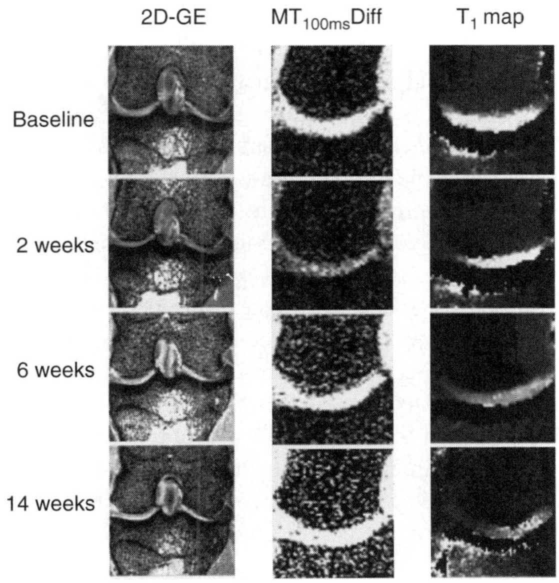

FIGURE 22.8 *In vivo* periodic assessment of macromolecular changes in the knee cartilage of a menisectomized goat. Note that while no obvious focal defect in the weight-bearing region of cartilage is observed in conventional 2D gradient echo (2D–GE) images, drastic changes in signal intensity occur in magnetization transfer (MT) and Gd(DTPA)$^{2-}$-enhanced images. Here MT contrast can be depicted from the difference (Diff) between two sets of images obtained with and without a saturation pulse of 100 msec (mixing time). In this particular goat, the corresponding MT rate constant first increased until 2 weeks postsurgery then decreased substantially until the end of the observation period, most likely indicative of a change in the collagen network. Gd(DTPA)$^{2-}$ diffusion in proteoglycan-depleted regions of cartilage is reflected by a decrease in T_1 relaxation time (bright for high T_1) of corresponding T_1 maps. In this particular goat, T_1 decreased substantially until 14-week postsurgery, sign of a loss in proteoglycan content.

due to the upright posture and rather active living style of the goats which in turn apply constant biomechanical stress on the knees, as opposed to a quieter species like the rabbit as the following data would suggest.

Early signs of cartilage degeneration were also detected in a surgical rabbit model of OA by combining MT–MRI and Gd(DTPA)$^{2-}$ MRI (unpublished data). Macromolecular changes occurred in the absence of obvious morphometric changes on MR images. Interestingly, beyond 6 weeks after meniscectomy, collagen damage, although subtle, progressed without a simultaneous increase in Gd(DTPA)$^{2-}$ diffusion. In fact, kinetics of Gd(DTPA)$^{2-}$ uptake were back towards baseline values at 12 weeks postsurgery, indicating that cartilage chondrocytes replenished PG posttrauma, while damage to the collagen framework was irreversible. Histological sections revealed only mild cartilage degeneration at 12 weeks postmedial meniscectomy surgery in adult rabbit knees. As suggested earlier, this may partly be due to the sedentary lifestyle of these animals, moderate exercise being well known to exacerbate articular cartilage lesions induced by meniscectomy [79]. Although progressive cartilage changes consistent with early OA developed over 6 weeks as judged by the decrease in the MT exchange and the increase in Gd(DTPA)$^{2-}$ uptake, the small cartilage thickness and mild pathology limits the utility of using rabbits for these studies.

22.7 MRI CONTRAST AGENTS IN ARTHRITIS

As pointed out earlier, actively inflamed synovitis is hypervascular with an increased vascular permeability. Vascular permeability is an important readout for monitoring disease progression and treatment response. Because they are approved for clinical use, Gd-containing small molecular contrast media are usually employed to this end. However, they have the inherent disadvantage to freely diffuse across even normal capillary membranes into the extracellular space. The permeability assessment would be improved through the use of macromolecular contrast media which are confined to the intravascular space in nonpathological tissues, however leak out leak out into the interstitium in case of pathology. Albumin-$(Gd-DTPA)_{30}$ is a 92-kDa blood pool contrast agent with a plasma half-life of approximately 3 h [80]. It was used to simultaneously derive, in rabbit arthritic knees, synovial tissue plasma-volume, fractional-leak-rate and permeability-surface-area-product by employing sequential T_1-weighted gradient-echo images [81]. A good correlation was found between the increased permeability detected with albumin-$(Gd-DTPA)_{30}$ and the inflammation in the synovium characterized by histology. Another albumin-binding blood pool contrast agent that has been successfully used in arthritis models is MS-325 [82].

In MR arthrography, the visualization of cartilage surface abnormalities after intraarticular application of Gd–DTPA is limited because of diffusion of the small molecular contrast agent into the cartilage. After injection of paramagnetic contrast agents (Gd–DTPA and manganese chloride) entrapped in liposomes into rabbit knees an excellent contrast between cartilage surface and joint space was achieved [83]. Diffusion of the contrast agent into the cartilage layer was prevented and the visualization of the cartilage surface was markedly improved. Small mechanically and enzymatically induced cartilage lesions could be reliably assessed, showing the potential of this approach to improve MR arthrography.

In inflammatory processes as occurring in RA, endothelial cells associated with the inflamed areas become activated during the process of leukocytic recruitment. These stimulated endothelial cells amplify several adhesion molecules, such as P-selectin, E-selectin, ICAM-1, and VCAM-1, to attract and bind inflammatory cells. In efforts towards improved detection of inflammatory processes, several contrast agents that target endothelial epitopes have been developed for ultrasound, MR, and radionuclide-based imaging. For instance, by adding avidin and biotinylated antibody to paramagnetic polymerized liposomes containing a Gd lipid chelator, antibody-conjugated paramagnetic liposomes have been constructed [84,85]. Another agent of potential interest for MRI involves the conjugation of monocrystalline iron oxide nanoparticles to antihuman E-selectin [86]. It remains to be shown if such MR agents indeed provide an earlier sensitive marker of inflammation in RA models that can be followed reliably as compared to those described before. For sensitivity reasons, the attachment of fluorescent labels to such agents enabling their detection by optical imaging methods as, for example, NIRF will probably be the more favorable avenue for detecting *in vivo* specific events in the inflammatory cascade using specially engineered probes.

22.8 DISCUSSION

From the pharmacological point of view, it is fundamental to find molecules that have structure-modifying properties in RA and OA. The previous discussion showed that MRI can play an active role in this search process, as elegantly demonstrated in a number of preclinical studies. The ability to noninvasively assess the effects of treatment in animal models by MRI can only benefit the development of therapies, especially because time-course studies can be easily performed. Morphological and functional measurements with MRI offer qualitative or quantitative readouts which turn out to be useful surrogate markers when testing compounds in animal models.

The inflammatory nature of RA gives rise to many opportunities to follow the pattern of the disease models by MRI. Inflammation is characterized by increased tissue perfusion and capillary permeability. Synovial uptake of Gd-containing contrast material, dependent on local tissue perfusion and microvascular permeability, results in leakage of i.v.-injected contrast medium into the interstitial space, leading to a signal increase in T_1-weighted MRI. One of the early characteristics of rheumatoid synovitis is the development of a new vascular network, for enhancing the delivery of cells and nutrients to the invading pannus. Assessing vascularity using imaging approaches, e.g., by applying bolus tracking MRI with the administration of an intravascular contrast agent, has the potential to evaluate or even predict bone destruction [43]. Another important marker is the infiltration of macrophages, which possess proinflammatory, destructive, and remodeling capabilities that contribute to the acute and chronic phases of RA [46]. Labeling macrophages with SPIO or USPIO administered i.v. 24 h before an MRI session is an important strategy to noninvasively follow the macrophage infiltration into sites of inflammation in animal models of RA [49,50]. MRI also has the capability of providing semiquantitative and quantitative information on bone erosion in such models [27,28,30,31].

As extensively discussed in Section 22.5.2, all these avenues have been successfully explored in preclinical studies aiming at the assessment of the efficacy of antiinflammatory compounds. The examination time, of the order of 20 min for a rat, enables a reasonable throughput for pharmacological studies. More important than that, MRI is a very practical tool in longitudinal studies since the data are usually analyzed on the same day of the measurement. Histology on the other hand is always a bottleneck in pharmacological studies; despite being able to deliver information at the cellular level with a very high anatomical resolution, it usually lags the experimental period by many months.

Of fundamental importance for translational research, in studies of Gd–DTPA uptake in the synovium of RA patients, the rate of synovial membrane enhancement has been demonstrated to be significantly correlated to histopathological features of synovitis like polymorphonuclear leukocyte infiltration, hyperemia, and fibrin deposition [35]. This technique can be used to grade the vascularity of proliferative synovitis [39]. It is thus to be expected that dynamic contrast-enhanced MRI with Gd–DTPA is going to play an important role in characterizing the efficacy of compounds both at the preclinical and clinical levels. The approaches aiming at assessing the vascularity or the macrophage infiltration still need to be characterized and validated in humans.

OA is a more subtle disease, in which focal and tiny lesions are expected. The main target of the disease is cartilage, which in animals has a thickness of less than 5 mm. The 3D nature of MRI is very useful when studying morphological changes at the level of, for example, the knee, which has a remarkably complicated structure. Nevertheless, time-consuming protocols are necessary to image at a fairly high resolution to generate good data. Thus, usually no more than five animals can be measured per day. Determining cartilage thickness or volume in models of OA has been found to be not reliable enough in longitudinal studies. However, assessing the biochemical status of cartilage has proven to be more promising, e.g., measurements of PG content by dGEMRIC or of cartilage integrity by MT–MRI. These approaches have been shown to be useful in animal models of OA [8,10,11]. Potentially they may provide information on the efficacy and mechanism of compounds.

The pharmaceutical industry is eager to develop new drugs that would not only treat for the pain in arthritis, but also restore joint function and overall mobility. Hence, the identification of new drug targets that are involved in the etiology of the disease is of high relevance for the development of structure-modifying therapies. Molecules that, in addition to controlling pain, influence the biochemical composition of cartilage and enhance its biomechanical stability have great potential as effective treatments for cartilage regeneration. For instance, compounds modulating molecular mechanisms allowing chondrocytes to counteract PG depletion and loosening of the collagen network early in the course of OA, are of interest [60]. However, in spite of considerable efforts, it has proved very difficult to develop new classes of therapeutic agents for arthritis. Although recently under pressure due to its side-effects, COX-2 inhibitors have been the only new class of drugs brought to the market in the past years. The ability to noninvasively assess the effect of treatment on the cartilage matrix can only be of benefit to the development of therapies aimed at providing chondroprotection. A dual imaging approach would be particularly justified on the basis of close proteoglycan/collagen interdependence and should help characterize these new compounds during efficacy studies on cartilage regeneration [87]. Along with morphological and functional assessments, MRI can potentially offer qualitative readouts which may be considered as useful surrogate markers of OA. While research focuses on drugs that can prevent unnecessary joint damage, such imaging biomarkers could also allow identification of patients who are more likely to develop OA.

The dGEMRIC and MT–MRI techniques have already been introduced into the clinics [70, 88–91]. As mentioned earlier, both techniques show potential in terms of detecting cartilage changes at the early state of osteoarthritic degeneration. Interestingly, it seems that human knee cartilage can adapt itself to a higher level of physical activity by increasing the glycosaminoglycan content [92]. As to MT–MRI, in spite of a certain variability between individuals, it seems clear that important information can be supplied from MT coefficients about the water content and collagen network in human cartilage [85]. In an attempt to better define *in vivo* surrogate markers of OA, an NIH/industry-sponsored initiative has recently been launched to look for possible signs of disease progression over a 4-year period in patients at risk of developing OA ($\sim$5000 patients in total, see www.niams.nih.gov/ne/oi/meetingsummary.htm). The MRI protocol in this initiative for the most part involves morphometric readouts like cartilage thickness and volume, or MRI markers of effusion and synovitis. Compositional markers of cartilage (i.e., MRI assessments of proteoglycan content and collagen organization) have not been excluded from the discussion. However, the scanning time which, for economical reasons, cannot exceed 1-h of magnet time, remains the main hurdle to these additional measurements. Of note, it is also intended in this initiative to compare the added value of MRI with conventional x-ray analysis. One should realize, however, that a recent study, which failed to identify loss of cartilage volume over 3 years in a cohort of patients with established knee OA using MRI, challenged the validity of this morphologic endpoint to assess structural changes in OA [93].

Although at present some information on the mechanism of drugs may be obtained indirectly using MRI (e.g., compounds aiming to suppress VEGF, or to protect chondrocytes), currently the sensitivity of the technique is not high enough to derive mechanistic information in general terms. It would be extraordinary to be able to identify noninvasively the effects of compounds on disease pathways in living animals. In the near future, we will witness the combination of MRI with other important imaging techniques, especially NIRF, which can visualize *in vivo* biological processes at the cellular and molecular levels. The administration of contrast agents tagged magnetically and fluorescently will be an important step in combining the high resolution provided by MRI with the high sensitivity of NIRF for obtaining mechanistic information of compounds in the same animal. Also, the combination of MRI with micro-CT will improve the readout of bony changes in small rodent disease models. Exciting activities are ahead of us, which are not only going to cement the role of imaging in arthritis research, but also hopefully lead to improved therapies which will improve the lives of millions of people suffering from these diseases.

APPENDIX 22.1 DELAYED GADOLINIUM-ENHANCED MRI

Since dGEMRIC is starting to be widely used both in the preclinical and the clinical context, some details on the methods used, starting with the pulse sequence to measure cartilage T_1 relaxation, are covered in this Appendix. The inversion-recovery pulse sequence is recognized to provide accurate cartilage T_1 data with little variation ($<8\%$ based on unpublished in-house data) between normal animals. It is combined with an imaging readout, typically a spin–echo sequence. Creating image series with varying inversion times (T_I) then allows calculation of T_1 maps from nonlinear regression analysis using a single exponential model function. T_1 measurements are usually time-consuming and this can be a problem for kinetic studies unless fast pulse sequences are considered. In order to apply dGEMRIC to a goat model of OA, we optimized pulse parameters on a 3 T system for a single T_1 measurement no longer than $\sim$20 min [11].

For rabbit experiments at 3 T involving a multipoint method with eight different TIs, acquisition times longer than 1 h would be necessary in order to calculate T_1 maps at high spatial resolution in the thin cartilage (<0.5 mm) [12]. Such conditions make it difficult to determine the optimal delay for cartilage $Gd(DTPA)^{2-}$ to reach the equilibrium concentration, and preclude kinetic assessments of $Gd(DTPA)^{2-}$ diffusion into cartilage. To account for these shortcomings, an *in vivo* two-point method may be considered as a good alternative to estimate T_1 relaxation time [94]. Besides its simplicity, the two-point method offers the main advantage of enough temporal resolution (~ 10 min for rabbits) to depict with precision kinetics of $Gd(DTPA)^{2-}$ diffusion across cartilage [12]. This is important considering that the delay for a full penetration of $Gd(DTPA)^{2-}$ may vary depending on the degree of PG loss. Image difference usually offers the best way to visualize time-course gadolinium uptake by cartilage. In the latter study cited, a gradual diffusion of $Gd(DTPA)^{2-}$ was observed from the cruciate ligament towards the medial region of articular cartilage and up to 1 h seemed necessary for a maximum decrease of T_1 in normal cartilage.

The two-point method uses reference data, obtained from the multipoint technique, for the pregadolinium cartilage T_1 value and assumes that a single postgadolinium measurement is sufficient. Signal intensities (S) are given by:

$$S_{pre} = S_0[1 - \exp(-TR/T_{1-pre})]\exp(-TE/T_2) \tag{22.A1}$$

$$S_{post} = S_0[1 - \exp(-TR/T_{1-post})]\exp(-TE/T_2) \tag{22.A2}$$

where S_0 is the signal at equilibrium, assuming that the contrast agent has no effect on T_2. Thus,

$$S_{post}/S_{pre} = [1 - \exp(-TR/T_{1-post})]/[1 - \exp(TR/T_{1-pre})] \tag{22.A3}$$

As a result T_{1-post} can be obtained by solving:

$$T_{1-post} = -TR/\{\ln[1 - (S_{post}/S_{pre})(1 - \exp(-TR/T_{1-pre})]\} \tag{22.A4}$$

with the T_{1-pre} value measured by the conventional multipoint inversion-recovery method in control studies. T_1 values determined by the inversion-recovery and the two-point methods are positively correlated. However, postcontrast T_1 values may be slightly overestimated by the latter method. Since the two-point method relies on historical data obtained from normal animals, possible variations in the baseline T_1 (precontrast value), due to cartilage degeneration, cannot be taken into account in further calculations which in turn may affect actual postcontrast T_1 values. For this reason, it may be worth considering the half-time of diffusion of $Gd(DTPA)^{-2}$, a kinetic variable independent of the precontrast T_1 value, as a more meaningful and reliable marker of PG degradation, as opposed to the amplitude of T_1 variations solely. The half-time ($t_{1/2}$) of T_1 decrease can be determined from the exponential fit as follows [12]:

$$T_1 = [T_{1-pre} - T_{1-final}]^* \exp^{(-kt)} + T_{1-final} \tag{22.A5}$$

where $k = \ln 2/t_{1/2}$. Finally, T_1 maps are usually computed using the single exponential model function

$$I = I_0[1 - (1 - \cos\theta).\exp(-TI/T_1)] \tag{22.A6}$$

where I_0 represents the initial (equilibrium) signal intensity within each pixel and θ accounts for the incomplete inversion ($0 < \cos\theta < 1$) and TI is the inversion time.

APPENDIX 22.2 MT SEQUENCE OPTIMIZATION

Magnetization transfer (MT) imaging probes the exchange of magnetization between bulk (mobile) water pool and the water pool bound to macromolecules, such as collagen, and hence shows promise as a method that can noninvasively examine the severity of cartilage abnormality. By selectively saturating the broad signal of macromolecule-bound water, the MRI observable resonance of the bulk water is attenuated, the degree of the signal reduction depending on the exchange rate and on T_1 spin-lattice relaxation. In practice, the amount of MT is generally quantified by calculating the MT ratio (MTR)

$$\mathrm{MTR} = (\mathrm{M_0} - \mathrm{M_S})/\mathrm{M_0} \qquad (22.\mathrm{A7})$$

which refers to signal intensities before (M_0) and after (Ms) saturation. Assuming a two-site exchange, the Ms/M_0 ratio decreases exponentially with increasing duration *t* of the saturation, i.e.,

$$\mathrm{MTR} = (\mathrm{M_0} - \mathrm{Ms})/\mathrm{M_0} = k\mathrm{T_{1a}}/(1 + k\mathrm{T_{1a}}) + k\mathrm{T_{1a}}/(1 + k\mathrm{T_{1a}})\exp\{-(k + 1/\mathrm{T_{1a}})t\} \qquad (22.\mathrm{A8})$$

which under steady-state conditions ($t \gg T_{1a}$) reduces to [95]:

$$\mathrm{MTR} = k\mathrm{T_{1a}}/(1 + k\mathrm{T_{1a}}) \qquad (22.\mathrm{A9})$$

where *k* is the rate constant for magnetization transfer and T_{1a} describes the relaxation of the water protons in the absence of exchange.

Usually MR parameters are selected so that a maximal saturation of the bound water can be obtained with minimal direct saturation of the bulk water. This has been verified in a preliminary study [10] where water signal intensities of physiological saline and low concentration of chondroitin sulfate (to mimic PG) and albumin solutions are not affected by the off-resonance MT pulse. The use of a rather narrow frequency bandwidth (5 $\mu T = 210$ Hz) as well as an optimized static magnetic field homogeneity should also help to minimize effects of direct saturation, especially when pulsing near the resonance frequency (1 to 3 kHz off resonance).

Since ultimately the method is intended to be applied to a live animal (or a patient), one other main constraint is to keep the total imaging time as short as possible. This limits the duration of the MT irradiation (the saturation pulse cannot exceed the repetition time), which ideally for efficient magnetization transfer is set to about 5 T_1 (i.e., $5 \times 1.3\ \mathrm{sec}^2$). Despite these restrictions, significant MT-induced signal attenuations have been measured in collagen phantoms from a validation study, whereas only negligible MT effects were observed in phantoms containing other macromolecules such as chondroitin sulfate and albumin [10]. Furthermore, analysis of MT images revealed a ~25, ~35, and ~30% signal attenuation in 10% w/v type I collagen gels, cartilage plugs, and cartilage from the weight-bearing areas of the goat knee, respectively. Biochemical data revealed that treatment of cartilage plugs with bacterial collagenase led to collagen depletion and correspondingly to a decrease of the MT response. In contrast, trypsin-induced proteoglycan loss in cartilage plugs did not alter the MT effect. A significant correlation was observed between the collagen content in these plugs and their respective MTRs. These data all led to the notion that the MT effect is largely governed by the collagen contribution. From a theoretical point of view, a dependence of the MT effect on the collagen concentration is not expected in a true saturation transfer experiment. The existence of a concentration dependence demonstrates that either there is no true saturation of the bound water pool or that the two-site exchange model is not strictly valid. Nevertheless, as variations in collagen content are small in osteoarthritic tissue, only on the order of 5% [96], any observed change in MTRs is likely to reflect a modification in collagen structure rather than a change in collagen concentration.

Why not measure *k* instead of MTR? The determination of the exchange rate constant *k* theoretically allows elimination of the contribution of T_1 relaxation, and as a true measure of the water exchange process, may be more sensitive in terms of detecting changes in collagen content or structure. We [10] derived the rate constant from the initial slope of the exponential decay (Equation 22.A8). The actual experiment was set up with varying saturation pulse lengths at a 1-kHz frequency offset and image parameters similar to the routine MT experiment. Each MT image was compared to a reference image recorded with a similar saturation delay and frequency offset, but the radio-frequency power set to zero. The whole measurement time for a rate constant determination was about 15 min/sample. Data obtained from type I collagen gels and cartilage plugs indicated that the sensitivity of k to changes in collagen concentrations is similar to that of MTRs for similar changes in concentration or treatment conditions [10]. The fact that the exchange rate k varies with the collagen concentration is a clear indication that structural changes occur within the collagen matrix, which likely alters the interaction to the water.

The high variability of *in vivo* MTR measurements could be a consequence of the pressure applied differently in the weight-bearing area of articular cartilage as a well-known inverse MTR-body weight correlation would suggest. This would agree with data obtained from normal volunteer studies, in which lowest values of MT coefficient were measured in the medial cartilage where compression forces are the greatest as opposed to the lateral and patellar cartilage [85]. The common assumption is that, as a result of pressure, free water extruded from cartilage has a reduced fluidity, which in turn may lower the relaxation time T_1 and affect the MTR. Taken together, these data suggest that, although slightly more time-consuming, the determination of the rate exchange k is worth pursuing as it may reflect collagen integrity in a more reliable manner than MT ratios.

REFERENCES

1. Brand, D. D., Kang, A. H., and Rosloniec, E. F., Immunopathogenesis of collagen arthritis, *Springer Semin. Immunopathol.*, 25, 3, 2003.
2. Moore, A. R., Collagen-induced arthritis, *Methods Mol. Biol.*, 225, 175, 2003.
3. Williams, R. O., Collagen-induced arthritis as a model for rheumatoid arthritis, *Methods Mol. Med.*, 98, 207, 2004.
4. Keystone, E. C., The utility of tumour necrosis factor blockade in orphan diseases, *Ann. Rheum. Dis.*, 63 (Suppl. 2), ii79, 2004.
5. Cooke, T., Antigen-induced arthritis, polyarthritis, and teno-synovitis, In *CRC Handbook of Animal Models for the Rheumatoid Diseases*, Greenwald, R. and Diamond, H., Eds., CRC Press, Boca Raton, pp. 53–81, 1988.
6. Moskowitz, R. W. et al., Experimentally induced degenerative joint lesions following partial meniscectomy in the rabbit, *Arthritis Rheum.*, 16, 397, 1973.
7. van den Berg, W. B., Lessons from animal models of osteoarthritis, *Curr. Opin. Rheumatol.*, 13, 452, 2001.
8. Laurent, D. et al., *Severity of Cartilage Degeneration in the Goat Knee After Meniscal Transection/Cartilage Groove Surgery as Measured by MT and Gd(DTPA)–MRI, ISMRM, 11th Scientific Meeting and Exhibition, Toronoto, Canada, May* 10–16, 2003.
9. Farkas, T., Bihari-Varga, M., and Biro, T., Thermoanalytical and histological study of intra-articular papain-induced degradation and repair of rabbit cartilage. I. Immature animals, *Ann. Rheum. Dis.*, 33, 385, 1974.
10. Laurent, D. et al., Quantitative and qualitative assessment of articular cartilage in the goat knee with magnetization transfer imaging, *Magn. Reson. Imaging*, 19, 1279, 2001.
11. Laurent, D. et al., In vivo assessment of macromolecular content in articular cartilage of the goat knee, *Magn. Reson. Med.*, 49, 1037, 2003.
12. Laurent, D. et al., In vivo qualitative assessments of articular cartilage in the rabbit knee with high-resolution MRI at 3 T, *Magn. Reson. Med.*, 50, 541, 2003.
13. Kikuchi, T., Sakuta, T., and Yamaguchi, T., Intra-articular injection of collagenase induces experimental osteoarthritis in mature rabbits, *Osteoarthritis Cartilage*, 6, 177, 1998.

14. Guzman, R. E. et al., Mono-iodoacetate-induced histologic changes in subchondral bone and articular cartilage of rat femorotibial joints: an animal model of osteoarthritis, *Toxicol. Pathol.*, 31, 619, 2003.
15. Sonderstrup, G., Development of humanized mice as a model of inflammatory arthritis, *Springer Semin. Immunopathol.*, 25, 35, 2003.
16. Helminen, H. J. et al., Transgenic mouse models for studying the role of cartilage macromolecules in osteoarthritis, *Rheumatology (Oxford)*, 41, 848, 2002.
17. Weissleder, R. and Mahmood, U., Molecular imaging, *Radiology*, 219, 316, 2001.
18. Faris, F. et al., Non-invasive in vivo near-infrared optical measurement of the penetration depth in the neonatal head, *Clin. Phys. Physiol. Meas.*, 12, 353, 1991.
19. Lai, W. F. et al., Early diagnosis of osteoarthritis using cathepsin B sensitive near-infrared fluorescent probes, *Osteoarthritis Cartilage*, 12, 239, 2004.
20. Hansch, A. et al., In vivo imaging of experimental arthritis with near-infrared fluorescence, *Arthritis Rheum.*, 50, 961, 2004.
21. Wunder, A. et al., In vivo imaging of protease activity in arthritis: a novel approach for monitoring treatment response, *Arthritis Rheum.*, 50, 2459, 2004.
22. Guglielmi, G. et al., Current methods and advances in bone densitometry, *Eur. Radiol.*, 5, 129, 1995.
23. Gasser, J. A., Quantitative assessment of bone mass and geometry by pQCT in rats in vivo and site specificity of changes at different skeletal sites, *J. Jpn. Soc. Bone Morphom.*, 7, 107, 1997.
24. Barck, K. H. et al., Quantification of cortical bone loss and repair for therapeutic evaluation in collagen-induced arthritis, by micro-computed tomography and automated image analysis, *Arthritis Rheum.*, 50, 3377, 2004.
25. Morenko, B. J. et al., In vivo micro computed tomography of subchondral bone in the rat after intra-articular administration of monosodium iodoacetate, *Contemp. Top. Lab. Anim. Sci.*, 43, 39, 2004.
26. Ford, N. L., Thornton, M. M., and Holdsworth, D. W., Fundamental image quality limits for microcomputed tomography in small animals, *Med. Phys.*, 30, 2869, 2003.
27. Beckmann, N. et al., Noninvasive 3D MR microscopy as a tool in pharmacological research: application to a model of rheumatoid arthritis, *Magn. Reson. Imaging*, 13, 1013, 1995.
28. Beckmann, N. et al., Effects of Sandimmune neoral on collagen-induced arthritis in DA rats: characterization by high resolution three-dimensional magnetic resonance imaging and by histology, *J. Magn. Reson.*, 131, 8, 1998.
29. Dawson, J., Gustard, S., and Beckmann, N., High-resolution three-dimensional magnetic resonance imaging for the investigation of knee joint damage during the time course of antigen-induced arthritis in rabbits, *Arthritis Rheum.*, 42, 119, 1999.
30. Faure, P., Doan, B. T., and Beloeil, J. C., In-vivo high resolution three-dimensional MRI studies of rat joints at 7 T, *NMR Biomed.*, 16, 484, 2003.
31. Jacobson, P. B. et al., A new spin on an old model: in vivo evaluation of disease progression by magnetic resonance imaging with respect to standard inflammatory parameters and histopathology in the adjuvant arthritic rat, *Arthritis Rheum.*, 42, 2060, 1999.
32. Harris, R. et al., ABT-963, a highly potent and selective disubstituted pyridazinone COX-2 inhibitor, *J. Pharmacol. Exp. Ther.*, 311, 904, 2004.
33. Badger, A. M. et al., Disease-modifying activity of SB 242235, a selective inhibitor of p38 mitogen-activated protein kinase, in rat adjuvant-induced arthritis, *Arthritis Rheum.*, 43, 175, 2000.
34. Badger, A. M. et al., Disease-modifying activity of SB 273005, an orally active, nonpeptide alphavbeta3 (vitronectin receptor) antagonist, in rat adjuvant-induced arthritis, *Arthritis Rheum.*, 44, 128, 2001.
35. Gaffney, K. et al., Quantification of rheumatoid synovitis by magnetic resonance imaging, *Arthritis Rheum.*, 38, 1610, 1995.
36. Ostergaard, M. et al., Quantification of synovistis by MRI: correlation between dynamic and static gadolinium-enhanced magnetic resonance imaging and microscopic and macroscopic signs of synovial inflammation, *Magn. Reson. Imaging*, 16, 743, 1998.
37. Ostergaard, M. et al., Quantitative assessment of synovial inflammation by dynamic gadolinium-enhanced MRI. A study of the effect of intraarticular methylprednisolone on the rate of early synovial enhancement, *Br. J. Rheumatol.*, 35, 50, 1996.

38. Jevtic, V. et al., Prognostic value of contrast enhanced Gd–DTPA–MRI for development of bone erosive changes in rheumatoid arthritis, *Br. J. Rheumatol.*, 35 (Suppl. 3), 26, 1996.
39. Gaffney, K. et al., Quantitative assessment of the rheumatoid synovial microvascular bed by gadolinium–DTPA enhanced magnetic resonance imaging, *Ann. Rheum. Dis.*, 57, 152, 1998.
40. Tofts, P. S. and Kermode, A. G., Measurement of the blood/brain barrier permeability and leakage space using dynamic MR imaging. 1. Fundamental concepts, *Magn. Reson. Med.*, 17, 357, 1991.
41. Singh, H. N. et al., Synovial fluid levels of tumor necrosis factor-alpha in the inflamed rat knee: modulation by dexamethasone and inhibitors of matrix metalloproteinase and phosphodiesterase, *Inflamm. Res.*, 46 (Suppl. 2), S153, 1997.
42. Yang, Y. et al., Antiinflammatory effect of lipocortin 1 in experimental arthritis, *Inflammation*, 21, 583, 1997.
43. Taylor, P. C., VEGF and imaging of vessels in rheumatoid arthritis, *Arthritis Res.*, 4 (Suppl. 3), S99, 2002.
44. Koch, A. E., Angiogenesis as a target in rheumatoid arthritis, *Ann. Rheum. Dis.*, 62 (Suppl. 2), ii60, 2003.
45. Polytarchou, C. and Papadimitriou, E., Antioxidants inhibit angiogenesis in vivo through down-regulation of nitric oxide synthase expression and activity, *Free Radic. Res.*, 38, 501, 2004.
46. Cutolo, M., Macrophages as effectors of the immunoendocrinologic interactions in autoimmune rheumatic diseases, *Ann. NY. Acad. Sci.*, 876, 32, 1999.
47. Weissleder, R. et al., Ultrasmall superparamagnetic iron oxide: characterization of a new class of contrast agents for MR imaging, *Radiology*, 175, 489, 1990.
48. Dardzinski, B. J. et al., MR imaging of murine arthritis using ultrasmall superparamagnetic iron oxide particles, *Magn. Reson. Imaging*, 19, 1209, 2001.
49. Beckmann, N. et al., Macrophage infiltration into the rat knee detected by MRI in a model of antigen-induced arthritis, *Magn. Reson. Med.*, 49, 1047, 2003.
50. Lutz, A. M. et al., Detection of synovial macrophages in an experimental rabbit model of antigen-induced arthritis: ultrasmall superparamagnetic iron oxide-enhanced MR imaging, *Radiology*, 233, 149, 2004.
51. Heinegard, D. and Oldberg, A., Structure and biology of cartilage and bone matrix noncollagenous macromolecules, *FASEB J.*, 3, 2042, 1989.
52. Torchia, D. A., Hasson, M. A., and Hascall, V. C., Investigation of molecular motion of proteoglycans in cartilage by 13C magnetic resonance, *J. Biol. Chem.*, 252, 3617, 1977.
53. Grushko, G., Schneiderman, R., and Maroudas, A., Some biochemical and biophysical parameters for the study of the pathogenesis of osteoarthritis: a comparison between the processes of ageing and degeneration in human hip cartilage, *Conn. Tissue Res.*, 19, 149, 1989.
54. Kempson, G. E. et al., The tensile properties of human femoral condyles related to the content of collagen and glycosaminoglycans, *Biochim. Biophys. Acta*, 297, 456, 1973.
55. Eckstein, F. et al., Quantitative relationships of normal cartilage volumes of the human knee joint — assessment by magnetic resonance imaging, *Anat. Embryol. (Berl.)*, 197, 383, 1998.
56. Burgkart, R. et al., Magnetic resonance imaging-based assessment of cartilage loss in severe osteoarthritis: accuracy, precision, and diagnostic value, *Arthritis Rheum.*, 44, 2072, 2001.
57. Peterfy, C. G., Applications of MRI for evaluating osteoarthritis, In *Advances in Osteoarthritis*, Tanaka, S. and Hamanishi, C., Eds., Springer, Tokyo, pp. 74–92, 1999.
58. Tessier, J. J. et al., Characterization of the guinea pig model of osteoarthritis by in vivo three-dimensional magnetic resonance imaging, *Osteoarthritis Cartilage*, 11, 841, 2003.
59. Calvo, E. et al., High-resolution MRI detects cartilage swelling at the early stages of experimental osteoarthritis, *Osteoarthritis Cartilage*, 9, 463, 2001.
60. Lohmander, L. S., Articular cartilage and osteoarthritis. The role of molecular markers to monitor breakdown, repair and disease, *J. Anat.*, 184, 477, 1994.
61. Bank, R. A. et al., The increased swelling and instantaneous deformation of osteoarthtitic cartilage is highly correlated with collagen degradation, *Arthritis Rheum.*, 43, 2202, 2000.
62. Fragonas, E. et al., Correlation between biochemical composition and magnetic resonance appearance of articular cartilage, *Osteoarthritis Cartilage*, 6, 24, 1998.
63. Borthakur, A. et al., Sensitivity of MRI to proteoglycan depletion in cartilage: comparison of sodium and proton MRI, *Osteoarthritis Cartilage*, 8, 288, 2000.

64. Burstein, D. et al., Diffusion of small solutes in cartilage as measured by nuclear magnetic resonance (NMR) spectroscopy and imaging, *J. Orthop. Res.*, 11, 465, 1993.
65. Lesperance, L. M., Gary, M. L., and Burstein, D., Determination of fixed charge density in cartilage using nuclear magnetic resonance, *J. Orthop. Res.*, 10, 1, 1992.
66. Shapiro, E. M. et al., ^{23}Na MRI accurately measures fixed charge density in articular cartilage, *Magn. Reson. Med.*, 47, 284, 2002.
67. Akella, S. V. et al., Proteoglycan-induced changes in T_1rho-relaxation of articular cartilage at 4 T, *Magn. Reson. Med.*, 46, 419, 2001.
68. Duvvuri, U. et al., T(1rho) relaxation can assess longitudinal proteoglycan loss from articular cartilage in vitro, *Osteoarthritis Cartilage*, 10, 838, 2002.
69. Bashir, A., Gray, M. L., and Burstein, D., Gd–DTPA^{2-} as a measure of cartilage degradation, *Magn. Reson. Med.*, 36, 665, 1996.
70. Bashir, A. et al., Nondestructive imaging of human cartilage glycosaminoglycan concentration depletion in articular cartilage, *Magn. Reson. Med.*, 41, 857, 1999.
71. Donahue, K. M. et al., Studies of Gd–DTPA relaxivity and proton exchange rates in tissue, *Magn. Reson. Med.*, 32, 66, 1994.
72. Kusaka, Y. et al., MR microimaging of articular cartilage and contrast enhancement by manganese ions, *Magn. Reson. Med.*, 24, 137, 1992.
73. Bacic, G. et al., MRI contrast enhanced study of cartilage proteoglycan degradation in rabbit knee, *Magn. Reson. Med.*, 37, 764, 1997.
74. Nissi, M. J. et al., Proteoglycan and collagen sensitive MRI evaluation of normal and degenerated articular cartilage, *J. Orthop. Res.*, 22, 557, 2004.
75. Menezes, N. M. et al., T_2 and T_1rho MRI in articular cartilage systems, *Magn. Reson. Med.*, 51, 503, 2004.
76. Kim, D. K. et al., Analysis of water–macromolecule proton magnetization transfer in articular cartilage, *Magn. Reson. Med.*, 29, 211, 1993.
77. Vahlensieck, M. et al., Magnetization transfer contrast (MTC) and MTC-substraction: enhancement of cartilage lesions and intra-cartilaginous degeneration in vitro, *Skeletal Radiol.*, 23, 535, 1994.
78. Gray, M. L. et al., Magnetization transfer in cartilage and its constituent macromolecules, *Magn. Reson. Med.*, 34, 319, 1995.
79. Armstrong, S. J. et al., Moderate exercise exacerbates the osteoarthritic lesions produced in cartilage by meniscectomy: a morphological study, *Osteoarthritis Cartilage*, 1, 89, 1993.
80. Schmiedl, U. et al., Albumin labeled with Gd–DTPA as an intravascular, blood pool enhancing agent for MR imaging: biodistribution of gadolinium, *Radiology*, 162, 205, 1987.
81. van Dijke, C. F. et al., MR imaging of the arthritic rabbit knee joint using albumin-(Gd–DTPA)30 with correlation to histopathology, *Magn. Reson. Imaging*, 17, 237, 1999.
82. Jiang, Y. et al., MRI of antigen-induced arthritis in rabbits: improved contrast and disease characterization with the blood pool agent MS-325, *Acad. Radiol.*, 9 (Suppl. 2), S480, 2002.
83. Grunder, W. et al., Improved nuclear magnetic resonance microscopic visualization of joint cartilage using liposome entrapped contrast agents, *Invest. Radiol.*, 33, 193, 1998.
84. Sipkins, D. A. et al., ICAM-1 expression in autoimmune encephalitis visualized using magnetic resonance imaging, *J. Neuroimmunol.*, 104, 1, 2000.
85. Mulder, W. J. et al., A liposomal system for contrast-enhanced magnetic resonance imaging of molecular targets, *Bioconjug. Chem.*, 15, 799, 2004.
86. Kang, H. W. et al., Magnetic resonance imaging of inducible E-selectin expression in human endothelial cell culture, *Bioconjug. Chem.*, 13, 122, 2002.
87. Hohe, J. et al., A technique for 3D in vivo quantification or proton density and magnetization transfer coefficients of knee joint cartilage, *Osteoarthritis Cartilage*, 8, 426, 2000.
88. Gasson, J. et al., Magnetic resonance imaging of rheumatoid arthritis in metacarpophalangeal joints, *Skeletal Radiol.*, 29, 324, 2000.
89. Burstein, D. et al., Protocol issues for delayed Gd(DTPA)(2 −)-enhanced MRI (dGEMRIC) for clinical evaluation of articular cartilage, *Magn. Reson. Med.*, 45, 36, 2001.
90. Gray, M. L. et al., Toward imaging biomarkers for osteoarthritis, *Clin. Orthop.*, 427, S175, 2004.

91. Williams, A. et al., Glycosaminoglycan distribution in cartilage as determined by delayed gadolinium-enhanced MRI of cartilage (dGEMRIC): potential clinical applications, *Am. J. Roentgenol.*, 182, 167, 2004.
92. Tiderius, C. J. et al., dGEMRIC (delayed gadolinium-enhanced MRI of cartilage) indicates adaptive capacity of human knee cartilage, *Magn. Reson. Med.*, 51, 286, 2004.
93. Gandy, S. J. et al., No loss of cartilage volume over three years in patients with knee osteoarthritis as assessed by magnetic resonance imaging, *Osteoarthritis Cartilage*, 10, 929, 2002.
94. Deichmann, R. and Haase, A., Quantification of T_1 values by SNAPSHOT–FLASH NMR imaging, *J. Magn. Reson.*, 96, 608, 1992.
95. Rudin, M. and Sauter, A., Measurement of reaction rates in vivo using magnetization transfer techniques, In *Basic Principles and Progress*, Vol. 27, Diehl, P., Ed., Springer, Heidelberg, 257, 1992.
96. Venn, M. and Maroudas, A., Chemical composition and swelling of normal and osteoarthritic femoral head cartilage. I. Chemical composition, *Ann. Rheum. Dis.*, 36, 121, 1977.

23 Rheumatoid and Osteoarthritis: Clinical Applications

Manish Kothari and Charles Peterfy

CONTENTS

23.1 INTRODUCTION

As more and more therapies for both rheumatoid arthritis (RA) and osteoarthritis (OA) become available, there is increased demand to evaluate both their appropriateness, and then their effectiveness on individual patients. As a result, the role of imaging in assessing and monitoring disease progress is on the rise, and is expected to grow significantly in the near future.

Although RA and OA are both major health problems, in which new therapies are being aggressively explored, the available treatments are in different stages of development. In RA, there is broad consensus on the nature of the disease. Established therapies are on the market for management of both clinical symptoms and structural modification. Structural modification via control of erosions and articular cartilage loss (radiographic joint-space narrowing) is already accepted as an endpoint and as an approved label. Osteoarthritis, on the other hand, has limited therapies available. Currently, no treatment exists that has been approved as a structure modifier. Also, the biochemical mechanism for disease progression is not yet well understood.

In spite of these differences, there is a number of overlapping needs and demands made on imaging for the assessment and monitoring of both RA and OA. Multiple components of the joints are involved. Three-dimensional visualization of tissue compartments is crucial to understand the extent of the disease and the interaction of the compartments. There is recognition with both RA and OA that earlier preventive treatment can improve joint performance before irreversible structural damage occurs.

This chapter outlines in detail the challenges facing imaging of RA and OA, present currently accepted practices in RA and OA, and finally, highlights promising techniques that are in development and that may have significant impact on future diagnosis and monitoring of these diseases.

23.2 IMAGING IN RHEUMATOID ARTHRITIS

The last decade has witnessed unprecedented advances in rheumatology, with the introduction of several new compounds capable of halting the relentless progression of joint destruction and functional disability in patients with RA. Many more compounds are currently in clinical trials. Prior to the introduction of effective therapy, the rheumatologist's demand for imaging joint structure was modest, at best. Although it was widely accepted that joint damage was a key driver of functional disability in RA, particularly in late disease [1–3], without effective therapies to prevent erosive destruction, there was limited need for detailed information about the integrity of joint structure. MRI promised to tell more about bone erosion, synovitis, and the integrity of cartilage, ligaments, and other articular tissues than radiography ever could, but the additional costs and inconveniences associated with MRI were not felt to be worth the extra performance. The information simply did not impact clinical management. Accordingly, most rheumatologists focused primarily on clinical and laboratory features of the disease, and used imaging only sparingly — if at all (see also Chapter 22, Section 22.3 and Section 22.4). The recent introduction of effective structure modifying therapies has changed the way that rheumatologists manage patients with RA, and this has created new demands on imaging both in clinical practice and in clinical research.

One important change is that it is no longer ethical to withhold effective therapy from patients, and therefore to conduct placebo-controlled clinical trials. This necessitates that putative new agents be tested against established therapies with known efficacy. Since such studies show much slower progression and smaller differences among treatment groups, they take substantially longer and require greater numbers of patients and clinical sites to achieve statistical significance. This increases the cost of clinical research and slows progress considerably. Unless more sensitive methods of predicting and monitoring treatment effects are developed the financial and practical ramifications of this problem will severely hinder further progress in therapeutics for RA.

Additionally, the availability of effective structure modifying therapy has stimulated a trend towards early, aggressive treatment prior to the development of joint damage [4,5] and associated irreversible functional disability [6–8]. During the first few years of disease, inflammation rather than structural damage accounts for the majority of functional disability in RA [1,9]. By eliminating inflammation at this stage, therefore, one can achieve full functional recovery. Indeed, inflammation is potentially reversible at any stage of the disease. However, as structural damage accumulates an increasing proportion of functional disability becomes irreversible. Accordingly, current treatment strategies target early disease to limit cumulative structural damage [5,6].

However, 30 to 40% of early RA cohorts do not progress, and therefore may not require aggressive therapy. Some have advocated treating all patients aggressively anyway in order to avoid missing those who might progress [10]. However, such a catch-all strategy carries significant financial and toxicity implications, as well as potential production challenges in some cases. Clearly, there is a need for better ways of identifying the aggressive phenotype of RA in early disease.

Absence of erosive damage on radiographs accurately identifies nonprogressors among patients with established disease ($>$ 18 months), but is only 41% accurate in patients with RA of less than 6 months duration [10]. Devauchelle Pensec et al. [11] found that radiographs acquired before one year of disease could not even reliably predict which patients would still have the diagnosis of RA 2 years later. Positive radiographs in their study were highly specific (96%) but diagnostically insensitive (17%). Others have reported similar findings [12–14]. Earlier reports by McQueen et al. [15,16] asserted that fewer than 20% of patients with RA of less than 6 months duration showed erosions on radiographs. In a different study by Machold et al. [17] fewer than 13% of RA patients showed radiographic erosions prior to 3 months. Accordingly, technical sensitivity for bone erosion is a critical performance requirement for imaging in early RA.

Conventional radiography has been the mainstay of RA imaging, with evaluation of both erosions and radiographic joint-space width (JSW) being used as disease markers. With careful attention to acquisition technique and reader training, radiography provides a reproducible technique for evaluating disease progression. Unfortunately, radiography's capacity for increased performance, as described earlier, is limited. Erosions that are not aligned tangentially to the x-ray beam (typically, erosions of dorsal and volar bone surfaces) are projected *en face* and can be obscured by superimposed bone. Penetrating erosions that are predominantly intramedullary and therefore surrounded by bone are also often obscured and difficult, if not impossible, to see. Additionally, joint flexion/contracture, subluxation or changes in x-ray beam centering can simulate joint-space narrowing (JSN) on radiographs. Periarticular osteoporosis may confound the interpretations of radiography. Finally, radiography is also unable to detect preerosive inflammation or directly visualize nonosseous components of the joint, such as articular cartilage, synovium, joint effusion, ligaments, tendons, discs, labra, menisci, or muscles.

In the following sections, we will outline the unparalleled ability of MRI to image arthritic joints. With its intrinsic tomographic nature, MRI can delineate features in all key tissue compartments, including the bone and the cartilage.

23.2.1 MRI of Erosion and Osteitis

Since it generates tomographic rather than projectional images, MRI can delineate erosions along all surfaces of bones, including the dorsal and volar surfaces, as well as the intramedullary component of penetrating erosions (Figure 23.1). Dozens of studies have shown MRI to be several times more sensitive than radiography [16,18–27] or ultrasound [27] for detecting bone erosions (see also Chapter 22, Section 22.5). This advantage of MRI has been demonstrated not only with conventional 1.5 T MRI but also with small, low-field (0.2 T) systems [27,28], which can image joints at a fraction of the cost of conventional MRI [29].

Baseline MRI revealed bone erosions in 42% of the early RA patients in a study by McQueen et al. [16], whereas radiography detected erosions in only 15% of these patients. Within one year, MRI was able to show the emergence of new erosions. Moreover, the baseline erosion score was

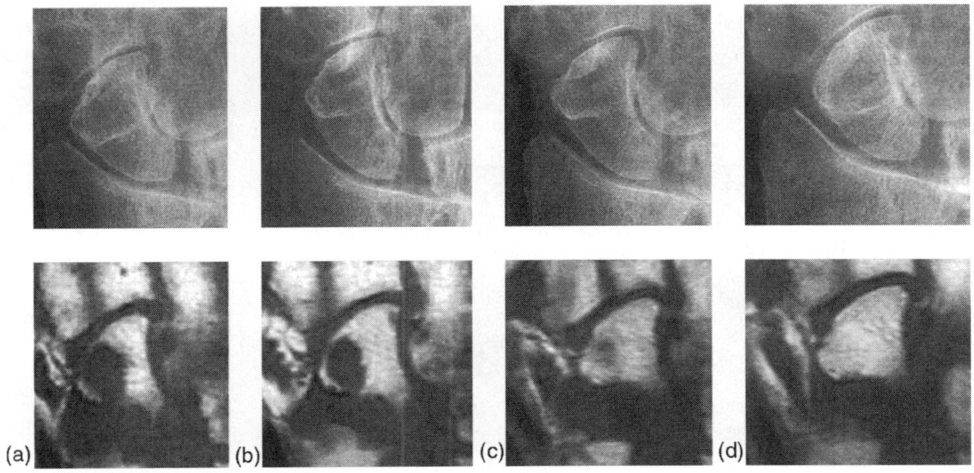

FIGURE 23.1 MRI is more sensitive than radiography to detect bone erosions. Radiographs (top) and coronal T_1-weighted images (bottom) at baseline (a), 3 months (b), 6 months (c), and 24 months (d) of a patient treated with methotrexate show a penetrating bone erosion in the distal pole of the scaphoid bone with a large intramedullary component. Despite the size of this erosion, it is barely visible with radiography. Follow-up images showed gradual filling in of the erosion over 2 years. (Reproduced from Peterfy, C. G., *Semin. Musculoskelet. Radiol.*, 5, 275, 2001. With permission. Copyright 2001 Georg Thieme Verlag KG, Stuttgart, New York.)

predictive of radiographic erosion score at 2 years ($p = .004$) [16]. Sixty-one percent of patients with erosions on MRI at baseline showed erosions on radiographs after 2 years, whereas only 18% of patients without baseline MRI erosions showed radiographic erosions in the same time interval. When bone marrow edema, synovitis, and tendonitis/tenosynovitis were also taken into account, MRI was even more predictive of subsequent radiographic erosion, offering optimized sensitivity and specificity values of 80 and 76%, respectively, and a negative predictive value of 86% [16]. Accordingly, in contrast to radiography, MRI can identify early RA patients who are unlikely to express an aggressively erosive phenotype and therefore less in need of aggressive, costly structure-modifying treatment. Excluding these individuals from clinical trials of putative new therapies can reduce the number of patients, study sites, and study duration required to test treatment efficacy.

There has been much debate about whether erosions depicted by MRI are truly erosions. Ganglion cysts, screw holes, some tumors, and surgical defects may display a similar appearance to individual erosions. What gives MRI specificity for the detection of bone erosions is the multiple character and anatomical distribution of synovitis, as well as the clinical setting of RA.

One of the most intriguing MRI features of active RA is what many have called bone marrow edema. This feature presents as free water signal in otherwise fatty marrow of articular bones, and is most conspicuous on fat-suppressed, T_2-weighted images (Figure 23.2). In contrast to bone erosions, which have sharply defined margins and contain only synovial fluid or synovial tissue, areas of marrow edema typically have poorly defined, feathery margins and contain residual trabeculae and marrow tissue, which are identified by the presence of magnetic susceptibility effects and T_1 contrast, respectively. Additionally, these areas enhance following intravenous injection of Gd-containing contrast material (Figure 23.2) [30], and correlate with clinical markers of inflammation, including C-reactive protein and disease activity score (DAS) [31] (see also Chapter 22, Section 22.5.2.1). Accordingly, osteitis may be a more appropriate term for this inflammatory feature [30].

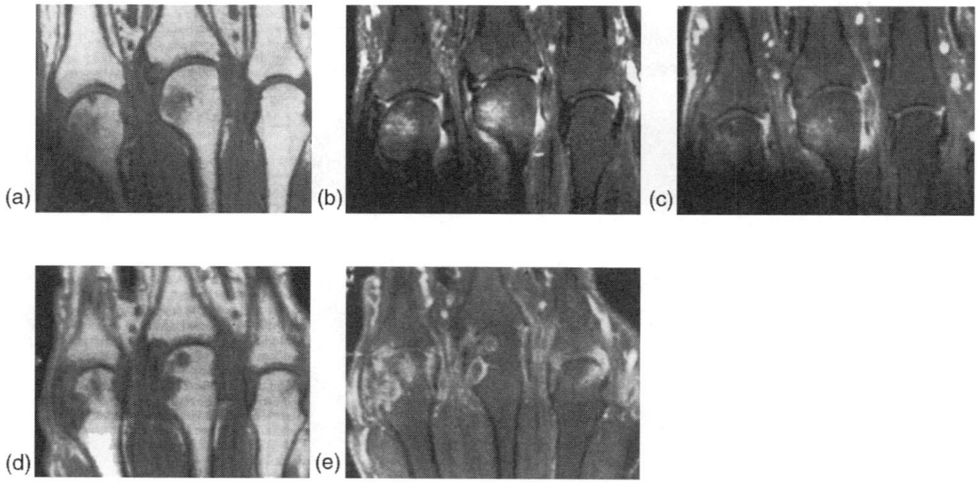

FIGURE 23.2 Preerosive osteitis. Coronal T_1-weighted (a) and fat-suppressed T_2-weighted (b) spin-echo images of the metacarpophalangeal joints of a patient with RA show areas of osteitis in the distal second and third metacarpals. The more sensitive fat-suppressed T_2-weighted images also show these changes in the adjacent proximal phalanges. Fat-suppressed T_1-weighted spin-echo with Gd-DTPA (c) shows enhancement of these areas consistent with inflammation. Follow up images 17 months later (T_1-weighted images without (d) and with (e) fat suppression and Gd-DTPA) show development of bone erosions with sharply defined rim enhancing margins at the sites of previous osteitis, and a new focus of osteitis in the previously quiescent fourth metacarpal head. (Reproduced from Peterfy, C. G., *Semin. Musculoskelet. Radiol.*, 5, 275, 2001. With permission. Copyright 2001 Georg Thieme Verlag KG, Stuttgart, New York.)

Several investigators have reported high prevalence of osteitis in the hands and wrists of RA patients, and presented evidence that osteitis can progress to bone erosions [15,19,24,32, 33]. Osteitis at baseline in patients with early RA was more predictive of bone erosions and functional outcome 6 years later than were any other MRI features, clinical features or C-reactive protein, alone or in combination [31]. Consistent with previous studies, erosive damage correlated with functional disability at 6 years but not in early disease, whereas osteitis correlated with disability in early disease, but not at 6 years. Interestingly, although DAS and the health assessment questionnaire improved mildly during the first two years of the study, presumably due to therapy, median osteitis score remained relatively constant throughout the 6 years, and bone erosion scores increased relentlessly and almost linearly over that same period.

Examples of osteitis resolving before the development of frank erosion have also been reported [15,33] (Figure 23.2). Accordingly, osteitis may be useful not only for predicting which patients are likely to progress, but also for monitoring antierosive treatment in these patients. In contrast to bone erosion, which is typically used as a negative marker, in that it indicates efficacy by not happening [34], recession of preexisting osteitis provides direct evidence that the process driving erosion has ceased, and thus offers a more rapid indication of therapeutic effects. Such a responsive marker would be useful for optimizing therapy in clinical practice, and for short proof-of-concept trials and other internal decision-making studies in clinical research.

Filling in, or healing, of preexisting erosions, a phenomenon which has been observed both with radiography [35] and MRI (Figure 23.1), similarly provides direct indication that the erosive process has stopped, and may thus also allow for a more rapid assessment of therapeutic efficacy. How frequently erosion healing occurs and whether or not it is accompanied by functional improvement is not known. It appears to be relatively uncommon on radiographs [35], but it is not an infrequent finding on MRI, at least anecdotally. The reason for this discrepancy may be technical. As for other osseous lesions, the majority of the radiographic lucency associated with RA erosions is attributable to cortical bone loss. The intramedullary component of bone erosions (Figure 23.1), unless associated with a calcified rim, is difficult to see with radiography. Penetrating erosions that have only small cortical components, therefore, are underestimated or occult on radiographs, particularly if the cortical defect is projected *en face*. These types of erosions, however, may be predisposed to reparative filling in, as they are surrounded by bone on all sides. Nonpenetrating erosions associated with extensive cortical bone loss may lack sufficient scaffolding to guide bone synthesis. Since MRI is disproportionately more sensitive to penetrating erosions, MRI would be expected to detect more healing erosions than radiography does. Again, erosion healing does not necessarily imply biomechanical recovery. However, it is a direct indication that the erosive process has stopped, and therefore it is a potentially useful marker of therapeutic efficacy. However, no reported studies have systematically examined erosion healing on MRI thus far.

23.2.2 Synovitis

Synovitis is another hallmark feature of RA that is visible with MRI. In the absence of fatty infiltration (lipoma arborescens) [36], fibrosis, or iron accumulation (hemosiderosis), however, thickened synovial tissue can be difficult to differentiate from adjacent synovial fluid with conventional MRI pulse sequences [37], and i.v. administration of Gd-containing contrast material is typically required [21,37–44]. Using various segmentation techniques, the volume of this enhancing, inflammatory compartment in the wrist or fingers can be quantified [45,46]. Savnik et al. [47] measured similar synovial volumes with low-field (0.2 T) dedicated extremity MRI as with conventional 1.5 T MRI. A number of studies have found synovial volume to correlate with joint swelling and tenderness [21,45,46,48,49], and to be predictive of bone erosion on follow-up images [15,21,28,33,50]. In one of these studies clinical examination detected only 49% of cases of synovitis demonstrable with low-field dedicated extremity MRI [28]. In the study by Benton et al. [31] synovitis scores did not correlate with clinical features at any time point, but it did predict erosions on MRI at 6 years.

In addition to volume, the rate and magnitude of synovial enhancement on sequential MR images following bolus i.v. injection of gadolinium- (Gd-) containing contrast material has been shown to correlate with the histological severity of inflammation in the synovium [51–53] and with clinical markers of disease activity [50]. Enhancement of synovium can be accurately quantified by dynamic MRI of single sections through the wrist [54]. In a recent randomized clinical trial, the knees of 34 RA patients were examined with dynamic, Gd-enhanced MRI at baseline and after 4 months of treatment with leflunomide [17] or methotrexate [17,55]. Despite the small number of patients and short study duration, measurements of the rate of synovial enhancement resolved a statistically significant difference between the two treatment groups, whereas the clinical examinations could not. In an earlier report, histological findings from synovial biopsies of the same joints correlated well with the MRI results [56]. Several other studies [21,49,50,57–60] have also shown synovial volume and synovial enhancement to decrease with therapy, but the follow-up interval in many of these was 6 months or longer.

Considerable work needs to be performed before dynamic contrast-enhanced MRI techniques can be imported to large-scale clinical trials and, ultimately, clinical service. Suitable equipment needs to be available at the sites for consistent acquisition, technologists need to be trained, validated software needs to be developed, etc. In dynamic studies of tumors, either a phantom or a T_1 calibration pulse sequence is used to correct for intrinsic T_1 effects on the uptake — the importance of this correction factor in RA needs to be addressed.

23.2.3 Cartilage, Ligaments, and Tendons

Another unique strength of MRI is its ability to directly visualize articular cartilage [61–64]. Direct imaging of this tissue is more specific than radiographic JSW, and tomography provides greater anatomical coverage of the joint surface than projection does. A number of morphological and compositional MRI markers of cartilage integrity have been developed [61,65–67], but most of this work derives from the knee, because the articular cartilage in the hand and wrist is extremely thin, and high-resolution imaging techniques are required.

In addition to monitoring changes in the bones, cartilage and synovium, MRI can directly visualize the full spectrum of tendon pathology, and has been shown to identify tendonitis and tendon rupture with greater accuracy than clinical examination [68,69]. In Benton's study [31], tendon scores were not themselves predictive of either bone erosion or functional disability, but when combined with bone erosion, both osteitis and synovitis were predictable. Ligaments and the triangular fibrocartilage complex can also be examined directly with MRI (see above). However, to date, very little attention has been given to imaging these structures in RA.

23.2.4 Low-Field Imaging in Rheumatoid Arthritis

While MRI is a relatively expensive procedure, its use in RA may prove cost-efficient if it can reduce unnecessary treatment of patients with costly biological therapies. As noted above, this may apply to more than 30% of RA patients on initial presentation. Nevertheless, conventional whole-body MRI is still relatively expensive and inconvenient, and although it is free of ionizing radiation, it is contraindicated in patients with pacemakers, aneurism clips, and other metal objects. Additionally, some patients find the experience unpleasant, and about 5% are unable to complete the examination because of claustrophobia. Recently, low-field strength extremity MRI systems were introduced as lower-cost alternatives in such circumstances [70,71]. Since these systems operate at lower magnetic field strength, typically 0.2 T, they can be made much smaller and operated less expensively. Also, whereas conventional 1.5 T magnets require placing the entire body into the bore, imaging with extremity MRI systems requires patients to insert only their limb into the magnet while sitting or lying next to the unit (Figure 23.3). This eliminates claustrophobia, and reduces risks associated with metal in the body or in the examination room. Owing to the small fringe-field, low weight, and small footprint of these systems, they can operate in environments that were previously inaccessible to MRI, such as medical offices. The smallest extremity MRI system that is currently available commercially is described by Crues et al. [70] (Figure 23.3b). This system can operate in as little as 4 m^2 of space, and is actually portable. The main disadvantage of extremity MRI systems is that their low magnetic field strength cannot support as much image resolution or as many image contrast mechanisms as conventional whole-body 1.5 T systems [28]. Additionally, the small size of these systems precludes imaging other body parts, such as the shoulders, hips, spine, chest, abdomen, and pelvis, which is a capability that most radiology services require. Owing to these limitations, extremity MRI systems were not initially felt by mainstream radiologists to provide sufficient performance for their needs. Higher-field strength (1.0 T) extremity systems that can support higher spatial resolution and broader contrast mechanisms, as well as larger low-field systems that can accommodate additional anatomical sites, such as the shoulders, have become available, but at the expense of larger space requirements and greater cost, and even these systems still offer some performance deficit in the eyes of many radiologists. It is important to bear in mind, however, that the needs of radiology are not the same as those of mainstream rheumatology. The circumstances and therefore the technical performance requirements for MRI in these two disciplines are very different. Rheumatologists do not need to image multiple body parts — at least, not in patients with RA. Imaging the hands, wrists, and feet is usually sufficient. They do not need, at this stage, highly sophisticated pulse sequences and contrast mechanisms. The ability to detect radiographically occult bone erosions, synovitis, and possibly osteitis and tendonitis would be good enough. A number of studies have already demonstrated that low-field MRI systems are technically capable of doing this [27,28,47,71–73]. In a study of 227 wrists of 132 patients with inflammatory arthritis, 95% of which had RA, Crues et al. [70] were able to identify roughly twice as many erosions using a small, portable 0.2 T MRI system than they could with radiography (Figure 23.4). Østergaard et al. [73] described similar findings in a different cohort of patients using a different low-field extremity system. In a study of 103 patients with inflammatory arthritis or noninflammatory arthralgia [25], Savnik et al. [47] found no significant difference in synovial volume measured by 0.2 T extremity MRI and that determined by 1.5 T conventional whole-body MRI. Cimmino et al. [72] found that the rate of synovial enhancement with Gd-containing contrast medium in 36 patients with RA and five healthy controls measured with 0.2 T extremity MRI correlated with clinical and laboratory markers of inflammation. Accordingly, low-field extremity

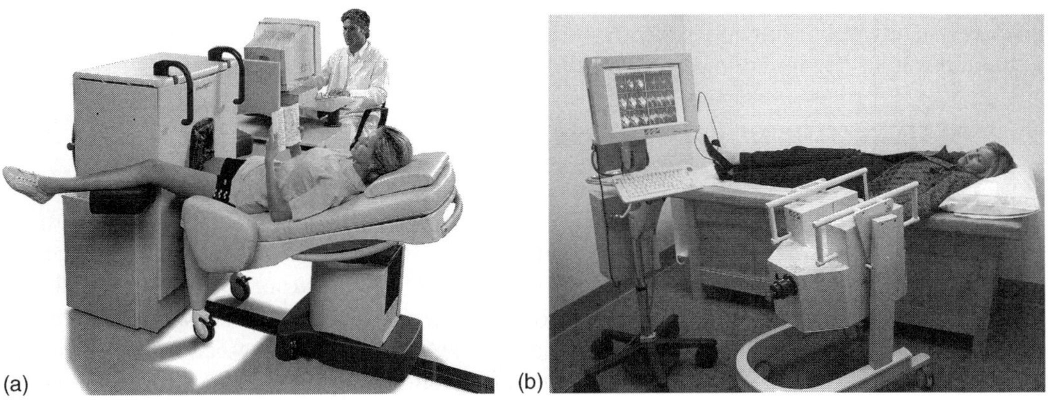

(a) (b)

FIGURE 23.3 Low-field extremity MRI. (a) Lunar (GE/Esaote) 0.2 T extremity MRI system. (b) MagneVu 0.2 T portable extremity MRI system.

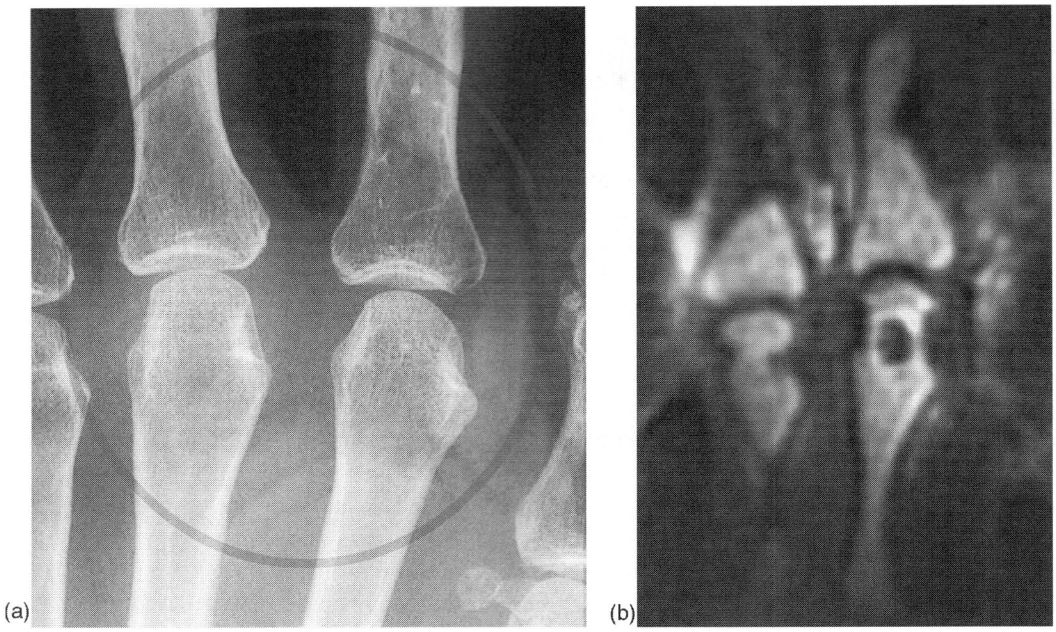

FIGURE 23.4 Low-field extremity MRI is more sensitive to detect bone erosion than radiography. (a) Radiograph of the second and third metacarpophalangeal joints shows no evidence of bone erosions. (b) Coronal extremity MRI image of the same region acquired with the portable extremity MRI system illustrated in Figure 23.3b shows a large intramedullary bone erosion in the distal end of the second metacarpal that is completely occult on radiographs. (Courtesy of N. Gaylis, Arthritis and Rheumatic Disease Specialties, Miami, Florida.)

MRI provides a promising solution for rheumatologists looking for sufficient diagnostic power to detect inflammation and erosive damage in early RA without the cost and inconvenience associated with conventional whole-body MRI. As experience with the use of MRI in RA increases among rheumatologists, their demand for technical performance can be expected to increase. Fueled by increasing utilization, extremity MRI systems can in turn be expected to improve their technical performance continuously in order to keep pace. If the trajectory of this improvement is steeper than that of mainstream radiology's demand for increasing technical performance in MRI, then at some point low-cost extremity MRI's performance may even satisfy some of mainstream radiology's needs, and thus begin displacing conventional MRI for certain applications. How quickly this process will advance is difficult to say. However, MRI is certainly expected to play an increasingly important role in day-to-day rheumatological practice over the next several years.

23.3 OSTEOARTHRITIS

Conventional radiography continues to be the primary imaging technique used to evaluate OA. This modality, however, is fundamentally limited by its inability to visualize directly articular cartilage, synovium, menisci, and other nonosseous structures involved in the pathophysiology of OA. Accordingly, cartilage loss in arthritis must be indirectly inferred from changes in the distance between opposing articular cortices, i.e., JSN. However, recent studies have shown that the menisci can also contribute to JSW and that meniscal subluxation [74,75] or resection [76] can cause radiographic JSN independently of cartilage thinning. Additionally, JSN probes cartilage loss only at the point where the two articular cartilage surfaces are in direct contact with each other. The location of this point on the tibia varies relatively little with knee flexion, but even minor changes in the position of the femur changes the corresponding point of articulation on the femoral surface.

Accordingly, the degree of flexion of the knee determines the regions of femoral and tibial cartilage included in JSW measurements. Since the intraarticular distribution of cartilage loss in OA is heterogeneous, the validity of JSN measurements depends on there being no change in the position of the femur relative to the tibia on serial examinations (Figure 23.5). Unfortunately, this condition

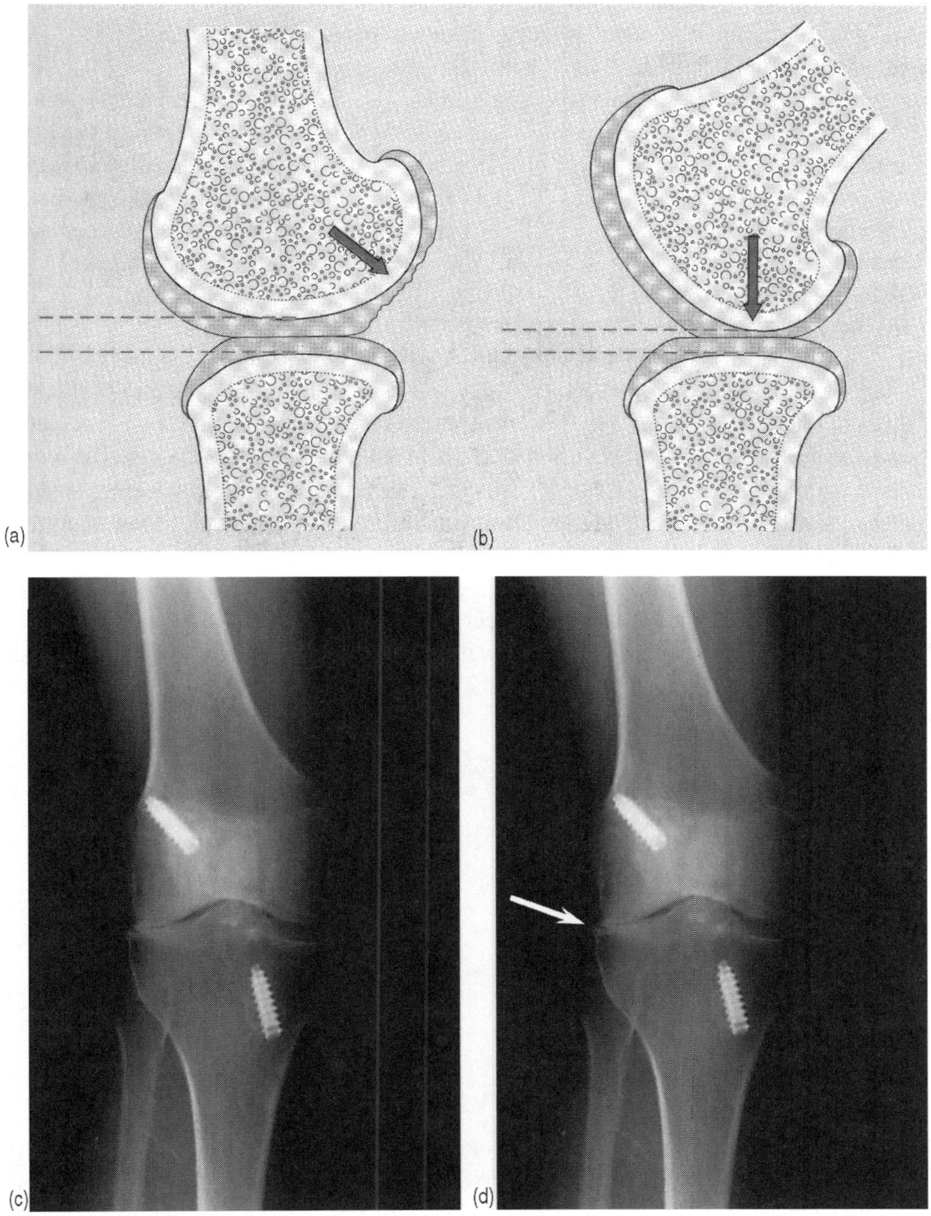

FIGURE 23.5 The importance of knee positioning in radiographic JSW measurement. The degree of flexion of the knee determines the region of femoral cartilage represented in JSW measurements. (a, b) Mild flexion articulates the central-posterior femoral cartilage, which tends to show thinning earlier. (c) Radiograph acquired in extension showing ample lateral femorotibial joint space. After mild flexion (d), this joint-space collapses to bone-on-bone contact. (a, b) (Adapted from Peterfy, C. G. et al., *Radiology*, 192, 485, 1994. With permission. Copyright 1994 Radiological Society of North America. (c, d) Courtesy of Synarc, Inc., San Francisco, CA. With permission.)

is not met with conventional standing radiography of the knee, and accordingly, the results of epidemiological studies and other investigations using this technique must be viewed with caution.

Several approaches have been proposed for improving the reproducibility of knee positioning for serial radiography, including the use of fluoroscopy, foot maps, and specially designed positioning devices (Figure 23.6). Fluoroscopic semiflexed radiography has been shown to provide good precision in single-site studies [77] but is difficult and costly to apply in multicenter research [78]. A number of nonfluoroscopic alternatives have also been developed, including the semiflexed metatarsophalangeal (MTP) technique [79,80] and the fixed-flexion technique [81]. Both these methods fix the rotation and angulation of the tibia. The fixed-flexion technique also fixes the angulation of the femur. Both techniques have been shown to offer cross-sectional reproducibility of JSW measurement comparable to that obtained with fluoroscopic semiflexed radiography. Both have also been used in large multicenter clinical trials and epidemiological studies. Although these techniques may improve the accuracy and the longitudinal precision of the measurements, they still suffer from the limitations of any radiographic approach.

MRI, in contrast, is well-suited for imaging diarthroidial joints. Not only does it offer a multiplanar tomographic viewing perspective, which eliminates projectional distortion and magnification and the problem of superimposition of overlapping structures, but it also provides unparalleled soft-tissue detail, allowing all components of the joint to be examined simultaneously and to view the joint as a whole organ [82]. Moreover, MRI is capable of probing not only the morphology of joint tissues but also a variety of compositional and functional parameters relevant to the arthritic process. Accordingly, of all the imaging modalities currently available, MRI holds the greatest promise for expanding our knowledge about OA and its causes, and for aiding clinicians in managing patients with the disease (see also Chapter 22, Section 22.6). Most of the attention in this regard has focused thus far on the knee, although there has been some work in the hip [83], shoulder [84], hands [85], lumbar facet joints [86], and temporomandibular joints [87].

MRI has played a central role in clinical evaluation of knee disorders for almost two decades. This experience has shown that damage to one tissue component within the joint can lead to damage

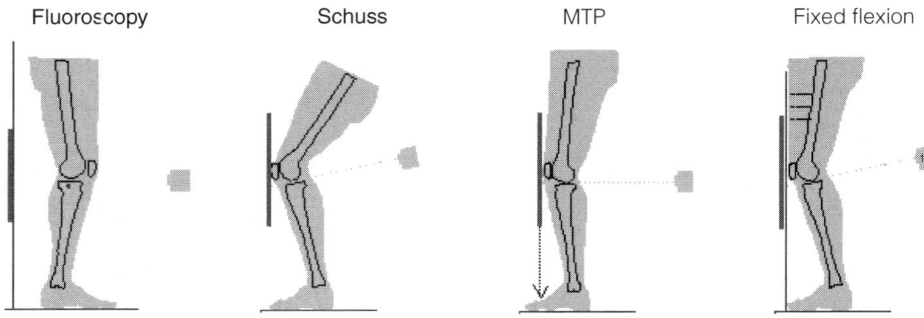

FIGURE 23.6 Techniques for serial radiography of the knee. (a) The fluoroscopic semiflexed technique provides good alignment and fixation of tibia, good fixation of the femur, but only minimal flexion of the knee. The knee-to-film distance is large and variable, and the source-to-knee distance is short and variable, leading to variable magnification, which must be corrected. The technique is more expensive than the three alternatives, and is difficult to perform in multicenter studies. (b) The Schuss view offers good alignment and fixation of the tibia, greater flexion of the knee (its main advantage), but poor fixation of the femur (its main limitation). The knee-to-film and source-to-knee distances are optimal and minimize magnification. Caudal beam angulation results in parallax error causing mild (3%) overestimation of JSW, but this cancels out on serial examinations. (c) The MTP technique offers good alignment and fixation of the tibia, but only minimal flexion of the knee, and only passive fixation of the femur. (d) The fixed-flexion technique provides good alignment and fixation of the tibia, good flexion of the knee, and active fixation of the femur (its main strength).

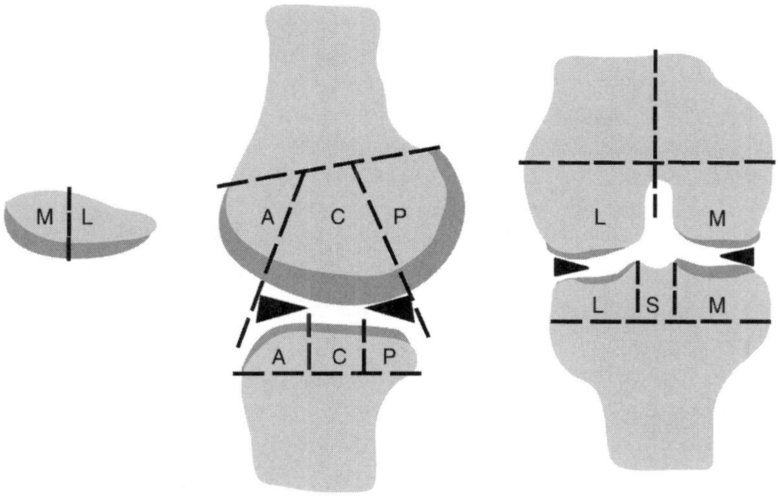

FIGURE 23.7 Regional subdivision of the articular surfaces. The patella (left image) is divided into medial (M) and lateral (L) regions, with the ridge considered part of the M region. The femur and tibia are also divided into M and L regions (right image), with the trochlear groove of the femur considered part of the M region. Region S represents the portion of the tibia beneath the tibial spines. The femoral and tibial surfaces are further subdivided into anterior (A), central (C), and posterior (P) regions (middle image). Region A of the femur corresponds to the patellofemoral articulation; region C is the weight bearing surface, and region P is the posterior convexity that articulates only in extreme flexion. Region C of the tibial surface corresponds to the uncovered portion between the anterior and posterior horns of the meniscus centrally and the portion covered by the body of the meniscus peripherally.

of other components, and that it is the collective impact of these abnormalities that leads to the pain and dysfunction experienced by the patient [88–91]. Accordingly, many feel that the knee is best evaluated as a whole organ, and that focusing on any individual structure, such as the meniscus or the articular cartilage, in isolation provides an oversimplified view of what is going on in the joint. A broader panel of imaging markers, i.e., a whole-organ evaluation, is needed to assess properly the structural integrity of joints affected by OA.

Peterfy et al. [92] presented a whole-organ MRI score (WORMS) technique of the knee joint. This system incorporates 14 independent articular features: cartilage signal and morphology, subarticular bone marrow abnormality, subarticular cysts, subarticular bone attrition, marginal osteophytes, medial and lateral meniscal integrity, anterior and posterior cruciate ligament integrity, medial and lateral collateral ligament integrity, synovitis, loose bodies, and periarticular cysts/bursae. Five of the features examined (cartilage signal and morphology, subarticular bone marrow abnormality, subarticular cysts, subarticular bone attrition, marginal osteophytes) related to the articular surfaces. These features are evaluated in 15 different regions subdivided by anatomical landmarks in the fully extended knee (Figure 23.7); 14 of these regions have articular surface.

Cartilage signal and morphology are scored with an eight-point scale (Figure 23.8) in each of the 14 articular-surface regions using fat-suppressed T_2-weighted fast spin-echo (FSE) images and fast fat-suppressed three-dimensional spoiled gradient-recalled images : 0 = normal thickness and signal; 1 = normal thickness but increased signal on T_2-weighted images; 2 = partial-thickness focal defect <1 cm in greatest width; 2.5 = full-thickness focal defect <1 cm in greatest width; 3 = multiple areas of partial-thickness (grade 2.0) defects intermixed with areas of normal thickness, or a grade 2.0 defect wider than 1 cm but $<75\%$ of the region; 4 = diffuse ($\geq 75\%$ of the region) partial-thickness loss; 5 = multiple areas of full-thickness

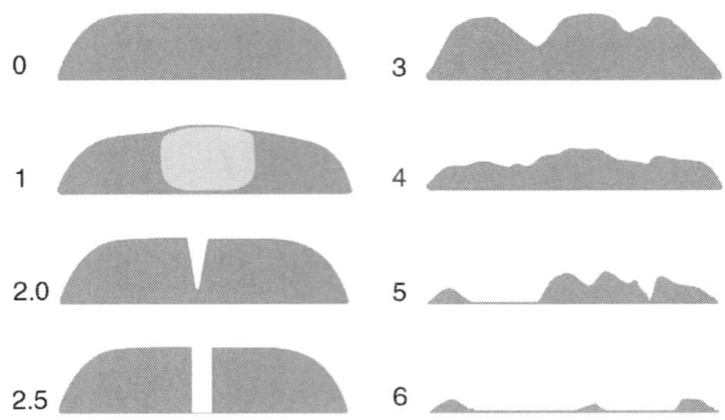

FIGURE 23.8 Eight-point scale for scoring articular cartilage signal and morphology. Each region of the knee surface is scored independently.

loss (grade 2.5) or a grade 2.5 lesion wider than 1 cm but <75% of the region; 6 = diffuse (≥75% of the region) full-thickness loss. This score combines several different constructs, including cartilage matrix integrity, cartilage thickness, articular surface coverage, cartilage surface smoothness, and the distribution of abnormalities.

Subarticular bone marrow abnormality is defined as poorly marginated areas of increased signal intensity in the normally fatty epiphyseal marrow on fat-suppressed T_2-weighted FSE images. This feature is graded in each of the 14 articular surface regions as well as the region of the tibia beneath the tibial spines (S) from 0 to 3 based on the extent of regional involvement (Figure 23.9): 0 = none; 1 = <25% of the region; 2 = 25 to 50% of the region; 3 = >50% of the region.

Subarticular cysts are identified as foci of markedly increased signal in the subarticular bone with sharply defined, rounded margins, and no evidence of internal marrow tissue or trabecular bone on fat-suppressed T_2-weighted FSE images. Bone cysts are graded in each region, including the subspinous region of the tibia (S), from 0 to 3 based on the extent of regional involvement, as for bone marrow abnormality: 0 = none; 1 = <25% of the region; 2 = 25 to 50% of the region; 3 = >50% of the region (Figure 23.10).

Flattening or depression of the articular surfaces is termed bone attrition and graded from 0 to 3 based on the subjective degree of deviation from the normal contour: 0 = normal; 1 = mild; 2 = moderate; 3 = severe. For example, the osseous articular surfaces of the medial and lateral femoral condyles and medial facet of the patella are all normally slightly convex. Accordingly, flattening = grade 1, slight concavity = grade 2, and marked concavity = grade 3. Figure 23.11 illustrates this for the lateral tibial plateau.

Osteophytes along 14 different margins of the knee, the anterior (A), central weight bearing (C), and posterior (P) margins of the femoral condyles and tibial plateaus, and the medial (M) and

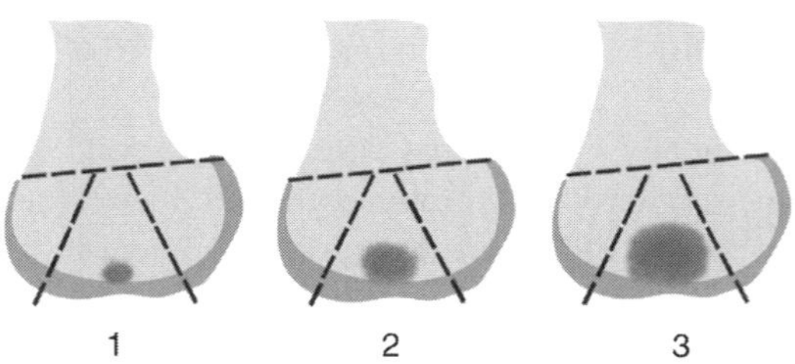

FIGURE 23.9 Subarticular marrow abnormality score. This score is based on the extent of regional marrow involvement by areas of free water signal with ill-defined margins.

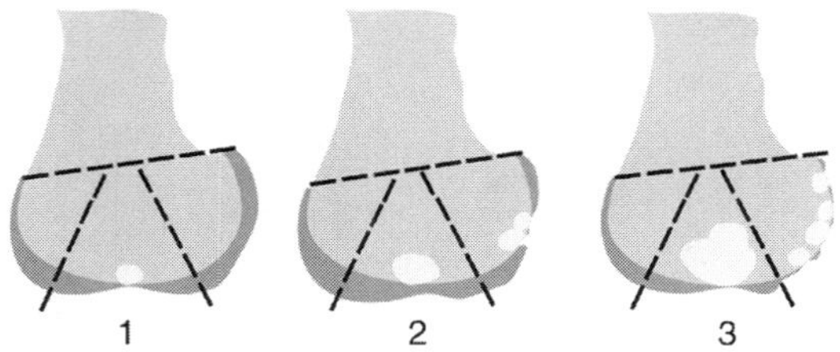

FIGURE 23.10 Subarticular cyst score. This score is based on the extent of focal bone loss through individual cysts (illustrated in the central region) or multiple cysts (illustrated in the posterior region) along the articular surface.

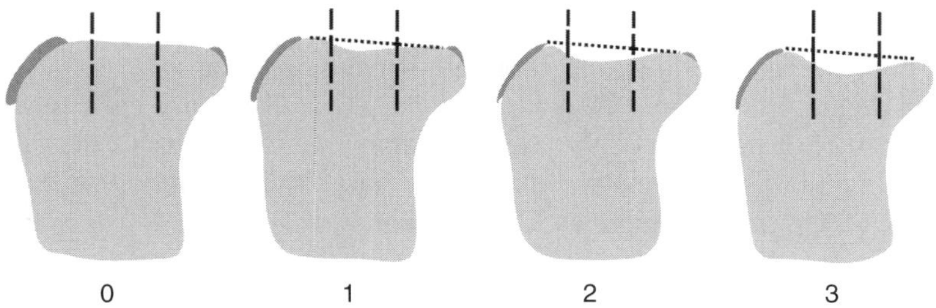

FIGURE 23.11 Subarticular bone attrition score. Bone attrition is scored on the basis of the degree of flattening or depression of the articular surface relative to normal.

lateral (L) margins of the patella, are graded from 0 to 7 using the following scale: 0 = none; 1 = equivocal; 2 = small; 3 = small to moderate; 4 = moderate; 5 = moderate to large; 6 = large; 7 = very large (Figure 23.12 and Figure 23.13).

The anterior cruciate ligament (ACL) and posterior cruciate ligament (PCL) are independently scored as intact (0) or torn (1) using sagittal T_2 FSE images. The medial collateral ligament (MCL) and lateral collateral ligament (LCL) are independently scored as intact (0), or torn (1) using coronal images. A combined ligament score is calculated by adding the sum of the ACL and PCL scores to half the sum of the MCL and LCL scores.

The anterior horn, body segment, and posterior horn of the medial and lateral menisci are graded separately from 0 to 4 on both sagittal and coronal images: 0 = intact; 1 = minor radial tear

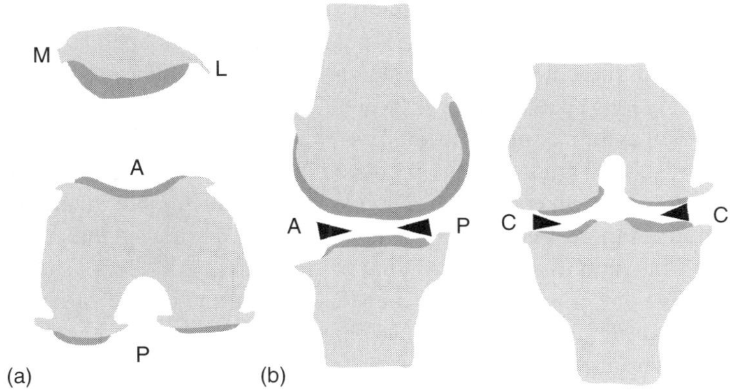

FIGURE 23.12 Regional subdivision of the articular margins. (a) Patellar medial (M) and lateral (L) margins are evaluated using axial images. (b) Femorotibial anterior (A) and posterior (P) margins are evaluated by combining information from both axial and sagittal (left panel) planes, whereas the central (C) femorotibial margins are evaluated using the coronal images (right panel).

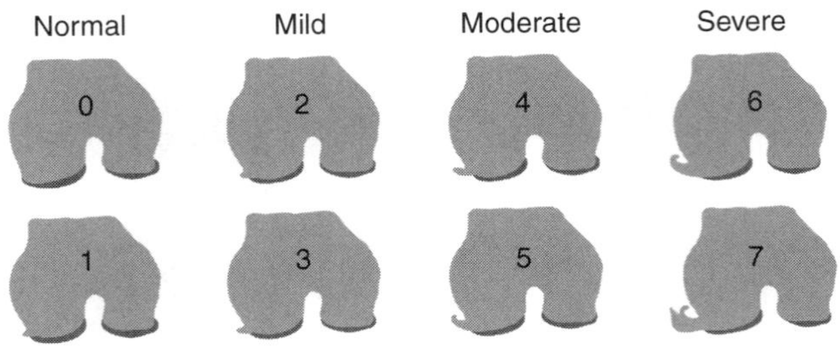

FIGURE 23.13 Eight-point scale for scoring marginal osteophytes. Osteophytes are scored on an eight-point scale based on size and the extent of margin involvement by the bone spur.

or parrot-beak tear; 2 = nondisplaced tear or prior surgical repair; 3 = displaced tear or partial resection; 4 = complete maceration/destruction or complete resection.

Synovial thickening and joint effusion are not distinguished from each other, but graded collectively from 0 to 3 in terms of the estimated maximal distention of the synovial cavity: 0 = normal; 1 = $<$33% of maximum potential distention; 2 = 33 to 66% of maximum potential distention; 3 = $>$66% of maximum potential distention.

Loose bodies in the synovial cavity are scored from 0 to 3 based on number: 0 = none; 1 = one loose body; 2 = two loose bodies; 3 = three or more loose bodies.

Synovial cysts or bursal collections about the knee are specified (e.g., popliteal, anserine, semimembranosis, meniscal, infrapatellar, prepatellar, tibiofibular, etc.) and graded 1 to 3 based subjectively on size. Any other findings (e.g., patellar tendon or quadriceps tendon abnormalities, avascular necrosis, stress fracture, insufficiency fracture, focal osteochondral fracture, bone or soft-tissue tumors) and technical limitations, such as failed fat suppression or metallic artifacts that interfere with the reliability of the scoring of a particular case, are also noted.

The final WORMS scores are tabulated as (1) independent values for each feature in each of the three compartments of the knee, (2) cumulative surface feature (cartilage, marrow abnormality, subarticular cysts, bone attrition, osteophytes) scores for each compartment, (3) cumulative scores for each feature throughout the knee, and (4) a total combined score for the entire knee.

A number of studies have indicated that the rate of cartilage volume loss in osteoarthritic patients ranges from 3 to 7% per year. Thus, techniques for quantifying the volume of articular cartilage and for mapping its thickness have also been developed and validated [65,93–98] (Figure 23.14). All these techniques rely on high image contrast and spatial resolution to achieve accurate and precise measurements [99]. The most commonly used pulse sequence for achieving this has been fat-suppressed, T_1-weighted, three-dimensional gradient-echo. One limitation of this pulse sequence, however, is its relatively long acquisition time (typically 12 min or more). This increases the costs of the examinations as well as the risk of deterioration of image quality by patient motion. Cicuttini et al. [96] reported that fast spoiled gradient-echo produced images of the knee with similar contrast and resolution to those acquired with conventional spoiled gradient-echo, but in approximately half the time (5.7 vs. 11.9 min). A more recent report by Glaser et al. [97] showed that using selective water excitation instead of fat-suppression offered similar time savings (7.2 vs. 16.5 min). Both these techniques are available on commercial, clinical MRI systems and are easy to use.

Most computer algorithms currently in use for quantifying cartilage volume and thickness require considerable user interaction and skill to achieve sufficient accuracy and precision. Even an experienced reader may take longer than an hour to segment the cartilage in a single knee. Recent advances in image segmentation, particularly the use of flexible electronic templates, promise to reduce this time and effort considerably.

In a cross-sectional study by Eckstein et al. [95] examining the variability of cartilage volume and thickness in the knees of 27 normal subjects, the coefficient of variation was greater than 20%,

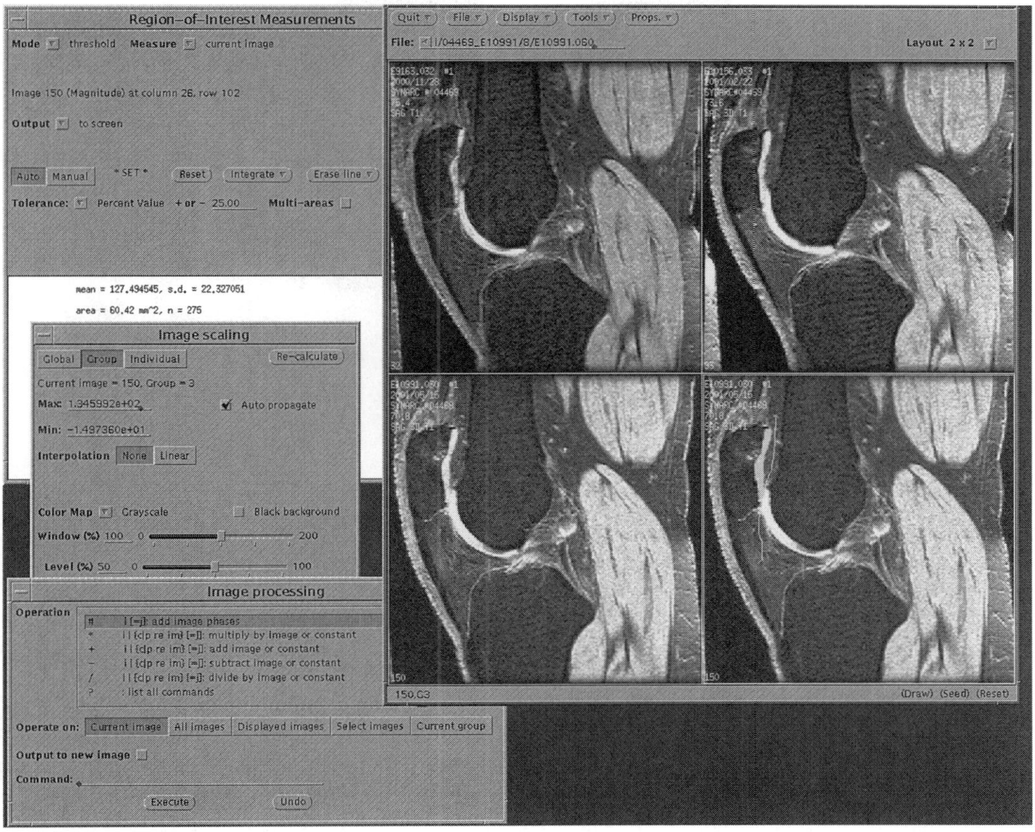

FIGURE 23.14 Quantifying articular cartilage volume. Lower right window of an MRI analysis workstation specialized for radiological clinical trials shows sagittal fat-suppressed, T_1-weighted three-dimensional gradient-echo image of the knee with the articular cartilage of the patella segmented using a seed-growing algorithm. A segmentation barrier is positioned where the patellar cartilage contacts the femoral cartilage to prevent the algorithm from crossing the interface between the two cartilage plates. (Figure courtesy of Synarc, Inc., San Francisco, CA. With permission.)

indicating that a loss of approximately one third of cartilage thickness would be needed to diagnose abnormality at a threshold of 2.5 standard deviations (SD) from normal. This argues against the feasibility of using t-score (2.5 SD below the young normal value) or z-score (2.5 SD lower than age-matched normal) to diagnose OA cross-sectionally, and supports subjects serving as their own controls in longitudinal assessments. Moreover, cartilage volume and thickness correlated poorly among the different cartilage plates within a single joint, or with anthropomorphic features, such as height, weight, and bone size. This suggests that it would not be possible to estimate premorbid cartilage volume or thickness at diseased articular surfaces based on measurements of normal cartilage plates elsewhere in the knee or by correcting against anthropomorphic features of the patient.

Unlike the knee, however, which has incongruent articular surfaces, the hip has a ball-in-socket configuration, and must be distracted in order to separate the femoral and acetabular surfaces on MRI. Nishii et al. [100] developed a specialized MRI-compatible distraction apparatus for this purpose. However, even with distraction, these articular surfaces are highly curved, giving rise to severe partial-volume effects in all planes unless extremely high spatial resolution is employed. Accordingly, cartilage thickness measurements in the hip have been challenging [101].

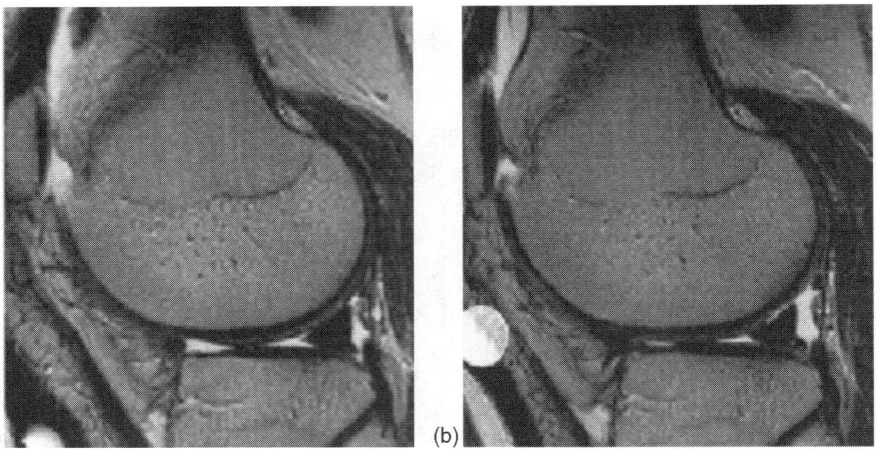

FIGURE 23.15 Progression of T_2 lesions in articular cartilage Serial sagittal T_2-weighted fast spin-echo images show a focal T_2 abnormality (arrows) in the femoral cartilage adjacent to the posterior horn of the lateral meniscus at baseline (a). Follow-up imaging 9 months later (b) shows a partial-thickness (grade 2.0) defect at that exact location. (Reproduced from Peterfy, C. G., *MRI Clin. N. Am.*, 8, 409, 2000. With permission from Elsevier, Inc. Copyright 2000.)

Even more intriguing than its ability to quantify cartilage morphology and geometry is MRI's unique capacity to probe noninvasively the compositional integrity of this tissue. Several studies showed that T_2 relaxation reflects the quantity and organization of fibrillar collagen in cartilage matrix [102–104]. Abnormal cartilage T_2 has been shown to correlate with areas of chondromalacia on arthroscopy, and although longitudinal studies using this MRI marker of matrix damage have yet to be published, some data suggest that abnormal T_2 is predictive of subsequent cartilage loss on follow-up MRI [105] (Figure 23.15). Reproducible quantification of cartilage T_2 has been demonstrated *in vivo* with conventional 1.5 T MRI, however, the dynamic range of this marker is still not known.

Other markers of cartilage matrix integrity include magnetization-transfer [106,107], water diffusion [67,108], Gd-DTPA uptake [66,109,110], and ^{23}Na MRI [111,112]. Further validation and characterization of these markers is needed to facilitate their use in clinical trials (see also Chapter 22, Section 22.6).

23.4 CONCLUSIONS

As effective structure-modifying therapies for RA begin to enter mainstream clinical practice, and early aggressive therapy becomes more widespread, the utility of conventional radiography for managing RA patients will continue to diminish. As Benton's report [31] demonstrates, MRI offers a powerful alternative to radiography in this circumstance. MRI is far more sensitive than radiography for detection of bone erosion in early RA patients, and is capable of detecting preerosive features, such as osteitis and synovitis, along with tendonitis and potentially other features that can be used to predict which patients will undergo severe destruction joint damage and irreversible functional disability. Being able to predict this accurately at the time of initial presentation is crucial to effective patient management [113,114].

MRI is also emerging as a tool of unprecedented power for evaluating joints with OA. Not only can it assess multiple articular structures simultaneously, but it can probe both the morphological and compositional integrity of these tissues. As structure-modifying therapies for OA are developed for clinical use, MRI will play an increasingly important role in the management of patients with this prevalent and debilitating disorder [115].

REFERENCES

1. Welsing, P. M. et al., The relationship between disease activity, joint destruction, and functional capacity over the course of rheumatoid arthritis, *Arthritis Rheum.*, 44, 2009, 2001.
2. Scott, D. L. et al., The links between joint damage and disability in rheumatoid arthritis, *Rheumatology (Oxford)*, 39, 122, 2000.
3. Clarke, A. E. et al., Radiographic damage in rheumatoid arthritis correlates with functional disability but not direct medical costs, *J. Rheumatol.*, 28, 2416, 2001.
4. Irvine, S., Munro, R., and Porter, D., Early referral, diagnosis, and treatment of rheumatoid arthritis: evidence for changing medical practice, *Ann. Rheum. Dis.*, 58, 510, 1999.
5. Emery, P., Evidence supporting the benefit of early intervention in rheumatoid arthritis, *J. Rheumatol.*, 29 (Suppl. 66), 3, 2002.
6. Landewe, R. B. et al., The benefits of early treatment in rheumatoid arthritis: confounding by indication, and the issue of timing no increased risk of malignancies and mortality in cyclosporin A-treated patients with rheumatoid arthritis, *Arthritis Rheum.*, 48, 1, 2003.
7. Bukhari, M. A. et al., Influence of disease-modifying therapy on radiographic outcome in inflammatory polyarthritis at five years: results from a large observational inception study, *Arthritis Rheum.*, 48, 46, 2003.
8. Emery, P. et al., Early referral recommendation for newly diagnosed rheumatoid arthritis: evidence based development of a clinical guide, *Ann. Rheum. Dis.*, 61, 290, 2002.
9. van der Heijde, D., Radiographic progression in rheumatoid arthritis: does it reflect outcome? Does it reflect treatment?, *Ann. Rheum. Dis.*, 60 (Suppl. 3), iii47, 2001.
10. Paulus, H. E. et al., Correlation of single time-point damage scores with observed progression of radiographic damage during the first 6 years of rheumatoid arthritis, *J. Rheumatol.*, 30, 705, 2003.
11. Devauchelle Pensec, V. et al., Ability of hand radiographs to predict a further diagnosis of rheumatoid arthritis in patients with early arthritis, *J. Rheumatol.*, 28, 2603, 2001.
12. Mau, W., Raspe, H. H., and Mersjann, H., Early arthritides: nosography, nosology, and diagnostic criteria, *Scand. J. Rheumatol. Suppl.*, 79, 3, 1989.
13. Nissila, M. et al., Prognosis of inflammatory joint diseases. A three-year follow-up study, *Scand. J. Rheumatol.*, 12, 33, 1983.
14. van der Horst-Bruinsma, I. E. et al., Diagnosis and course of early-onset arthritis: results of a special early arthritis clinic compared to routine patient care, *Br. J. Rheumatol.*, 37, 1084, 1998.
15. McQueen, F. et al., Magnetic resonance imaging of the wrist in early rheumatoid arthritis reveals progression of erosions despite clinical improvement, *Ann. Rheum. Dis.*, 58, 156, 1999.
16. McQueen, F. M. et al., What is the fate of erosions in early rheumatoid arthritis? Tracking individual lesions using x-rays and magnetic resonance imaging over the first two years of disease, *Ann. Rheum. Dis.*, 60, 859, 2001.
17. Machold, K. P. et al., Very recent onset arthritis-clinical, laboratory, and radiological findings during the first year of disease, *J. Rheumatol.*, 29, 2278, 2002.
18. Jorgensen, C. et al., Sensitivity of magnetic resonance imaging of the wrist in very early rheumatoid arthritis, *Clin. Exp. Rheumatol.*, 11, 163, 1993.
19. McQueen, F. et al., Magnetic resonance imaging of the wrist in early rheumatoid arthritis reveals a high prevalence of erosions at four months after symptom onset, *Ann. Rheum. Dis.*, 57, 350, 1998.
20. Peterfy, C. et al., Comparison of MRI and X-ray for monitoring erosive changes in rheumatoid arthritis, *Arthritis. Rheum.*, 41 (Suppl), S51, 1998.
21. Østergaard, M. et al., Magnetic resonance imaging-determined synovial membrane volume as a marker of disease activity and a predictor of progressive joint destruction in the wrists of patients with rheumatoid arthritis, *Arthritis Rheum.*, 42, 918, 1999.
22. Klarlund, M. et al., Wrist and finger joint MR imaging in rheumatoid arthritis, *Acta Radiol.*, 40, 400, 1999.
23. Foley-Nolan, D. et al., Magnetic resonance imaging in the assessment of rheumatoid arthritis — a comparison with plain film radiographs, *Br. J. Rheumatol.*, 30, 101, 1991.
24. McGonagle, D. et al., The relationship between synovitis and bone changes in early untreated rheumatoid arthritis: a controlled magnetic resonance imaging study, *Arthritis Rheum.*, 42, 1706, 1999.

25. Østergaard, M. et al., Scoring of synovial membrane hypertrophy and bone erosions by MR imaging and clinically active and inactive rheumatoid arthritis of the wrist, *Scand. J. Rheumatol.*, 24, 212, 1995.
26. Emery, P. and Luqmani, R., The validity of surrogate markers in rheumatic disease, *Br. J. Rheumatol.*, 32 (Suppl. 3), 3, 1993.
27. Backhaus, M. et al., Prospective two year follow up study comparing novel and conventional imaging procedures in patients with arthritic finger joints, *Ann. Rheum. Dis.*, 61, 895, 2002.
28. Lindegaard, H. et al., Low field dedicated magnetic resonance imaging in untreated rheumatoid arthritis of recent onset, *Ann. Rheum. Dis.*, 60, 770, 2001.
29. Peterfy, C. G., Roberts, T., and Genant, H. K., In *Dedicated Extremity MRI: An Emerging Technology*, *Radiol. Clin. N. Am.*, Kneeland, J. B., Ed., Saunders, Philadelphia, pp. 1–20, 1996.
30. Peterfy, C. G., Magnetic resonance imaging of the wrist in rheumatoid arthritis, *Semin. Musculoskelet. Radiol.*, 5, 275, 2001.
31. Benton, N. et al., MRI of the wrist in early rheumatoid arthritis can be used to predict functional outcome at 6 years, *Ann. Rheum. Dis.*, 63, 555, 2004.
32. McQueen, F. M., Magnetic resonance imaging in early arthritis: what is its role?, *Rheumatology (Oxford)*, 39, 700, 2000.
33. Savnik, A. et al., MRI of the wrist and finger joints in inflammatory joint diseases at 1-year interval: MRI features to predict bone erosions, *Eur. Radiol.*, 12, 1203, 2002.
34. van der Heijde, D. M., How to read radiographs according to the Sharp/van der Heijde method, *J. Rheumatol.*, 26, 743, 1999.
35. Sharp, J. T. et al., Repair of erosions in rheumatoid arthritis does occur. Results from 2 studies by the OMERACT subcommittee on healing of erosions, *J. Rheumatol.*, 30, 1102, 2003.
36. Feller, J. F., Rishi, M., and Hughes, E. C., Lipoma arborescens of the knee: MR demonstration, *Am. J. Roentgenol.*, 163, 162, 1994.
37. Peterfy, C. G. et al., MR imaging of the arthritic knee: improved discrimination of cartilage, synovium and effusion with pulsed saturation transfer and fat-suppressed T_1-weighted sequences, *Radiology*, 191, 413, 1994.
38. Smith, H. J., Larheim, T. A., and Aspestrand, F., Rheumatic and nonrheumatic disease in the temporomandibular joint: gadolinium-enhanced MR imaging, *Radiology*, 185, 229, 1992.
39. Yamato, M. et al., MRI of the knee in rheumatoid arthritis: Gd-DTPA perfusion dynamics, *J. Comput. Assist. Tomogr.*, 17, 781, 1993.
40. Drape, J. L. et al., Intraarticular diffusion of Gd-DOTA after intravenous injection in the knee: MR imaging evaluation, *Radiology*, 188, 227, 1993.
41. Winalski, C. S. et al., Enhancement of joint fluid with intravenously administered gadopentetate dimeglumine: technique, rationale, and implications, *Radiology*, 187, 179, 1993.
42. Jevtic, V. et al., Precontrast and postcontrast (Gd-DTPA) magnetic resonance imaging of hand joints in patients with rheumatoid arthritis, *Clin. Radiol.*, 48, 176, 1993.
43. Jevtic, V. et al., Distinctive radiological features of small hand joints in rheumatoid arthritis and seronegative spondyloarthritis demonstrated by contrast-enhanced (Gd-DTPA) magnetic resonance imaging, *Skeletal Radiol.*, 24, 351, 1995.
44. Klarlund, M. et al., Dynamic magnetic resonance imaging of the metacarpophalangeal joints in rheumatoid arthritis, early unclassified polyarthritis and healthy controls, *Scand. J. Rheumatol.*, 29, 108, 2000.
45. Østergaard, M. et al., Quantitative assessment of the synovial membrane in the rheumatoid wrist: an easily obtained MRI score reflects the synovial volume, *Br. J. Rheumatol.*, 35, 965, 1996.
46. Østergaard, M. et al., Magnetic resonance imaging-determined synovial membrane and joint effusion volumes in rheumatoid arthritis and osteoarthritis: comparison with the macroscopic and microscopic appearance of the synovium, *Arthritis Rheum.*, 40, 1856, 1997.
47. Savnik, A. et al., MRI of the arthritic small joints: comparison of extremity MRI (0.2 T) vs high-field MRI (1.5 T), *Eur. Radiol.*, 11, 1030, 2001.
48. Palmer, W. E. et al., Quantification of inflammation in the wrist with gadolinium-enhanced MR imaging and PET with 2-[F-18]-fluoro-2-deoxy-D-glucose, *Radiology*, 196, 645, 1995.
49. Sugimoto, H., Takeda, A., and Kano, S., Assessment of disease activity in rheumatoid arthritis using magnetic resonance imaging: quantification of pannus volume in the hands, *Br. J. Rheumatol.*, 37, 854, 1998.

50. Huang, J. et al., A 1-year follow-up study of dynamic magnetic resonance imaging in early rheumatoid arthritis reveals synovitis to be increased in shared epitope-positive patients and predictive of erosions at 1 year, *Rheumatology (Oxford)*, 39, 407, 2000.
51. Tamai, K. et al., Dynamic magnetic resonance imaging for the evaluation of sunovitis in patients with rheumatoid arthritis, *Arthritis Rheum.*, 37, 1151, 1994.
52. Stiskal, M. A. et al., Rheumatoid arthritis of the craniocervical region by MR imaging: detection and characterization, *Am. J. Roentgenol.*, 165, 585, 1995.
53. Østergaard, M. et al., Quantification of synovistis by MRI: correlation between dynamic and static gadolinium enhanced magnetic resonance imaging and microscopic and macroscopic signs of synovial inflammation, *Magn. Reson. Imaging*, 16, 743, 1998.
54. Østergaard, M., Different approaches to synovial membrane volume determination by magnetic resonance imaging: manual versus automated segmentation, *Br. J. Rheumatol.*, 36, 1166, 1997.
55. Reece, R. J. et al., Comparative assessment of leflunomide and methotrexate for the treatment of rheumatoid arthritis, by dynamic enhanced magnetic resonance imaging, *Arthritis Rheum.*, 46, 366, 2002.
56. Kraan, M. C. et al., Modulation of inflammation and metalloproteinase expression in synovial tissue by leflunomide and methotrexate in patients with active rheumatoid arthritis: findings in a prospective, randomized, double-blind, parallel design clinical trial in thirty nine patients at two centers, *Arthritis Rheum.*, 43, 1820, 2000.
57. Østergaard, M. et al., Quantitative assessment of synovial inflammation by dynamic gadolinium-enhanced magnetic resonance imaging. A study of the effect of intra-articular methyl-prednisolone on the rate of early synovial enhancement, *Br. J. Rheumatol.*, 35, 50, 1996.
58. Kalden-Nemeth, D. et al., NMR monitoring of rheumatoid arthritis patients receiving anti-TNFalpha monoclonal antibody therapy, *Rheumatol. Int.*, 16, 249, 1997.
59. Lee, J. et al., Magnetic resonance imaging of the wrist in defining remission of rheumatoid arthritis, *J. Rheumatol.*, 24, 1303, 1997.
60. Huh, Y. M. et al., Role of the inflamed synovial volume of the wrist in defining remission of rheumatoid arthritis with gadolinium-enhanced 3D-SPGR MR imaging, *J. Magn. Reson. Imaging*, 10, 202, 1999.
61. Peterfy, C. G., Scratching the surface: articular cartilage disorders in the knee, *MRI Clin. N. Am.*, 8, 409, 2000.
62. Disler, D., Fat-suppressed three-dimensional spoiled gradient-recalled MR imaging: assessment of articular and physeal hyaline cartilage, *Am. J. Roentgenol.*, 169, 1117, 1997.
63. Recht, M. P. et al., Accuracy of fat-suppressed three dimensional spoiled gradient-echo FLASH MR imaging in the detection of patellofemoral articular cartilage abnormalities, *Radiology*, 198, 209, 1996.
64. Bredella, M. et al., Accuracy of T2-weighted fast spin-echo MR imaging with fat saturation in detecting cartilage defects in the knee: comparison with arthroscopy in 130 patients, *Am. J. Roentgenol.*, 172, 1073, 1999.
65. Peterfy, C. G. et al., Quantification of articular cartilage in the knee by pulsed saturation transfer and fat-suppressed MRI: optimization and validation, *Radiology*, 192, 485, 1994.
66. Bashir, A., Gray, M. L., Hartke, J., and Burstein, D., Nondestructive imaging of human cartilage glycosaminoglycan concentration by MRI, *Magn. Reson. Med.*, 41, 857–865, 1999.
67. Burstein, D. et al., Diffusion of small solutes in cartilage as measured by nuclear magnetic resonance (NMR) spectroscopy and imaging, *J. Orthop. Res.*, 11, 465, 1993.
68. Rubens, D. J. et al., Rheumatoid arthritis: evaluation of wrist extensor tendons with clinical examination versus MR imaging — a preliminary report, *Radiology*, 187, 831, 1993.
69. Valeri, G. et al., Tendon involvement in rheumatoid arthritis of the wrist: MRI findings, *Skeletal Radiol.*, 30, 138, 2001.
70. Crues, J. V. et al., Identification of wrist and metacarpophalangeal joint erosions using a portable magnetic resonance system compared to conventional radiographs, *J. Rheumatol.*, 31, 676, 2004.
71. Peterfy, C. G., Roberts, T., and Genant, H. K., Dedicated extremity MR imaging. An emerging technology, *Radiol. Clin. N. Am.*, 35, 1, 1997.

72. Cimmino, M. et al., Dynamic gadolinium-enhanced magnetic resonance imaging of the wrists in patients with rheumatoid arthritis can discriminate active from inactive disease, *Arthritis Rheum.*, 48, 1207, 2003.
73. Østergaard, M. et al., New radiographic bone erosions in the wrists of patients with rheumatoid arthritis are detectable with magnetic resonance imaging a median of two years earlier, *Arthritis Rheum.*, 48, 2128, 2003.
74. Gale, D. R. et al., Meniscal subluxation: association with osteoarthritis and joint space narrowing, *Osteoarthritis Cartilage*, 7, 526, 1999.
75. Breitenseher, M. J. et al., MR imaging of meniscal subluxation in the knee, *Acta Radiol.*, 38, 876, 1997.
76. Messner, K. et al., Radiographic joint space narrowing and histologic changes in a rabbit meniscectomy model of early knee osteoarthrosis, *Am. J. Sports Med.*, 29, 151, 2001.
77. Buckland-Wright, J. C. et al., Quantitative microfocal radiographic assessment of osteoarthritis of the knee from weight bearing tunnel and semiflexed standing views, *J. Rheumatol.*, 21, 1734, 1994.
78. Mazzuca, S. et al., Field test of the reproducibility of automated measurements of medial tibiofemoral joint space width derived from standardized knee radiographs, *J. Rheumatol.*, 26, 1359, 1999.
79. Buckland-Wright, J. et al., Substantial superiority of semiflexed (MTP) views in knee osteoarthritis: a comparative radiographic study, without fluoroscopy, of standing extended, semiflexed (MTP), and schuss views, *J. Rheumatol.*, 26, 2664, 1999.
80. Mazzuca, S. A. et al., Field test of the reproducibility of the metatarsophalangeal view with repeated radiographic examinations of subjects with osteoarthritis of the knee, *Arthritis Rheum.*, 46, 109, 2002.
81. Peterfy, C. et al., Nonfluoroscopic method for flexed radiography of the knee that allows reproducible joint-space width measurement, *Arthritis Rheum.*, 41, S361, 1998.
82. Peterfy, C., Imaging Techniques, *Rheumatology 2E*, Vol. 1, Klippel, J. and Dieppe, P., Eds., Mosby, Philadelphia, pp. 14.1–14.18, 1997.
83. Nishii, T. et al., Articular cartilage abnormalities in dysplastic hips without joint space narrowing, *Clin. Orthop.*, 383, 183, 2001.
84. Peterfy, C. et al., Evaluating arthritic changes in the shoulder with MRI, In *Shoulder Magnetic Resonance Imaging*, Steinbach, L., Tirman, P., Peterfy, C. et al.,, Eds., Lippencott-Raven, Philadelphia, PA, pp. 221–237, 1998.
85. Robson, M. et al., A combined analysis and magnetic resonance imaging technique for computerised automatic measurement of cartilage thickness in the distal interphalangeal joint, *Magn. Reson. Imaging*, 13, 709, 1995.
86. Fujiwara, A. et al., Orientation and osteoarthritis of the lumbar facet joint, *Clin. Orthop.*, 385, 88, 2001.
87. Bertram, S. et al., Diagnosing TMJ internal derangement and osteoarthritis with magnetic resonance imaging, *J. Am. Dent. Assoc.*, 132, 753, 2001.
88. Hochberg, M. C. et al., Epidemiologic associations of pain in osteoarthritis of the knee: data from the national health and nutrition examination survey and national health and nutrition examination-I epidemiologic follow-up survey, *Semin. Arthritis Rheum.*, 18, 4, 1989.
89. Summers, M. et al., Radiographic assessment and psychologic variables as predictors of pain and functional impairment in osteoarthritis of the knee or hip, *Arthritis Rheum.*, 31, 204, 1988.
90. Felson, D. T. et al., The association of bone marrow lesions with pain in knee osteoarthritis, *Ann. Intern. Med.*, 134, 541, 2001.
91. Hirasawa, Y. et al., Nerve distribution to the human knee joint: anatomical and immunohistochemical study, *Int. Orthop.*, 24, 1, 2000.
92. Peterfy, C. G., Whole-organ magnetic resonance imaging score (WORMS) of the knee in osteoarthritis, *Osteoarthritis Cartilage*, 12, 177, 2004.
93. Pilch, L. et al., Assessment of cartilage volume in the femorotibial joint with magnetic resonance imaging and 3D computer reconstruction, *J. Rheumatol.*, 21, 2307, 1994.
94. Eckstein, F. et al., Assessment of articular cartilage volume and thickness with magnetic resonance imaging (MRI), *Trans. Orthop. Res. Soc.*, 20, 194, 1995.
95. Eckstein, F. et al., Interindividual variability and correlation among morphological parameters of knee joint cartilage plates: analysis with three-dimensional MR imaging, *Osteoarthritis Cartilage*, 9, 101, 2001.

96. Cicuttini, F. et al., Comparison and reproducibility of fast and conventional spoiled gradient-echo magnetic resonance sequences in the determination of knee cartilage volume, *J. Orthop. Res.*, 18, 580, 2000.
97. Glaser, C. et al., Optimization and validation of a rapid high-resolution T_1-w 3D FLASH water excitation MRI sequence for the quantitative assessment of articular cartilage volume and thickness, *Magn. Reson. Imaging*, 19, 177, 2001.
98. Cohen, Z. A. et al., Knee cartilage topography, thickness, and contact areas from MRI: in-vitro calibration and in-vivo measurements, *Osteoarthritis Cartilage*, 7, 95, 1999.
99. Hardy, P. A. et al., The influence of the resolution and contrast on measuring the articular cartilage volume in magnetic resonance images, *Magn. Reson. Imaging*, 18, 965, 2000.
100. Nishii, T. et al., Articular cartilage evaluation in osteoarthritis of the hip with MR imaging under continuous leg traction, *Magn. Reson. Imaging*, 16, 871, 1998.
101. Hodler, J. et al., Width of the articular cartilage of the hip: quantification by using fat-suppression spin-echo MR imaging in cadavers, *Am. J. Roentgenol.*, 159, 351, 1992.
102. Dardzinski, B. et al., Spatial variation of T_2 in human articular cartilage, *Radiology*, 205, 546, 1997.
103. Mosher, T., Dardzinski, B., and Smith, M., Human articular cartilage: influence of aging and early symptomatic degeneration on the spatial variation of T_2-preliminary findings at 3 T, *Radiology*, 241, 259, 2000.
104. Xia, Y. et al., Quantitative in situ correlation between microscopic MRI and polarized light microscopy studies of articular cartilage, *Osteoarthritis Cartilage*, 9, 393, 2001.
105. Zaim, S. et al., Early cartilage degeneration of the knee after meniscal surgery: MRI findings, *Osteoarthritis Cartilage*, 9, S37, 2001.
106. Kim, D. K. et al., Analysis of water-macromolecule proton magnetization transfer in articular cartilage, *Magn. Reson. Med.*, 29, 211, 1993.
107. Hohe, J. et al., A technique for 3D in vivo quantification of proton density and magnetization transfer coefficients of knee joint cartilage, *Osteoarthritis Cartilage*, 8, 426, 2000.
108. Xia, Y. et al., Diffusion and relaxation mapping of cartilage-bone plugs and excised disks using microscopic magnetic resonance imaging, *Magn. Reson. Med.*, 31, 273, 1994.
109. Bashir, A., Gray, M. L., and Burstein, D., Gd-DTPA as a measure of cartilage degradation, *Magn. Reson. Med.*, 36, 665, 1996.
110. Burstein, D., Bashir, A., and Gray, M. L., MRI techniques in early stages of cartilage disease, *Invest. Radiol.*, 35, 622, 2000.
111. Reddy, R. et al., Sodium MRI of human articular cartilage in vivo, *Magn. Reson. Med.*, 39, 697, 1998.
112. Shapiro, E. M. et al., 23Na MRI accurately measures fixed charge density in articular cartilage, *Magn. Reson. Med.*, 47, 284, 2002.
113. Peterfy, C. G., Imaging of the disease process, *Curr. Opin. Rheumatol.*, 14, 590, 2002.
114. Peterfy, C. G., Is there a role for extremity magnetic resonance imaging in routine clinical management of rheumatoid arthritis?, *J. Rheumatol.*, 31, 640, 2004.
115. Peterfy, C. G., Scratching the surface: articular cartilage disorders in the knee, *MRI Clin. N. Am.*, 8, 409, 2000.

Editorial Comments

Organ transplantation is the generally preferred medical procedure of treatment for patients with end-stage organ failure. In the late 1950s, the early years of transplantation, corticosteroids, together with azathioprine, provided the basis of maintenance immunosuppression. At that time, steroids were not only the primary immunosuppressive agents for maintenance regimens, but virtually stood alone as the treatment for acute rejection. With the advent of calcineurin inhibitors such as cyclosporine or tacrolimus in the early 1980s, the major role of corticosteroids in maintenance began to lessen. Currently, steroids are used primarily as adjunctive therapy together with immunosuppressants as calcineurin inhibitors, or targeted immunosuppressive agents as mycophenolate mofetil or rapamycin. Therapies developed in the past two decades have definitively improved the short-term survival of organ allografts.

Despite improvements in one-year allograft survival rates, the incidence of chronic allograft loss has remained high. Moreover, a significant drawback of current antirejection therapies is that recipients require life-long treatment on an immunosuppressive regimen and are thus potentially left at risk of side effects. Therefore, immunosuppressive protocols are optimized to minimize long-term complications, e.g., by avoiding, reducing, or withdrawing one or more medications from the multidrug regimens. In addition, the search for, and the development of, novel immunotherapeutic strategies with less side effects proceeds.

Finding biomarkers to noninvasively follow the status of allografts is fundamental in this research area. For instance, to determine which patients maintain functional organs despite discontinuation of an immunosuppressant. Or to find out if a new drug is enabling an allograft to function properly. Chapter 24 reviews the application of MR methods in the field of transplantation, highlighting their role for the noninvasive characterization of grafts *in situ*.

Cellular loss is common to many disease conditions. Recent evidence that these cells can be replaced has generated huge excitement over possible clinical applications. The use of stem or progenitor cells, which can differentiate into site-appropriate phenotypes required to repair the damaged tissue, has already demonstrated potential in animal models. However, many aspects of this novel therapeutic strategy require further elucidation, especially issues regarding the safety of cellular transplants.

Despite their importance, histological methods are limited in what concerns the examination of the dynamic of transplant-induced recovery. Ideally, the survival, migration, and functional consequences of transplanted cells should be probed noninvasively. In Chapter 25, Piotr Walczak and Jeff Bulte discuss how MRI is being used to serially visualize and monitor cellular transplants in intact living animals. These efforts are likely to provide important insights into the dynamics of *in vivo* cell biology, as well as to enable the monitoring of therapies based on the use of stem cells and progenitors.

24 *In Vivo* Magnetic Resonance Techniques in Transplantation Research

Nicolau Beckmann and Detlef Niese

CONTENTS

24.1 INTRODUCTION

Organ transplantation is nowadays the preferred and accepted treatment option in end-stage organ disease. The patient and transplant survival time following organ transplantation has improved substantially over the last decades. Several factors contributed to this development: progress in organ procurement, more stringent criteria for the selection of suitable donors and recipients, a better understanding of the biology, treatment and prevention of acute graft rejection, improved diagnosis and treatment of infectious complications, and better monitoring of transplanted patients.

The success rate of solid organ transplantation in terms of recipient actuarial survival has increased dramatically since the introduction of cyclosporine immunosuppressive therapy. Thanks to the fact that acute rejection can now be managed, chronic rejection remains the main complication. This involves both the reaction of the host to the graft (mainly T-cell mediated and also antibody — B-lymphocyte-driven) and reactions in the graft towards injury (vasculopathy or graft vessel disease in, e.g., kidney and heart grafts, *bronchiolitis obliterans* in lung grafts). Acute graft rejection requires highly active and tolerable immunosuppressants with an optimal side effect profile including tolerance-inducing approaches. However, treatment of chronic rejection still represents a major challenge. Protection of the graft (e.g., endothelial cells) from damage like ischemia/reperfusion injury or treatment of endothelial proliferation and vasculopathy are options which are being discussed [1–3].

Today, transplant recipients are being followed using many invasive and noninvasive diagnostic procedures, e.g., physical examination, biopsy, immunological monitoring, electrocardiography, ultrasound, radionuclide imaging, computerized tomography (CT), MRI, and MRS. Among those, noninvasive techniques for the diagnosis of graft rejection are particularly essential as they can provide information about the anatomical and functional status of the graft without exposing the patients to major risks. On the other hand, graft biopsy, the current gold standard in heart, kidney and liver transplantation, is not free of risk and subject to potential error of sampling.

The application of MR methods in the field of transplantation, highlighting their role for the noninvasive characterization of grafts *in situ* as compared to other available imaging techniques, has already been extensively reviewed earlier [4,5]. In this chapter, we focus on recent developments aiming at simplifying preclinical and clinical studies in solid organ transplantation.

24.2 CURRENT CRITERIA FOR CHARACTERIZING REJECTION OF GRAFTS

In general, allograft rejection can be defined as "an immunological reaction to the presence of a foreign tissue or organ, which has the potential to result in graft dysfunction and failure" [6]. Biopsies continue to be the gold standard to evaluate the state of rejection of a graft. Real-time ultrasound-guided allograft biopsy in conjunction with adoption of the Banff criteria [7] or of the Chronic Allograft Disease Index [8] for histological evaluation, are routinely performed to characterize kidney grafts [9]. Thus, acute rejection detected by biopsy, identified as a marker of long-term graft survival [8,10], is used together with actuarial graft and patient survival as an endpoint in kidney transplantation. Invasive endomyocardial biopsies, classified according to The International Society for Heart and Lung Transplantation grading system [11], are employed for cardiac transplant rejection surveillance. Percutaneous biopsies, classified according to Banff [12] or Birmingham criteria [13], are used to characterize liver allografts. Transbronchial biopsy is used for diagnosing rejection in lung and heart–lung transplantation patients, as the presence of inflammatory cell findings in biopsy specimens is highly specific for rejection. Biopsy specimens are graded according to the International Society for Heart and Lung Transplantation criteria [11].

The invasive nature, expenses, resources required, and the low but definite risks limit serial sampling, a serious disadvantage in clinical drug development. In addition, false–negative results can be obtained because of sampling errors, e.g., if a pattern of rejection shows a focal distribution.

These reasons have motivated investigators to search for less invasive procedures, as shown in the following sections.

24.2.1 Kidney Transplantation

Actuarial patient and graft survival remain the standard clinical endpoints in renal transplantation. Although initially graft failure at 1-year was used as an endpoint in clinical trials, improvements in graft survival in the past two decades shifted the endpoint from graft survival to acute rejection rates [14,15]. Ironically, the reduction achieved in acute rejection rates has limited the ability to assess the efficacy of newer immunosuppressive agents, calling for alternative short-term surrogate endpoint markers capable of predicting long-term renal transplant survival. Potential surrogate markers are clinical parameters such as renal function, renal histological findings of fibrosis, and immunological markers (see [16,17] and references within). Posttransplant renal function, estimated by serum creatinine within 1-year, has been shown to correlate with long-term survival. In clinical trials, the more accurate renal function assessment by clearance studies and cystatin C may be even more useful. Immunological markers, such as antidonor antibodies, levels of blood and urine cytokines, real time PCR, ELISPOT, and microarrays, may provide more insight into the immunological reaction of the host to the graft and *vice versa* [18]. Such data have been proposed as markers for diagnosis and monitoring of acute and chronic graft rejection.

Intense monitoring and radiological imaging are fundamental to ensure a successful outcome for renal transplantation. Several imaging techniques are routinely used to detect posttransplantation complications, including standard radiology, Doppler ultrasound (both gray-scale and color-flow Doppler), CT, conventional angiography, and perfusion urography.

24.2.2 Heart Transplantation

Acturial graft- and patient survival are also broadly accepted endpoints for the evaluation of the success of heart transplantation. The diagnosis of acute rejection is usually based on cardiac function parameters and confirmed by histological evaluation of endomyocardial biopsies. Chronic rejection manifests as coronary vessel disease with subendothelial thickening and reduction of coronary blood flow. The exact quantification of the process requires invasive techniques such as endovascular ultrasound. The search for noninvasive surveillance techniques for cardiac rejection has centered on measurements of cardiac function (e.g., analysis of heart rate variability [19], pulsed Doppler tissue imaging [20], acoustic quantification echocardiography [21], intragraft electrical events, peripheral proteomic markers of graft micronecrosis, immune activation, and nonimmune signs of rejection; for overviews, see [17,22,23]). Although several investigations indicated a reasonable negative predictive value of such monitoring, the specificity still remains poor. Scintigraphic methods aiming at the early and specific detection of graft necrosis and apoptosis seem to be one of the most promising approaches. However, well-planned studies are required to define the predictive values of these noninvasive techniques and to evaluate their clinical safety.

24.2.3 Liver Transplantation

Serum liver tests (bilirubin, alkaline phosphatase, and aspartate transaminase) may suggest the presence of acute rejection but are nonspecific. This is of particular relevance because these tests do not allow differentiation between graft rejection and infection, be it as a consequence of immunosuppression (e.g., *Cytomegalovirus* infection) or recurrence of hepatitis which may have been the reason for transplantation. Several inflammatory parameters in the bile or peripheral blood (e.g., cytokines as IL-2, IL-6, IL-8 or IL-10, ICAM-1, sIL-2R, sTNF-RII) are being investigated as potential markers of graft rejection, or to distinguish infection from acute rejection early after liver transplantation [24–26].

Imaging techniques are becoming essential in the management of orthotopic liver transplantation (for an overview, see [27,28]), fulfilling an important role in the preoperative evaluation and selection of suitable candidates. At the same time, they are essential in the early detection of postoperative complications, which can lead to clinical symptoms similar to those of acute rejection. Color Doppler ultrasonography [29] and CT [30] have been considered valuable tools for monitoring normal liver transplantation and biliary postoperative complications. T-tube cholangiography or invasive procedures, such as endoscopic retrograde cholangiography and percutaneous transhepatic cholangiography, are as well suited to assess biliary complications [31]. These techniques are also being used for therapeutic purposes. Despite being able to diagnose hepatic artery complications, digital subtraction angiography is not appropriate for screening because of its high costs and invasive nature with the associated risks and potential complications [32]. Doppler ultrasound is the primary modality used to evaluate the hepatic artery in the posttransplantation period [29].

24.2.4 Lung Transplantation

Cellular changes associated with rejection, as mild peripheral blood basophilia as well as increased proportions of lymphocytes in early and neutrophils in later-occurring rejection, observed in broncho-alveolar lavage fluid, are not considered specific for rejection but may warrant clinical suspicion of rejection [33,34]. Among imaging methods, high resolution CT and 18F-fluorodeoxyglucose (18FDG) positron emission tomography (PET) provide the potential for characterizing the rejection of lung transplants. In addition to bronchodilatation, CT allows monitoring of the diminution of peripheral bronchovascular markings, thickening of septal lines, and volume reduction, which usually precede the establishment of obliterating bronchiolitis, the equivalent of chronic rejection following lung transplantation [35]. 18FDG-PET enables to discriminate between infection and rejection in lung transplant recipients [36].

24.3 MR in Animal Studies of Transplantation

Many methods for minimizing the immunosuppressive requirements following allotransplantation have been proposed based on a growing understanding of physiological and allospecific immunity. Major reasons for these efforts are the clinical risks associated with immunosuppression as well as the specific safety concerns of the molecules used (e.g., nephrotoxicity, diabetogenicity, etc.). Before these regimens can be developed for clinical application, they require validation in models that are reasonably predictive of their performance in humans. Several animal models are available to develop organ transplant protocols and to test the effects of immunomodulatory compounds [37]. These models are also essential for identifying and validating possible biomarkers of acute and chronic rejection in view of translational research. Here, we address recent efforts in using MR techniques for the noninvasive characterization of solid organ grafts in animal studies of transplantation.

24.3.1 Kidney Transplantation

Orthotopic kidney transplantation models are adopted in rodents to study renal allograft rejection [38]. One of the recipient's kidneys is nephrectomized and replaced with a kidney from a syngeneic or from an allogeneic animal. The graft may have a life-supporting function, in which case the contralateral kidney from the recipient animal is also removed. However, the recipient's contralateral kidney may as well remain in place, and the entire rejection process may be followed with minimal physiological alterations.

24.3.1.1 Macrophage Infiltration into Kidney Grafts

Macrophages are key cells in the immunological defense system. They have the ability to ingest all kinds of material, foreign and self, and therefore play a key role in both the innate and adaptive immune responses. Their ability to act independently, or in concert with other cellular or humoral constituents of the immune system, allows them to play a vital role in host defense. Leukocyte infiltration, predominantly recipient-derived lymphocytes and macrophages, is a prominent feature of allograft rejection [39].

Detection of macrophage infiltration into allografts by MRI in combination with the administration of superparamagnetic iron oxide (SPIO) preparations has been proposed as a strategy to noninvasively characterize the graft rejection status in several rat models of transplantation. As mentioned in previous chapters, iron oxide particles of mean diameter of the order of 100 nm are not immediately trapped by the mononuclear phagocytic system, but can be taken up in the blood by monocytes through absorptive endocytosis [40]. The influx of iron loaded macrophages into the grafts may lead to detectable signal changes due to magnetic susceptibility effects.

Macrophage infiltration during the acute rejection process of kidney grafts has been demonstrated in the Dark Agouti (DA) to Brown Norway (BN) model [41,42]. Administration of ultrasmall superparamagnetic iron oxide (USPIO) particles, of mean diameter of the order of 30 nm, at day 4 posttransplantation led to distinct signal attenuation in the cortex of allogeneic kidneys one day later. Immunohistological staining for ED1 + macrophages and CD4 + and CD8 + T cells in allogeneic transplanted kidneys indicated the accumulation of these immune cells as acute rejection occurred. Morphological studies by electron microscopy confirmed the existence of iron particles inside the lysosomes of macrophages of rejecting kidneys, while Prussian blue staining detected the presence of iron plaques in macrophages. However, no signal reduction was observed in isografts and allografts of recipients receiving triple immunosuppressant treatment with daily subcutaneous injections of Methylprednisolone (2 mg/kg), Rapamycin (1 mg/kg) and Cyclosporine A (CsA) (5 mg/kg) [41].

Although numerous experimental and human studies have emphasized their presence during acute renal allograft rejection [39,43], early infiltration by macrophages is considered to be a poor prognostic sign for allograft survival [44]. Nevertheless, several studies support the hypothesis that macrophage-derived inflammation is a cofactor for chronic allograft nephropathy [45–47], monocytes/macrophages and T cells being the predominant graft-invading cells of rat renal allografts with chronic rejection [48–50]. In view of the fact that chronic graft dysfunction represents the leading cause for the still-unsatisfactory long-term results after organ transplantation, investigating macrophage infiltration into allografts during chronic rejection constitutes an important paradigm.

In the less stringent Fisher 344 to Lewis model, starting 12 weeks posttransplantation, MR images from grafts of untreated recipients that had received SPIO contrast agent (mean size of particles 150 nm) exhibited distinctive signal attenuation in the cortex [51]. Animals treated with CsA (Neoral 1.5 mg/kg/day p.o. by gavage for 10 days after transplantation) to prevent acute rejection showed a signal attenuation in the cortex at 33 weeks posttransplantation, while kidneys from rats treated additionally with everolimus (Certican 1.25 mg/kg/day p.o. by gavage until the end of the study), a rapamycin-derivative, had no changes in anatomical appearance (Figure 24.1). A significant negative correlation was found between the MRI cortical signal intensity and the histologically determined iron content in macrophages located in the cortex. Moreover, a very strong and highly significant negative correlation was found between the MRI signal in the cortex and the rejection scores according to the Banff classification [52], suggesting that this method might be considered as an alternative to histologic evaluation. Renography (see Section 24.3.1.3) revealed a significantly reduced functionality of the kidneys of untreated controls 33 weeks after transplantation, while no significant changes in perfusion were observed in any group of rats.

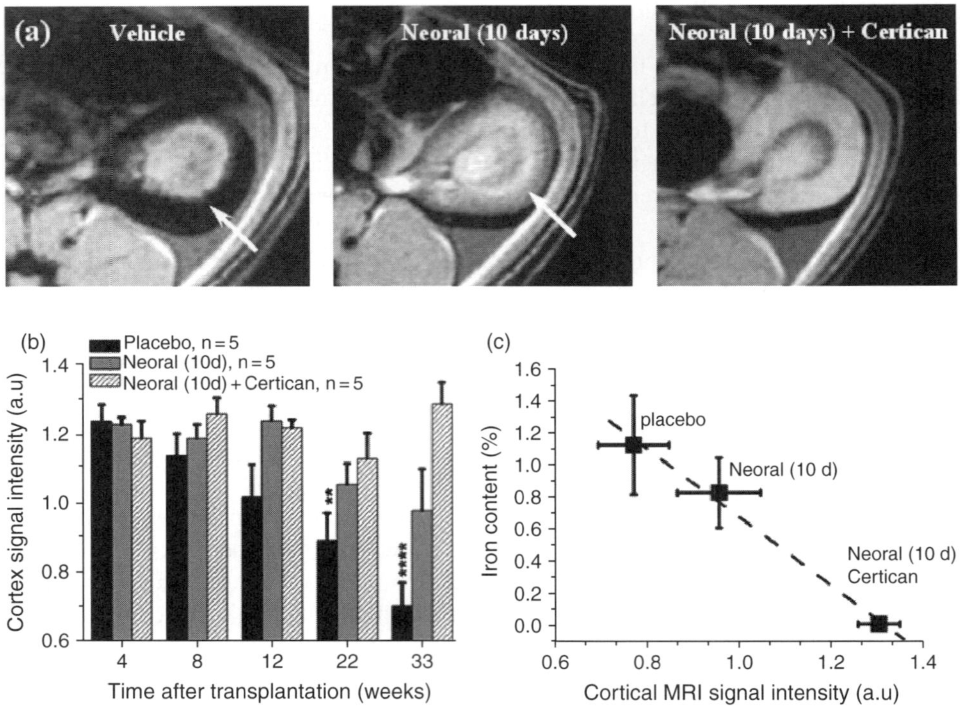

FIGURE 24.1 Macrophage infiltration into kidney grafts in the Fisher to Lewis transplantation model of chronic rejection. (a) Gradient-echo images (TR 16.8 msec, TE 8.4 msec, field of view 6×6 cm^2, matrix 256×128, slice 1.5 mm, number of averages 20) acquired at week 33 after transplantation from the grafts of an untreated control recipient, and of recipients treated with either CsA (Neoral 1.5 mg/kg/day p.o. for 10 days) or with CsA (Neoral 1.5 mg/kg/day p.o. for 10 days) and Certican (1.25 mg/kg/day p.o. during the whole study). No respiratory gating was applied during image acquisition. (b) Significant signal attenuation was observed in the cortex of grafts starting at week 12 after transplantation. SPIO (Endorem 0.5 ml/kg, Guerbet, France) was administered at a minimum interval of 4 weeks before image acquisition. (c) Mean ($\pm$ s.e.m. for five animals in each group) percentage of iron in the kidney cortex vs. mean ($\pm$ s.e.m. for five animals in each group) cortical MRI signal intensity. A significant negative correlation ($r = -0.86$, $p < 0.0001$) was found between the iron content in macrophages determined histologically and the MRI signal intensity. (Reproduced from Beckmann et al., *Magn. Reson. Med.*, 49, 459, 2003. With permission of John Wiley & Sons, Inc. Copyright 2003.)

Thus, graft nephropathy was detected significantly earlier than changes in graft function occurred by labeling macrophages with SPIO. Analysis of biochemical parameters in the urine and the blood revealed proteinuria starting at 16 weeks in CsA-treated recipients. However, creatinine and the glomerular filtration rate calculated from the amount of urine collected in a 24-h-period remained unchanged up to week 28 [52].

24.3.1.2 Kidney Perfusion

Transplanted organs frequently develop graft vessel disease, a form of accelerated arteriosclerosis that is a critical element of chronic rejection [53], which is responsible for over 50% of organ failure. Vascular changes are seen in 40 to 60% of the grafts within the first 5 years after transplantation, with typical persistent perivascular inflammation and concentric neointima formation often combined with medial thinning and necrosis [54].

Graft first-pass perfusion with a bolus tracking method based on the administration of intravascular contrast agents, e.g., SPIO [4,55–57] or USPIO [58], has been shown to be a reliable method to noninvasively detect vascular changes associated with the rejection process in rat kidney allografts (Figure 24.2). The superparamagnetic contrast agent induces local changes in susceptibility which result in a signal attenuation proportional to the perfusion of the kidney. Determination of absolute perfusion rates is not feasible due to fundamental problems in the assessment of the mean transit time or the mean residence time of the tracer in the tissue [59]. Nevertheless, it is possible to determine relative perfusion rates, which is perfectly acceptable considering that, in many cases, a native kidney can be used as reference. Perfusion indexes can be determined from the mean values of the ratios [60]

$$-\ln[S(t)/S(0)] \propto \mathrm{TE}Vc_T(t) \tag{24.1}$$

over a number of images following injection of the contrast agent (typically covering the first pass of the bolus), where $S(t)$ is the signal intensity in a given region at a time point t, $S(0)$ is the mean signal intensity in the same region at baseline (before injection of the contrast agent), TE is the echo time, V the blood volume, and c_T the concentration of contrast agent.

24.3.1.3 Renography

Extracellular contrast agents such as Gd-DTPA are predominantly cleared in the kidney. Therefore, dynamic changes of the T_1 relaxivity in the various kidney structures may provide information on its functionality. Renography involves a rapid intravenous bolus injection of a paramagnetic contrast agent (e.g., Gd-DTPA). Using T_1-weighted pulse sequences, the passage of the contrast agent through the renal system can be monitored in a time-resolved manner (Figure 24.3). Functional information is derived by analyzing the signal or the tracer concentration profiles [61,62]. Detection of compromised graft functionality by MRI renography has been demonstrated for the DA to Lewis [4] and for the Fisher to Lewis [51] models of kidney transplantation.

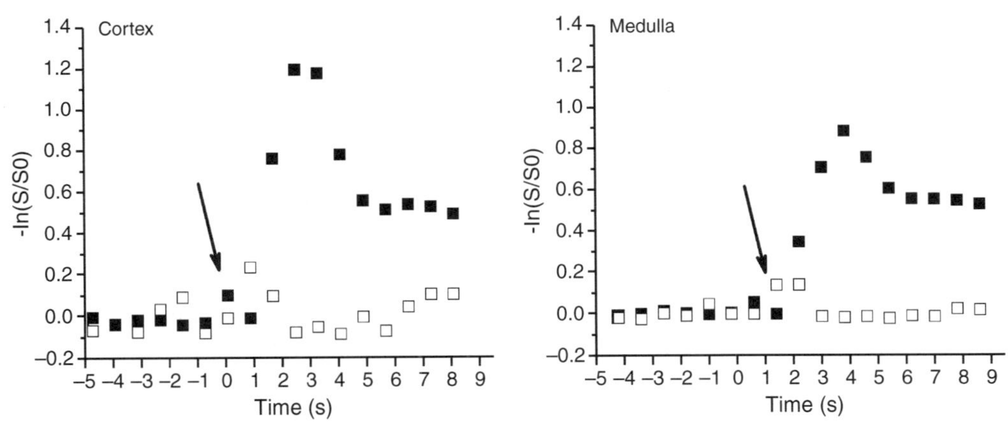

FIGURE 24.2 Graft perfusion assessments in Lewis recipients of DA kidneys using a bolus tracking approach at day 60 after transplantation. Gradient-echo images (TR 6.25 msec, TE 3.8 msec, matrix 128 × 64, pixel size = 470 × 940 μm^3, slice 2 mm, 2 averages) were acquired consecutively with a time resolution of 0.8 sec/image. After the acquisition of a number of baseline images, SPIO (Endorem 0.5 ml/kg) was injected i.v. as a bolus, during 1 sec (arrows). Position of the ROI's for signal evaluation was carefully chosen to ensure that they covered only either the cortex or the medulla, despite movements of the kidney caused by respiration. For the same amount of contrast agent injected, perfusion is proportional to the area under the curve. The results correspond to signal evaluation in the grafts of vehicle — (open symbols) and CsA (Neoral 7.5 mg/kg p.o. for 14 days)-treated (closed symbols) recipients. The graft of the vehicle-treated animal was severely rejected.

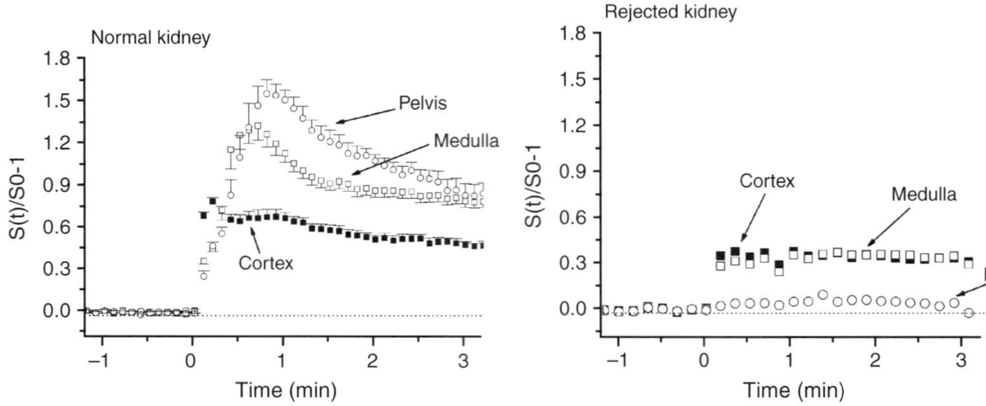

FIGURE 24.3 MRI renography of the rat kidney, assessing the clearance of an extracellular contrast agent (Gd-DOTA, 500 μl/kg, 0.25 mmol/ml) injected i.v. as a bolus, following the acquisition of ten baseline images. Prominent signal enhancement is seen in normal kidneys (left; mean values for five animals), first in the cortex, then in the medulla and in the pelvis. In the case of a rejected allograft (kidney from a DA rat transplanted into a Lewis rat, 90 days after transplantation), the signal enhancements achieved for the same amount of contrast agent are significantly reduced, indicating an impaired organ function. Gradient-echo images (TR 10 msec, TE = 2.4 msec, matrix = 128 × 64, pixel size = 400 × 800 μm^3, 2 mm slice, 16 averages) were acquired consecutively with a time resolution of 6 sec/image.

24.3.2 Heart Transplantation

Heterotopic heart or heterotopic heart and lung transplantation models are usually adopted in animal studies. This enables the rejection process to be studied without many physiological alterations, since the grafts do not have a life-supporting function. In these models, the recipient receives another heart (or heart and lung) outside the chest, for instance in the abdominal region, while the native organs are kept in place [63–65].

24.3.2.1 Macrophage Infiltration into Cardiac Grafts

Similarly to kidney transplantation, gradient-echo MRI in combination with the administration of USPIO 24 h before image acquisition was shown to offer promise as a noninvasive method for detecting acute cardiac transplant allograft rejection. In a DA to BN rat model of heart transplantation, at postoperative day 7 a significant reduction in MR signal intensity was observed in allotransplanted hearts, which developed moderate rejection. Syngeneic transplants showed no differences in MR signal intensities before and after USPIO injections. After injection of USPIO particles at postoperative day 6, a group of allotransplanted rats were treated with CsA (3 mg/kg). Recipients treated with CsA for 7 days showed no reduction in MR signal intensity after USPIO reinjection at day 14, whereas animals treated for 4 days showed a significant decrease in MR signal intensity in the transplanted hearts indicative of acute allograft rejection. Pathological analysis of these animals revealed that dextran-coated USPIO particles were taken up by the infiltrating macrophages that accumulated within the rejecting cardiac graft [66].

24.3.2.2 Permeability of Microvasculature in Cardiac Grafts

USPIO or SPIO particles constitute blood pool contrast agents which normally remain within the vascular space. However, they might leak into the interstitial space in areas of inflammation associated with rejection, where vascular permeability is increased. Following this reasoning, it has been shown in the PVG to Wistar/Kyoto model that acutely rejecting heart transplants can be distinguished from nonrejecting ones using MRI in combination with the administration of an USPIO contrast agent [67]. On the 2nd and 6th postoperative days, USPIO (2 mg iron/kg body weight) was injected i.v., followed for 44 min by three-dimensional T_1-weighted MRI of the heart grafts, with an imaging time of 2 min per image. At day 6, there was a significant increase of the signal intensity in the myocardium in allografts compared to that in syngeneic controls, indicating an increased leakage of the contrast agent. Furthermore, in the allogeneic group, the histologically determined degree of rejection correlated positively with the relative MRI signal enhancement [67].

24.3.2.3 Cardiac Contractile Function

Tagging is a powerful tool to assess the mechanical function of the heart. Grid-like tags, composed of planes of saturated signals intersecting the myocardium, are generated by, for example, SPAMM schemes [68] applied prior to the imaging sequence, thus providing points for tracking regional wall motion and contractility. Tags are applied as close as possible to the R wave to enable tracking motion throughout the whole systole and diastole phases. Losses in mechanical function at early acute rejection has been detected in a heterotopic working heart model in rats [5].

24.3.3 Lung Transplantation

As pointed out before, intraabdominal heterotopic heart and lung transplantation models in small rodents are usually adopted [63–65]. To avoid interference of abdominal gases and bowel and respiratory movements during acquisition of MR images, Kanno et al. [69] developed a new model of heterotopic heart and lung transplantation into the inguinal region.

As in kidney and heart transplantation models, gradient-echo MRI in combination with USPIO administration has been shown to be of value for monitoring macrophage infiltration into allogeneic lung grafts in the DA to BN model [69]. At day 5 after transplantation, allografts in animals without CsA treatment were severely rejected as revealed by histology. Correspondingly, USPIO led to a significant signal attenuation in images of allografts 24 h after being administered. Syngeneic transplants showed no evidence of rejection and no differences in MRI signals between the images before and after injection of USPIO. Allotransplants in animals treated with CsA showed mild rejection. USPIO-induced MRI signal changes in CsA-treated animals were smaller than those observed in untreated allografts. Immunohistochemistry and iron staining of the allografts indicated that USPIO particles were taken up by the infiltrating macrophages that accumulated at the rejection site [69].

24.4 MR IN CLINICAL STUDIES

In order to evaluate the feasibility of incorporating MR techniques into clinical trials in transplantation, it is important to understand what they can contribute to patient care following organ transplantation. The following sections will explore recent applications of MR in the pre- and posttransplantation phases.

24.4.1 Kidney Transplantation

Because of its direct multiplanar capability, superb soft tissue contrast and ability to obtain dynamic 3D angiograms using contrast agents lacking nephrotoxicity, MRI and especially MR angiography (MRA) are ideal techniques for evaluating pre- and posttransplant kidneys [70,71].

24.4.1.1 Pretransplant Assessment of Donors and Graft Viability

Renal angiography is the final step in the work-up of potential kidney donors. This method is used to identify the number of renal arteries for each kidney, to determine the presence of early first order renal artery branches, and to diagnose abnormalities of the renal arteries such as stenoses. The findings can influence the choice of which kidney will be harvested or exclude a donor.

Conventional angiography is costly and risky for the evaluation of healthy living kidney donors. As an alternative, contrast-enhanced 3D MRA has been demonstrated to be not only a reliable, noninvasive tool for the preoperative evaluation of potential living renal donors [72–74], but even superior to digital subtraction angiography (DSA) in assessing the renal vasculature in living kidney donors [75] (Figure 24.4).

Using a decision-analytic model, Liem et al. [76] evaluated the societal cost-effectiveness of DSA, gadolinium-enhanced MRA, contrast material-enhanced spiral CT angiography, and

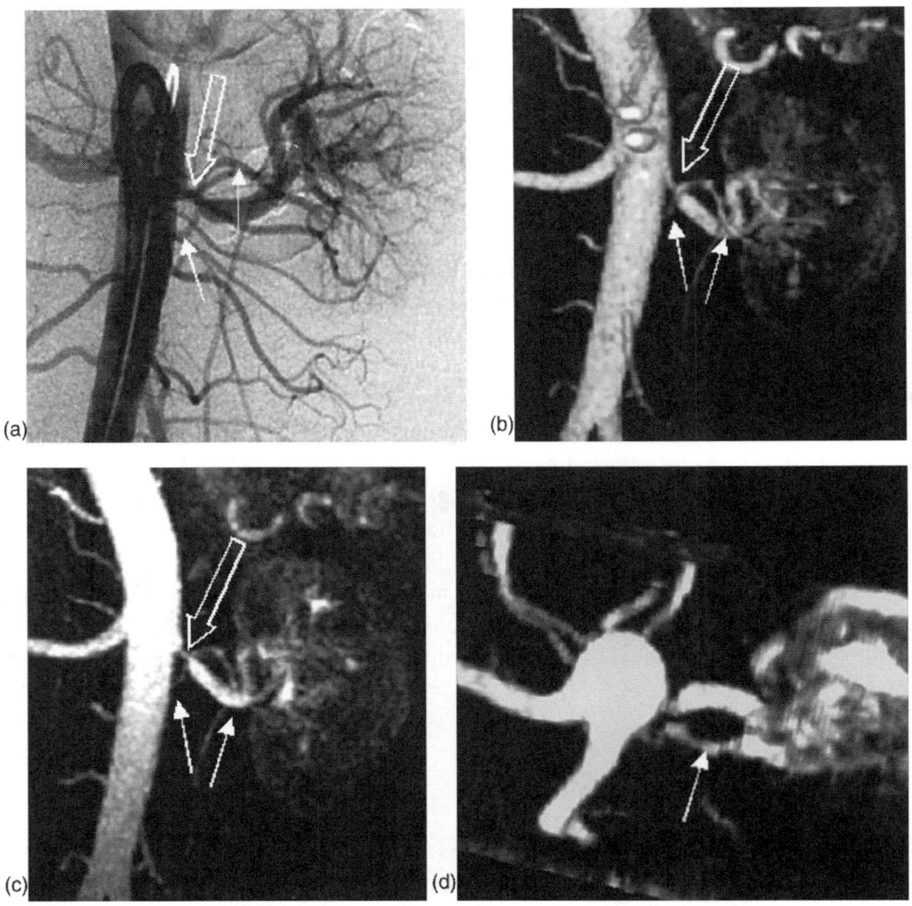

FIGURE 24.4 A 58-year-old male potential living renal donor. (a) DSA suffering from overlay by branches of superior mesenteric artery. The accessory renal artery (arrows) was initially not identified and misdiagnosed as a branch of the superior mesenteric artery. Additional findings of a stenosis (~70%) of left main renal artery (open arrow). (b) Volume rendering and (c) maximum intensity projection (MIP) of a contrast-enhanced 3D MRA data set clearly visualizes accessory renal artery (arrows) and stenosis of left main renal artery (open arrow). (d) Volume rendering of a contrast-enhanced 3D MRA data set (cranial view) clearly demonstrates small accessory renal artery (arrow) originating ventrally to the main renal artery. (Reproduced from Fink et al., *Eur. Radiol.*, 13, 794, 2003. Courtesy of Dr. C. Fink. With permission of Springer, Heidelberg. Copyright 2003.)

combinations of these imaging techniques. For preoperative imaging in a potential renal donor, DSA is the most cost-effective strategy if it has a specificity greater than 99% for detection of renal disease; otherwise, MRA combined with CT angiography is the most cost-effective strategy.

The diagnostic value of MR urography in detecting abnormalities of the urinary tract for the preoperative evaluation of living renal donors was assessed by Bakker et al. [77]. MR urography is performed by pursuing two different imaging strategies [78]. In the first case, heavily T_2-weighted turbo spin-echo sequences are employed to obtain unenhanced static images of the urinary tract. In the second approach imitating conventional intravenous pyelography, referred to as excretory MR urography, a gadolinium contrast agent is injected i.v. and, after its renal excretion, the gadolinium-enhanced urine is imaged with fast T_1-weighted gradient-echo sequences. Both MR urographic techniques can be combined for a comprehensive examination of the upper urinary tract. Image quality was found to be inadequate to evaluate the calyces and pelvis for small filling defects or deformities in approximately 25% of the patients; however, the technique was accurate in detecting abnormalities of the urinary collecting system as needed for the preoperative evaluation of living renal donors [77]. It may replace invasive procedures such as antegrade pyelography in the preoperative work-up.

As acute tubular necrosis is still an important cause for postoperative malfunction of renal grafts, it is desirable to have a method predicting such a complication. The ratio of phosphomonoesters (PME, largely consisting of adenosine monophosphate) and inorganic phosphate (Pi) in the renal tissue, assessed using 31P MRS during the cold ischemia period, had been proposed earlier as an indicator of graft quality [79]. The PME/Pi ratio calculated from chemical shift imaging (CSI) spectra has recently been shown to be a reliable indicator of viability of renal grafts [80]. Early knowledge of graft quality may allow preservation of the graft and postoperative therapy to be adapted to the conditions of the organ, for example, by initial withholding of nephrotoxic calcineurin inhibitors (see also Section 24.5) in patients with a high risk of delayed graft function.

24.4.1.2 Posttransplant Assessment of Complications

Certain complications are inevitable during long-term follow up of transplanted patients: peritransplant fluid collections, vascular and urologic problems, infection, rejection, malignancy, and nephrotoxicity [81]. Although Doppler ultrasound is helpful to detect most vascular conditions of the renal allograft, sonographic findings are occasionally nonspecific [82]. MRI and gadolinium-enhanced 3D MRA are the safest method to assess suspected complications associated with allograft renal vasculature, despite the fact that ultrasound and CT scans are still largely chosen for renal allograft evaluation. Contrast-enhanced 3D MRA has been demonstrated to be a reliable method for identifying postoperative arterial stenoses after kidney transplantation [83]. In addition, dynamic MR angiography can be helpful in detecting venous complications and perfusion defects in kidney allografts.

The diagnostic work-up of renal transplants with impaired function due to urological problems can be difficult. Contrast-enhanced MR urography has been found to be a highly sensitive and specific noninvasive method to evaluate patients suspected of having typical posttransplant urological complications [84].

Automated parametric quantification of cortical and medullary enhancement is feasible and allows the accurate detection of nonsurgical complications in renal transplants by MR renography [85]. The mean medullary nephronal washout rate and cortical arterial blood volume have been found to be lower in diseased renal transplants. The combination of these parameters is thus a strong predictor of renal transplant disease.

31P MRS has been considered as a noninvasive technique to determine long-term posttransplant renal prognosis. Using the ISIS sequence for spectral localization, Seto et al. [86] found that a beta-adenosine triphosphate/inorganic phosphate (beta-ATP/Pi) ratio larger than

1.2 had a sensitivity of 93%, specificity of 100%, and accuracy of 95% in predicting 3-year renal survival; a beta-ATP/Pi ratio larger than 1.2 had a sensitivity of 91%, specificity of 67%, and accuracy of 77% for predicting 5-year renal survival.

24.4.2 Heart Transplantation

Only few clinical studies employing MR techniques to detect heart rejection in humans have been published to date. Nevertheless, cardiac MRI has been shown to be a promising technique for the detection of graft rejection [87]. In a prospective study in which cardiac MRI was performed at the same time as the scheduled endomyocardial biopsies, the aim was to assess the value of Gd-enhanced cardiac MRI to detect rejection (necrosis) and its ability to discriminate it from other pathologic alterations (edema and fibrosis). Pre- and postcontrast white and black-blood anatomic sequences (breathhold fast spin-echo T_1-weighted images), as well as myocardial cine, perfusion, and viability sequences, were used to determine ejection fraction, ventricular volumes, pericardial effusion, hypertrophy, and myocardial contrast agent uptake. Patients with myocyte necrosis showed increased myocardial uptake, while interstitial fibrosis has been associated with decreased levels of uptake [87].

Transplant arteriopathy often lacks clinical symptoms and is the reason for frequent surveillance angiography in heart transplant recipients. MR perfusion imaging based on the administration of a Gd-chelate allows the noninvasive assessment of transmural and selective endomyocardial and epimyocardial perfusion. It has been demonstrated that the technique is able to detect cardiac graft arteriopathy reflected in a decreased myocardial perfusion rate [88]. After the exclusion of left ventricular hypertrophy and prior rejection, the resting endomyocardial/epimyocardial perfusion ratio might be sufficient to indicate arteriopathy.

Animal studies suggested an increase of T_2 values during rejection [89]. Marie et al. [90] evaluated if myocardial T_2, determined using a black-blood MRI sequence (an original inversion-recovery/spin-echo sequence), could predict acute heart transplant rejection. The use of such sequences allows suppression of the confusing influence of blood signal when myocardial T_2 is calculated to detect edema. The technique was found to be not only sufficiently sensitive to identify most of the moderate acute rejections documented with biopsy at the same time, but to be also able to predict the subsequent occurrence of such biopsy-defined rejections.

P31 MRS was used to measure ratios of various high-energy phosphate metabolites and the intracellular pH in grafts *ex vivo*. The ratio PCr/Pi and the intracellular pH as markers of ischemic injury before transplantation can be considered as an objective and accurate criterion for the decision to accept or refuse heart grafts for transplantation [91]. Under *in vivo* conditions and using a P31 CSI protocol, Buchthal et al. [92] showed that, although significantly lower than in normal control subjects, resting myocardial PCr/ATP ratios of transplant subjects are not useful in assessing the level of cardiac rejection. Perhaps this measurement may be more predictive in mildly exercised myocardium.

24.4.3 Liver Transplantation

Improvements in immunosuppression have increased 5-year survival rates of patients after liver transplantation to greater than 70%. Thus, liver transplantation is now considered a curative therapeutic option for patients with end-stage liver disease. MRI techniques, in particular MR arteriography, venography, and cholangiography, allow a comprehensive noninvasive investigation of anatomic and pathologic features in pre- and postoperative liver transplant patients, and may eventually replace many, if not all, of the numerous diagnostic examinations performed in this patient population [93,94].

24.4.3.1 Pretransplant Assessments

Potential liver donors must undergo an extensive and costly preharvest assessment, during which the majority of candidates are eliminated, mostly because of an unfavorable hepatic parenchymal or vascular morphological state. The current evaluation protocol proceeds in a stepwise fashion and includes CT for liver planimetry and exclusion of parenchymal lesions, endoscopic retrograde cholangiopancreatography for assessment of the biliary anatomy in selected cases, and DSA for depiction of the hepatic vascular system [95]. Knowledge of the hepatic parenchymal and vascular anatomy is crucial to reduce the incidence of complications after transplantation [96].

The combination of contrast-enhanced MRA (CE-MRA) with MR anatomical imaging involving the administration of Gd-containing contrast material was shown to have superior diagnostic value than intraarterial DSA (i.a.DSA) to examine liver transplantation candidates [97,98]. Although both approaches furnish similar results concerning the arterial part of the vascular supply to the liver, CE-MRA is significantly better for the detection of collaterals and for the assessment of the inferior vena cava, the hepatic and the renal veins. CE-MRA in combination with MR anatomical imaging is also superior to i.a.DSA in the detection of liver malignancy [97].

The same technique was also found to be more sensitive than helical CT for the detection of hepatocellular carcinoma [99], the fifth most common neoplasm in the world and the leading cause of death among cirrhotic patients [100]. MR may offer an advantage over CT in the detection of focal parenchymal lesions in patients awaiting liver transplantation [101].

Ferumoxides in combination with gradient-echo sequences may improve the diagnostic accuracy and the sensitivity to detect malignant hepatic lesions in patients with end-stage cirrhosis of the liver. However, the specificity is not improved even after the administration of ferumoxides because of the false–positive lesions that are mainly the result of fibrotic changes [102].

In summary, MR volumetry, venography, angiography, and cholangiography with three-dimensional reconstruction is sufficient for all major imaging evaluation [95,103]. A comprehensive assessment of the hepatic parenchyma, biliary and pancreatic ductal system, and hepatic arterial, portal, and venous systems can be accomplished using a single MR protocol [104]. This may replace the traditional conventional catheter angiography, computed tomography, sonography, and endoscopic retrograde cholangiography as a single investigation in the evaluation of the potential liver transplant donors.

24.4.3.2 Posttransplant Assessments

Kim et al. [105] evaluated the efficacy of CE-MRA for detecting vascular complications in patients who have undergone living-related liver transplantation. The study demonstrated that MRA was sensitive, but not specific, in the detection of significant vascular stenosis after transplantation. At least, MRA findings reliably excluded the possibility of significant stenosis.

24.4.4 Lung Transplantation

Although CT is the standard imaging procedure in the follow-up after lung transplantation, it suffers from serious disadvantages. Unfortunately, CT often shows few or even no changes despite clinical deterioration of the patient's condition. Furthermore, it is considered to be an insensitive technique for the diagnosis of obliterating bronchiolitis, the equivalent of chronic rejection following lung transplantation. The evidence of air trapping is frequently used as a diagnostic hint [106].

MRI of the lungs using hyperpolarized ^{3}He gases (see also Chapter 18 and Chapter 19) has been shown to be well suited to detect ventilation defects in lung-transplant recipients [107]. The technique is clearly superior to morphologic imaging with CT. However, it still remains to be determined if ventilation defects in clinically asymptomatic lung-transplant recipients are early signs of obliterating bronchiolitis. Also, the specificity of ^{3}He-MRI needs to be evaluated.

Mismatch in ventilation and perfusion is a pronounced phenomenon in recipients of lung transplants due to pulmonary vascular disease [108]. Conventional nuclear ventilation/perfusion (V/Q) scanning is limited in spatial resolution and requires exposure to radioactivity. The sequential use of ^{3}He-MRI and perfusion imaging provides a tool for studying V/Q relationships in lung transplant patients [109]. Perfusion images can be acquired without the use of contrast agents, applying for instance arterial spin-labeling techniques [110]. It has been shown that ^{3}He distribution and blood perfusion appeared uniform in normal subjects and throughout nonrejected lung allografts, while the gas distribution and perfusion in emphysematous lungs were nonuniform and paralleled radiographic abnormalities [109].

Techniques based on imaging hyperpolarized gases are likely to become very valuable tools for assessing ventilation defects in transplanted lungs. However, despite the excellent contrast achieved in imaging hyperpolarized gases, the cost and technical demands in producing them still restrict the general applicability of this method. Oxygen-enhanced approaches, which make use of molecular oxygen as contrast agent [111], are significantly easier to implement and could become an interesting alternative in the near future (see also Chapter 18 and Chapter 19).

24.5 TOXIC EFFECTS OF COMPOUNDS

Besides eventually detecting the positive effects of compounds, MR techniques might also be used to study their toxicity (see also Chapter 26). For instance, fluid-attenuated inversion-recovery (FLAIR) and diffusion-weighted MRI have been used to investigate tacrolimus (FK-506)-induced encephalopathy [112,113]. The techniques were shown to be useful in predicting the outcome of tacrolimus-induced neurotoxicity. It has been suggested that FK-506 encephalopathy may be triggered by the disturbance of the electrolyte and/or fluid equilibrium, given a certain serum level of the compound.

Also, CsA is infrequently associated with an acute encephalopathy including seizures and alterations in mental status. The areas involving a presumed CsA toxicity are similar to those seen in FK-506 toxicity. Gleeson et al. [114] reviewed the clinical history, electroencephalogram (EEG), and neuroimaging findings in 19 children with CsA-induced acute encephalopathy and seizure syndrome over a 10-year period, in order to delineate clinical characteristics, imaging features, and to determine the risk of seizure recurrence in this population. It appears that a significant risk of seizure recurrence exists following CsA-induced acute encephalopathy and seizure syndrome, primarily in those children with persistent EEG or imaging abnormalities.

For over two decades, calcineurin inhibitors have been the mainstay of immunosuppressive therapy following solid organ transplantation. However, calcineurin inhibitor nephrotoxicity is one of the main contributors to chronic kidney allograft dysfunction. A novel class of immunosuppressants that inhibit the kinase mammalian target of rapamycin (mTOR), although not nephrotoxic themselves, enhance calcineurin inhibitor nephrotoxicity. *Ex vivo* studies using an MRS-based metabonomic approach revealed that calcineurin inhibitor toxicity is caused by drug-induced mitochondrial dysfunction and that mTOR inhibitors enhance the negative effects of calcineurin inhibitors on cell energy metabolism [115].

Muromonab-CD3 (OKT3), a mouse monoclonal antibody directed against human T lymphocytes, is a potent immunosuppressive agent used to reverse and prevent allograft rejection, mostly in cardiac transplant recipients [116]. Neurotoxicity from OKT3 usually manifests itself as transient aseptic meningitis and remains uncommon. A dramatic neurologic syndrome after orthotopic heart transplant characterized by akinetic mutism, blepharospasm, anomic aphasia, and delirium has been recently described [117]. MRI showed meningeal enhancement and single-photon emission computed tomography (SPECT) showed markedly reduced tracer uptake. Discontinuation of OKT3 resulted in resolution of this neuropsychiatric syndrome, and reversal of abnormalities on neuroimaging that coincided with normalization of CD3 + lymphocyte count.

MRI and cerebral perfusion studies may help support the diagnosis of encephalopathic signs to toxicity of immunosuppressive drugs.

24.6 MR TECHNIQUES FOR PHARMACEUTICAL RESEARCH IN TRANSPLANTATION

Table 24.1 provides an overview of the present use of MR techniques in the area of transplantation. Because of its good spatial resolution and versatility, MRI already has a significant role in preclinical drug studies in small rodents. Repetitive measurements are feasible, and allow the easy collection of time series data. This is very important, since transplantation studies usually have a long duration (weeks to months). Moreover, MR readouts are readily available, allowing flexible and adaptable experimental protocol designs. For instance, one may conceive changing therapeutic regimens or terminating a study according to changes detected in MR signatures. The use of MR in animal studies of transplantation may also impact the design of clinical studies (see below). Evidently, histology will continue to be essential in preclinical activities. However, despite its obvious advantages concerning spatial resolution and staining capabilities, it is a terminal and time consuming procedure.

In clinical transplantation studies, however, MR is at present a less prominently used diagnostic procedure. Depending on the transplanted organ, other imaging modalities as well as biopsies and histological evaluations are routinely being employed. Therefore, it is important to determine for which applications MR may offer advantages compared to other techniques, and to properly validate the methodology in such cases. Only then will MR be considered for clinical trials in transplantation by clinical researchers, clinicians, and authorities. Also, possible adverse effects on transplanted organs of contrast agents used in MR studies need to be excluded. Major promises of MR technology include less or no invasiveness, speed, fast availability of readouts, standardization, documentation, and the possibility to investigate functional rather than just structural changes. These promises are even more critical as more and more organs — mostly kidneys but now also livers with increasing frequency — are obtained from living donors. Here, a careful and extensive screening is not only of relevance for ensuring the quality of the graft but also for the safety of the organ donor. It should be noted that animal studies can be very useful to validate MR compared to other imaging techniques and to other parameters of rejection [57]. Furthermore, such studies may be important in the search and validation of new noninvasive markers of rejection. Validation studies can be optimized and performed much easier in rodents before being transferred to the clinical situation.

Despite the many promises of MR, cost has been a major hurdle for the broader introduction of this technology into transplantation diagnostics. Today, the impact of a given technology on general health care cost is an important aspect which cannot be ignored. A solid organ transplantation in human costs between, approximately, US$60,000 and 90,000, not including long-term immunosuppression and patient monitoring. Evidently, in addition to the stress on the patients, especially in view of the chronic shortage in donor organs, graft loss imposes major costs. Therefore, any monitoring method that improves the chances of graft survival while increasing the safety of the patients is also highly attractive from an economic point of view. Such a procedure includes donor selection, graft characterization prior to transplantation, and close patient monitoring following transplantation (e.g., detection of complications, patient management). In this sense, even expensive diagnostic methods, such as MRI, are clearly attractive from a health economics point-of-view.

These aspects are also of interest when considering the use of MR in clinical transplantation trials. As mentioned above, many factors determine the success of a transplantation procedure, amongst which the immunosuppressive therapy is only one. Other factors include the condition of the donor before explantation, quality and preservation of the graft, duration of

TABLE 24.1
Summary of Recent Studies Involving the Use of MR Techniques in Transplantation Research

Organ	Approach	Comments	References
Kidney	Macrophage infiltration with SPIO or USPIO	Preclinical; clinical use needs to be shown	[41,42,51,52]
	Perfusion	Preclinical	[4,55–58]
	Renography with Gd-containing contrast agents	Preclinical and clinical studies available; however, careful clinical validation still lacking. Detection of nonsurgical complications of renal transplants	[4,51,56,85]
	Contrast-enhanced 3D MRA	Clinical; preoperative evaluation of living renal donors; identification of postoperative arterial stenoses	[72–75,83]
	MR urography	Clinical; preoperative evaluation of living renal donors; evaluation of patients having posttransplant urological complications	[77,78,84]
	31P MRS	PME/Pi ratio as an indicator of viability of renal grafts. Determination of long-term posttransplant renal prognosis based on beta-ATP/Pi ratio	[79,80,86]
Heart	Macrophage infiltration with USPIO	Preclinical	[66]
	Vessel permeability with USPIO	Preclinical	[67]
	Contractile function	Preclinical	[5]
	Gd-enhanced cardiac MRI	Clinical; detection of necrosis (rejection)	[87]
	Perfusion MRI with Gd-chelates	Clinical; detection of cardiac graft arteriopathies	[88]
	Assessment of myocardial T_2 using black-blood MRI sequences	Determination of acute heart rejection	[90]
Liver	Contrast-enhanced MRA	Clinical; examination of liver transplantation candidates; detection of postoperative vascular complications	[97,98,105]
	MR volumetry, venography, angiography, and cholangiography	Clinical; comprehensive assessment of the hepatic parenchyma, biliary and pancreatic ductal system, and hepatic arterial, portal, and venous systems accomplished using a single MR protocol	[95,103,104]
Lung	Macrophage infiltration with USPIO	Preclinical	[69]
	3He-MRI	Clinical; detection of ventilation defects; in combination with perfusion MRI, assessments of ventilation/perfusion mismatch	[107–109]

More comprehensive studies are necessary to validate the use of these techniques in the context of drug trails.

explantation procedure and transport, and general condition and morbidity of the recipient. Efficient characterization and selection of donors and grafts prior to transplantation, as well as clear differentiation between surgical complications and those with an immunological origin, are therefore critical to derive meaningful data from a clinical trial with an immunosuppressive drug. Thus, MRI may play an important role to better define the quality of the grafts and the patient population to be included in a clinical trial. After proper validation, it may also be possible to use MRI technologies to reduce the need for biopsies and histological evaluations. This would be of particular relevance in heart and lung transplantation where routine serial biopsies, invasive ultrasound techniques, or functional evaluations are needed to identify emerging graft rejections or chronic rejection early enough. Chronic graft rejection is the major reason for graft loss in all organs. Once established, it is considered a nonreversable condition. Early detection of chronic rejection is therefore a critical need. Transplantation is typically performed in large centers or university hospitals, which usually have MR systems. Still, the costs of approximately US$ 1000 for a clinical imaging session might be an issue when considering the use of MRI in phase 3 and 4 studies. However, aside of the cost for the procedure, when making such decisions one also has to calculate the cost for alternative techniques, their diagnostic value, and costs caused by diagnostics related morbidity [76].

As a further diagnostic tool, proteomics/genomics biomarkers in the blood and urine are currently in development with the hope of being able to distinguish patients without a rejection from those with an acute rejection [118–120]. However, such biomarkers will also have to be properly validated. Furthermore, lack of specificity still appears to be an issue with these important markers. Imaging, on the other hand, provides the potential for monitoring the status of a graft *in situ*. It is not unlikely that, in the future, a combination of imaging, proteomics/genomics biomarkers, and clinical diagnosis tools will enable characterization of a transplant without the need of biopsies. This would benefit patients and improve drug trials in transplantation. To reach this development, a strong collaborative work of researchers in experimental laboratories and clinics is necessary.

ACKNOWLEDGMENTS

We are greatefully indebted to Maddeleine Tanner, Dr. Christian Bruns, Akiko Hof, Prof. Robert Hof, Prof. Randall Morris (Stanford), and Charles Pally for the support on transplantation, to Catherine Cannet for her histological work, and to Stefan Zurbruegg for technical aid.

REFERENCES

1. Lietz, K. and Miller, L. W., Current understanding and management of allograft vasculopathy, *Semin. Thorac. Cardiovasc. Surg.*, 16, 386, 2004.
2. Patel, J. K. and Kobashigawa, J. A., Immunosuppression, diagnosis, and treatment of cardiac allograft rejection, *Semin. Thorac. Cardiovasc. Surg.*, 16, 378, 2004.
3. Ponticelli, C., Renal transplantation : where do we stand today?, *Nephrol. Dial. Transplant.*, 19, 2937, 2004.
4. Beckmann, N., Hof, R. P., and Rudin, M., The role of magnetic resonance imaging and spectroscopy in transplantation: from animal models to man, *NMR Biomed.*, 13, 329, 2000.
5. Wu, Y. J. et al., MRI investigations of graft rejection following organ transplantation using rodent models, *Methods Enzymol.*, 386, 73, 2004.
6. International Working Party, Terminology for hepatic allograft rejection, *Hepatology*, 22, 648, 1995.
7. Racusen, L. C. et al., The Banff 97 working classification of renal allograft pathology, *Kidney Int.*, 55, 713, 1999.

8. Yilmaz, S. et al., Protocol core needle biopsy and histologic Chronic Allograft Damage Index (CADI) as surrogate end point for long-term graft survival in multicenter studies, *J. Am. Soc. Nephrol.*, 14, 773, 2003.
9. Fisher, J. S., Woodle, E. S., and Thistlethwaite, J. R. Jr., Kidney transplantation: graft monitoring and immunosuppression, *World J. Surg.*, 26, 185, 2002.
10. Hariharan, S. et al., Improved graft survival after renal transplantations in recipient in the United States, 1988 to 1996, *N. Engl. J. Med.*, 342, 605, 1999.
11. Winters, G. L., Marboe, C. C., and Billingham, M. E., The international society for heart and lung transplantation grading system for heart transplant biopsy specimens: clarification and commentary, *J. Heart Lung Transplant.*, 17, 754, 1998.
12. Demetris, A. J. et al., Banff schema for grading liver allograft rejection: an international consensus document, *Hepatology*, 25, 658, 1997.
13. Mirza, D. F. et al., Timing and candidacy for transplantation in acute liver failure: the European experience, *Liver Transpl. Surg.*, 1, 182, 1995.
14. Kahan, B. D., Efficacy of sirolimus compared with azathioprine for reduction of acute renal allograft rejection: a randomized multicenter study. The rapamune US study group, *Lancet*, 356, 194, 2000.
15. Mcdonald, A. S., A worldwide, phase III, randomized, controlled, safety and efficacy study of a sirolimus/cyclosporine regimen for the prevention of acute rejection in recipients of primary mismatched renal allografts, *Transplantation*, 71, 271, 2001.
16. Hariharan, S. et al., Surrogate markers for long-term renal allograft survival, *Am. J. Transplant.*, 4, 1179, 2004.
17. Hartono, C., Dadhania, D., and Suthanthiran, M., Noninvasive diagnosis of acute rejection of solid organ transplants, *Front. Biosci.*, 9, 145, 2004.
18. Hutchinson, P. et al., Laboratory assessment of immune function in renal transplant patients, *Nephrol. Dial. Transplant.*, 18, 983, 2003.
19. Izrailtyan, I. et al., Early detection of acute allograft rejection by linear and nonlinear analysis of heart rate variability, *J. Thorac. Cardiovasc. Surg.*, 120, 737, 2000.
20. Fabregas, R. I. et al., Usefulness of pulsed doppler tissue imaging for noninvasive detection of cardiac rejection after heart transplantation, *Transplant. Proc.*, 31, 2545, 1999.
21. Moidl, R. et al., Noninvasive monitoring of peak filling rate with acoustic quantification echocardiography accurately detects acute cardiac allograft rejection, *J. Heart Lung Transplant.*, 18, 194, 1999.
22. Cook, D. J., Bishay, E. S., and Yamani, M., The use and misuse of immunologic monitoring after transplantation: approaches that have proved useful, *Curr. Opin. Cardiol.*, 15, 104, 2000.
23. Mehra, M. R. et al., Anything but a biopsy: noninvasive monitoring for cardiac allograft rejection, *Curr. Opin. Cardiol.*, 17, 131, 2000.
24. Umeshita, K. et al., Determination of the presence of interleukin-6 in bile after orthotopic liver transplantation. Its role in the diagnosis of acute rejection, *Ann. Surg.*, 223, 204, 1996.
25. Lun, A. et al., Diagnostic value of peripheral blood T-cell activation and soluble IL-2 receptor for acute rejection in liver transplantation, *Clin. Chim. Acta*, 320, 69, 2002.
26. Warle, M. C. et al., Early differentiation between rejection and infection in liver transplant patients by serum and biliary cytokine patterns, *Transplantation*, 76, 146, 2003.
27. Garcia-Criado, A. et al., Radiology in liver transplantation, *Semin. Ultrasound CT MR*, 23, 114, 2002.
28. Boraschi. P. and Donati, F., Complications of orthotopic liver transplantation: imaging findings, *Abdom. Imaging*, 2004.
29. Crossin, J. D., Muradali, D., and Wilson, S. R., US of liver transplants: normal and abnormal, *Radiographics*, 23, 1093, 2003.
30. Yeh, B. M. et al., Biliary tract depiction in living potential liver donors: comparison of conventional MR, mangafodipir trisodium-enhanced excretory MR, and multi-detector row CT cholangiography-initial experience, *Radiology*, 230, 645, 2004.
31. Keogan, M. T. et al., The role of imaging in the diagnosis and management of biliary complications after liver transplantation, *AJR*, 173, 215, 1999.
32. Brancatelli, G. et al., Three-dimensional multislice helical computed tomography with the volume rendering technique in the detection of vascular complications after liver transplantation, *Transplantation*, 73, 237, 2002.

33. Tikkanen, J. et al., Cytological monitoring of peripheral blood, bronchoalveolar lavage fluid, and transbronchial biopsy specimens during acute rejection and cytomegalovirus infection in lung and heart–lung allograft recipients, *Clin. Transplant.*, 15, 77, 2001.
34. Lau, C. L. and Patterson, G. A., Current status of lung transplantation, *Eur. Respir. J. Suppl.*, 47, 57s, 2003.
35. Ikonen, T. et al., High-resolution CT in long-term follow-up after lung transplantation, *Chest*, 111, 370, 1997.
36. Jones, H. A. et al., Use of 18FDG-pet to discriminate between infection and rejection in lung transplant recipients, *Transplantation*, 15(77), 1462, 2004.
37. Schuurman, H.-J. et al., Preclinical models of chronic rejection: promises and pitfalls, *Transplant. Proc.*, 29, 2624, 1997.
38. Engelbrecht, G. et al., New rapid technique for renal transplantation in the rat, *Microsurgery*, 13, 340, 1992.
39. Rocha, P. M. et al., Effector mechanisms in transplant rejection, *Immunol. Rev.*, 196, 51, 2003.
40. Weissleder, R. et al., Ultrasmall superparamagnetic iron oxide: characterization of a new class of contrast agents for MR imaging, *Radiology*, 175, 489, 1990.
41. Zhang, Y. et al., Magnetic resonance imaging detection of rat renal transplant rejection by monitoring macrophage infiltration, *Kidney Int.*, 58, 1300, 2000.
42. Ye, Q. et al., In vivo detection of acute rat renal allograft rejection by MRI with USPIO particles, *Kidney Int.*, 61, 1124, 2002.
43. Grau, V., Herbst, B., and Steiniger, B., Dynamics of monocytes/macrophages and T lymphocytes in acutely rejecting rat renal allografts, *Cell. Tissue Res.*, 291, 117, 1998.
44. Grimm, P. C. et al., Clinical rejection is distinguished from subclinical rejection by increased infiltration by a population of activated macrophages, *J. Am. Soc. Nephrol.*, 10, 1582, 1999.
45. Croker, B. P. et al., Macrophages and chronic renal allograft nephropathy, *Kidney Int.*, 57, S42, 1996.
46. Azuma, H. et al., Hepatocyte growth factor prevents the development of chronic allograft nephropathy in rats, *J. Am. Soc. Nephrol.*, 12, 1280, 2001.
47. Herrero-Fresneda, I. et al., Do alloreactivity and prolonged cold ischemia cause different elementary lesions in chronic allograft nephropathy?, *Am. J. Pathol.*, 162, 127, 2003.
48. Ziai, F. et al., Renal allograft protection with losartan in Fisher–Lewis rats: hemodynamics, macrophages, and cytokines, *Kidney Int.*, 57, 2618, 2000.
49. Hamar, P. et al., Involvement of interleukin-2 and growth factors in chronic kidney allograft rejection in rats, *Transplant. Proc.*, 33, 2160, 2001.
50. Yang, J. et al., Targeting of macrophage activity by adenovirus-mediated intragraft overexpression of TNFRp55-Ig, IL-12p40, and vIL-10 ameliorates adenovirus-mediated chronic graft injury, whereas stimulation of macrophages by overexpression of IFN-gamma accelerates chronic graft injury in a rat renal allograft model, *J. Am. Soc. Nephrol.*, 14, 214, 2003.
51. Beckmann, N. et al., Macrophage labeling by SPIO as an early marker of allograft chronic rejection in a rat model of kidney transplantation, *Magn. Reson. Med.*, 49, 459, 2003.
52. Beckmann, N. et al., Macrophage infiltration in rat kidney allografts detected by MRI: early marker of chronic rejection that strongly correlates with histology, *Radiology*, in press, 2006.
53. Cook, N. S. et al., Chronic graft loss: dealing with the vascular alterations in solid organ transplantation, *Transplant. Proc.*, 30, 2413, 1998.
54. Davis, C. et al., The role of inflammation in vascular injury and repair, *J. Thromb. Haemost.*, 1, 1699, 2003.
55. Beckmann, N. et al., Magnetic resonance imaging for the evaluation of rejection of a kidney allograft in the rat, *Transpl. Int.*, 9, 175, 1996.
56. Beckmann, N. et al., From anatomy to the target: contributions of magnetic resonance imaging to preclinical pharmaceutical research, *Anat. Rec.*, 265, 85, 2001.
57. Gaschen, L. et al., MRI and ultrasonographic detection of morphologic and hemodynamic changes in chronic renal allograft rejection in the rat, *J. Magn. Reson. Imaging*, 13, 232, 2001.
58. Yang, D. et al., USPIO-enhanced dynamic MRI: evaluation of normal and transplanted rat kidneys, *Magn. Reson. Med.*, 46, 1152, 2001.
59. Weisskoff, R. M. et al., Pitfalls in MR measurement of tissue blood flow with intravascular tracers: which mean transit time?, *Magn. Reson. Med.*, 29, 553, 1993.

60. Rosen, B. R. et al., Perfusion imaging with contrast agents, *Magn. Reson. Med.*, 14, 249, 1990.
61. Taylor, J. et al., Magnetic resonance renography: optimisation of pulse sequence parameters and Gd-DTPA dose, and comparison with radionuclide renography, *Magn. Reson. Imaging*, 15, 637, 1997.
62. Baumann, D. and Rudin, M., Quantitative assessment of rat kidney function by measuring the clearance of the contrast agent Gd(DOTA) using dynamic MRI, *Magn. Reson. Imaging*, 18, 587, 2000.
63. Lee, S. et al., Heterotopic heart and lung transplantation in the rat, *Am. J. Pathol.*, 59, 279, 1970.
64. Fox, U and Montorsi, M., A technical modification of heart–lung transplantation in rats, *J. Microsurg.*, 1, 377, 1980.
65. Chung, W. S. et al., Review of significant microvascular surgical breakthroughs involving the heart and lungs in rats, *Microsurgery*, 19, 71, 1999.
66. Kanno, S. et al., Macrophage accumulation associated with rat cardiac allograft rejection detected by magnetic resonance imaging with ultrasmall superparamagnetic iron oxide particles, *Circulation*, 104, 934, 2001.
67. Johansson, L. et al., Acute cardiac transplant rejection: detection and grading with MR imaging with a blood pool contrast agent-experimental study in the rat, *Radiology*, 225, 97, 2002.
68. Young, A. A. et al., Validation of tagging with MR imaging to estimate material deformation, *Radiology*, 188, 101, 1993.
69. Kanno, S. et al., A novel approach with magnetic resonance imaging used for the detection of lung allograft rejection, *J. Thorac. Cardiovasc. Surg.*, 120, 923, 2000.
70. Fang, Y. C. and Siegelman, E. S., Complications of renal transplantation: MR findings, *J. Comput. Assist. Tomogr.*, 25, 836, 2001.
71. Zapletal, C. et al., Critical view of imaging techniques for donor evaluation in living donor kidney transplantation, *Transplant. Proc.*, 35, 948, 2003.
72. Fink, C. et al., Preoperative evaluation of living renal donors: value of contrast-enhanced 3D magnetic resonance angiography and comparison of three rendering algorithms, *Eur. Radiol.*, 13, 794, 2003.
73. Hussain, S. M. et al., MR imaging: a one-stop shop modality for preoperative evaluation of potential living kidney donors, *Radiographics*, 23, 505, 2003.
74. Subramaniam, M., Mizzi, A., and Roditi, G., Magnetic resonance angiography in potential live renal donors: a joint radiological and surgical evaluation, *Clin. Radiol.*, 59, 335, 2004.
75. Giessing, M. et al., Gadolinium-enhanced three-dimensional magnetic resonance angiography versus conventional digital subtraction angiography: which modality is superior in evaluating living kidney donors?, *Transplantation*, 76, 1000, 2003.
76. Liem, Y. S. et al., Living renal donors: optimizing the imaging strategy–decision- and cost-effectiveness analysis, *Radiology*, 226, 53, 2003.
77. Bakker, J. et al., MR urography for the preoperative evaluation of living renal donors, *Eur. Radiol.*, 12, 2021, 2002.
78. Nolte-Ernsting, C. C. et al., MR urography today, *Abdom. Imaging*, 28, 191, 2003.
79. Hene, R. J. et al., Pre-transplantation assessment of renal viability with 31P magnetic resonance spectroscopy, *Kidney Int.*, 46, 1694, 1994.
80. Niekisch, M. B. et al., Improved pretransplant assessment of renal quality by means of phosphorus-31 magnetic resonance spectroscopy using chemical shift imaging, *Transplantation*, 77, 1041, 2004.
81. Vazquez, M. A. et al., Long-term outcomes of renal transplantation: a result of the original endowment of the donor kidney and the inflammatory response to both alloantigens and injury, *Curr. Opin. Nephrol. Hypertens.*, 9, 643, 2000.
82. Baxter, G. M., Ultrasound of renal transplantation, *Clin. Radiol.*, 56, 802, 2001.
83. Huber, A. et al., Contrast-enhanced MR angiography in patients after kidney transplantation, *Eur. Radiol.*, 11, 2488, 2001.
84. Cohnen, M. et al., Contrast-enhanced MR urography in the evaluation of renal transplants with urological complications, *Clin. Nephrol.*, 58, 111, 2002.
85. de Priester, J. A. et al., Automated quantitative evaluation of diseased and nondiseased renal transplants with MR renography, *J. Magn. Reson. Imaging*, 17, 95, 2003.
86. Seto, K. et al., Long-term assessment of posttransplant renal prognosis with 31 P magnetic resonance spectroscopy, *Transplantation*, 72, 627, 2001.
87. Almenar, L. et al., Utility of cardiac magnetic resonance imaging for the diagnosis of heart transplant rejection, *Transplant. Proc.*, 35, 1962, 2003.

88. Muehling, O. M. et al., Reduced myocardial perfusion reserve and transmural perfusion gradient in heart transplant arteriopathy assessed by magnetic resonance imaging, *J. Am. Coll. Cardiol.*, 42, 1054, 2003.
89. Walpoth, B. H. et al., Assessment of cardiac rejection and immunosuppression by magnetic resonance imaging and spectroscopy, *Transplant. Proc.*, 27, 2088, 1995.
90. Marie, P. Y. et al., Detection and prediction of acute heart transplant rejection with the myocardial T_2 determination provided by a black-blood magnetic resonance imaging sequence, *J. Am. Coll. Cardiol.*, 37, 825, 2001.
91. Kober, F. et al., Objective and noninvasive metabolic characterization of donor hearts by phosphorous-31 magnetic resonance spectroscopy, *Transplantation*, 74, 1752, 2002.
92. Buchthal, S. D. et al., 31P-magnetic resonance spectroscopy studies of cardiac transplant patients at rest, *J. Cardiovasc. Magn. Reson.*, 2, 51, 2000.
93. Freedman, B. J., Lowe, S. C., and Saouaf, R., MR imaging in hepatic transplantation, *Magn. Reson. Imaging Clin. N. Am.*, 9, 821, 2001.
94. Hussain, H. K. and Nghiem, H. V., Imaging of hepatic transplantation, *Clin. Liver Dis.*, 6, 247, 2002.
95. Chen, Y. S. et al., Evaluation of living liver donors, *Transplantation*, 75(3 Suppl), S16, 2003.
96. Tzakis, A. G. et al., Renal artery reconstruction for harvesting injuries in kidney transplantation with particular reference to the use of vascular allografts, *Transpl. Int.*, 1, 80, 1988.
97. Boeve, W. J. et al., Superior diagnostic strength of combined contrast enhanced MR-angiography and MR-imaging compared to intra-arterial DSA in liver transplantation candidates, *Magn. Reson. Imaging*, 19, 609, 2001.
98. Carr, J. C. et al., Preoperative evaluation of the entire hepatic vasculature in living liver donors with use of contrast-enhanced MR angiography and true fast imaging with steady-state precession, *J. Vasc. Interv. Radiol.*, 14, 441, 2003.
99. Burrel, M. et al., MRI angiography is superior to helical CT for detection of HCC prior to liver transplantation: an explant correlation, *Hepatology*, 38, 1034, 2003.
100. Parkin, D. M. et al., Estimating the world cancer burden: globocan 2000, *Int. J. Cancer*, 94, 153, 2001.
101. Eubank, W. B. et al., Preoperative evaluation of patients awaiting liver transplantation: comparison of multiphasic contrast-enhanced 3D magnetic resonance to helical computed tomography examinations, *J. Magn. Reson. Imaging*, 16, 565, 2002.
102. Mori, K. et al., Detection of malignant hepatic lesions before orthotopic liver transplantation: accuracy of ferumoxides-enhanced MR imaging, *Am. J. Roentgenol.*, 179, 1045, 2002.
103. Cheng, Y. F. et al., Single imaging modality evaluation of living donors in liver transplantation: magnetic resonance imaging, *Transplantation*, 72, 1527, 2001.
104. Goyen, M. et al., Right-lobe living related liver transplantation: evaluation of a comprehensive magnetic resonance imaging protocol for assessing potential donors, *Liver Transpl.*, 8, 241, 2002.
105. Kim, B. S. et al., Vascular complications after living related liver transplantation: evaluation with gadolinium-enhanced three-dimensional MR angiography, *Am. J. Roentgenol.*, 181, 467, 2003.
106. Lee, E. S. et al., Early bronchiolitis obliterans following lung transplantation: accuracy of expiratory thin-section CT for diagnosis, *Radiology*, 216, 472, 2000.
107. Gast, K. K. et al., MRI in lung transplant recipients using hyperpolarized 3He: comparison with CT, *J. Magn. Reson. Imaging*, 15, 268, 2002.
108. Ross, D. J. et al., Regional distribution of lung perfusion and ventilation at rest and during steady-state exercise after unilateral lung transplantation, *Chest*, 104, 130, 1993.
109. Lipson, D. A. et al., Pulmonary ventilation and perfusion scanning using hyperpolarized helium-3 MRI and arterial spin tagging in healthy normal subjects and in pulmonary embolism and orthotopic lung transplant patients, *Magn. Reson. Med.*, 47, 1073, 2002.
110. Roberts, D. A. et al., Pulmonary perfusion: respiratory-triggered three-dimensional MR imaging with arterial spin tagging-preliminary results in healthy volunteers, *Radiology*, 212, 890, 1999.
111. Edelman, R. R. et al., Noninvasive assessment of regional ventilation in the human lung using oxygen-enhanced magnetic resonance imaging, *Nat. Med.*, 2, 1236, 1996.
112. Furukawa, M. et al., MRI in seven cases of tacrolimus (FK-506) encephalopathy: utility of FLAIR and diffusion-weighted imaging, *Neuroradiology*, 43, 615, 2001.
113. Shimono, T. et al., MR imaging with quantitative diffusion mapping of tacrolimus-induced neurotoxicity in organ transplant patients, *Eur. Radiol.*, 13, 986, 2003.

114. Gleeson, J. G. et al., Cyclosporin a acute encephalopathy and seizure syndrome in childhood: clinical features and risk of seizure recurrence, *J. Child Neurol.*, 13, 336, 1998.
115. Serkova, N. and Christians, U., Transplantation: toxicokinetics and mechanisms of toxicity of cyclosporine and macrolides, *Curr. Opin. Investig. Drugs*, 4, 1287, 2003.
116. Renders, L. and Valerius, T., Engineered CD3 antibodies for immunosuppression, *Clin. Exp. Immunol.*, 133, 307, 2003.
117. Pittock, S. J. et al., OKT3 neurotoxicity presenting as akinetic mutism, *Transplantation*, 75, 1058, 2003.
118. Clarke, W. et al., Characterization of renal allograft rejection by urinary proteomic analysis, *Ann. Surg.*, 237, 660, 2003.
119. Borozdenkova, S. et al., Use of proteomics to discover novel markers of cardiac allograft rejection, *J. Proteome Res.*, 3, 282, 2004.
120. Schaub. S. et al., Proteomic-based detection of urine proteins associated with acute renal allograft rejection, *J. Am. Soc. Nephrol.*, 15, 219, 2004.

25 MR Imaging and the Development of Stem Cell-Based Therapies

Piotr Walczak and Jeff W. M. Bulte

CONTENTS

25.1 INTRODUCTION

Technological advancements in recent years have introduced various *in vivo* imaging modalities for the study of living organisms, including those suitable for cellular imaging. Positron emission tomography (PET) [1], bioluminescent imaging [2], single photon emission tomography (SPECT) [3], and MRI [4] are all suitable to track labeled cells, with MRI having superior temporal and spatial resolution. Tracking cells using MRI relies on biocompatible MR contrast agents allowing repetitive monitoring of targeted cells. The rapidly growing stem cell field has recognized *in vivo* cell visualization as a valuable tool to study the biology of stem cells, as well as a noninvasive method for *in vivo* monitoring, which may also facilitate proper translation of stem cell-based therapies into the clinical setting. Stem cell therapy is currently being evaluated as a possible treatment for numerous diseases, with an emphasis on brain or cardiac disorders for which an effective therapy is lacking.

The term stem cell refers to a cell of indefinite or prolonged self-renewal capacity that is capable of multiple descendent cell type generations (Figure 25.1). The preservation of stem cells in adult organisms reflects the necessity for cellular turnover in certain organs (i.e., the intestine, skin epithelium). It also provides a quiescent cellular pool, which, in case of injury or malfunction, can lead either to regeneration (hepatic, bone, and hematopoietic cells) or tissue repair (e.g., in the brain, heart, and skin). Even organs previously thought incapable of regeneration, such as the brain or the heart, contain cells capable of generating appropriate phenotypes following injury [5]. It has also been shown that cells derived from the adult heart [6] or brain [7] are able to generate cardiomyocytes or neurons, respectively. In animals, the phenomenon of robust regeneration (e.g., frog leg regrowth) is understood as a basic, fairly uncomplicated regeneration. The highly refined function of (abstract) thinking in humans, however, requires that the cellular and functional plasticity of neural circuitries be highly controlled, which makes the capacity and/or likelihood of regeneration extremely limited [8]. At the postdevelopmental stage, cellular–neuronal plasticity (neurogenesis) in the adult is preserved only in two distinct brain regions: the subgranular layer of the dentate gyrus [9] and the subventricular zone-rostral migratory system [10]. These limitations of neogenesis can be overcome either by transplantation of appropriate cells, or by modulation of regulatory mechanisms acting on endogenous progenitors (once these mechanisms are sufficiently understood).

The history of stem cell therapy began with a naturally regenerating system — the blood. Under physiological conditions, hematopoietic lineages are populated by constantly dividing bone marrow stem cells. When these cells malfunction or are ablated, they must be quickly replaced by transplantation to ensure the survival of the individual. Bone marrow transplantation was used clinically for the first time in the late 1950s in France, when bone marrow cells were used as a treatment for accidentally irradiated individuals [11]. Since then, significant progress has been made in stem cell therapy, which is now recommended as a treatment for numerous hematological [12] or oncological [13] conditions. However, to date, only stem cell therapies based on bone marrow replacement have proved to be clinically effective, but much work is underway to extend stem cell therapy to other pathological conditions. Reports of results from animal models of such diseases as Parkinson's disease [14], stroke [15], spinal cord motor neuron disease [16], multiple sclerosis [17], or myocardial infarction [18] show that disease symptoms may be substantially alleviated using a stem cell transplantation approach.

Stem cell therapy does not necessarily need to be implemented through transplantation of exogenous cells. The *in situ* manipulation of endogenous progenitors and their amplification and recruitment for the replenishment of missing cellular phenotypes has also shown therapeutic promise in experiments in the rat brain. These experiments showed that subventricular zone neural progenitors could be recruited and directed to replace neurons, which were eliminated earlier by targeted apoptosis [19].

Although there has been some progress in stem cell research, there are significant technical limitations in our ability to further characterize stem cells. Most of the current scientific methods assess the function of cells by detecting their gene products postmortem, while other methods are based on the *in vitro* observation of explants in usually unfavorable conditions far from their natural milieu inside the organism. The challenge of these methodological limitations can only be addressed by modern imaging techniques that will provide *in vivo* cell monitoring, either of the transplants or transgenically tagged endogenous cell populations.

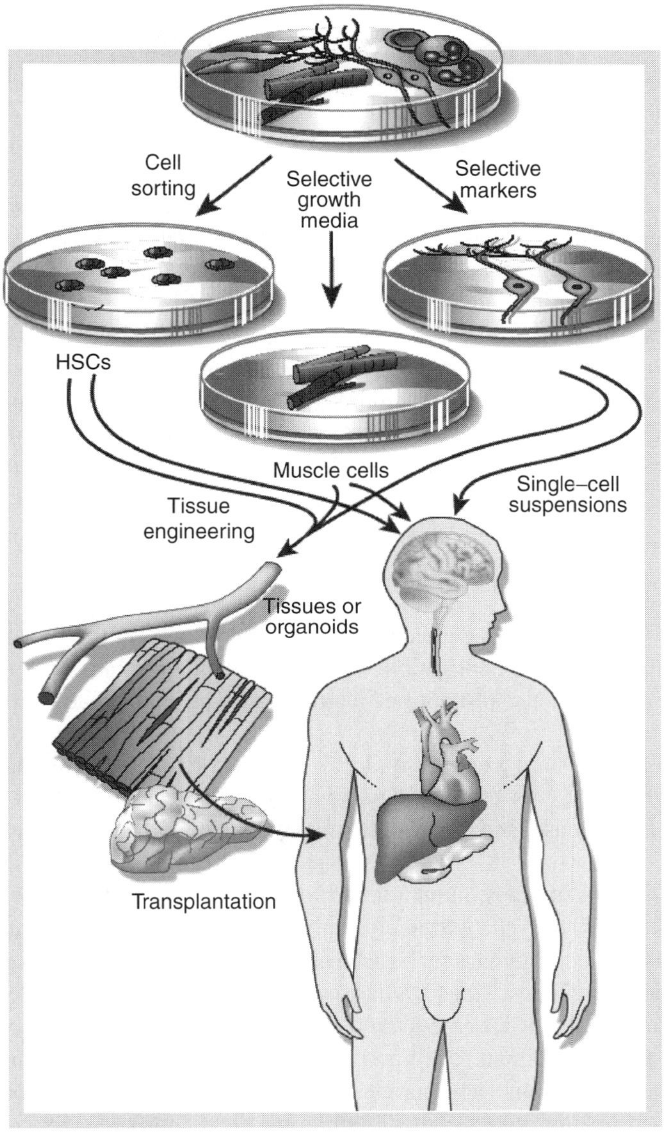

FIGURE 25.1 Therapeutic use of stem cells and progenitors. Stem cells are pluripotent cells, i.e., they have the ability to generate multiple different phenotypes. The principle of stem cell-based therapy is based on the selective differentiation of stem cells into, for example, muscle cells or hematopoietic stem cells (HSCs), and their further purification and transplantation in order to facilitate regeneration of damaged organs. In the near future, perhaps more complex tissue constructs can be generated *in vitro* for replacement tissue fragments or even whole organs. (From Donovan, P. J. and Gearhart, J., *Nature*, 414, 92, 2001. With permission of Nature Publishing Group. Copyright 2001.)

25.2 STEM CELL-BASED THERAPY FOR THE CNS

25.2.1 Parkinson's Disease

Parkinson's disease (PD) is a common chronic neurological disorder of unknown etiology, typically affecting people over the age of 65. Approximately 1% of Americans live with PD and the incidence is growing as society ages. PD is characterized by a loss of dopamine-producing neurons (DA neurons) within the substantia nigra, which are responsible for control and modulation of movements. Consequently, disruption of this regulatory mechanism results in the primary symptoms of Parkinson's syndrome: hypokinesia, rigidity, postural instability, resting tremor, and difficulty in motion initiation.

Current treatment of PD is based on administration of a dopamine precursor (levodopa). This drug significantly decreases morbidity and mortality in most patients, but the disease progresses and, over time, higher doses of the drug are required. Long-term therapy with this drug is complicated by serious side effects (on–off phenomena, dystonia, or dyskinesias) [20]. Clearly, there is an urgent need for novel effective treatment of PD, and cell transplantation to replace lost DA neurons is considered a possible option. Cell transplantation in a PD model was successfully implemented and reported for the first time in 1979 by Bjorklund and collaborators [21]. In their study, fetal neural tissue was transplanted into a rodent PD model, resulting in significant improvement of motor function. This successful experiment attracted the attention of both clinicians and researchers to further explore the nature of the benefits and apply these benefits to humans.

25.2.1.1 Experiments in Animal Models

Intensive research using rodent and nonhuman primate models of PD are designed to address critical issues for the successful application of cell transplantation, including the identification of easily accessible cell types, the promotion of graft survival, and broad, uniform dopaminergic innervation.

Animal models of PD are created by local pharmacological destruction of dopaminergic neurons [22,23], which does not reflect the pathogenesis of PD in humans but sufficiently mimics the late stage of the disease and is a good model to study therapeutic effects in transplant experiments.

In the first trials in PD models, human fetal brain tissue was used; the positive effect of these experiments was diminished by the extremely limited access to that cell source. While work using fetal neural tissue is still continuing, it is clear that this source of cells will never be available for a large population of PD patients. Thus, finding alternative cell sources that can be amplified to virtually unlimited quantities is a prerequisite for broad clinical application. It has been shown that stem cells derived from the human fetal brain can be expanded and, after transplantation into the rodent brain, migrate and acquire appropriate neuronal phenotypes [24]. Another source of stem cells that can be used for transplantation are embryonic stem cells (ES). ES can be obtained from the blastocyst inner cell mass. It has been shown that ES can give rise to functional dopaminergic neurons in the rat brain [25]. However, ethical concerns, as well as the risk of tumor formation, argue for the utilization of other, more differentiated cell types, such as fetal organ-specific progenitors, bone marrow, umbilical cord blood-derived cells, or even progenitors derived from adult tissues.

In addition to appropriate cell source selection, the promotion of graft survival is an important consideration; transplantation of cells or tissue into the postdevelopmental brain yields as low as 3 to 20% of initially injected cells. Improvement of cell survival can be achieved by scavenging of toxic free radicals [26] or by administration of growth factors [27]. Another factor that determines successful transplantation is the brain area innervated by the graft, which is closely related to migration and axonal outgrowth. The adult brain lacks most of the developmental signals leading to migration and axonal sprouting; thus, it is critical to maintain not only the brain's supply of these signals, but also to ensure the survival of the cell graft. In experiments addressing this concept, pretransplant treatment of neuronal precursors with glial cell line-derived neurotrophic factor (GDNF) resulted in robust graft survival, distribution, and innervation [28].

25.2.1.2 Clinical Studies

Cellular grafts in experimental animal models of PD not only survived, innervated host striatum, produced missing neurotransmitter dopamine, and reduced motor deficits, but also, importantly, produced no adverse symptoms, which led to prompt clinical application of this approach (Figure 25.2). Clinical trials with human fetal neural tissue grafts began in the mid 1980s [29,30]. Initial studies showed a modest improvement of motor function and an increase in fluorodopa uptake, both indications of graft survival, as well as no adverse effect of the therapy. Preliminary open-label trials on a small number of patients were followed by a more objective double-blind controlled study [31]. In this study, improvement was observed among younger patients, but there was no significant overall improvement for all age groups between the placebo and the transplant group. Modest improvement in PD patients encourages therapeutic stem cell research, but there is still work to be done at the bench before more complete recovery in PD patients can be achieved.

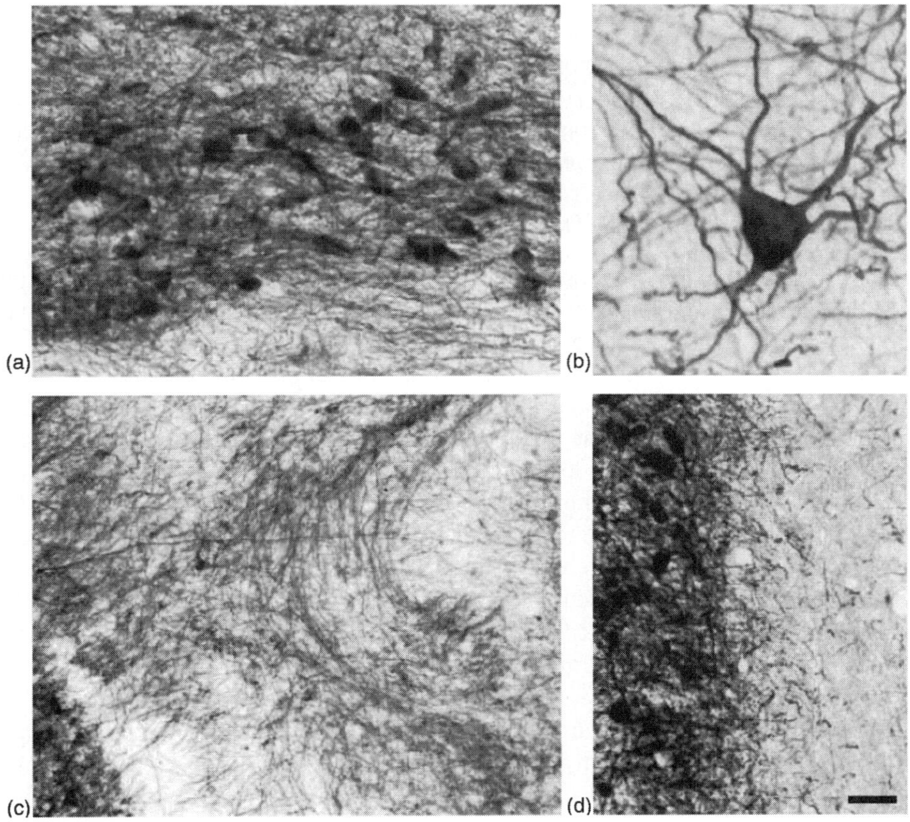

FIGURE 25.2 Cell grafting in Parkinson's disease. Histology of the striatum of a Parkinson's patient, who underwent fetal ventral mesencephalon tissue transplantation and died 18 months later for reasons unrelated to his neurological condition. The striatum of patients with advanced Parkinson's disease is usually devoid of tyrosine hydroxylase (TH)-positive dopaminergic neurons. In this particular case, large amounts of dopaminergic neurons were detected throughout the striatum by anti-TH immunohistochemistry (a–d). Transplanted cells developed a cellular morphology similar to endogenous dopamine-producing neurons and incorporated within the tissue architecture. The grafted striata with their innervation projections, resembled normal brain. (Reproduced from Kordower, J. H. et al., *N. Engl. J. Med.*, 332, 1118, 1995. With permission of The Massachusetts Medical Society. Copyright 1995.)

25.2.2 Spinal Cord Injury

According to the National Spinal Cord Injury Association, spinal cord injury affects approximately 11,000 Americans a year, with a total of up to 400,000 individuals living with spinal cord injury (SCI) in the U.S.A. Currently, there is no effective consensus treatment for SCI that significantly improves the prognosis. All recommended therapeutic approaches focus on limiting secondary damage. It has been observed that intensive resuscitative therapy following injury leads to improved recovery [32], and further modest benefits may be achieved if, within 8 h of the injury, high-dose-corticosteroid [33] and/or MG-1-ganglioside therapy [34] is administered. The efficacy of these drugs was broadly reviewed by the Congress of Neurological Surgeons [35] and, because of controversial outcomes, both drugs are currently optional, but not the recommended treatment for acute SCI. While ongoing clinical trials aim to evaluate the effectiveness of steroids and MG-1 ganglioside in the treatment of acute SCI, it is clear that only modest, if any, improvement can be achieved with these drugs and further, more efficacious therapeutic approaches need to be developed.

The repair of damaged spinal cord was not even an issue several decades ago, when few spinal injury victims survived the acute phase of injury, and those who survived usually died soon after as a result of sepsis [36]. Since then, there has been major progress in medical and rehabilitative care, which allows for long-term survival of individuals affected by SCI and, as a result, there is an increasing interest in new therapeutic strategies for spinal cord regeneration to help these thousands of SCI sufferers. Research in SCI therapy is focused on two complementary directions: limiting or preventing secondary damage and regeneration of damaged neurons.

25.2.2.1 Prevention of Secondary Damage

Total damage of all axonal connections during the initial injury occurs in only approximately 20% of cases [37]. The primary injury usually severs only a fraction of neural tissue, primarily the center of the spinal cord with its gray matter and adjacent white matter tracts. However, further damage of the spared axons and neurons begins as soon as several minutes after the primary insult. Stem cell-based therapies are more suited to the regenerative approach, which will be further discussed below, but these therapies may also help to maintain the function of challenged axons or prevent apoptosis. An understanding of the mechanisms leading to secondary damage allows therapeutic strategies to be targeted to these areas, including transplanted cells as carriers of trophic factors. The window of opportunity for limiting secondary damage is narrow, and therapeutic interventions must be applied within approximately 8 h of injury to have a chance for success.

A series of experiments performed on animal models of SCI supported this approach. It has been shown that transplanted stem cells, engineered to over-express neurotrophin-3 and nerve growth factor, rescue axotomized neurons [38]. Fetal spinal cord tissue transplants also effectively protected neurons from apoptosis in a rat SCI model [39], and genetically engineered fibroblasts that over-express brain-derived neurotrophic factor protected Red Nucleus neurons from apoptosis or atrophy [40]. The SCI-related demyelinization process has been managed, to some extent, by transplantation of peripheral myelin makers — Schwann or olfactory-ensheathing cells, which myelinate axons and improve their function. All of these examples suggest that treatment with engineered stem cells might have an important role in minimizing the secondary damage associated with SCI.

25.2.2.2 Regeneration of Spinal Cord

Recovery of neurological function depends on limiting the extent of the lesion by preventing secondary damage. There is usually a large amount of irreversibly lost neurons and completely separated axons, which will never reconnect spontaneously. In these cases, treatment is required that will either induce endogenous neurons to extend their axons and recreate neural connections, or, alternatively, transplant native or engineered progenitor cells, which will participate in the recreation of neural circuitries themselves, or will provide an environment that can support regeneration (Figure 25.3).

For more than a century, scientists have been interested in the regenerative processes in the CNS. Santiago Ramón y Cajal, who was the first to describe regeneration in the peripheral nervous system (PNS), wrote about the CNS: "Once development was ended, the founts of growth and regeneration of the axons and dendrites dried up irrevocably. In adult centers the nerve paths are something fixed, ended, immutable. Everything may die, nothing may be regenerated" [41]. However, he observed regeneration in the CNS, demonstrated by the sprouting of growth cones. Cajal noted that the regeneration was interrupted for unknown reasons. In the last decades, substantial progress has been made in understanding the mechanism of action of the molecules

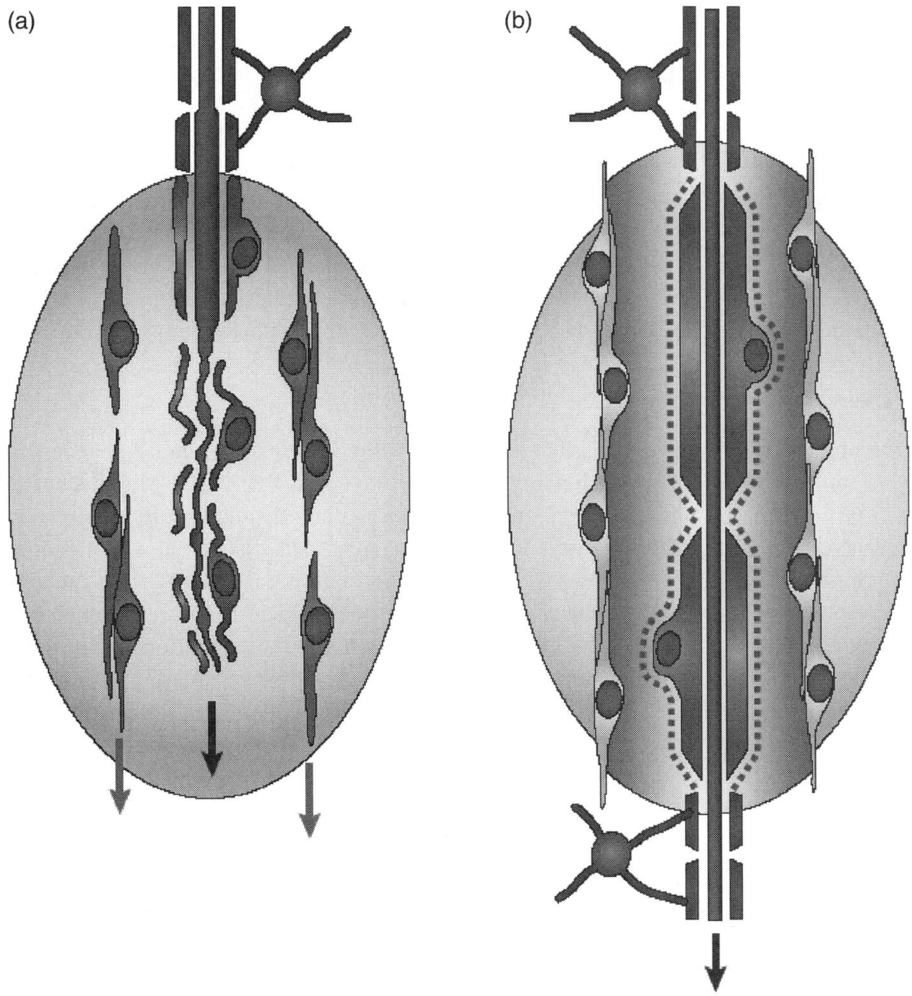

FIGURE 25.3 Regeneration of damaged corticospinal tract induced by olfactory ensheathing cell transplantation. Soon after transplantation (a) degenerating axons are surrounded by elongated Schwann-like cells. Four weeks postgrafting (b) regenerating axons are enwrapped with new myelin sheaths, covered by basal lamina. At the periphery of the damaged neuronal tract, another cell type forms a tubular space limiting the lesion area. Outside the lesion, endogenous oligodendrocytes form myelin sheaths that are continuous with the myelin sheaths formed by the grafted cells. (Reproduced from Li, Y., Field, P. M., and Raisman, G., *J. Neurosci.*, 18, 10514, 1998. With permission of the Society for Neuroscience. Copyright 1998.)

responsible for this inhibition. Among factors detrimental to CNS regeneration are myelin degradation products (myelin associated glycoprotein, oligodendrocyte–myelin glycoprotein, and Nogo-A). The idea that myelin is a major obstacle in regeneration is even more justified when one considers that all neuroregenerative processes in the CNS dry up at approximately the same time as myelin sheaths are formed [42]. Research has shown that targeting the above-mentioned molecules can result in successful, at least to some extent, rewiring of the injured spinal cord [43,44]. Achievements in the field of SCI (improved medical care in the acute phase, better understanding of secondary damage processes, and mechanisms prohibiting regeneration) and the tremendous progress in stem cell research provide an unprecedented opportunity for the application of stem cell-based therapies in the treatment of SCI.

The feasibility of a stem cell transplantation approach for SCI regeneration was demonstrated in a series of animal studies. It has been shown that human fetal spinal cord tissue grafted onto the rat SCI model integrates with the host spinal cord, and grafted neurons extend their processes far into the host tissue [45]. Significant behavioral improvement, accompanied by regeneration on a microscopic level, was also observed after intraspinal transplantation of mouse embryonic stem cell-derived neural cells [46]. Since access to fetal tissue is limited, and the use of both fetal tissue and embryonic stem cells is hindered by serious ethical issues, investigators are searching for noncontroversial sources of readily available and/or expandable pluripotent cells. Stem cells derived from the skin, for example, were induced *in vitro* to generate neurons or glia after transplantation into the SCI model [47]. Promising results in animal models of SCI encourage clinical applications. Few of the clinical trials performed to date [47,48], however, haven't shown significant alleviation of symptoms, but have proved the safety and feasibility of the method and prepared the basis for further, more successful therapeutic approaches with stem cells.

25.2.3 De- and Dysmyelination

Among the numerous types of genetic and acquired myelin diseases (e.g., multiple sclerosis (MS), progressive multifocal leukoencephalopathy, encephalomyelitis, Pelizaeus–Merzbacher disease), MS is the most common. It affects over 2 million people worldwide and unfortunately no effective treatment is available. This inflammatory, demyelinating disease is associated with an autoimmune reaction against myelin, manifested by perivascular inflammation, focal demyelination, and axonal loss with astrocytic scarring. MS is characterized by episodes of deterioration followed by periods of remission, as a result of repeated cycles of demyelination and remyelination within the plaques. In the late stages of the disease, the demyelination process takes over completely with no periods of remission. This can be explained by the presence of oligodendroglial progenitors in the brain, which initially effectively remyelinate the lesions [49], but have limited proliferative and migratory abilities that are quickly exhausted by the chronic course of the disease [50].

The concept described above also applies to many other demyelinating diseases. Thus, these pathologies can be effectively addressed by transplantation of exogenous cells with the ability to differentiate toward myelin-producing cells that recreate myelin sheaths. Several cell types are considered good candidates, after being evaluated in numerous models of genetic, chemical, or autoimmune-induced demyelinization. Oligodendrocyte precursors were expanded *in vitro* and, after injection into the demyelinated rat spinal cord, restored myelin architecture [51]. In addition, the cells migrated further distances and remyelinated faster than endogenous cells [52]. Schwann cells derived from the PNS are an alternative source of cells that can effectively myelinate CNS axons and improve nerve conduction [17]. The advantage of Schwann cells is that they can be easily obtained, expanded *in vitro*, and used in the same individual for autotransplantation. Olfactory ensheathing cells derived from the peripheral nervous system are able to produce myelin and remyelinate large axons [53], but stem cells are preferable with their advantage of expandability and nearly unlimited cell access [54]. Neural stem cells derived from neonatal mouse cerebellum, transplanted into a genetic mouse model of dysmyelination, have been shown to distribute widely, myelinate large brain areas, and decrease symptoms of the disease (Figure 25.4) [55]. ES are considered to have the highest differentiation potential and were shown to differentiate toward oligodendrocytes upon transplantation into the demyelinated brain [56]. However, many graft

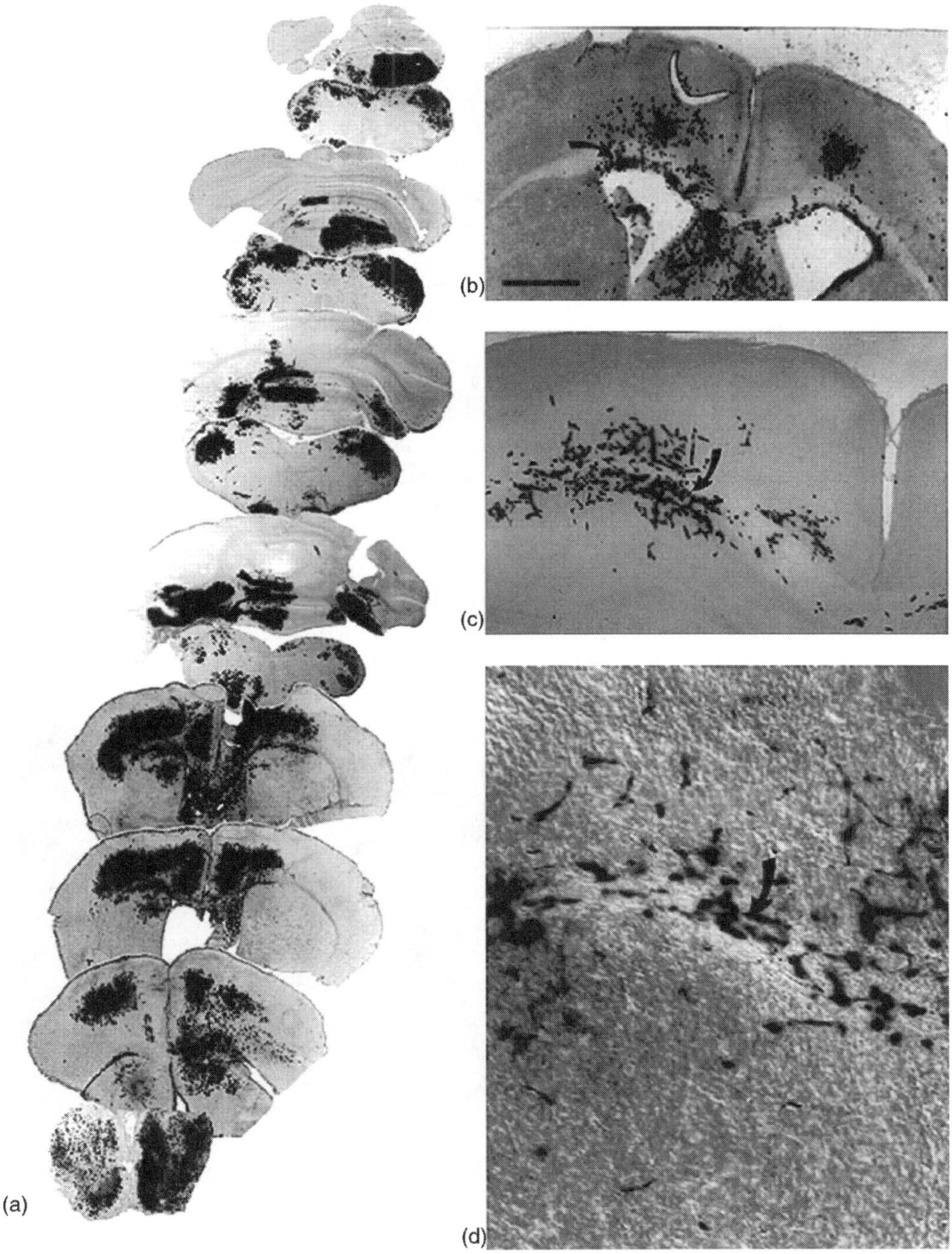

FIGURE 25.4 Cell grafting in dysmyelinated disease. Neural stem cells derived from a neonatal mouse 8 weeks after intraventricular transplantation into dysmyelinated (shiverer) mouse brain as detected by X-gal staining for the LacZ reporter gene. Grafted cells distributed widely throughout the entire mouse brain (a), with higher magnification in b–d. Cells differentiated into myelin-producing oligodendrocytes and reduced the tremor present in this transgenic model. (Reproduced from Yandava, B. D., Billinghurst, L. L., and Snyder, E. Y., et al., *Proc. Natl Acad. Sci. USA*, 96, 7029 1999. With permission. Copyright 1999. National Academy of Sciences.)

experiments using ES resulted in teratoma formation, raising major safety concerns [57]. Control over stem cell proliferation and differentiation will allow using the full potential of cell transplantation in functional restoration in de- and dysmyelinating diseases.

25.2.4 Other CNS Disorders

PD, SCI and Demyelinating diseases are not the only CNS pathologies that could benefit from cell transplantation. Stroke, for example, is the third leading cause of death in the U.S.A. In the last decade, cell transplantation in stroke attracted the attention of many researchers and clinicians. Two therapeutic strategies were developed with the use of stem cells: replacement of lost neurons and trophic support rescuing and rescuing challenged neurons in the lesion penumbra. Human fetus-derived neural stem cells, upon transplantation into a rat stroke model, survived, migrated specifically to the lesion, and differentiated toward both neuronal and glial elements [58]. Rats transplanted with fetal progenitors, homotopic to the lesion, showed improved limb motor function [59]. An interesting new approach for stroke therapy with cell transplantation emerged a few years ago: it was discovered that umbilical cord blood derived stem cells long used for hematological disorders could alleviate stroke symptoms [15]. In addition, it has been observed that, following bone marrow transplantation, donor-derived cells are found in most organs, including the brain, and these cells acquire the phenotypes of many cell types, including microglia or neurons (Figure 25.5) [60]. An immortalized cell line, NT2-N, resembling neuronal progenitors, was used in patients with basal ganglia strokes [61]. The transplantation procedure was not associated with any adverse cell-related effects and, moreover, half the patients (6 out of 12) showed improvement in the total stroke scale score.

Huntington's disease (HD), is considered a good target for cell transplantation, similar to Parkinson's disease, since a strictly defined population of neurons (GABA-producing neurons) is

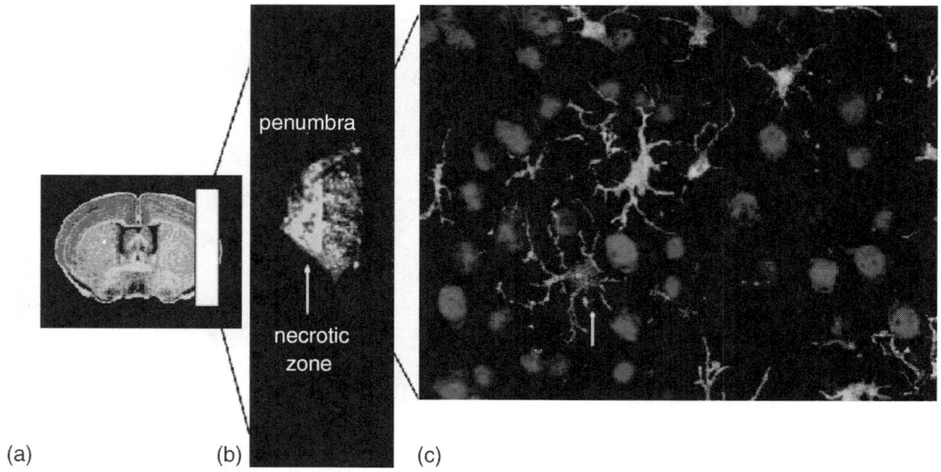

FIGURE 25.5 (See color insert following page 328.) Transdifferentiation of bone marrow stem cells. Histological images of adult mouse brain following lethal irradiation and rescue with a bone marrow transplant from a transgenic green fluorescent (GFP) mouse. Four months later the animal underwent a middle cerebral artery occlusion to induce a stroke lesion. Three months after stroke induction, histological analysis revealed infiltration of GFP + (green) donor derived cells into the stroke lesion (b). Most of the cells differentiated into glial cells, but a low percentage also expressed neuronal nuclear antigens (C: red cells = anti-NeuN; blue = nuclei (DAPI)) suggesting that circulating stem cells originating from bone marrow can contribute to brain remodeling. (Reproduced from Szentirmai, O. and Carter, B. S., *Neurosurgery*, 55, 283, 2004. With permission. Copyright 2004. Lippincott Williams and Wilkins.)

lost in a limited brain area. The use of intrastriatal transplantation of fetal neural tissue has shown promise in a number of animal studies [62,63], in which complete and persistent recovery in a frontal-type cognitive task was achieved in a primate HD model. An initial clinical study in HD patients showed good differentiation and histological integration of the fetal graft [64].

Numerous studies have addressed the correction of genetic defects with transplantation of engineered cells. Neural progenitors over-expressing beta-glucuronidase transplanted in a mouse model of mucopolysaccharidosis, a lysosomal storage disease, were able to correct the metabolism of glycosaminoglycans [65]. Neural progenitors expressing a beta-hexosaminidase alpha subunit, upon implantation into the mouse brain, produced significant amounts of the enzyme [66], opening up treatment possibilities for Tay–Sachs disease [66].

Undoubtedly, stem cell-based therapy has great potential and offers hope for individuals with untreatable brain diseases. However, we are still a long way from effective restoration of lost neurological function. The efforts of researchers and clinicians, as well as the determination of patients to participate in novel promising trials, will ensure progress in this area. Improved knowledge about cellular graft survival, migration, graft–host interactions, and appropriate innervation will amplify beneficial results, while a better understanding of the developmental mechanisms leading to proliferation and functional differentiation of progenitor cells will allow for manufacturing of large amounts of standardized transplantable cells.

25.3 STEM CELL-BASED THERAPY FOR THE INFARCTED MYOCARDIUM

Cardiac disease is the leading cause of death in the U.S.A., but, with the improved medical management of acute cases of cardiac disease in recent years, survival rates have increased, which, consequently, produced a large number of people living with various degrees of heart failure (see also Chapter 17). Like the brain, heart tissue has limited, if any, regenerative capacity. Loss of cardiac myocytes, whether due to heart infarct, hypertension, or cardiomyopathies, can to a certain degree be compensated for by the hypertrophy of the remaining cardiac cells, but, at some point, these compensatory cells are replaced by nonfunctional connective tissue. Progress in stem cell research has opened new therapeutic avenues for the treatment of cardiac failure; transplantation of cells able to replenish damaged cardiomyocytes has been recognized as a valuable tool to enhance cardiac regeneration.

Interest in cardiac regeneration with stem cells increased after a series of reports showed that if a heart derived from female donor is transplanted into a male, after some time, male-derived cardiomyocytes, detected by the presence of the Y chromosome, appear in the heart in mice [67] as well as in humans [68]. Although formation of new cardiomyocytes naturally does not lead to significant functional improvement, this was an important stimulus to explore the nature of cardiac regeneration and find ways to enhance it, e.g., by cell transplantation. Several different cell types have been successfully used in myocardial infarction in animal models and humans, including skeletal muscle-derived satellite cells, bone marrow-derived hematopoietic and mesenchymal stem cells, and embryonic and fetal stem cells. Intracardial transplantation of skeletal muscle progenitors was first tested and proved effective in animals [69], which resulted in their use in severe cardiac infarction in humans [70]. This trial produced mixed results when major concerns were raised after several patients developed arrhythmias; larger placebo-controlled trials are necessary to address this issue.

Bone marrow, another attractive source of transplantable cells, consists of two major components: hematopoietic and mesenchymal stem cells, which have attractive features for cardiac repair. Mesenchymal stem cells were shown to generate cardiomyocytes *in vitro* [71] and *in vivo* [72]. Furthermore, transplantation of bone marrow-derived cells improved cardiac function in infarcted rodent hearts [67,73]. In the bone marrow transplantation study, where female patients received a gender-mismatched graft, Y chromosome-positive cardiomyocytes were found posttransplantation [74], providing evidence that bone marrow has the capacity to repopulate the cardiomyocytes. Thus, direct intracardial bone marrow stem cell transplantation may be used to augment this process. In a recent randomized controlled clinical trial of intracoronary transfer of autologous bone marrow-derived cells, the procedure proved to effectively improve cardiac function in a transplanted, compared to a conventionally treated, group of patients [75]. One advantage of using either skeletal muscle or bone marrow cells is easy access to a relatively large amount of cells, which could be used in an autologous grafting system, thus avoiding the problem of graft rejection and life-long immunosuppressive treatment. In addition to the two cell sources described above, fetal cardiomyocytes and smooth muscle or fibroblasts [76,77] have also shown to effectively improve function in the infarcted heart. Although ESCs were proved to be functional in a rodent heart infarct model [78], their developmental regulatory mechanisms are still not completely understood and transplantation is often associated with the formation of teratomas [79].

In summary, there is strong evidence from basic and clinical research that stem cell-based therapies can be successfully implemented for diseases of a variety of organ systems; however, to date, little is known about the mechanisms leading to functional improvement. These mechanisms are currently indirectly deduced by performing retrospective postmortem histological analysis. The disadvantage of these conventional approaches is that they lack dynamic characterization and measurement. A great step forward in the understanding of the dynamics of stem cell biology may be found in the noninvasive *in vivo* visualization of the transplanted cells. The ability to follow the spatio-temporal distribution and trafficking is of great importance for basic scientists, as well as clinicians, who will eventually be able to noninvasively monitor and optimize the course of treatment.

25.4 NEED FOR NONINVASIVE MONITORING OF STEM CELL-BASED THERAPIES

Due to the development of advanced imaging equipment, the overall progress in cell biology, and the invention of new labels and contrast agents, cellular imaging has emerged as a new field, which can be broadly defined as the dynamic observation of cellular elements in a living organism. While MR tracking of transplanted cells is now an established method [4], other attractive applications of modern imaging techniques are under way to allow visualization of cellular and molecular processes, such as gene expression [80] and receptor–ligand or protein–protein interactions. All these tools offer valuable data for cell biology in general, and for the emerging stem cell imaging field in particular. The objective of *in vivo* cell monitoring is to facilitate observation of cells in their native environment — the living organism, allowing interactive adjustments and optimization of experimental protocols. Most methods currently used to determine the fate of transplanted cells are based on postmortem detection, using reporter signals (vital dyes, reporter genes, or the nucleotide analog BrdU). These detection procedures require laborious tissue preparation that are often plagued with quantitative and qualitative misjudgments. Furthermore, data obtained from conventional processing reflects the endpoint of the experiment, leaving a large information gap about the events that occur during the course of the study. The application of novel *in vivo* cell tracking methods will not only help to reduce the number of experimental animals required for the overall study, but additionally, each serially imaged animal will, over time, serve as its own baseline control. One of the primary applications for noninvasive cell tracking may be in the use of therapeutic stem cells, as their utilization in humans will require a method for repeatable, reliable monitoring, without the need for invasive tissue biopsy. MRI is ideally suited for noninvasive, high-resolution visualization of transplanted stem cells. The application of MR for the *in vivo* visualization of transplanted cells in experimental disease models does not only allow for graft detection, but can also show the speed and extent of cell migration.

25.5 PREPARATION OF MAGNETICALLY LABELED STEM CELLS

In order to detect cells with MRI, the cytoplasm does need to contain a suitable MR contrast agent. Most currently used contrast agents for *in vivo* cell detection are based on superparamagnetic iron oxide (SPIO). An important advantage of the iron oxides is their biocompatibility: even if released from the endosomal compartment, they will eventually undergo biodegradation into biologically available iron [81]. Most SPIO-based particles consist of micro (mono) crystalline iron oxide cores coated with dextrans. SPIOs provide the targeted cell with a large magnetic moment that creates substantial disturbances in the local magnetic field, leading to a rapid dephasing of protons, including those surrounding the labeled cell. MR imaging techniques, such as gradient echo sequences, that do not compensate for dephasing, are particularly sensitive to detect the presence of iron oxide magnetic nanoparticles.

For efficient magnetic labeling of nonphagocytic cells, the outer surface of the contrast agent must be modified and prepared for various mechanisms of cellular internalization. Internalization of the SPIO particles agent is important, as particles attached to the outer cell membrane may interfere with cell signaling, or may easily be detached and transferred to other cells. Efficient internalization of SPIOs has been achieved by several methods, including peptide or antibody coating and the use of transfection agents.

25.5.1 PEPTIDES AND ANTIBODY COATING

An example of peptide-induced transmembrane transport of SPIO colloids is the HIV-derived tat peptide, which, due to its membrane-translocating signal, efficiently transports conjugated molecules, leading to their nuclear accumulation [82]. To achieve efficient linking with the tat peptide, the dextran of the magnetic colloid is incubated with epichlorydin followed by ammonia, which creates reactive amino groups suitable for peptide binding [82,83]. The cellular iron oxide uptake is proportional to the number of tat peptides per iron oxide particle [84]. The tat peptide method has been successfully implemented in various experimental paradigms, and SPIO-tat-labeled T cells injected systemically were detected with MRI to home preferentially to the liver and spleen [85,86]. In an animal model of autoimmune diabetes, labeled antigen-specific T lymphocytes were detected specifically in the pancreas [87]. The feasibility of this labeling method was also confirmed by cytological studies showing that the method does not affect cellular function [85].

Antibody coating is another technique for intracellular contrast agent delivery, taking advantage of receptor-based transmembrane transport. An example of a receptor involved in the internalization process is the transferrin receptor [88], present on virtually every cell. In order to use this system for SPIO delivery, the particles were covalently bound to antitransferrin receptor monoclonal antibodies. Oligodendrocyte progenitors or neural precursor cells labeled this way and transplanted in the spinal cords of myelin-deficient animals or in the brains of mice could be detected 2 weeks after injection, using high resolution *ex vivo* MR imaging, being visible as hypointense streaks as far as 1 cm from the injection site [89]. Immunohistochemical staining against proteolipid protein, an essential component of myelin, precisely confirmed distribution of grafted cells detected by MR.

Receptor targeting, or the use of monoclonal antibodies for magnetic labeling, has the distinct advantage of allowing labeling of distinct cell subset populations, but, on the other hand, introduces some limitations. Monoclonal antibodies usually have species-restricted specificity, which causes laborious antibody generation for virtually every experimental paradigm, as well as complex approval procedures that are an important consideration before these agents can be introduced into the clinical setting.

25.5.2 Use of Transfection Agents

Heat-activated dendrimers have been used as transfection agents for over a decade and are commercially available. Magnetodendrimers consist of polycrystalline iron oxide particles coated on the surface with multiple dendrimers [90]. In contrast to the antibody-mediated transport described earlier, this mechanism allows for efficient intracellular magnetic labeling of cells regardless of their antigenic profile. An example of magnetodendrimers is MD-100, which binds to the cell membrane, as induced by its dendrimer coating, and causes membrane invagination and subsequent endocytosis. Internalized magnetodendrimers are eventually deposited in endosomes. Multiple cell types of human and animal origin, including human neural and mesenchymal stem cells [91], have been efficiently labeled with MD-100 by simple 24 to 48 h cell culture incubation. Regardless of the origin or animal species, incubated cells show a comparable degree of particle uptake into endosomes (9 to 14 pg of iron per cell), demonstrating the nonspecific nature of the magnetodendrimer uptake. MD-100-labeled oligodendroglial progenitors, intraventricularly transplanted into neonatal dysmyelinated Long Evans Shaker rats, were visualized using high resolution *in vivo* MRI. Migration (confirmed by classical LacZ staining) was followed along the course of 6 weeks, and, at later time points, contrast began to fade, presumably caused by biodegradation of iron oxide particles [91]. The major disadvantage of the magnetodendrimers is that they are not commercially, and thus not widely, available.

The next generation of more convenient magnetic labeling methods is based on the use of polycationic transfection agents (TAs), e.g., poly L-lysine (PLL) [92] and protamine sulfate [93]. Polycationic TAs have zeta potentials that vary from 1 to 65 mV, whereas dextran-coated Ferumoxides with carboxyl groups on the surface of the nanoparticle have zeta potentials of approximately −41 mV [94]. Combining negatively charged dextran-coated SPIO particles with positively charged TAs in a test tube in appropriate ratios results in complex formation through van der Waals interactions, which in turn results in a decrease in the T_2 relaxivity of the SPIO [94]. The alteration of the T_1 and T_2 relaxation rates indicates that the TAs coat the SPIO, preventing solvent water protons from normal exchange with the paramagnetic sites on iron oxide nanoparticles and thus no effective dipole–dipole T_1 relaxation [94]. The increase in the T_2 relaxation rate indicates that there is an appreciable outer sphere relaxation effect that is enhanced through TA-mediated clustering of SPIO particles. However, the shielding of water from the surface of the SPIO nanoparticles does not necessarily translate into cellular magnetic labeling efficiency, and results indicate that cellular labeling requires a balance between positive and negative charges on the surface of the nanoparticles.

The adaptation of the commercially available SPIO compound Feridex® (an FDA-approved contrast agent for hepatic imaging) to magnetically label nonphagocytes, e.g., stem cells, has been an important development in cellular imaging enabling a quick and easy labeling of cells regardless of their phenotypic characteristics. PLL opsonizes iron particles and, similar to dendrimers, alleviates transmembrane transport and the formation of endosomes. Following Feridex–PLL labeling, no toxic effects are observed, and the proliferation and differentiation capacity are unaffected for most cell types. The amount of cellular iron uptake (10 to 20 pg Fe per cell) is comparable to the results obtained with magnetodendrimer labeling.

An attractive approach for magnetic cell labeling in a clinical setting is the combination of two FDA-approved compounds, Feridex and protamine sulfate [93]. This may facilitate further clinical applications of MRI cell tracking. Protamine sulfate is a low molecular weight polycation, clinically used to reverse the anticoagulative action of heparin, being also an effective transfection agent. Similar to other polycations, protamine sulfate reverses the negative zeta potential of ferumoxides and shuttles them into the cellular endosomal compartment. Another advantage of protamine sulfate is a good toleration by cells with a higher window of tolerance than, for example, PLL.

25.5.3 Other Magnetic Labeling Methods

Other approaches for (nonspecific) magnetic cell labeling have recently been developed; these include the use of dextran-conjugated gadolinium or large magnetic microspheres. Gadolinium chelates, commonly used as extracellular MR contrast agents, have been complexed to dextran and the fluorescent compound rhodamine in order to magnetically label cells. Such complexes have been shown to generate sufficient contrast changes to visualize transplanted cells *in vivo* and follow their migration in a rat stroke model. The fluorescent label of the compound is useful to validate the obtained results using conventional fluorescent microscopy methods [95]. Magnetic labeling with large styrene/divinyl benzene-coated magnetic microspheres, unlike all of the previously described methods, is not based on the spontaneous uptake of particles. Microspheres are actively shot into the cells using a helium-propelled gene gun. Particles, close to 1 μm in size, were efficiently used for labeling and imaging of subventricular zone neural progenitor cells in a rat stroke model. Migration of grafted cells over time could be observed using a 7 T spectrometer. Labeled cells migrated over a significant distance, took on the properties of neurons as assessed histologically, and induced improvement in neurological function, thus suggesting that this labeling method is safe and does not affect the function of cells [96].

25.6 MONITORING OF STEM CELL-BASED THERAPY BY MR

The *ex vivo* MR analysis of the global or local distribution of transplanted stem cells is now a routinely used method that complements conventional histological techniques. This method allows for 3D whole body or organ imaging and presentation of data in any desired anatomical plane — features that are impossible or extremely difficult to achieve using conventional microscopy. Postmortem (*ex vivo*) imaging is not subject to the MR technique limitations associated with living organism imaging (limited acquisition time or motion artifacts); thus, the spatial resolution, signal-to-noise ratio, and sensitivity are much better. The MRI cell tracking technique, however, offers far more valuable data when used in a living organism, allowing for dynamic evaluation of cell migration. From a clinical perspective, it also offers a noninvasive means of monitoring cell-based therapy that enables determining the cell fate without the need for tissue biopsy. Recently, numerous studies have been published describing *in vivo* cell visualization using MR (micro) imaging. SPIO-based intracellular magnetic contrast agents induce sufficient signal changes to detect very small groups of labeled cells using an image resolution of approximately 100 μm. Brain and cardiac disorders have so far received the most attention for the potential application of MRI stem cell tracking techniques.

25.6.1 CNS Disorders

As described earlier, the adult brain contains neuronal progenitors, which, under physiological conditions, proliferate, migrate, and differentiate into the appropriate lineages [9,97]. When transplanted into disease models, these cells were shown to distribute widely in the early (i.e., neonatal) developmental stage [55]. To meet the challenge of *in vivo* imaging of transplanted cells in neurological disease models, several groups have used different imaging modalities, including transcranial bioluminescence [98] and MRI [89,99–103], and were able to successfully perform longitudinal studies visualizing the distribution of cells over time. Using the bioluminescence approach, transplanted neural stem cells engineered to express the reporter gene luciferase were shown to migrate long distances to reach a tumor mass in the hemisphere contralateral to their implantation site [98]. The advantage of bioluminescence studies is the relative simplicity of the procedure, the low cost of equipment, the permanent reporter gene labeling (i.e., no dilution of label upon cell division), and the ability to assess whole body distribution without background signal; unfortunately, poor resolution and limited tissue transparency seriously restrict broader applications for this technique. Unlike bioluminescence, MRI, with its nearly cellular resolution and 3D data acquisition capabilities, can precisely localize transplanted neural stem cells with close correlation to histological data [91].

One example of an application for MR cell tracking and cell-based therapy is in MS [99], which can potentially be treated by transplantation of cells that are capable of repopulating exhausted endogenous myelin-producing oligodendrocytes. A key issue in this approach is to achieve wide distribution of grafted cells. MRI cell tracking was successfully implemented in a rat model of MS, following induction of experimental allergic encephalomyelitis (EAE), which closely resembles the pathology observed in MS (see also Chapter 12). In rats with EAE, inflammatory cells are activated to migrate into the white matter of the brain, thereby inducing the targeted migration of transplanted neural precursor cells [104]. When MD-100-labeled neurospheres were transplanted into the ventricles of EAE rats at the peak of their disease, migration into white matter structures could be observed on the MR images, with a close correlation to conventional histological analysis (Figure 25.6) [99].

In vivo MRI has been used to demonstrate the extent of the distribution of neural stem cell derived oligodendrocytes in a dysmyelinated rat model. Magnetodendrimer-labeled

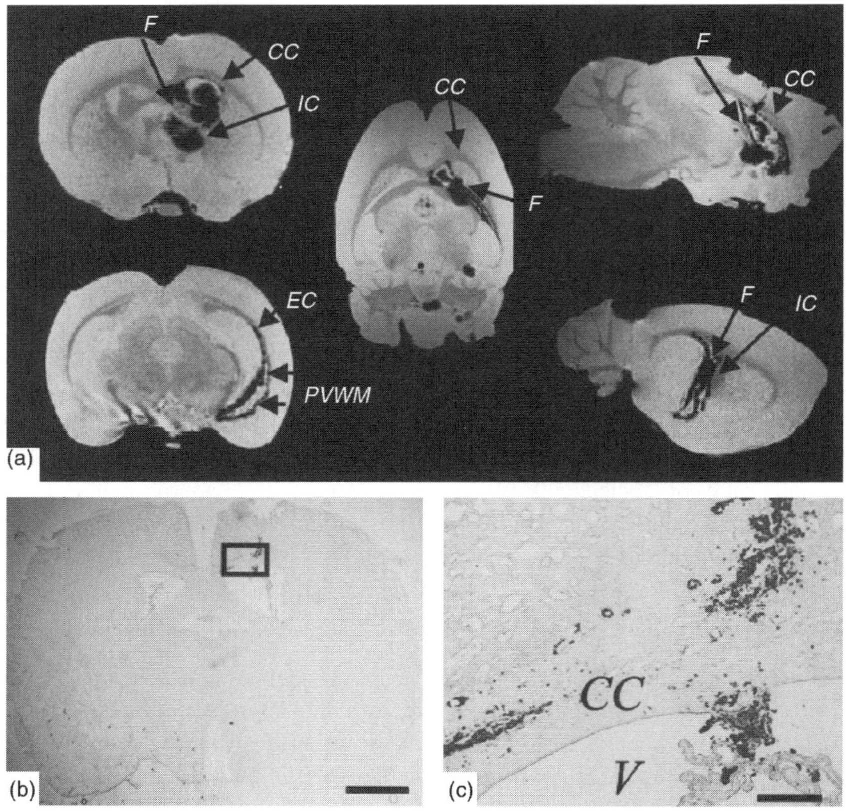

FIGURE 25.6 Magnetically labeled neural progenitor cells transplanted in the ventricles of rats with EAE. *Ex vivo* images were obtained 1 week after transplantation. (a) MR microscopy demonstrating hypointense signal induced by SPIO (magnetodendrimer)-labeled cells. Arrows indicate white matter brain structures containing grafted cells. (b, c) Prussian Blue staining for iron of histological section corresponding to the top left MR image validates the MR imaging findings. CC = corpus callosum, EC = external capsule, IC = internal capsule, F = fimbria, PVWM = periventricular white matter, V = ventricle. Scale bar = 2 mm (b) and 200 μm (c). (Reproduced from Bulte, J. W. et al., *Magn. Reson. Med.*, 50, 201, 2003. With permission of Wiley-Liss, Inc., a subsidiary of John Wiley & Sons. Copyright 2003.)

oligodendrocyte progenitors transplanted into the neonatal rat allowed for *in vivo* detection for up to 4 weeks. Gradual signal fading beyond that time point was most likely caused by biodegradation of the contrast agent [91]. The migratory properties of oligodendrocyte progenitors are naturally stronger in the early developmental stage, and their application in adult or aged subjects is more challenging. Several molecules, however, are known to induce oligodendrocyte progenitor migration (reviewed in [105]). MR cell tracking would be even more valuable if migration could be extended and its direction could be controlled, e.g., by exogenous mediators.

Stroke is an example of another brain disorder where restorative cell therapy may be even more challenging than that in MS, and will likely require sophisticated monitoring methods as can be provided by *in vivo* MRI cell tracking. Migration of SPIO-labeled embryonic stem cells toward the stroke lesion from one hemisphere to the other has been demonstrated on high resolution MRI scans. The extensive migratory behavior was confirmed by conventional green fluorescent protein (GFP) reporter gene fluorescent microscopy [100]. Similar results were obtained when gadolinium–rhodamine labeled neural progenitors were injected in the contralateral hemisphere, with cells invading the penumbra [95] (Figure 25.7). Targeted migration of SPIO-labeled neural stem cells could also be visualized following a different administration route, i.e., intracisternal injection [96]. The difficulty in regenerating damaged neural circuitries is largely attributed to the lack of appropriate developmental signals. Thus, hope for the treatment of brain diseases such as stroke relies on the ability to control migration and differentiation-inducing signals and, most importantly, molecules that direct axon sprouting, allowing for new transplanted neurons to reach targets as distant as 1 m (in the case of human cortico-spinal tracts or motor neuron axons). It is

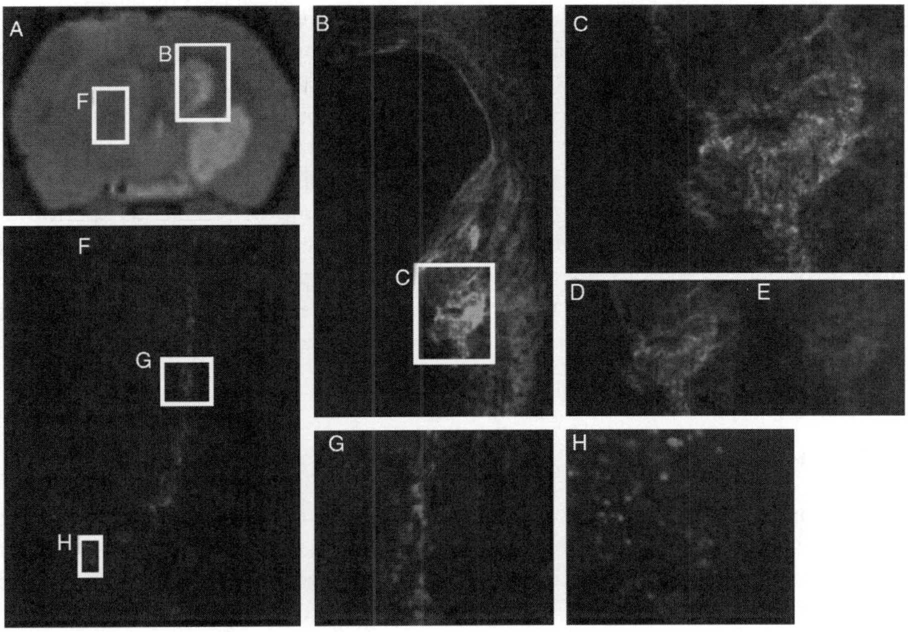

FIGURE 25.7 (See color insert following page 328.) MRI of cellular migration in a rat stroke model. Neural stem cells labeled with gadolinium- and rhodamine-containing dextran polymers were transplanted into the brain hemisphere contralateral to the stroke lesion 3 months after induction. T_2-weighted MRI, obtained 14 days after injection, revealed hypointense regions in proximity to the stroke lesion, indicating infiltration by grafted cells (A). Fluorescent microscopy (C–H) confirmed the presence of rhodamin labeled cells (red) within or close to the lesion, which was filled with astrocytic scar tissue (green, anti-GFAP staining). This labeling strategy allows for convenient bimodal imaging of transplanted cells. (Reproduced from Modo, M. et al., *Neuroimage*, 21, 311, 2004. With permission. Copyright 2004. Elsevier.)

possible that technological and methodological advancements will soon enable the use of MRI to visualize sprouting axons of labeled neurons as well as interactive redirection to reach appropriate targets. Finally, other MR tracking studies in the CNS have been performed, including the demonstration of brain tumor infiltration of microsphere-labeled neural stem cells [106].

25.6.2 Infarcted Myocardium

Cardiac tissue almost completely lacks regenerative capacity. Thus, interest in restoration of lost or limited heart function with stem cell-based therapies has been a major research focus, in particular for initiating clinical trials. As mentioned previously, there is a large body of evidence based on animal research, as well as on initial clinical trials, that cell-based therapy may effectively delay or prevent congestive heart failure. It is believed that the therapeutic effect of stem cell transplantation can be further optimized if the posttransplant cell fate could be evaluated *in vivo*. This would help to determine the appropriate cell delivery route, to assess the accuracy of injection, and to correlate the cell distribution with the functional performance of the heart muscle.

MR cell tracking has proved to be suitable in the detection of intramyocardial as well as peripheral cell injection in animal infarct models. The distribution of Feridex–PLL labeled swine mesenchymal stem cells, for example, was studied upon direct intramyocardial injection into a swine infarct model [107]. In MR images, grafts were seen 24 h after cell injection as hypointense areas, surrounded by hyperintense delayed-enhanced infarct tissue with a sharp delineation of the cellular biodistribution borders. The hypointense regions gradually expanded at later time points to reach 115% of volume (as compared to 24 h) at 1 week postgrafting, when the infarct area was considerably reduced. Postmortem histological analysis confirmed the presence of transplanted cells, corresponding to the hypointense areas on MRI. In another study, large, micron-size magnetic beads were used to label swine mesenchymal stem cells for intramyocardial injection. As little as 10^5 labeled cells were detected on MRI scans [108]. The advantage of the use of larger beads is enhanced signal loss, allowing the detection of lower cell numbers *in vivo*; however, these beads are not biodegradable preventing their use in the clinic.

MRI can be helpful in other aspects associated with cell-based therapy of cardiac infarction. The initial estimation of infarct size and localization can be efficiently performed with noninvasive, delayed contrast-enhanced MRI [109]. This provides critical data for the estimation of the number of cells needed for therapy and to plan the optimal delivery route (transthoracic vs. transvascular). In addition, with the use of recently developed MR-compatible injection catheters [110,111], injection of labeled cells can be precisely targeted within or near the periphery of the infarct.

25.7 CONCLUSIONS

MRI cell tracking has become an important tool for studying the in vivo behavioral properties of stem cells. The strength of this method, unlike any other, is that it enables the noninvasive observation of cells in their native environment — a living organism — with high resolution and whole body penetration. This provides the opportunity to correlate behavioral observations or physiological measures with the distribution of administered cells. MRI cell tracking may expedite the clinical application of cell therapies by contributing to our understanding of stem cell biology, as well as offering the potential as a safe and suitable monitoring tool.

ACKNOWLEDGMENTS

The authors are supported by NIH RO1 NS045062, and are grateful to Mary McAllister for editorial suggestions.

REFERENCES

1. Koehne, G. et al., Serial in vivo imaging of the targeted migration of human HSV–TK-transduced antigen-specific lymphocytes, *Nat. Biotechnol.*, 21(405), 413, 2003.
2. Hardy, J. et al., Extracellular replication of Listeria monocytogenes in the murine gall bladder, *Science*, 303, 851, 2004.
3. Chin, B. B. et al., In-111-oxime labeled mesenchymal stem cell SPECT imaging after intravenous administration in myocardial infarction, *J. Nucl. Med.*, 44, 192, 2003.
4. Bulte, J. W. M., Duncan, I. D., and Frank, J. A., In vivo magnetic resonance tracking of magnetically labeled cells after transplantation, *J. Cereb. Blood Flow Metab.*, 22, 899, 2002.
5. Kernie, S. G., Erwin, T. M., and Parada, L. F., Brain remodeling due to neuronal and astrocytic proliferation after controlled cortical injury in mice, *J. Neurosci. Res.*, 66, 317, 2001.
6. Beltrami, A. P. et al., Evidence that human cardiac myocytes divide after myocardial infarction, *N. Engl. J. Med.*, 344, 1750, 2001.
7. Doetsch, F. et al., Subventricular zone astrocytes act as neural stem cells, *J. Neurol.*, 246, 747, 1999.
8. Rakic, P., Neuroscience — immigration denied, *Nature*, 427, 685, 2004.
9. Kornack, D. R. and Rakic, P., Continuation of neurogenesis in the hippocampus of the adult macaque monkey, *Proc. Natl Acad. Sci. USA*, 96, 5768, 1999.
10. Alvarez-Buylla, A. and Lim, D. A., For the long run: maintaining germinal niches in the adult brain, *Neuron*, 41, 683, 2004.
11. Bortin, M. M., A compendium of reported human bone marrow transplants, *Transplantation*, 9, 571, 1970.
12. Passweg, J. R. et al., Bone marrow transplantation for severe aplastic anemia: has outcome improved?, *Blood*, 90, 858, 1997.
13. Gratwohl, A. et al., Hematopoetic stem cell transplantation for solid tumors in Europe, *Ann. Oncol.*, 15, 653, 2004.
14. Steece-Collier, K. et al., Embryonic mesencephalic grafts increase levodopa-induced forelimb hyperkinesia in Parkinsonian rats, *Mov. Disord.*, 18, 1442, 2003.
15. Willing, A. E. et al., Intravenous versus intrastriatal cord blood administration in a rodent model of stroke, *J. Neurosci. Res.*, 73, 296, 2003.
16. Kerr, D. A. et al., Human embryonic germ cell derivatives facilitate motor recovery of rats with diffuse motor neuron injury, *J. Neurosci.*, 23, 5131, 2003.
17. Kohama, I. et al., Transplantation of cryopreserved adult human Schwann cells enhances axonal conduction in demyelinated spinal cord, *J. Neurosci.*, 21, 944, 2001.
18. Pittenger, M. F. and Martin, B. J., Mesenchymal stem cells and their potential as cardiac therapeutics, *Circ. Res.*, 95, 9, 2004.
19. Magavi, S. S. and Macklis, J. D., Manipulation of neural precursors in situ: induction of neurogenesis in the neocortex of adult mice, *Neuropsychopharmacology*, 25, 816, 2001.
20. Schrag, A. and Quinn, N., Dyskinesias and motor fluctuations in Parkinson's disease. A community-based study, *Brain*, 123, 2297, 2000.
21. Bjorklund, A. and Stenevi, U., Reconstruction of the nigrostriatal dopamine pathway by intra-cerebral nigral transplants, *Brain Res.*, 177, 555, 1979.
22. Mendez, J. S. and Finn, B. W., Use of 6-hydroxydopamine to create lesions in catecholamine neurons in rats, *J. Neurosurg.*, 42, 166, 1975.
23. Langston, J. W. et al., Selective nigral toxicity after systemic administration of 1-methyl-4-phenyl-1,2,5,6-tetrahydropyrine (MPTP) in the squirrel monkey, *Brain Res.*, 292, 390, 1984.
24. Liker, M. A. et al., Human neural stem cell transplantation in the MPTP-lesioned mouse, *Brain Res.*, 971, 168, 2003.
25. Kim, J. H. et al., Dopamine neurons derived from embryonic stem cells function in an animal model of Parkinson's disease, *Nature*, 418, 50, 2002.
26. Brundin, P. et al., Improving the survival of grafted dopaminergic neurons: a review over current approaches, *Cell Transplant.*, 9, 179, 2000.
27. Helt, C. E. et al., Neuroprotection of grafted neurons with a GDNF/caspase inhibitor cocktail, *Exp. Neurol.*, 170, 258, 2001.

28. Apostolides, C. et al., Glial cell line-derived neurotrophic factor improves intrastriatal graft survival of stored dopaminergic cells, *Neuroscience*, 83, 363, 1998.
29. Lindvall, O., Transplantation into the human brain: present status and future possibilities, *J Neurol Neurosurg Psychiatry*, (Suppl), 39, 1989.
30. Kordower, J. H. et al., Neuropathological evidence of graft survival and striatal reinnervation after the transplantation of fetal mesencephalic tissue in a patient with Parkinson's disease, *N. Engl. J. Med.*, 332, 1118, 1995.
31. Olanow, C. W. et al., A double-blind controlled trial of bilateral fetal nigral transplantation in Parkinson's disease, *Ann. Neurol.*, 54, 403, 2003.
32. Levi, L., Wolf, A., and Belzberg, H., Hemodynamic parameters in patients with acute cervical cord trauma: description, intervention, and prediction of outcome, *Neurosurgery*, 33, 1007, 1993.
33. Bracken, M. B., Methylprednisolone and acute spinal cord injury: an update of the randomized evidence, *Spine*, 26, S47, 2001.
34. Geisler, F. H., Dorsey, F. C., and Coleman, W. P., Recovery of motor function after spinal-cord injury-a randomized, placebo-controlled trial with GM-1 ganglioside, *N. Engl. J. Med.*, 324, 1829, 1991.
35. Hadley, M. N., Pharmacological therapy after acute cervical spinal cord injury, *Neurosurgery*, 50, S63, 2002.
36. DeVivo, M. J. et al., Cause of death for patients with spinal cord injuries, *Arch. Intern. Med.*, 149, 1761, 1989.
37. Bunge, R. P. et al., Observations on the pathology of human spinal cord injury. A review and classification of 22 new cases with details from a case of chronic cord compression with extensive focal demyelination, *Adv. Neurol.*, 59, 75, 1993.
38. Himes, B. T. et al., Transplants of cells genetically modified to express neurotrophin-3 rescue axotomized Clarke's nucleus neurons after spinal cord hemisection in adult rats, *J. Neurosci. Res.*, 65, 549, 2001.
39. BernsteinGoral, H. and Bregman, B. S., Axotomized rubrospinal neurons rescued by fetal spinal cord transplants maintain axon collaterals to rostral CNS targets, *Exp. Neurol.*, 148, 13, 1997.
40. Murray, M. et al., Transplantation of genetically modified cells contributes to repair and recovery from spinal injury, *Brain Res. Brain Res. Rev.*, 40, 292, 2002.
41. Ramón y Cajal, S. and May, R. M., *Degeneration and Regeneration of the Nervous System*, Oxford University Press, Humphrey Milford, London, 1928.
42. Keirstead, H. S. et al., Suppression of the onset of myelination extends the permissive period for the functional repair of embryonic spinal cord, *Proc. Natl Acad. Sci. USA*, 89, 11664, 1992.
43. Brosamle, C. et al., Regeneration of lesioned corticospinal tract fibers in the adult rat induced by a recombinant, humanized IN-1 antibody fragment, *J. Neurosci.*, 20, 8061, 2000.
44. Harper, J. M. et al., Axonal growth of embryonic stem cell-derived motoneurons in vitro and in motoneuron-injured adult rats, *Proc. Natl Acad. Sci. USA*, 101, 7123, 2004.
45. Giovanini, M. A. et al., Characteristics of human fetal spinal cord grafts in the adult rat spinal cord: influences of lesion and grafting conditions, *Exp. Neurol.*, 148, 523, 1997.
46. McDonald, J. W. et al., Transplanted embryonic stem cells survive, differentiate and promote recovery in injured rat spinal cord, *Nat. Med.*, 5, 1410, 1999.
47. Gorio, A. et al., Fate of autologous dermal stem cells transplanted into the spinal cord after traumatic injury (TSCI), *Neuroscience*, 125, 179, 2004.
48. Sykova, E. et al., Bone marrow stromal cells — a promising tool for therapy of brain and spinal cord injuries, *Exp. Neurol.*, 187, 220, 2004.
49. Murray, P. D. et al., Spontaneous remyelination following extensive demyelination is associated with improved neurological function in a viral model of multiple sclerosis, *Brain*, 124, 1403, 2001.
50. Wolswijk, G., Oligodendrocyte precursor cells in the demyelinated multiple sclerosis spinal cord, *Brain*, 125, 338, 2002.
51. Groves, A. K. et al., Repair of demyelinated lesions by transplantation of purified O-2A progenitor cells, *Nature*, 362, 453, 1993.
52. Blakemore, W. F., Gilson, J. M., and Crang, A. J., Transplanted glial cells migrate over a greater distance and remyelinate demyelinated lesions more rapidly than endogenous remyelinating cells, *J. Neurosci. Res.*, 61, 288, 2000.

53. Imaizumi, T., Lankford, K. L., and Kocsis, J. D., Transplantation of olfactory ensheathing cells or Schwann cells restores rapid and secure conduction across the transected spinal cord, *Brain Res.*, 854, 70, 2000.
54. Imaizumi, T. et al., Xenotransplantation of transgenic pig olfactory ensheathing cells promotes axonal regeneration in rat spinal cord, *Nat. Biotechnol.*, 18, 949, 2000.
55. Yandava, B. D., Billinghurst, L. L., and Snyder, E. Y., Global cell replacement is feasible via neural stem cell transplantation: evidence from the dysmyelinated shiverer mouse brain, *Proc. Natl Acad. Sci. USA*, 96, 7029, 1999.
56. Brustle, O. et al., Embryonic stem cell-derived glial precursors: a source of myelinating transplants, *Science*, 285, 754, 1999.
57. Bjorklund, L. M. et al., Embryonic stem cells develop into functional dopaminergic neurons after transplantation in a Parkinson rat model, *Proc. Natl Acad. Sci. USA*, 99, 2344, 2002.
58. Kelly, S. et al., Transplanted human fetal neural stem cells survive, migrate, and differentiate in ischemic rat cerebral cortex, *Proc. Natl Acad. Sci. USA*, 101, 11839, 2004.
59. Riolobos, A. S. et al., Functional recovery of skilled forelimb use in rats obliged to use the impaired limb after grafting of the frontal cortex lesion with homotopic fetal cortex, *Neurobiol. Learn. Mem.*, 75, 274, 2001.
60. Szentirmai, O. and Carter, B. S., Genetic and cellular therapies for cerebral infarction, *Neurosurgery*, 55, 283, 2004.
61. Kondziolka, D. et al., Transplantation of cultured human neuronal cells for patients with stroke, *Neurology*, 55, 565, 2000.
62. Kordower, J. H., Isacson, O., and Emerich, D. F., Cellular delivery of trophic factors for the treatment of Huntington's disease: is neuroprotection possible?, *Exp. Neurol.*, 159, 4, 1999.
63. McBride, J. L. et al., Human neural stem cell transplants improve motor function in a rat model of Huntington's disease, *J. Comp. Neurol.*, 475, 211, 2004.
64. Freeman, T. B. et al., Transplanted fetal striatum in Huntington's disease: phenotypic development and lack of pathology, *Proc. Natl Acad. Sci. USA*, 97, 13877, 2000.
65. Snyder, E. Y., Taylor, R. M., and Wolfe, J. H., Neural progenitor cell engraftment corrects lysosomal storage throughout the MPS VII mouse brain, *Nature*, 374, 367, 1995.
66. Lacorazza, H. D. et al., Expression of human beta-hexosaminidase alpha-subunit gene (the gene defect of Tay–Sachs disease) in mouse brains upon engraftment of transduced progenitor cells, *Nat. Med.*, 2, 424, 1996.
67. Jackson, K. A. et al., Regeneration of ischemic cardiac muscle and vascular endothelium by adult stem cells, *J. Clin. Invest.*, 107, 1395, 2001.
68. Quaini, F. et al., Chimerism of the transplanted heart, *N. Engl. J. Med.*, 346, 5, 2002.
69. Taylor, D. A. et al., Regenerating functional myocardium: improved performance after skeletal myoblast transplantation, *Nat. Med.*, 4, 929, 1998.
70. Menasche, P., Cell transplantation for the treatment of heart failure, *Semin. Thorac. Cardiovasc. Surg.*, 14, 157, 2002.
71. Makino, S. et al., Cardiomyocytes can be generated from marrow stromal cells in vitro, *J. Clin. Invest.*, 103, 697, 1999.
72. Liechty, K. W. et al., Human mesenchymal stem cells engraft and demonstrate site-specific differentiation after in utero transplantation in sheep, *Nat. Med.*, 6, 1282, 2000.
73. Kocher, A. A. et al., Neovascularization of ischemic myocardium by human bone-marrow-derived angioblasts prevents cardiomyocyte apoptosis, reduces remodeling and improves cardiac function, *Nat. Med.*, 7, 430, 2001.
74. Deb, A. et al., Bone marrow-derived cardiomyocytes are present in adult human heart: a study of gender-mismatched bone marrow transplantation patients, *Circulation*, 107, 1247, 2003.
75. Wollert, K. C. et al., Intracoronary autologous bone-marrow cell transfer after myocardial infarction: the BOOST randomised controlled clinical trial, *Lancet*, 364, 141, 2004.
76. Li, R. K. et al., In vivo survival and function of transplanted rat cardiomyocytes, *Circ. Res.*, 78, 283, 1996.
77. Sakai, T. et al., Fetal cell transplantation: a comparison of three cell types, *J. Thorac. Cardiovasc. Surg.*, 118, 715, 1999.

78. Hodgson, D. M. et al., Stable benefit of embryonic stem cell therapy in myocardial infarction, *Am. J. Physiol. Heart Circ. Physiol.*, 287, H471, 2004.
79. Asano, T. et al., Engraftment and tumor formation after allogeneic in utero transplantation of primate embryonic stem cell, *Transplantation*, 76, 1061, 2003.
80. Louie, A. Y. et al., In vivo visualization of gene expression using magnetic resonance imaging, *Nat. Biotechnol.*, 18, 321, 2000.
81. Weissleder, R. et al., Superparamagnetic iron-oxide — pharmacokinetics and toxicity, *Am. J. Roentgenol.*, 152, 167, 1989.
82. Lewin, M. et al., Tat peptide-derivatized magnetic nanoparticles allow in vivo tracking and recovery of progenitor cells, *Nat. Biotechnol.*, 18, 410, 2000.
83. Josephson, L. et al., High-efficiency intracellular magnetic labeling with novel superparamagnetic–Tat peptide conjugates, *Bioconjug. Chem.*, 10, 186, 1999.
84. Zhao, M. et al., Differential conjugation of tat peptide to superparamagnetic nanoparticles and its effect on cellular uptake, *Bioconjug. Chem.*, 13, 840, 2002.
85. Dodd, C. H. et al., Normal T-cell response and in vivo magnetic resonance imaging of T cells loaded with HIV transactivator–peptide-derived superparamagnetic nanoparticles, *J. Immunol. Methods*, 256, 89, 2001.
86. Schoepf, U. et al., Intracellular magnetic labeling of lymphocytes for in vivo trafficking studies, *Biotechniques*, 24, 642, 1998.
87. Moore, A. et al., Non-invasive imaging of antigen-specific T cells in insulitic lesions, *Diabetes*, 51, A109, 2002.
88. Jefferies, W. A. et al., Transferrin receptor on endothelium of brain capillaries, *Nature*, 312, 162, 1984.
89. Bulte, J. W. et al., Neurotransplantation of magnetically labeled oligodendrocyte progenitors: magnetic resonance tracking of cell migration and myelination, *Proc. Natl Acad. Sci. USA*, 96, 15256, 1999.
90. Strable, E. et al., Synthesis and characterization of soluble iron oxide–dendrimer complexes, *Chem. Mater.*, 13, 2201, 2001.
91. Bulte, J. W. et al., Magnetodendrimers allow endosomal magnetic labeling and in vivo tracking of stem cells, *Nat. Biotechnol.*, 19, 1141, 2001.
92. Frank, J. A. et al., Clinically applicable labeling of mammalian and stem cells by combining superparamagnetic iron oxides and transfection agents, *Radiology*, 228, 480, 2003.
93. Arbab, A. S. et al., Efficient magnetic cell labeling with protamine sulfate complexed to ferumoxides for cellular MRI, *Blood*, 104, 1217, 2004.
94. Kalish, H. et al., Combination of transfection agents and magnetic resonance contrast agents for cellular imaging: relationship between relaxivities, electrostatic forces, and chemical composition, *Magn. Reson. Med.*, 50, 275, 2003.
95. Modo, M. et al., Mapping transplanted stem cell migration after a stroke: a serial, in vivo magnetic resonance imaging study, *Neuroimage*, 21, 311, 2004.
96. Zhang, Z. G. et al., Magnetic resonance imaging and neurosphere therapy of stroke in rat, *Ann. Neurol.*, 53, 259, 2003.
97. Luskin, M. B., Restricted proliferation and migration of postnatally generated neurons derived from the forebrain subventricular zone, *Neuron*, 11, 173, 1993.
98. Tang, Y. et al., In vivo tracking of neural progenitor cell migration to glioblastomas, *Hum. Gene Ther.*, 14, 1247, 2003.
99. Bulte, J. W. et al., MR microscopy of magnetically labeled neurospheres transplanted into the Lewis EAE rat brain, *Magn. Reson. Med.*, 50, 201, 2003.
100. Hoehn, M. et al., Monitoring of implanted stem cell migration in vivo: a highly resolved in vivo magnetic resonance imaging investigation of experimental stroke in rat, *Proc. Natl Acad. Sci. USA*, 99, 16267, 2002.
101. Zhang, R. L. et al., Migration and differentiation of adult rat subventricular zone progenitor cells transplanted into the adult rat striatum, *Neuroscience*, 116, 373, 2003.
102. Jendelova, P. et al., Imaging the fate of implanted bone marrow stromal cells labeled with superparamagnetic nanoparticles, *Magn. Reson. Med.*, 50, 767, 2003.
103. Hawrylak, N. et al., Nuclear magnetic resonance (NMR) imaging of iron oxide-labeled neural transplants, *Exp. Neurol.*, 121, 181, 1993.

104. Ben-Hur, T. et al., Transplanted multipotential neural precursor cells migrate into the inflamed white matter in response to experimental autoimmune encephalomyelitis, *Glia*, 41, 73, 2003.
105. Jarjour, A. A. and Kennedy, T. E., Oligodendrocyte precursors on the move: mechanisms directing migration, *Neuroscientist*, 10, 99, 2004.
106. Zhang, Z. et al., In vivo magnetic resonance imaging tracks adult neural progenitor cell targeting of brain tumor, *Neuroimage*, 23, 281, 2004.
107. Kraitchman, D. L. et al., In vivo magnetic resonance imaging of mesenchymal stem cells in myocardial infarction, *Circulation*, 107, 2290, 2003.
108. Hill, J. M. et al., Serial cardiac magnetic resonance imaging of injected mesenchymal stem cells, *Circulation*, 108, 1009, 2003.
109. Simonetti, O. P. et al., An improved MR imaging technique for the visualization of myocardial infarction, *Radiology*, 218, 215, 2001.
110. Lederman, R. J. et al., Catheter-based endomyocardial injection with real-time magnetic resonance imaging, *Circulation*, 105, 1282, 2002.
111. Karmarkar, P. V. et al., MR trackable intramyocardial injection catheter, *Magn. Reson. Med.*, 51, 1163, 2004.
112. Donovan, P. J. and Gearhart, J., The end of the beginning for pluripotent stem cells, *Nature*, 414, 92, 2001.
113. Li, Y., Field, P. M., and Raisman, G., Regeneration of adult rat corticospinal axons induced by transplanted olfactory ensheathing cells, *J. Neurosci.*, 18, 10514, 1998.

Editorial Comments

The use of *in vivo* MRI techniques in pharmaceutical safety studies is surprisingly far behind their utilization in drug efficacy testing. The reason for this situation is rather related to organizational issues than to the properties of MRI. Toxicological studies are performed under strict Good Laboratory Practice guidelines, which demand special preparation of the laboratories. Most imaging units in pharmaceutical industry probably do not meet the required standards of those guidelines. On the other hand, toxicology is often carried out in separate areas, outside the research settings where the imaging laboratories are located. Transportation of animals during toxicological assessments is avoided as much as possible in order to minimize potential influences of stress on the outcomes. Nonetheless, it is conceivable that imaging studies accomplished on separate groups of animals could support toxicological studies performed for regulatory purposes.

In Chapter 26, David Reid provides compelling evidence that the excellent diagnostic capabilities of MRI for the detection of pathological alterations in soft tissues can be explored not only to detect drug effects, but also to follow the origin, progression, and regression of chemically induced lesions in the same live animal. Of particular interest in this context is the detection of the effects of chemicals on organ function since this information cannot be derived using histology.

26 MRI in Pharmaceutical Safety Assessment

David Reid

CONTENTS

26.1 INTRODUCTION

This chapter is not an overview of the sciences of toxicology and pharmaceutical safety assessment, which are thoroughly reviewed in standard textbooks [1,2]. Rather, it examines those elements of these disciplines that are, or should be, amenable to productive investigation by MRI approaches.

26.1.1 Advantages of MRI

The use of *in vivo* MRI in preclinical studies of basic physiology, anatomical structure, and pharmacology, is now common and routine in a number of industrial and academic laboratories. Features of MRI which make it so attractive in *in vivo* studies of direct drug action also offer new ways of addressing the causes, mechanisms, and consequences of the unwanted side effects of pharmacological agents. It does not use ionizing radiation (unlike x-ray CT), or require the administration of radioactive tracer substances (unlike PET, gamma scintigraphy, or SPECT), so there are essentially no practical limits to how frequently scans may be performed. The scanning procedure itself has only slight, if any, harmful or physiologically perturbing effects on the organism. Structure and function of organs and tissues are studied *in situ* and *in vivo* without the potentially confounding influences of surgical insertion of probes, or *post mortem* tissue dissection, fixation, sectioning, and staining. In toxicology studies, animals can be scanned before dosing begins, so randomization to groups is possible from baseline scans and each animal can be used as its own control; both factors favor increased statistical power and thereby reduction in the use of experimental animals, and refinement of experimental procedures. Longitudinal studies of toxicity progression and regression, and crossover designs, are straightforward to design and implement if necessary. Unlike the exciting new optical and radiotracer methods which are becoming available for the imaging of toxicologically induced changes in gene expression, MRI methods do not require genetic manipulation of animals to insert reporter genes to reflect transcriptional activity, nor the administration of radiolabeled or optical probe molecules. In fact, apart from the obvious constraints around access to MRI facilities and expertise, the ability to conduct investigations in practically any species, at any stage of testing, invests the approach with an attractive simplicity and universality.

There are, however, down sides. Firstly, it is necessary to anesthetize animals for scanning. This is a potential confounding factor in toxicology due to the possibility of drug–anesthetic metabolic interactions, but can be controlled for by, for instance, the inclusion of satellite animals or groups which receive all treatments in life, except anesthesia and scanning, and which then undergo the same *post mortem* assessments (e.g., histopathology, organ weight) as the anesthetized, scanned animals. Secondly, it requires skill, insight, and experience to identify and optimize MRI methodologies for addressing unfamiliar problems in toxicological pathology although, once set up, a new method can generally be used in a push button routine manner by relatively inexperienced staff. Thirdly, MRI is not a sensitive detection modality, which is generally not a problem in anatomical imaging where the target structure is delineated by abundant water and fat. However, it will limit the use of molecular targeted contrast agents which require local concentrations orders of magnitude higher than those needed for nuclear imaging to influence their environment to a measurable extent. It also limits the usefulness of spectroscopic imaging of the distribution of less abundant metabolites, the levels of which may be useful toxicity biomarkers.

26.1.2 Pathologies Observable by MRI

In spite of its attractions [3], the application of MRI to pharmaceutical safety assessment as an end in its own right has lagged behind its use in pharmacological model development and drug efficacy testing. Thus, there are numerous published examples of MRI scanning of lesions induced chemically for pharmacological purposes, e.g., excitotoxin injections into the brain to model neurodegenerative processes, the administration of bacterial endotoxins or allergens to provoke inflammatory responses in lung, joints, or brain, to mimic asthma, arthritis, or multiple sclerosis, respectively, or the topical application of vasoconstrictors to provoke regional ischemia. However, the potential for the use of MRI in toxicology investigations is considerable, as born out by the larger body of literature dealing with its use in the study of environmental and industrial toxins and drugs of abuse.

A straightforward but nevertheless potentially extremely valuable application of MRI is measuring longitudinal changes in organ size. While this can generally be cheaply and quickly measured *post mortem*, imaging avoids possible errors in dissection and organ removal and, of course, enables serial measurements in the same animals. It may thus make longitudinal studies in large, expensive, or highly sentient animals such as primates, practical and ethically acceptable when they would not be so if *post mortem* methods had to be used.

Beyond straightforward anatomical imaging, MRI image contrast can be tailored to reflect different molecular properties of tissue and cellular water, and thereby underlying pathology. The extent and nature of water–macromolecule interactions govern T_1 and T_2 relaxation processes, and magnetization transfer (MT) contrast. Differential water molecular diffusion rates, and anisotropies, make diffusion-weighted imaging (DWI) a powerful probe of water compartmentation, and hence cell swelling and lysis, and axonal demyelination. MRI is an ideal technique for measuring tissue edema in response to toxicological necrotic processes, pathological kidney function or vascular changes, and inflammatory or irritant challenges. It is a method-of-choice for detection and quantification of solid tumors in most organs due to the distinctive relaxation times of neoplastic and cancerous tissue. To some extent, it is possible to predict the MRI acquisition technique, or stain as it has been referred to [4], which will best reflect a given toxicological pathology. Nevertheless, it is usual to use an empirical approach to establishing the best acquisition protocol to highlight a new pathology in an MR image, and pilot studies using model systems are valuable in establishing the methodology prior to imaging the effects of test compounds. It is advisable and usual to substantiate *in vivo* MRI findings with conventional *post mortem* histopathological and/or gravimetric/volumetric measurements, especially as the microscopic approaches provide opportunities to gather complementary information based on, for instance, immunohistochemistry and high resolution light or electron microscopy. In this way, correlations between *in vivo* MRI and conventional pathology toxicity biomarkers are being built up and validated.

In terms of physiological function, MRI is an ideal approach to measuring cardiac ejection fraction and output (as well as cardiac hypertrophy) and studying toxic insults which alter these. Dynamic MRI contrast enhancement using paramagnetic tracer reagents has great potential for elucidating toxicological derangement of perfusion in organs such as kidney and testis, toxicological disruption of the blood brain barrier, and vascular permeability in inflammation. Finally, blood oxygen level dependent (BOLD) MRI is a promising approach to investigating toxicological compromise of metabolic activity, and angiography to investigating toxicological changes in arterial and venous structure.

This chapter will review literature reports and present examples of applications of MRI in toxicology, with an emphasis on pharmaceutical side effects. Some organ systems have been the subject of numerous toxicological imaging studies (liver, heart, central nervous system, kidneys); imaging markers of toxicology in several others (endocrine and reproductive organs) have not been well characterized although it is quite possible to envisage applications of great value.

26.2 ORGAN SPECIFIC TOXICITY

26.2.1 Liver

As it is the first organ to encounter ingested drugs, and plays a major role in their metabolism, the liver is a frequent site of pharmaceutical side effects and industrial chemical toxicity. Several common forms of liver toxicity are amenable to observation and study by MRI. These include steatosis (fatty liver), defined biochemically as a 5% increase in liver fat, cirrhosis, an end stage of chronic liver disease in which destroyed hepatocytes become replaced by fibrotic scar-like tissue, chemically induced neoplasia leading to MRI-visible tumors, and hypertrophy, which is provoked by a number of compounds, such as barbiturates, and the widely used antihyperlipidaemic fibrates.

MRI has been used to study fat infiltration and cirrhosis [5], hepatic edema [6,7], and interactions with ethanol [8] associated with the model hepatotoxin carbon tetrachloride. Chronic ethanol ingestion causes liver T_2W and manganese dipyridoxal diphosphate contrast enhancement changes [9]. T_1W scans show areas of low signal intensity corresponding to areas of bromobenzene induced liver necrosis in rats [10]. Cell specific superparamagnetic contrast agents are useful in characterizing experimentally induced liver cirrhosis and fibrosis [11]. T_2W and water chemical shift imaging methods show edema proximal to the hepatic portal vein induced by microcystin-LR [12]. MRI T_1 and T_2 parameters and the degree of cirrhosis and fibrosis induced in rat liver by carbon tetrachloride and thioacetamide correlate well [13]. T_2W imaging shows hyperintense

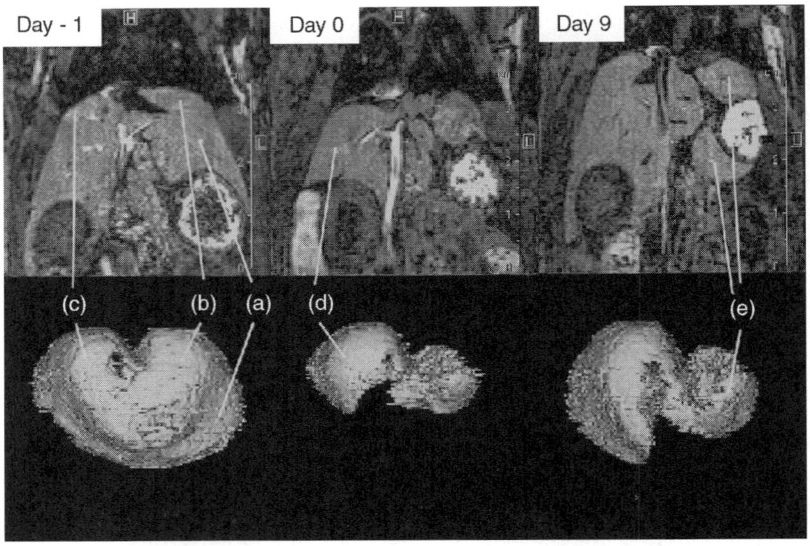

FIGURE 26.1 Liver regeneration after partial hepatectomy. The top panels depict typical coronal slices through 3D respiratory and cardiac gated spin echo images through the upper abdomen of a rat before (left), immediately after (middle), and 9 days after surgical removal of the left lateral and left median lobes of the liver. The bottom panels show surface rendered views of the digitally segmented and reconstructed liver at the same time points. The reconstructions clearly convey how a functional liver regenerates by a process of hypertrophy of the relict lobes. The lobes are identified as follows: a — Left lateral, b — median (left), c — median (right), d — right lateral, e — caudate. Experimental details: 7 T 3D fat suppressed inversion recovery-prepared segmented multi-spin echo, NEchoes 16, TI 950 msec TE_{eff} 25 msec TR ca. 3,000 msec determined by respiratory triggering. (Reproduced from Hockings et al., *Toxicol. Pathol.*, 30, 606, 2002. With permission of Society of Toxicologic Pathology. Copyright 2002 Taylor and Francis.)

edema in rats after intraperitoneal injection of the cyanobacterial toxin nodularin [14]. Image guided spectroscopy of fat has been used to study hepatic steatosis (fatty liver) [15].

The response of the rapidly regenerating liver to test compounds after surgical partial hepatectomy is used in mechanistic toxicology to predict hepatotoxic or hepatocarcinogenic potential. A study using MRI to track liver regeneration in rats exemplifies the attractions of the imaging approach [16]. Figure 26.1 shows representative coronal image slices through 3D datasets from the same animal before, and 1 and 9 days after, partial hepatectomy. Image segmentation, reconstruction, and surface- or volume-rendering techniques provide the investigator with a 3D depiction of the organ, and the changes it undergoes in response to surgery and regeneration, which are comparable with those available by *post mortem* dissection; the process also yields quantitative volumetric data for statistics, reduces animal use and surgery time, and enhances study power through each subject acting as its own control.

Figure 26.2 shows MRI and image-guided MRS being used to investigate fatty liver. The image is an axial slice through the liver of a rat on a steatotic regime, while the image-localized proton NMR spectrum reflects the fat content of the liver by virtue of the signals between 0.9 and 3 ppm from methyl and methylene functional groups in acyl lipid chains; the spectrum from a control nonsteatotic liver (not shown) comprises only the signal from tissue water around 4.8 ppm.

26.2.2 Heart and Cardiovascular System

Numerous preclinical imaging studies of the heart in experimental models of myocardial disease suggest MRI would be a useful way of studying cardiac myopathies and myocardial necrosis

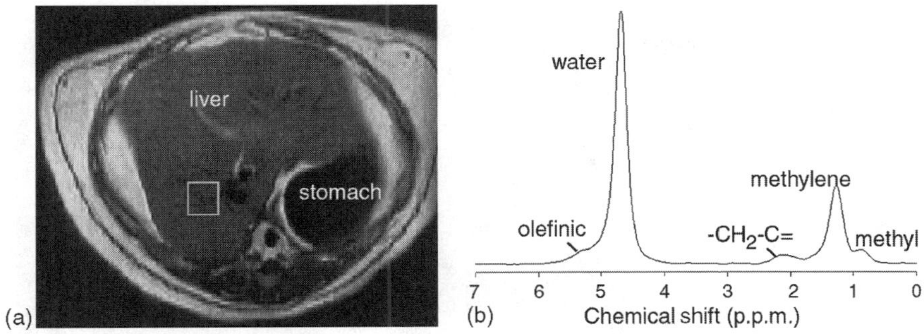

FIGURE 26.2 MR of hepatic steatosis and abnormal fat distribution. Image guided ^{1}H MR spectrum from the region of interest shown in the upper axial image from the liver of a rat undergoing a treatment which produces fatty liver. Apart from the signal from water (which in normal animals is the only substance observable by ^{1}H spectroscopy in the liver), several signals from various chemical functional groups in lipids are clearly observed and quantifiable. Note the prominent hyperintense deposits of subcutaneous and visceral fat visible in the MR image. Localized spectroscopy of this type allows hepatic steatosis to be tracked over time. Experimental details: 2 T, PRESS, TE/TR 20/2000 msec). (Reproduced from Hockings, P.D. et al., *Diabetes Obes. Metab*, 5, 234, 2003. With permission of Blackwell Publishing. Copyright 2003.)

induced by, for instance, catecholamines and the antineoplastic anthracycline antibiotics. Because of the high oxygen requirements by the functioning myocardium, heart muscle is particularly vulnerable to anoxic injury, sometimes provoked by what are in effect exaggerated pharmacological responses. Atherosclerotic plaques in arteries resulting from hyperlipidemia are detectable by MRI. Noncardiac gated time-averaged fast gradient echo imaging of the rat heart has been used to assess ventricular hypertrophy induced by carbon monoxide [17]. Iron overload in the myocardium has been measured using a signal intensity correlation method [18].

Figure 26.3 exemplifies the use of MRI to measure cardiac hypertrophic side effects of the vasodilator minoxidil, mediated by plasma volume increase and consequent preload, followed by ventricular lumen and total myocardial volume increase without significant myocardial wall thickening [19]. MRI also calls attention to another side effect, probably also related to plasma volume increase, namely pericardial effusion, which was confirmed at *post mortem* examination.

26.2.3 Kidneys and Urinary System

The kidneys are important drug and xenobiotic metabolism sites, receiving approximately 25% of the cardiac output. Morphological lesions generally occur in specific cells or regions (cortex, medulla), which in extreme cases can lead to misshapen organs. Other MRI-observable toxicology mediated events include vascular mineralization and thrombosis, and tubular degeneration, hypertrophy, mineralization and necrosis. T_1 and T_2 changes reflect a variety of processes underlying different nephrotoxic mechanisms including the action of gentamicin [20], bromoethanamine, hexachloro-1, 3-butadiene, and puromycin aminonucleoside [21], and mercuric chloride [22]. BOLD MRI shows the decline in renal oxygen content via T_2^* decrease in rats treated with nitric oxide synthase inhibitors, or radiocontrast agents [23]. Experiments in uninephrectomized rats treated with diatrizoate suggest negatively enhancing superparamagnetic iron oxide particles are useful in delineating renal toxicity [24].

Figure 26.4 suggests two related approaches to the use of MRI in the study of nephrotoxicty, one based on straightforward T_2W anatomical imaging, the other on dynamic contrast enhancement. The top three frames contrast a pair of kidneys from a control animal (left) with the appearance on T_2W images, of the kidneys of animals treated with model regiospecific nephrotoxins. The coronal

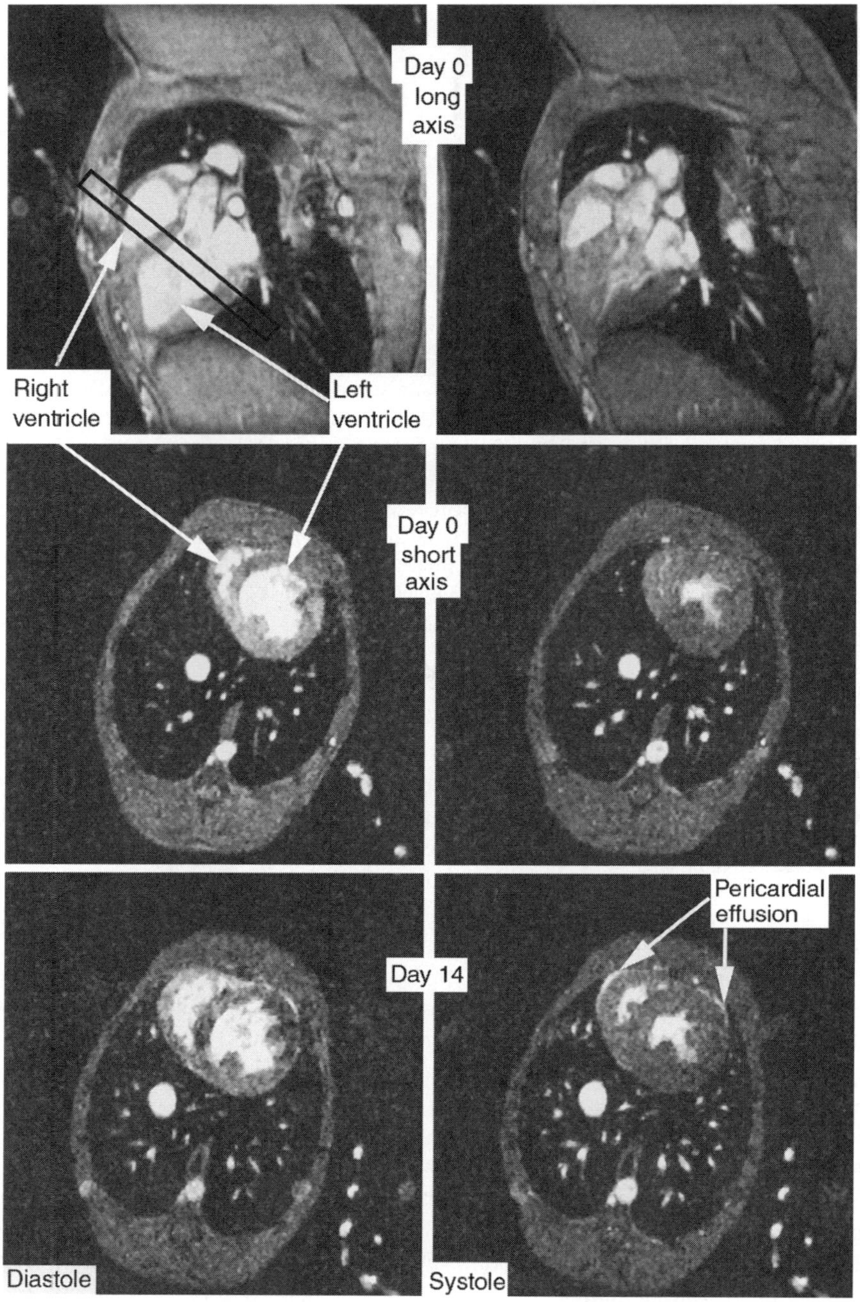

FIGURE 26.3 Cardiac hypertrophy and pericardial effusion. Long axis views (top) through the heart of a dog at end diastole (left) and end systole (right). The short axis views were acquired before (middle) and after (bottom) dosing with a peripheral vasodilator which produces a reflex plasma volume overload. Each view is typical of multiple slices which are acquired to cover the entire volume of the heart; functional measures (cardiac output and ejection fraction) are calculated from diastolic and systolic chamber volumes. Note the marked enlargement of the cardiac ventricles, with minimal thickening of the ventricular muscle walls — a hallmark of a plasma volume overload-induced cardiac hypertrophy. Pericardial effusion — plasma leak into the space between pericardium and myocardium — is highlighted in the posttreatment images. Experimental details: 2 T, Cardiac and respiratory triggered cine imaging, segmented gradient echo α 20°, NEchoes 4, TE 3 msec, TR 8 ms, 32 msec/cine frame.

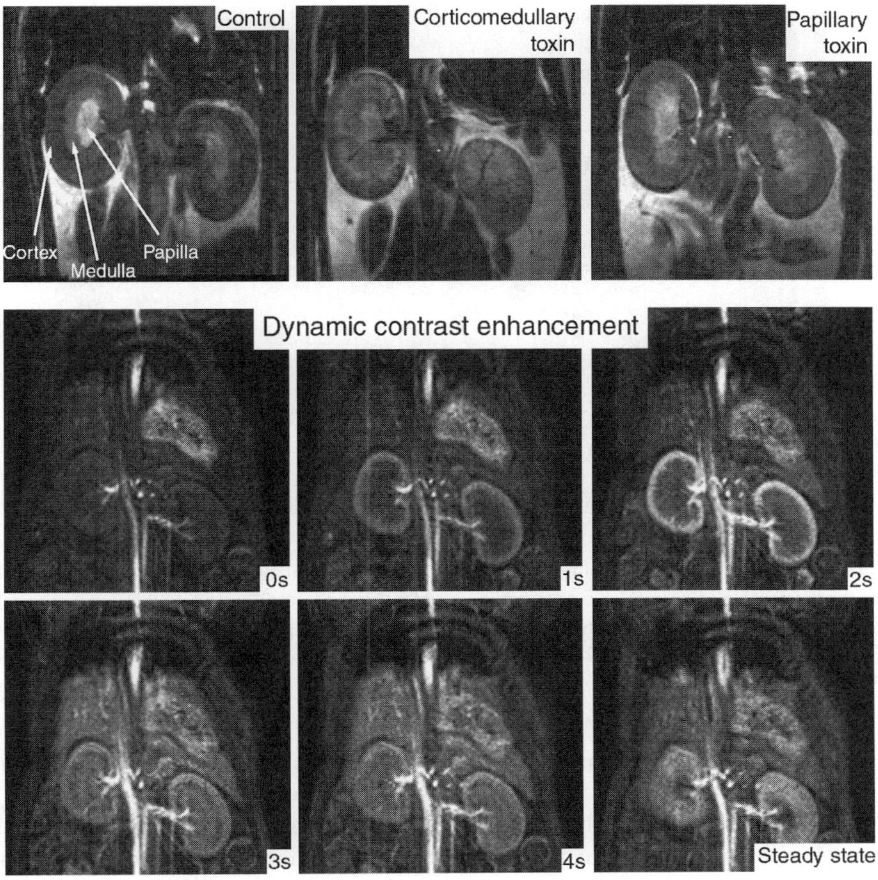

FIGURE 26.4 Imaging of kidney toxicity and function. Top: Coronal slices through T_2 weighted 3D images of the kidneys of a control rat (left), and of rats treated with toxins specific for the S3 region of the renal cortex at the cortico-medullary boundary (hexachlorobutadiene, HCBD, middle), and for the renal papilla (bromoethanamine, BEA, right). In the control animal the cortex, medulla, and papilla are well differentiated. In the HCBD treated animal (middle) there is a distinct bright band of edema; in the BEA treated animal image contrast between medulla and papilla is lost. In both treated animals the organs are measurably enlarged. Experimental details: 7 T, Respiratory triggered, multi-spin echo, NEchoes 32, TE_{eff} 240 msec, TR ca. 2 sec. Middle and bottom rows: A time series of rapid coronal T_1-weighted images through the kidneys of a rat prior to (top left) and at 1 sec intervals after intravenous (tail vein) injection of a bolus of Gd (DTPA) contrast agent. The passage of the agent through the kidneys, to a final steady state distribution (bottom right panel), is clearly visualized and quantifiable. Nephrotoxin induced compromise of kidney structure and function can be clearly identified by derangement of these perfusion dynamics, and is potentially a powerful and precise way of studying the functional consequences of nephrotoxic insult. Experimental details: 7 T, Ungated, fast gradient echo SNAP, α 25°, TE/TR 2/8 msec, 1 sec/cine frame.

sections in the middle and bottom rows show rapid (1 sec per image) T_1W images through the kidneys of a normal rat prior to, and after, passage through the kidneys of an intravenous bolus of a gadolinium based (Gd DTPA) contrast agent. The kinetics of signal enhancement throughout the kidneys can be quantified and correlated with regiospecific toxic effects.

26.2.4 Lung

The lung is the site of direct toxic action of inhaled substances, including environmental pollutants, as well as being vulnerable to exposure to blood-born intoxicants via the pulmonary circulation.

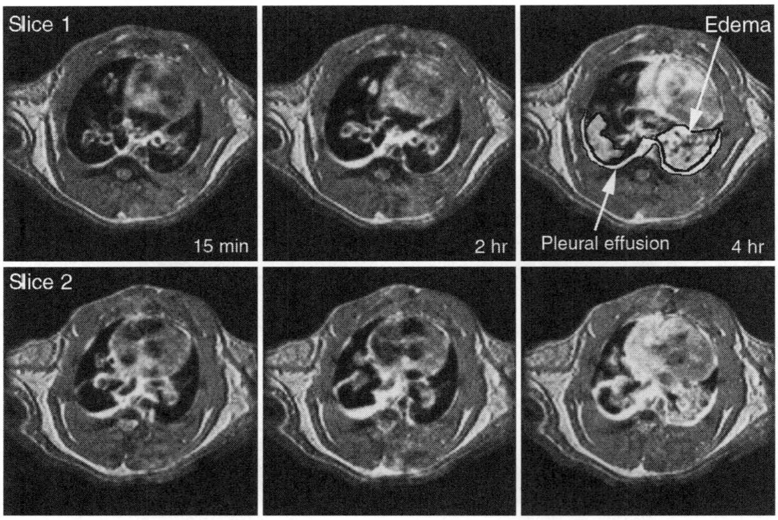

FIGURE 26.5 Pleural effusion and pulmonary edema. Axial slices at two different levels (top and bottom) through the thorax of a rat after systemic administration of a thiourea compound which evokes pleural effusion and pulmonary edema. Both responses are easily identified and quantifiable, as illustrated by the panel in which the boundaries of the effusion, and edema, are outlined. Experimental details: 7 T, Multislice gradient echo, α 20°, TE/TR 4/200 msec.

MRI detects inflammatory pulmonary edema [25,26] and mucous secretions [27], which are common acute responses to lung injury conventionally detected *post mortem* by lung weight, histopathology, or inflammatory cell counting. Acute inflammation [28] and subsequent fibrosis, a chronic response to lung injury characterized by the deposition of collagen fibrils (typified by silicosis) and resultant tissue stiffening, are reflected in lung relaxation time changes [29], and increased vascular permeability of gadolinium chelates [30,31]. High molecular oxygen levels also increase pulmonary capillary permeability, which is detectable using signal enhancement by a polylysine-Gd-DTPA macromolecular blood pool contrast agent [32].

Bronchoprovocation is used to test the potential of compounds to induce bronchoconstriction, using a variety of measures of pulmonary function and gas exchange. Emphysema is provoked by cigarette smoke and some other agents and is characterized by alveolar enlargement and wall destruction without significant fibrosis. The use of hyperpolarized noble gas (He-3, Xe-129) MRI to explore the effects of pulmonary toxins on ventilation and lung structural remodeling is an exciting future prospect [33,34].

Pleural effusion can be induced by compounds which contain, or are metabolized to, thioureido or benzamide chemical groups, reactive derivatives which appear to selectively increase pulmonary vascular permeability. Figure 26.5 shows the progression of pleural effusion in a rat after intraperitoneal injection of a test compound which produces thiourea; in the representative axial slices shown, pleural effusion is clearly visible in the T_2 weighted images as hyperintense masses in the dorsal portion of the lung which increase with time. Some pulmonary vascular edema is also visible and characterized by a more diffuse signal. The volumes of effusate and edema can be readily quantified as a function of time.

26.2.5 Brain and Nervous System

Although protected to some extent by the blood–brain barrier, numerous compounds do nevertheless exert toxicity in the brain, broadly definable as neuronopathies, axonopathies, myelinopathies, and toxicity associated with disruption of neuronal transmission mechanisms.

Many of these pathologies should be detectable by MRI, in addition to manifesting as functional impairments in appropriate behavioral assays. Cholinesterase inhibitors cause changes in brain relaxation and apparent diffusion coefficients (ADCs) which appear to reflect cellular degradation followed by remodeling [35]. Changes in T_2 and tissue ADCs induced by oral 2-L-chloropropionic acid parallel the onset of clinical behavioral signs [36]. Anatomical MRI shows a decrease in the cerebral cortical surface area of rats chronically exposed to toluene [37]. In humans, MRI shows demyelination in patients being treated for chronic lymphocytic leukemia with the cytotoxic agent fludaribine [38], cerebral white matter lesions in cyclosporine-A treated patients [39], and diffuse changes [40] and generalized atrophy and ventricular enlargement [41] in workers chronically exposed to industrial solvents. Vigabatrine induced cerebellar white matter lesions are visible by MRI in rats [42], as are the cortical effects of methyl mercury in marmosets [43] and rats [44]. MRI showed hippocampal atrophy in the brains of year-old monkeys which had been treated *in utero* with dexamethasone [45]. MRI effectively detects estrogen induced pituitary changes and tumorogenesis in rats [46,47]. High dose vigabatrine microvacuolation in dogs causes changes in T_2 intensity *ex vivo* [48], and the use of high resolution *ex vivo* MR microscopy has been proposed as a tool in neurotoxicology [49,50].

A practical illustration of longitudinal imaging in neurotoxicity is depicted in Figure 26.6, which shows representative axial slices through the brain of a rat 10 days (left) and 10 weeks (right) after administration of a model neurotoxin 3-nitropropionic acid, which is specifically toxic to the striatal projection neurons. At 10 days, diffuse hyperintense striatal lesions are visible by T_2W (TE = 70 msec) image; by 10 weeks these are localized to the lateral zones of the striatum where gliotic scarring is apparent, and appear to be involved with cerebrospinal fluid (CSF). CSF is also distinguished, as hypo-intense, in the T_1W images.

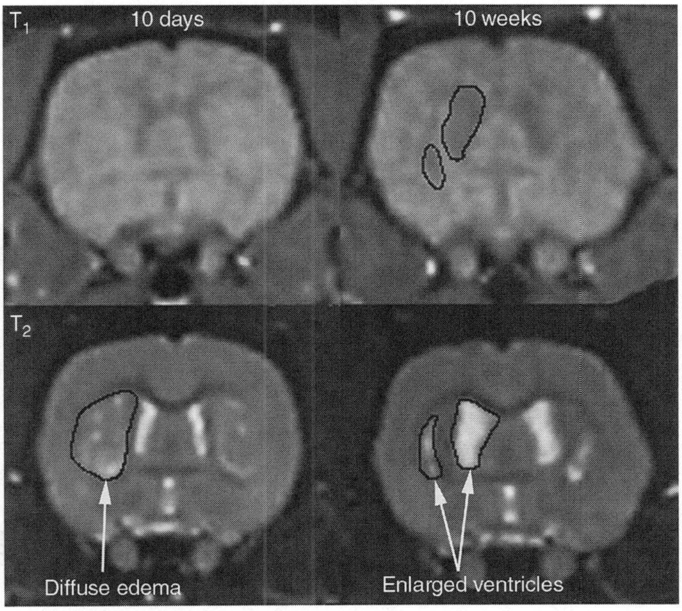

FIGURE 26.6 Chronic neurotoxicity. Representative axial slices through the brain of a rat 10 days (left) and 10 weeks (right) after systemic treatment with the model neurotoxin 3-nitropropionic acid, which causes selective degeneration of the striatal projection neurons. Acute effects are manifested as localized hyperintensity in the striatum, probably due to edema, in the 10 day T_2 image. More chronic effects — enlarged cerebral ventricles and abnormal CSF distribution — show in T_1 and T_2 scans as hypo-intense and hyperintense regions, respectively. (Courtesy of T. Roberts and S. Williams, King's College London, U.K.)

26.2.6 Endocrine Organs

The adrenals are among the endocrine glands most susceptible to toxicologic insult, with both cortical and medullary zones being affected by a pharmacologically highly diverse range of compounds, provoking atrophy, hypertrophy, degeneration, and vacuolation. Clinical MRI is widely used to detect adrenal structural abnormalities and cancer [51–53]. The adrenals are readily distinguished by MRI in several species, including dog [54] and mouse [55], but there are few literature reports of its use to study adrenal toxicity experimentally. Other endocrine organs such as the pancreas, thyroid and parathyroid glands, and pituitary, are also prone to toxicological changes such as atrophy or necrosis but are not as readily imaged because of irregular shape, involvement with the gastrointestinal tract, or small size.

Figure 26.7 shows a series of contiguous coronal slices exemplifying the tractability of the rat adrenal glands to MRI observation. These anatomical images readily distinguish cortex and medulla, and it is easy to appreciate how some of the common adrenal toxicities which lead to morphological changes could be studied.

26.2.7 Reproductive System

There are few reports of the use of MRI in the study of reproductive system toxicology, in spite of the fact that both female and male reproductive systems are highly amenable to MRI. Toxicity-linked testicular and epidydimal atrophy is not unusual, while the seminiferous tubules of the testes are susceptible to chemically induced damage leading to vacuolation and necrosis. The prostate gland is susceptible to toxicological atrophy or hypertrophy. While clinical MRI is used to detect and diagnose fetal abnormalities in humans, its potential to study the effects of teratogens preclinically *in vivo*, *in utero*, is largely unexplored, although retinoic acid-induced developmental abnormalities have been imaged *ex vivo* in mouse embryos [56]. The high level of detail available from MRI of preclinical species is illustrated in Figure 26.8, which shows typical axial spin echo image slices through the lower abdomen of a male rat. Clearly visible are the testes themselves and their large surface blood vessels, the epididimydes, and portions of the spermatic cords.

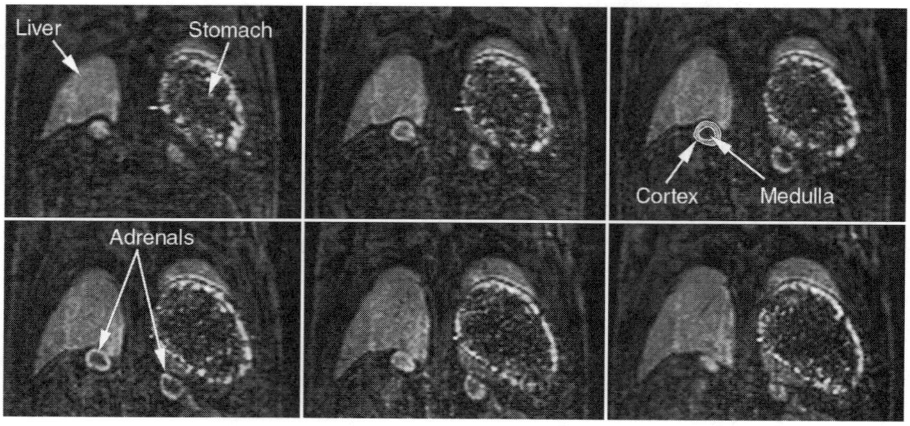

FIGURE 26.7 Endocrine system. Coronal cardiac- and respiratory-gated spin echo MR image slices through a normal live rat abdomen, highlighting the good definition of the adrenal glands, and differentiation between cortical and medullary zones. The potential of MRI for characterizing the evolution of adrenal hypertrophy, atrophy, or medulla- or cortex-specific toxicities, is readily appreciated. Experimental details as for Figure 26.1.

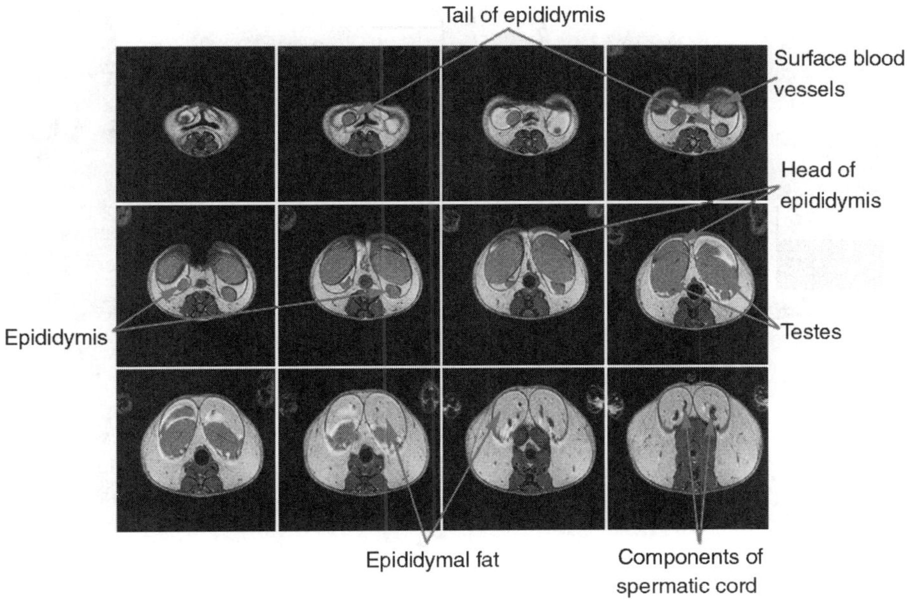

FIGURE 26.8 Reproductive system. A series of axial multislice spin echo proton density images through the lower abdomen of a normal, live male rat, exemplifying the anatomical detail provided around testicular structures which are common toxicity sites, such as the testes themselves, testicular blood vessels, the epididymis, and the spermatic cords. The seminiferous tubules, also commonly affected toxicologically, are below the resolution of this *in vivo* scan. Experimental details: 2 T, Multislice spin echo TE/TR 17/2000 msec.

Approaches to longitudinal studies of testicular hypertrophy or atrophy, more structure — specific pathologies, and perfusion abnormalities using contrast agent tracking, are obvious and attractive, but little reported.

26.2.8 Other Organs and Tissues

Although MRI-visible arthritic or synovitic lesions are not common in toxicology, the power of MRI in studying these pathologies in preclinical and clinical joint disease suggests it could be useful in such cases. MRI can detect early cartilage degeneration in response to interleukin-1 infusion in rabbit knees [57], and vesiculation and erosions in response to fluoroquinoline antibiotics in rabbits [58] and dogs [59]. Ocular cataract formation is an occasional toxic response, and has been imaged in dogs in response to dietary galactose [60]. MRI has been used to study the effects on skin morphology of irritant jet aircraft fuels [61].

26.2.9 Carcinogenesis

As discussed extensively in Chapter 13 through Chapter 15, MRI is prominent in the clinical diagnosis and laboratory study of cancers and other tumors. Its use in the study of chemical carcinogenesis has not been so widespread. However, hepatic neoplasms in rats induced by diethylnitrosamine and subsequent 17-α-ethynylestradiol treatments are detected by T_2W MRI [62]. Superparamagnetic iron oxide contrast agents facilitate the differentiation of experimental liver tumors provoked by thioacetamide in rats from a background of advanced cirrhosis [63].

Figure 26.9 illustrates the potential of MRI to characterize experimental chemical carcinogenesis [64]; it shows a murine mammary tumor which has arisen after systemic injection of carcinogenic methylnitrosourea (MNU). The image set presents an interesting example of

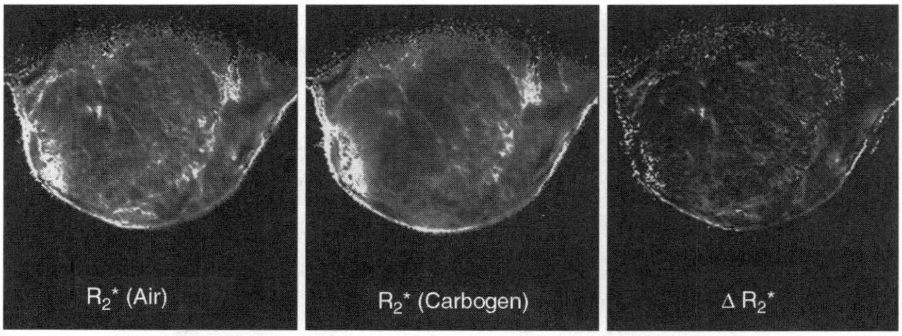

FIGURE 26.9 Chemical carcinogenesis. R_2^* maps depicting metabolic activity in mammary tumors induced in rats by systemic injection of the model carcinogen methylnitrosourea (MNU). Switching the animal from breathing air to carbogen reduces R_2^* in areas of the tumor which are well vascularized, best illustrated in the difference ΔR_2^* map. Such approaches could be used to study the rate of onset, evolution, and metabolic characteristics, of drug induced carcinogenesis and tumors in any organ. Courtesy of Dr. Simon Robinson and Professor John Griffiths, St. George's Hospital Medical School, London, U.K. (Reproduced from Robinson et al., *J. Magn. Reson. Imaging*, 17, 445, 2003. With permission of John Wiley & Sons. Copyright.)

combined application of BOLD imaging, and vasodilatation induced by carbogen (5% carbon dioxide) breathing. The images are maps of the inhomogeneous R_2^* relaxation rate (equal to the reciprocal of the T_2^* relaxation time) across the tumor; areas of high intensity in the air-breathing map correspond to tissue with large R_2^* rates, i.e., tissue where paramagnetic deoxyhemoglobin is abundant. As the animal is switched to breathing carbogen, the blood supply to well-vascularized areas of the tumor mass increases, paramagnetic deoxyhemoglobin declines, and the R_2^* values fall. The difference (ΔR_2^*) map thus shows high intensity for the well-vascularized tissue. The example illustrates the potential for MRI in studying not only the anatomical architecture, but also the metabolic activity of carcinogen provoked tumors.

26.2.10 *Ex Vivo* and Whole Body MRI

While the use of MRI to image isolated fixed tissues and organs may appear pointless when histopathological techniques are so well established and widely accepted, and provide spatial resolution orders of magnitude beyond what MRI can deliver, there are occasions when the MRI scan can offer unique insights and understandings. In large part this arises from the versatility of 3D MR imaging approaches: isotropic resolution 3D datasets can be reformatted so that any viewing plane can be interrogated; 3D feature segmentation, reconstruction and surface- or volume-rendered displays of diseased organs and structures can alert the investigator to the unexpected, and in any case are valuable tools for presentation and display. After scanning, of course, tissue is still available for conventional histopathology.

Some of the attractions of high resolution 3D imaging of fixed tissues and organs are exemplified in Figure 26.10, which depicts different visualizations of a fixed testis from a rat. The 3D nature of the dataset allows one to section the image at any angle to emphasize and interrogate different structures. For instance, the planar short axis MR image view (Figure 26.10a) illustrates the bright (fixative-filled) seminiferous tubules at good resolution, in recognizable correspondence with their histological appearance (Figure 26.10b). Such presentations give no impression of the overall architecture of the organ, however, but this is provided by the longitudinal sections exemplified in Figure 26.10c. These approaches may also save time and contribute information in the examination of embryos and fetuses required for the assessment of teratogenic potential.

Another interesting extension of MRI, offering the investigator a unique view of a target organ in the wider context of overall anatomy, is whole-body imaging. Thus, Figure 26.11

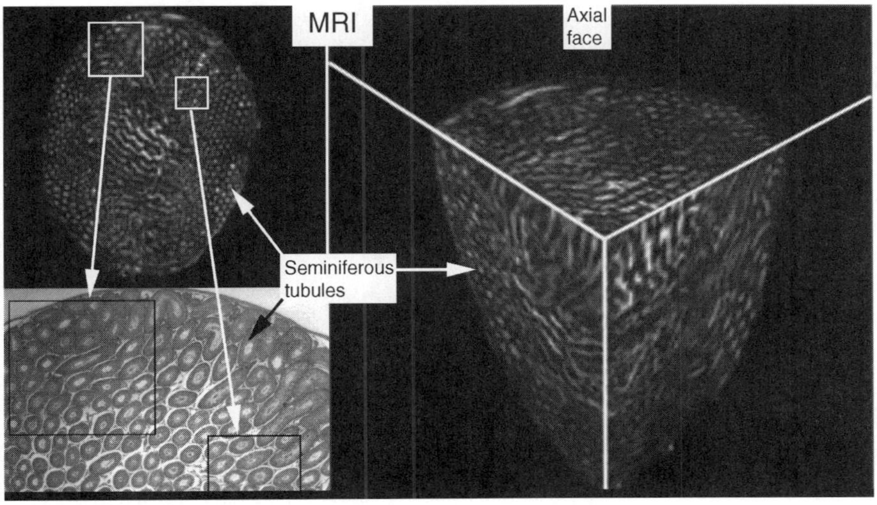

FIGURE 26.10 3D MRI of fixed tissue. Different depictions of the microstructure of a fixed rat testis, the MR images being derived from a high resolution (100 μm isotropic) spin echo image acquired over a scan time of several hours. There is good correspondence between the MRI and the histological sections across the seminiferous tubules. The overall 3D architecture of the organ, however, is best appreciated by a composite view in which virtual slices are displayed in both cross and longitudinal section relative to the tubules (c) (using the image processing and presentation software Amira). MRI experimental details: 7 T 3D segmented RARE spin echo, NEchoes 16, TE_{eff}/TR 60/600 msec, 20 signal averages, 256 cubic matrix, FoV 2.56 cm^3.

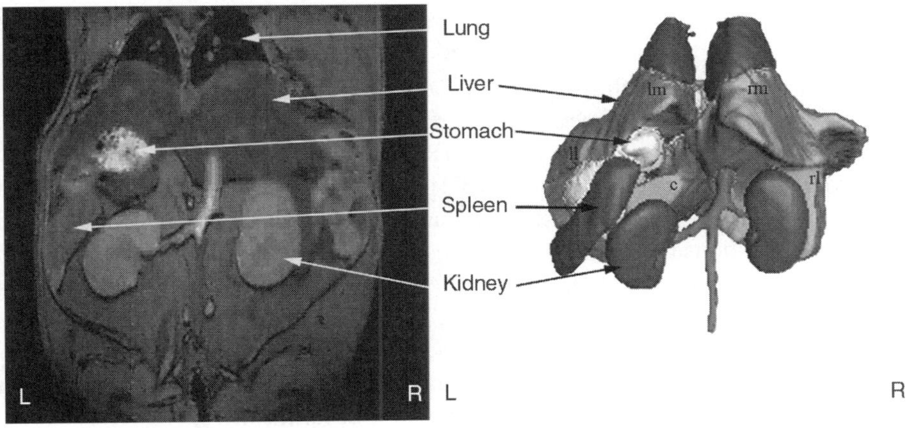

FIGURE 26.11 Towards whole body in vivo MRI. Nondisruptive 3D MRI not only provides the opportunity of interrogating toxicological changes in the structure of entire organs *in situ*, but also enables the investigator to visualize the organ or structure of interest in its broader anatomical context in the living animal. The left hand panel shows a characteristic coronal slice from a 3D gradient echo image through the abdomen of a mouse. A number of organs are clearly visible in the section, which typifies the raw data output from the scanner. The overall relationship between the organs, however, is most successfully conveyed in the 3D organ-by-organ reconstruction (using Amira) shown on the right. The perspective is dorsal to ventral, i.e., reversed relative to the normal anatomical convention, as if one were viewing the reconstruction through the animal's spine. Lobes of the liver are labeled as follows: rm — right median, lm — left median, rl — right lateral, ll — left lateral, c — caudate.

(right hand panel) shows a digital partial reconstruction (excluding the lower gastrointestinal tract, and spine) of the major abdominal organs of a mouse, extracted and surface rendered from a 3D isotropic volume dataset, typified by the single slice shown to the left. While such presentations may not offer any more analytical value than measures such as organ volume, they can prove valuable presentation and conceptualization tools.

26.3 MRI IN REGULATED STUDIES

The applications of MRI cited and exemplified so far would have a place in investigative safety assessment around a compound or pharmacological class, driven by a need to better understand a toxicological phenomenon or mechanism. If, however, such studies are to be used to support a primary safety endpoint prior to administration to humans, they will be reportable to regulatory agencies, such as the Food and Drug Administration (FDA) in the U.S.A. Such studies must follow Good Laboratory Practice (GLP) guidelines, which require experimental procedures, instrument calibration, and data analysis and retention, to be performed according to Standard Operating Procedures (SOPs), with processes and compliance subject to regular inspections by national agencies such as the FDA. Regulated GLP studies in which MRI is or has been used are to date extremely rare, but some of the relevant issues can be considered. Many of these are common to optical and other imaging techniques which rely on digital data capture, analysis, and storage.

There is some guidance in the FDA's "CFR 21 Part 11 Electronic records; Electronic signatures" publication (see website entry http://www.fda.gov/ora/compliance_ref/part11/). In some respects, necessary measures may simply constitute formalizing and documenting procedures which are already in place in a laboratory. For instance, for volumetric studies, calibration of MRI instruments against geometric phantoms, preferably standards supplied by a manufacturer, should be conducted and documented in an instrument maintenance logbook prior to and during studies, at intervals defined by an SOP. Studies involving more complex types of imaging, such as distinguishing necrotic or cancerous from healthy tissue on the basis of relaxation or diffusion properties, will prove more challenging to standardize, with a requirement for regular calibration of the relevant parameters against standards for the parametric properties. Some manufacturers of analytical instrumentation which is used in GLP and other regulated activities such as manufacturing, including NMR spectrometers, do offer periodic calibration and certification as part of service agreements. Changing hardware (RF and gradient coils, amplifiers), or versions of data capture software, during a study is to be avoided. Records of training to a competent standard, if possible certified by a relevant instrument manufacturer, or software supplier, for anyone involved in data generation and analysis, are to be established, maintained, and eventually archived in the organization's regulatory compliance archive. The biological phase of the study — species, gender, strain, source, body weight range, dosing routes and schedules, scanning points, blood sampling etc. — must accord with a defined protocol under the control of a Study Director, who ensures adherence to the protocol and documentation of any deviations and their reasons, and with the approval of the organization's regulatory compliance department.

There should be an SOP in which the nature of the experimental raw data is defined, and the time period for which this is to be retained. To be exempt from the need to retain digital images, it may be possible to define one's raw data as numbers representing, say, MRI organ volumes. However, the continuing development of robust, backed-up data storage, archival and retrieval systems, which will audit trail data to the extent of documenting any analysis carried out on it, and by whom, make the prospect of defining and storing the entire digital output from the scanner as raw data much less daunting than it used to be. Given the long periods for which raw digital data retention may be necessary (50 years is a possibility), however, one of the greatest challenges to the archivist is likely to be the refreshing of historical image file formats so that they remain readable by current software, rather than mere storage and tracking of large volumes of digital data.

26.4 FUTURE DEVELOPMENTS

So far, the story of MRI in practical pharmaceutical safety assessment is one of promise rather than fulfillment. There is widespread interest in its potential (and that of other noninvasive imaging techniques) in nonregulated studies aimed at investigating mechanisms of pharmaceutical toxicity, although it is noticeable that, for several target organs, it is still easier to propose hypothetical, rather than cite actual, applications. Also, it must be admitted that many literature examples relate to rather severe toxicities induced by distinctly nonpharmaceutical compounds and toxins. In reality, the desire will be to study more relevant effects than the ones observed in these instances. New developments in MRI hardware and methodology will increase sensitivity and discriminating power, as will the use of contrast agents targeted to biomolecules which represent markers of specific toxicities and processes. The invention and commercialization of pathology-specific contrast agents for clinical diagnosis could help toxicological imaging become more sensitive and refined, permitting the identification of more subtle pathology, and more confident and earlier discrimination between healthy and affected tissue. (The more sensitive nuclear imaging techniques will also play a significant role here). MRI offers unique insights into some of those physiological processes which might precede full-blown toxicity, especially through function-sensitive techniques. One thinks of BOLD to measure tissue oxygenation, and dynamic contrast enhancement to measure compromised blood flow, tissue perfusion, and prenecrotic inflammatory activity.

It is unlikely that a slow-turnaround, analysis-intensive technique such as MRI will serve a screening function in bringing unknown or unanticipated toxicities to light. However, 3D *post mortem* whole body imaging, providing comprehensive coverage of all organ systems at extremely high spatial resolution, has compelling potential applications in anatomical phenotyping of transgenic mice [65], as exemplified in Figure 26.12. It is easy to conceive how these comprehensive views of the entire organism and the interrelationships between anatomical structures might refine the detection of toxicological pathology, as well as phenotypic abnormalities which are genetically based. There is a strong drive in the transgenic animal field to automate and multiplex the image acquisition processes, and the interrogation of images for abnormal features

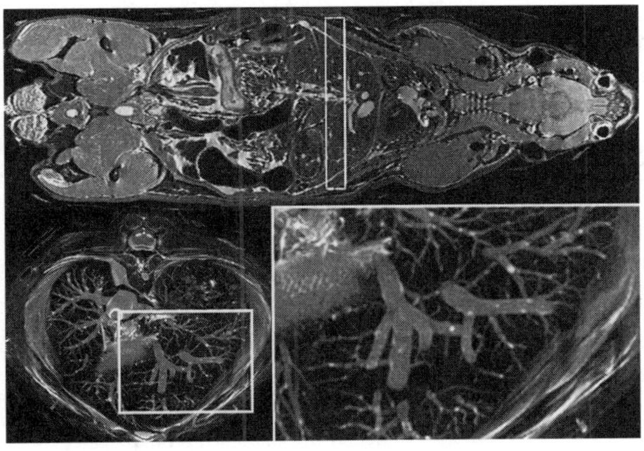

FIGURE 26.12 Whole body *post mortem* MRI. A representative coronal slice (top) through a high resolution image (512 × 512 × 2048 data matrix array providing 50 μm isotropic resolution) of a mouse cadaver fixed with formalin doped with a gadolinium based T_1 enhancement agent. The box indicates the volume which has been reformatted to the transverse slice at bottom left; the bottom right maximum intensity projection (MIP) emphasizes the exquisite detail with which the technique is able to delineate organ vasculature, in this case of the liver. (Courtesy of Prof. G. A. Johnson, Duke University.)

(see also Chapter 5). Such approaches are likely to be at least tested in the use of MRI to detect anatomical markers of hitherto unknown or unpredicted toxicologic pathology.

Nevertheless, in the foreseeable future MR imaging's most powerful and compelling applications will be in the elucidation of physiological mechanisms underlying pharmaceutical toxicity, especially where no other convenient *in vivo* biomarkers exist, and/or where enhanced precision and the statistical power usually conferred by longitudinal designs are necessary. With the increasing availability of clinical scanners, and the development of clinical molecular-targeted contrast agents, it may also become practical to use MRI for early, precise, detection of adverse side effects with simple image signatures such as organ size changes, in humans, especially in the absence of other convenient biomarkers.

ACKNOWLEDGMENTS

Tim Bertram, Jeff Birmingham, Dan Bradley, Keith Brooks, Robin Buckingham, Albert Busza, Joanne Byrne, Simon Campbell, Kumar Changani, John Connolly, Ana Criado-Gonzalez, Heather Elliott, Colin Fish, Bob Greenhill, Paul Hockings, Kerstin Kramer, Heather Lloyd, Paul Mullins, Dennis Murphy, Janette Osborne, Anisha Patel, Bela Patel, Steve Polley, Peter Reid, Toby Roberts, Nadeem Saeed, Mark Slaughter, Sean Smart, Gemma Taylor, David Templeton, Greg Whelan, Alan White.

REFERENCES

1. Klaassen, C. D., Ed., *Casarett & Doull's Toxicology*, 6th ed., McGraw-Hill, New York, 2004.
2. Gopinath, C., Prentice, D. E., and Lewis, D. J., Atlas of experimental toxicological pathology, *Current Histopathology Series*, Vol. 13, Gresham, G. A., Ed., MTP Press, Lancaster, 1987.
3. Dixon, D. et al., Magnetic resonance imaging (MRI): a new tool in experimental toxicologic pathology, *Toxicol. Pathol.*, 16, 386, 1988.
4. Delnomdedieu, M. et al., Magnetic resonance microscopy — a new tool for the toxicologic pathologist, *Toxicol. Pathol.*, 24, 36, 1996.
5. Hazle, J. D., Narayana, P. A., and Dunsford, H. A., Chronic carbon tetrachloride and phospholipase D hepatotoxicity in rat: in vivo 1H magnetic resonance, total lipid analysis, and histology, *Magn. Reson. Med.*, 15, 211, 1990.
6. Towner, R. A. et al., MRI study of the inhibitory effect of new spin traps on in vivo CCl4-induced hepatotoxicity in rats, *Free Radic. Biol. Med.*, 14, 677, 1993.
7. Towner, R. A. et al., In vivo magnetic resonance imaging study of Kupffer cell involvement in CCl4-induced hepatotoxicity in rats, *Can. J. Physiol Pharmacol.*, 72, 441, 1994.
8. Towner, R. A. et al., Enhancement of carbon tetrachloride-induced liver injury by a single dose of ethanol: proton magnetic resonance imaging (MRI) studies in vivo, *Biochim. Biophys. Acta*, 1096, 222, 1991.
9. Sidhu, M. K. et al., Manganese dipyridoxal diphosphate-enhanced magnetic resonance imaging in the evaluation of hepatocyte function, *Invest Radiol.*, 28, 903, 1993.
10. Zhou, X. et al., Studies on bromobenzene-induced hepatotoxicity using in vivo MR microscopy with surgically implanted RF coils, *Magn. Reson. Med.*, 31, 619, 1994.
11. Kreft, B. et al., Diagnostic value of a superparamagnetic iron oxide in MR imaging of chronic liver disease in an animal model, *Am. J. Roentgenol.*, 170, 661, 1998.
12. Sturgeon, S. A. and Towner, R. A., In vivo assessment of microcystin-LR-induced hepatotoxicity in the rat using proton nuclear magnetic resonance (1H-NMR) imaging, *Biochim. Biophys. Acta*, 1454, 227, 1999.
13. Kreft, B. et al., Evaluation of different models of experimentally induced liver cirrhosis for MRI research with correlation to histopathologic findings, *Invest Radiol.*, 34, 360, 1999.
14. Towner, R. A. et al., In vivo assessment of nodularin-induced hepatotoxicity in the rat using magnetic resonance techniques (MRI, MRS and EPR oximetry), *Chem. Biol. Interact.*, 139, 231, 2002.

15. Hockings, P. D. et al., Rapid reversal of hepatic steatosis, and reduction of muscle triglyceride, by rosiglitazone: MRI/S studies in Zucker fatty rats, *Diabetes Obes. Metab.*, 5, 234, 2003.
16. Hockings, P. D. et al., Longitudinal magnetic resonance imaging quantitation of rat liver regeneration after partial hepatectomy, *Toxicol. Pathol.*, 30, 606, 2002.
17. Bambach, G. A., Penney, D. G., and Negendank, W. G., In situ assessment of the rat heart during chronic carbon monoxide exposure using nuclear magnetic resonance imaging, *J. Appl. Toxicol.*, 11, 43, 1991.
18. Jensen, P. D. et al., Indirect evidence for the potential ability of magnetic resonance imaging to evaluate the myocardial iron content in patients with transfusional iron overload, *MAGMA.*, 12, 153, 2001.
19. Hockings, P. D. et al., Validation of MRI measurement of cardiac output in the dog: the effects of dobutamine and minoxidil, *Toxicol. Mech. Methods*, 13, 39, 2003.
20. Iaina, A., Abrashkin, S., and Weininger, J., Proton MR study of different types of experimental acute renal failure in rats, *Magn. Reson. Imaging*, 4, 241, 1986.
21. Finney, J. S. et al., The application of proton nuclear magnetic resonance imaging for the in vivo characterisation of chemically induced renal lesions in rats over a prolonged time study, *Magn. Reson. Imaging*, 8, 713, 1990.
22. Farmer, T. H. et al., Implanted coil MR microscopy of renal pathology, *Magn. Reson. Med.*, 10, 310, 1989.
23. Prasad, P. V. et al., Changes in intrarenal oxygenation as evaluated by BOLD MRI in a rat kidney model for radiocontrast nephropathy, *J. Magn. Reson. Imaging*, 13, 744, 2001.
24. Laissy, J. P. et al., Reversibility of experimental acute renal failure in rats: assessment with USPIO-enhanced MR imaging, *J. Magn. Reson. Imaging*, 12, 278, 2000.
25. Beckmann, N. et al., Pulmonary edema induced by allergen challenge in the rat: noninvasive assessment by magnetic resonance imaging, *Magn. Reson. Med.*, 45, 88, 2001.
26. Tigani, B. et al., Pulmonary inflammation monitored noninvasively by MRI in freely breathing rats, *Biochem. Biophys. Res. Commun.*, 292, 216, 2002.
27. Beckmann, N. et al., Noninvasive detection of endotoxin-induced mucus hypersecretion in rat lung by MRI, *Am. J. Physiol. Lung Cell Mol. Physiol.*, 283, L22, 2002.
28. Shioya, S. et al., Acute and repair stage characteristics of magnetic resonance relaxation times in oxygen-induced pulmonary edema, *Magn. Reson. Med.*, 8, 450, 1988.
29. Taylor, C. R. et al., Proton relaxation times in bleomycin-induced lung injury, *Invest. Radiol.*, 22, 621, 1987.
30. Suga, K. et al., Altered clearance of gadolinium diethylenetriaminepentaacetic acid aerosol from bleomycin-injured dog lungs: initial observations, *Am. J. Respir. Crit. Care Med.*, 167, 1704, 2003.
31. Kersjes, W. et al., Differentiation of alveolitis and pulmonary fibrosis in rabbits with magnetic resonance imaging after intrabronchial administration of bleomycin 2, *Invest. Radiol.*, 34, 13, 1999.
32. Brasch, R. C. et al., Pulmonary oxygen toxicity: demonstration of abnormal capillary permeability using contrast-enhanced MRI, *Pediatr. Radiol.*, 23, 495, 1993.
33. Chen, X. J. et al., Detection of emphysema in rat lungs by using magnetic resonance measurements of 3He diffusion, *Proc. Natl. Acad. Sci. U.S.A*, 97, 11478, 2000.
34. Ward, E. R. et al., Proton and hyperpolarized helium magnetic resonance imaging of radiation-induced lung injury in rats, *Int. J. Radiat. Oncol. Biol. Phys.*, 58, 1562, 2004.
35. Bhagat, Y. A. et al., Magnetic resonance imaging predicts neuropathology from soman-mediated seizures in the rodent, *Neuroreport*, 12, 1481, 2001.
36. Williams, R. E. et al., MRI studies of the neurotoxic effects of L-2-chloropropionic acid on rat brain, *Magn. Reson. Imaging*, 19, 133, 2001.
37. von Euler, M. et al., Inhalation of low concentrations of toluene induces persistent effects on a learning retention task, beam-walk performance, and cerebrocortical size in the rat, *Exp. Neurol.*, 163, 1, 2000.
38. Gonzalez, H. et al., Progressive multifocal leukoencephalitis (PML) in three patients treated with standard-dose fludarabine (FAMP), *Hematol. Cell Ther.*, 41, 183, 1999.
39. Shbarou, R. M., Chao, N. J., and Morgenlander, J. C., Cyclosporin A-related cerebral vasculopathy, *Bone Marrow Transplant.*, 26, 801, 2000.
40. Thuomas, K. A. et al., MR imaging in solvent-induced chronic toxic encephalopathy, *Acta Radiol.*, 37, 177, 1996.

41. Bernsen, H. J. et al., Magnetic resonance studies on brain dysfunction induced by organic solvents, *Acta Neurol. Belg.*, 92, 207, 1992.
42. Jackson, G. D. et al., Vigabatrin-induced lesions in the rat brain demonstrated by quantitative magnetic resonance imaging, *Epilepsy Res.*, 18, 57, 1994.
43. Eto, K. et al., Methylmercury poisoning in common marmosets — a study of selective vulnerability within the cerebral cortex, *Toxicol. Pathol.*, 29, 565, 2001.
44. Kinoshita, Y. et al., Apparent diffusion coefficient on rat brain and nerves intoxicated with methylmercury, *Environ. Res.*, 80, 348, 1999.
45. Uno, H. et al., Neurotoxicity of glucocorticoids in the primate brain, *Horm. Behav.*, 28, 336, 1994.
46. van Nesselrooij, J. H. et al., Magnetic resonance imaging compared with hormonal effects and histopathology of estrogen-induced pituitary lesions in the rat, *Carcinogenesis*, 12, 289, 1991.
47. van Nesselrooij, J. H. et al., Rat pituitary changes observed with magnetic resonance imaging following removal of estrogen stimulus: correlation with histopathology and immunohistology, *Carcinogenesis*, 13, 277, 1992.
48. Peyster, R. G. et al., Use of ex vivo magnetic resonance imaging to detect onset of vigabatrin-induced intramyelinic edema in canine brain, *Epilepsia*, 36, 93, 1995.
49. Lester, D. S. et al., Virtual neuropathology: three-dimensional visualization of lesions due to toxic insult, *Toxicol. Pathol.*, 28, 100, 2000.
50. Lester, D. S. et al., 3-Dimensional visualization of lesions in rat brain using magnetic resonance imaging microscopy, *Neuroreport*, 10, 737, 1999.
51. Krestin, G. P., Steinbrich, W., and Friedmann, G., Adrenal masses: evaluation with fast gradient-echo MR imaging and Gd-DTPA-enhanced dynamic studies, *Radiology*, 171, 675, 1989.
52. Krestin, G. P., Genitourinary MR: kidneys and adrenal glands, *Eur. Radiol.*, 9, 1705, 1999.
53. Yamada, T. et al., Adrenal carcinoma with a signal loss on chemical shift magnetic resonance imaging, *J. Comput. Assist. Tomogr.*, 27, 606, 2003.
54. Llabres-Diaz, F. J. and Dennis, R., Magnetic resonance imaging of the presumed normal canine adrenal glands, *Vet. Radiol. Ultrasound*, 44, 5, 2003.
55. Beckmann, N. et al., Non-invasive, quantitative assessment of the anatomical phenotype of corticotropin-releasing factor-overexpressing mice by MRI, *NMR Biomed.*, 14, 210, 2001.
56. Sugimoto, M. et al., Availability of NMR microscopic observation of mouse embryo disorder: examination in malformations induced by maternal administration of retinoic acid, *J. Vet. Med. Sci.*, 64, 427, 2002.
57. Wilson, D. et al., Magnetic resonance imaging and morphometric quantitation of cartilage histology after chronic infusion of interleukin 1 in rabbit knees, *Proc. Soc. Exp. Biol. Med.*, 203, 30, 1993.
58. Gough, A. et al., Quinolone arthropathy in immature rabbits treated with the fluoroquinolone, PD 117596, *Exp. Toxicol. Pathol.*, 48, 225, 1996.
59. Yabe, K. et al., Diagnosis of quinolone-induced arthropathy in juvenile dogs by use of magnetic resonance (MR) imaging, *J. Vet. Med. Sci.*, 59, 597, 1997.
60. Mori, K. et al., Magnetic resonance imaging of the galactosemic dog eye using magnetization transfer contrast, *Curr. Eye Res.*, 14, 1035, 1995.
61. Kanikkannan, N., Locke, B. R., and Singh, M., Effect of jet fuels on the skin morphology and irritation in hairless rats, *Toxicology*, 175, 35, 2002.
62. Johnson, G. A. et al., Magnetic resonance imaging of hepatic neoplasms in the rat, *Vet. Pathol.*, 26, 303, 1989.
63. Bachmann, R. et al., Enhanced tumor detection in the presence of liver cirrhosis: experimental study on the diagnostic value of a superparamagnetic iron oxide MR imaging contrast agent (NSR 0430), *J. Magn. Reson. Imaging*, 9, 251, 1999.
64. Robinson, S. P. et al., Tumor vascular architecture and function evaluated by non-invasive susceptibility MRI methods and immunohistochemistry, *J. Magn. Reson. Imaging*, 17, 445, 2003.
65. Johnson, G. A. et al., Morphologic phenotyping with MR microscopy: the visible mouse, *Radiology*, 222, 789, 2002.

27 *In Vivo* MR in Pharmaceutical Research: Essential or Nice to Have?

Nicolau Beckmann and Jeffrey Evelhoch

CONTENTS

27.1 IN FAVOR OF IMAGING

It cannot be denied that the ability to noninvasively derive structural, functional, metabolic, and meanwhile also cellular and targeted information at high resolution, renders MR highly relevant for pharmacological studies. Nevertheless, because the establishment and operation of an imaging facility is costly, it is essential to address issues concerning the relevance of imaging contributions for decision making. It is fundamental that questions such as "Could similar information be generated more economically and/or more efficiently using other methods, like established pharmacological techniques or '-omics' technologies?" or "What is the added value of sophisticated imaging procedures?" be addressed when MR methods are being considered for use in drug research.

Possible answers for these questions depend, among others, on the organ and the pharmacological problem being tackled. Evidently, imaging applications will not be questioned as long as they provide unique information, or when data can be obtained more efficiently and/or less expensively than using standard analytical methods. Treatment efficacy can be evaluated over extended periods of time, allowing analysis of morphological and physiological changes with respect to a pretreatment reference state. Intraindividual variability is thereby reduced and thus statistical significance may be obtained with smaller groups. Imaging can also be applied for stratification of treatment groups: prior to therapy administration, individuals can be classified into homogenous treatment groups which should translate into data with improved statistical relevance.

In particular, functional information is difficult, if not impossible, to be obtained employing conventional approaches; thus, this is an area in which MRI becomes essential. Cardiac MRI, and pharmacological fMRI of the brain or of the lung are good examples. Purely anatomical readouts can be relevant as well, especially in the context of chronic diseases. Of course, MRI derived anatomical information becomes essential even in acute studies when the aim is to obtain volumes of organs or of responses elicited by a given insult.

For instance, edema volumes determined by MRI in stroke (Chapter 8, Section 8.6.2) or in pulmonary inflammation models (Chapter 18, Section 18.4.1) have been extensively used to characterize the effects of compounds. These applications are successful since routine assessment of edema volumes by histology would require significant human resources and time, whereas MRI values can be provided almost immediately following image acquisition using semiautomatic segmentation procedures. Moreover, after the imaging experiments, animals can be used for additional experiments, e.g., for behavioral tests in the case of stroke or for analysis of lung fluid.

High resolution (3D) imaging becomes particularly relevant when examining heterogeneous structures such as cancers. The technique may provide important mechanistic information on compounds not accessible, for example, when assessing tumor sizes using microcalipers. Furthermore, biopsies for histological analysis are always prone to sampling errors when collecting tissue specimens. On the other hand, histology provides highly specific information rarely available to a global imaging technique. In fact, the two readouts are complementary: histological analysis is required for validation of the imaging approaches, while tissue sampling guided by imaging may enhance the specificity of the specimens.

An important advantage of imaging is that tissue is analyzed in its host environment. Possible artifacts generated during tissue collection, fixation, or processing are thereby avoided. Tissue collection is invariably linked to a period of global ischemia for a specimen, which affects the levels of energy metabolites. Similarly, histological processing may lead to morphological distortions that can affect morphometric measurements.

A final main argument in favor of using imaging methods to characterize animal models of human disease is that they definitely may facilitate the translation between preclinical and clinical drug development. Once potential biomarkers are identified and qualified, similar study designs can be applied to preclinical and clinical studies. Moreover, studies in animals can serve as the basis to rationalize experimental findings in humans through the use of analogous biomedical readouts. Of note, clinically approved MRI contrast agents are either paramagnetic agents derived from the open chain DTPA or from the macrocyclic chelate DOTA, or superparamagnetic iron oxides for contrast-enhanced MRI of the liver. Thus, at least in the near future, it will be difficult to translate into the clinics cellular or even targeted imaging applications in animals based on the use of functionalized contrast agents (see Chapter 4).

27.2 ROOM FOR IMPROVEMENTS ON MR TECHNIQUES

Several improvements from the technical side are expected to enhance the value of MR techniques in biomedical research. Throughput is certainly an issue. The time required for the acquisition of a data set is the rate-limiting step in morphological studies. It is expected that parallelization of data acquisition [1] to reduce *k*-space sampling frequency will have a major impact on throughput in animal and clinical imaging. For cancer, whole body MRI, also in combination with PET, may play a significant role since metastases are often spread throughout the body [2–5]. Procedures to acquire images from several animals simultaneously are also going to impact throughput (see Chapter 5).

Sensitivity is always a matter for MR. Despite a general trend towards higher magnetic fields, the body is often the largest source of noise under such conditions. One interesting alternative is the development of cryogenic RF probes for low magnetic fields. Operation at low fields has the advantage of less noise contribution from lossy samples. Cooled coil materials, such as copper, and low- or high-temperature superconductors are being extensively investigated with the aim of increasing the sensitivity in biomedical MR applications [6,7]. Another important avenue involves the design of contrast agents (see also Chapter 4). For instance, proton exchange processes between water and solutes containing exchangeable protons, known as chemical exchange-dependent saturation transfer (CEST), have recently become of interest for monitoring pH effects, detecting cellular mobile proteins and peptides, and enhancing the detection sensitivity of various low-concentration endogenous and exogenous species [8,9]. Paramagnetic lanthanide complexes are the prototypes of a novel class of CEST contrast agents [10]. The modulation of the magnetic properties along the lanthanide series allows an in-depth understanding of the determinants of saturation transfer effects and provides useful insights for the design of more efficient agents (see also Chapter 4, Section 4.7). Other important developments include pH-sensitive lanthanides [11] and gadofullerenes [12], and parahydrogen-induced polarization. Initially known as PASADENA [13] and ALTADENA [14], these experiments are based on the discovery that the hydrogenation of small organic molecules with parahydrogen leads to a highly ordered spin state conspicuously showing up by the observation of very large MR signals for the corresponding protons. The transfer of spin order to heteronuclei as ^{13}C and ^{15}N by field-cycling is being explored as a means to improve the sensitivity of these nuclei. The maximum ^{13}C polarization achieved is about 2×10^5 times the thermal equilibrium value, with T_1 of approximately 60 sec [15]. The major challenge will be to make such techniques work for molecules of interest in tissues. It remains to be shown that long enough ^{13}C hyperpolarization can be achieved for metabolic studies.

Further improvements are also needed in the area of quantification of imaging data. A detailed understanding of the underlying biochemical and biophysical processes and the development of improved tissue models are going to be necessary to derive truly quantitative physiological values of, for example, tissue perfusion, oxygenation levels, or tracer concentrations. Certainly a lot can be learned and adapted from the elegant models developed for PET quantitative analyses [16–19]. Also, improved standardization to facilitate the comparison of data acquired at different centers, irrespective of the MR equipment, is mandatory. Two examples of efforts on standardization are a core within the Alzheimer's Disease Neuroimaging Initiative (ADNI, see below), the NIH-funded longitudinal AD study, focussed on this issue and the recent workshop sponsored by the National Cancer Institute [20] providing consensus recommendations for MR measurement methods at 1.5 T and endpoints for use in Phase 1/2*a* trials of anticancer therapeutics affecting tumor vascular function (http://imaging.cancer.gov/reportsandpublications/ReportsandPresentations/MagneticResonance)

27.3 IMAGING BIOMARKERS

A central aspect in pharmaceutical research is the availability of biomarkers to improve early decision making on safety and efficacy in drug discovery (see Chapter 3 for a thorough discussion). Of course, biomarkers are not confined to imaging, and techniques such as genomics, proteomics, and metabonomics [21] are becoming highly relevant for translational applications. However, these approaches either require a tissue biopsy or provide only a systemic assessment (i.e., from blood, plasma, or urine samples).

In order to develop MR-based biomarkers it is essential to put them in the context of current readouts to characterize a certain disease or disease model. If well-established readouts with a clear link to disease outcome or the biological characteristic of interest exist, comparison of MR responses to such readouts is mandatory. When available, it is highly recommendable to use clinically accepted readouts as standards since that will facilitate translation into clinical trials. For instance, in the case of kidney transplantation, clinical Banff criteria have been introduced as reference in preclinical studies (see Chapter 24, Section 24.3.1.1). The highly significant negative correlation between MR signals reflecting the infiltration of iron-labeled macrophages into kidney allografts and the Banff scores for the same organs provided the basis for an early assessment of chronic rejection [22].

There has been considerable confusion regarding the meaning of the term validation in the context of biomarkers, primarily due to the implication of an either/or status irrespective of the intended use of the biomarker (see also Chapter 3, Section 3.2). In order to recognize that demonstrating a biomarker is suitable for use in drug development is a process rather than an endpoint, the FDA recently introduced the concept of qualification of biomarkers for their intended use(s) [23]. Biomarkers have multiple uses in drug development including: making decisions regarding the progression of a drug to the next stage of development; selecting patients for clinical trials who are best candidates for the drug's target; choosing the optimal dose for later stage trials; and documenting the efficacy and/or safety of a drug as required to gain regulatory approval to market the drug.

As one would expect, given the motivation for the FDA to introduce the term qualification, the rigor required to qualify a biomarker depends on its intended function. If the biomarker is used for internal preclinical decision-making, qualification includes establishing that the method accurately measures the desired information and is technically reliable (i.e., reproducible and precise). Qualification of biomarkers used for internal decision-making in clinical studies requires that the clinical technical reliability and the value added are documented by a combination of preclinical studies, clinical studies using no experimental drug, and the biomedical literature. If biomarkers are used for regulatory licensure decisions, in addition to the requirements for internal decision-making, qualification requires a broad-based demonstration of the performance in late-stage clinical trials (e.g., Phase 2–3), generally conducted by more than one company.

When biomarkers are used for internal decision-making, individual companies might consider a biomarker qualified based on their own experience before the drug development community generally accepts it. However, qualification of a biomarker for regulatory licensure decisions requires evaluation by independent panels advising the regulatory bodies. While individual companies may be able to complete the initial phases of developing and evaluating MR biomarkers alone, efforts similar to the Single Nucleotide Polymorphism (SNP) Consortium (http://snp.cshl.org/) should both reduce the cost and speed the process of developing and qualifying MR biomarkers. The SNP Consortium, which originated in 1999 and was funded by 10 major pharmaceutical companies and the Wellcome Trust, brought together academic, government and industry researchers to map at least 150,000 SNPs in the human genome. As is the case with the SNP Consortium, the development of MR biomarkers is an area of precompetitive research where only a critical mass of effort will produce the results that are needed.

The Critical Path Initiative (http://www.fda.gov/oc/initiatives/criticalpath/whitepaper.html) introduced by the FDA in 2004 lays the foundation for public–private partnerships among industry, public bodies (such as the Medical Research Council, National Institutes of Health, FDA), and not-for-profit organizations (such as the Wellcome Trust, Cancer Research U.K., and the Critical Path Institute). The FDA, several biopharmaceutical companies, and various biomarker companies are already collaborating on the application of a cross-platform RNA standard for assessing microarray data comparability [24]. In the area of MR, there are two public–private partnerships between the NIH and the pharmaceutical industry: the Osteoarthritis Initiative (OAI) (http://www.niams.nih.gov/ne/oi/index.htm) and the Alzheimer's Disease Neuroimaging Initiative (ADNI) (http://www.nia.nih.gov/) (http://www.loni.ucla.edu/ADNI/About/About_Funding.shtml). The OAI is a multi-center, 5-year-observational study of knee osteoarthritis (OA) started in February 2004 that collects information on potential biomarkers for OA, including MRI, and trends in OA onset and progression. The OAI recruits and follows for at least a four-year period participants who have knee OA or are at high risk for developing knee OA. The ultimate goal is to identify biomarkers of OA risk or progression, which could also help assess the effectiveness of disease modifying treatments. ADNI is a $60 million, 5-year public–private partnership started in October 2004 aiming to test whether serial MRI, PET, other biological markers, and clinical and neuropsychological assessments can be combined to measure the progression of mild cognitive impairment and early Alzheimer's disease. The study will compare neuroimaging, biological, and clinical information from study participants seeking correlations among the data that will track the progress of memory loss from its earliest stages.

As similar public–private partnerships (including regulatory input) are established to develop and qualify biomarkers, including MR biomarkers, more powerful diagnostic and prognostic tools should be a by-product. Not only will the biopharmaceutical industry benefit from such an effort, but also medical practice and public health, in general.

REFERENCES

1. Pruessmann, K. P., Parallel imaging at high field strength: synergies and joint potential, *Top. Magn. Reson. Imaging*, 15, 237, 2004.
2. Antoch, G. et al., Whole-body dual-modality PET/CT and whole-body MRI for tumor staging in oncology, *JAMA*, 290, 3199, 2003.
3. Gaa, J., Rummeny, E. J., and Seemann, M. D., Whole-body imaging with PET/MRI, *Eur. J. Med. Res.*, 9, 309, 2004.
4. Goehde, S. C. et al., Full-body cardiovascular and tumor MRI for early detection of disease: feasibility and initial experience in 298 subjects, *Am. J. Roentgenol.*, 184, 598, 2005.
5. Schlemmer, H. P. et al., Fast whole-body assessment of metastatic disease using a novel magnetic resonance imaging system: initial experiences, *Invest. Radiol.*, 40, 64, 2005.
6. Darrasse, L. and Ginefri, J. C., Perspectives with cryogenic RF probes in biomedical MRI, *Biochimie*, 85, 915, 2003.
7. Lee, K. H. et al., Performance of large-size superconducting coil in 0.21 T MRI system, *IEEE Trans. Biomed. Eng.*, 51, 2024, 2004.
8. Snoussi, K. et al., Sensitive CEST agents based on nucleic acid imino proton exchange: detection of poly(rU) and of a dendrimer-poly(rU) model for nucleic acid delivery and pharmacology, *Magn. Reson. Med.*, 49, 998, 2003.
9. Zhou, J. et al., Quantitative description of proton exchange processes between water and endogenous and exogenous agents for WEX, CEST, and APT experiments, *Magn. Reson. Med.*, 51, 945, 2004.
10. Terreno, E. et al., Ln(III)-DOTAMGly complexes: a versatile series to assess the determinants of the efficacy of paramagnetic chemical exchange saturation transfer agents for magnetic resonance imaging applications, *Invest. Radiol.*, 39, 235, 2004.
11. Woods, M. et al., pH-sensitive modulation of the second hydration sphere in lanthanide(III) tetraamide-DOTA complexes: a novel approach to smart MR contrast media, *Chemistry*, 9, 4634, 2003.
12. Toth, E. et al., Water-soluble gadofullerenes: toward high-relaxivity, pH-responsive MRI contrast agents, *J. Am. Chem. Soc.*, 127, 799, 2005.
13. Bowers, C. R. and Weitekamp, D. P., Parahydrogen and synthesis allow dramatically enhanced nuclear alignment, *J. Am. Chem. Soc.*, 109, 5541, 1987.
14. Pravica, M. G. and Weitekamp, D. P., Net alignment by adiabatic transport of parahydrogen addition products to high magnetic field, *Chem. Phys. Lett.*, 145, 255, 1998.
15. Goldman, M. et al., Hyperpolarization of 13C through order transfer from parahydrogen: a new contrast agent for MRI, *Magn. Reson. Imaging*, 23, 153, 2005.
16. Acton, P. D., Zhuang, H., and Alavi, A., Quantification in PET, *Radiol. Clin. North Am.*, 42, 1055, 2004.
17. Cunningham, V. J., Gunn, R. N., and Matthews, J. C., Quantification in positron emission tomography for research in pharmacology and drug development, *Nucl. Med. Commun.*, 25, 643, 2004.
18. Horwitz, B., Relating fMRI and PET signals to neural activity by means of large-scale neural models, *Neuroinformatics*, 2, 251, 2004.
19. Van den Hoff, J., Principles of quantitative positron emission tomography, *Amino Acids*, 29, 341, 2005.
20. Evelhoch, J. et al., Expanding the use of magnetic resonance in the assessment of tumor response to therapy: workshop report, *Cancer Res.*, 65, 7041, 2005.

21. Nicholson, J. K. et al., Metabonomics: a platform for studying drug toxicity and gene function, *Nat. Rev. Drug Discov.*, 1, 153, 2002.
22. Beckmann, N. et al., Macrophage infiltration in rat kidney allografts detected by MRI: early marker of chronic rejection that strongly correlates with histology, *Radiology*, in press, 2006.
23. Baker, M., In biomarkers we trust?, *Nat. Biotechnol.*, 23, 297, 2005.
24. Pine, P.S. et al., Application of a Cross-Platform Rna Standard for Assessing Microarray Data Comparability, 2005 FDA Science Forum, D-14, Washington, DC, April 2005.

Index

C

D

E

F

G

H

I

J

K

L

O

P

Q

R

S

T

U

V

W

X

Z